Cardiac Drug Development Guide

METHODS IN PHARMACOLOGY AND TOXICOLOGY

Y. James Kang, MD, SERIES EDITOR

METHODS IN PHARMACOLOGY AND TOXICOLOGY

Cardiac Drug Development Guide

Edited by

Michael K. Pugsley

Department of Pharmacology, Forest Research Institute,
Jersey City, NJ

HUMANA PRESS 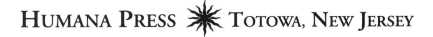 TOTOWA, NEW JERSEY

Production Editor: Jessica Jannicelli.

Cover design by Patricia F. Cleary.

For additional copies, pricing for bulk purchases, and/or information about other Humana titles, contact Humana at the above address or at any of the following numbers: Tel.: 973-256-1699; Fax: 973-256-8341; E-mail: humana@ humanapr.com or visit our website: http://humanapress.com

This publication is printed on acid-free paper. ∞
ANSI Z39.48-1984 (American National Standards Institute) Permanence of Paper for Printed Library Materials.

Photocopy Authorization Policy:
Authorization to photocopy items for internal or personal use, or the internal or personal use of specific clients, is granted by Humana Press Inc., provided that the base fee of US $20.00 per copy is paid directly to the Copyright Clearance Center at 222 Rosewood Drive, Danvers, MA 01923. For those organizations that have been granted a photocopy license from the CCC, a separate system of payment has been arranged and is acceptable to Humana Press Inc. The fee code for users of the Transactional Reporting Service is: [1-58829-097-2/03 $20.00].

Printed in the United States of America.   10 9 8 7 6 5 4 3 2 1

Library of Congress Cataloging-in-Publication Data

Cardiac drug development guide / edited by Michael K. Pugsley.
     p. ; cm. -- (Methods in pharmacology and toxicology)
Includes bibliographical references and index.
  ISBN 1-58829-097-2 (alk. paper) eISBN: 1-59259-404-2
 1. Cardiovascular agents. 2. Drug development.
  [DNLM: 1. Cardiovascular Agents--pharmacology. 2. Drug Design. 3.
Drug Evaluation, Preclinical--methods. QV 150 C2633 2003] I. Pugsley,
Michael K. II. Series.
  RM345.C34 2003
  615'.71--dc21
                                    2003012876

Preface

Cardiac Drug Development Guide outlines, in detail, the therapeutics of cardiac medicine currently at the cutting edge of scientific research and development around the world. This volume integrates basic and clinical cardiac pharmacology by combining, for the first time, both classical and molecular aspects of therapeutic drug development. The chapters comprise a broad spectrum of therapeutic areas and hence involve a comprehensive discussion of molecular, biochemical, and electrophysiological concepts based on years of in vitro as well as in vivo pharmacological studies. In addition, the latter part of the book includes comprehensive clinical cardiac chapters that describe important topics in molecular medicine. These chapters also discuss current clinical therapeutic trends in medicine and provide an evaluation of the efficacy of novel drugs in these areas.

Cardiac Drug Development Guide has many distinctive and outstanding features that set it apart from other cardiac pharmacology books. This book introduces topics in an easily understandable format for researchers in many varying disciplines by integrating and thereby simplifying concepts not usually discussed across a broad range of cardiac disciplines and in a highly technical field. Each chapter not only introduces and describes the physiology, pharmacology, and pathophysiology of the disease, but also overviews the clinical implications of drug development, what stages these areas are currently in, and also reviews some of the methodologies involved in drug discovery and development. As a result, this book provides a comprehensive overview of the most advanced procedures in cardiac pharmacology today. It is hoped that *Cardiac Drug Development Guide* provides useful information to graduate students, academic scientists, clinicians, and those researchers in the pharmaceutical and biotechnology sectors of the drug industry.

Cardiac Drug Development Guide was fashioned from my many years of experience both learning pharmacology as a graduate student in Canada and as an MRC postdoctoral research fellow and applying that knowledge in industry as a senior pharmacological scientist. I wish to thank all my colleagues around the world for contributing to this book and to my family, especially my loving wife, Suzanne, for all their support.

Michael K. Pugsley

Contents

Contributors

FRED S. APPLE • *Clinical Laboratories, Hennepin County Medical Center and Department of Laboratory Medicine and Pathology, University of Minnesota, School of Medicine, Minneapolis, MN*

MIROSLAV BARANCIK • *Department of Cardiovascular Physiology, Institute for Heart Research, Slovak Academy of Sciences, Slovak Republic*

JOEL S. BENNETT • *Hematology-Oncology Division, Department of Medicine, University of Pennsylvania School of Medicine, Philadelphia, PA*

NEIL E. BOWLES • *Department of Pediatrics, Baylor College of Medicine, Houston, TX*

MARIAROSARIA BUCCI • *Department of Experimental Pharmacology, Faculty of Pharmacy, University of Naples, Naples, Italy*

GIUSEPPE CIRINO • *Department of Experimental Pharmacology, Faculty of Pharmacy, University of Naples, Naples, Italy*

HUGH CLEMENTS-JEWERY • *Centre for Cardiovascular Biology and Medicine, King's College London, London, UK*

MICHAEL J. CURTIS • *Centre for Cardiovascular Biology and Medicine, King's College London, London, UK*

AMIT DESAI • *Department of Pharmacy Practice, School of Pharmacy, University of the Pacific, Stockton, CA*

ANDREA D. ECKHART • *Department of Surgery, Duke University Medical Center, Durham, NC*

ENE ETTE • *Vertex Pharmaceutical Corporation, Cambridge, MA*

DAVID FEDIDA • *Department of Physiology, University of British Columbia, Vancouver, Canada*

LEON J. GUPPY • *Department of Pharmacology and Therapeutics, University of British Columbia, Vancouver, Canada*

LASZLO HEJJEL • *Division of Cardiac Surgery, Heart Institute, Medical Faculty, University of Pecs, Pecs, Hungary*

J. CHRISTIAN HESKETH • *Department of Experimental Medicine, Cardiome Pharma Corporation, Vancouver, Canada*

MORRIS KARMAZYN • *Department of Physiology and Pharmacology, University of Western Ontario, Ontario, Canada*

WALTER J. KOCH • *Department of Surgery, Duke University Medical Center, Durham, NC*

DAVID J. LEFER • *Department of Molecular and Cellular Physiology, Louisiana State University Health Sciences Center, Shreveport, LA*

HUA LI • *Department of Pediatrics, Baylor College of Medicine, Houston, TX*

JEANNE M. NERBONNE • *Department of Molecular Biology and Pharmacology, Washington University Medical School, St. Louis, MO*

JAMES PARRATT • *Department of Physiology and Pharmacology, University of Strathclyde, Strathclyde Institute for Biomedical Sciences, Glasgow, Scotland*

INMACULADA POSADAS MAYO • *Department of Experimental Pharmacology, Faculty of Pharmacy, University of Naples, Naples, Italy*

MICHAEL K. PUGSLEY • *Department of Pharmacology, Forest Research Institute, Jersey City, NJ*

TANYA RAVINGEROVA • *Department of Cardiovascular Physiology, Institute for Heart Research, Slovak Academy of Sciences, Slovak Republic*

ELIZABETH ROTH • *Department of Experimental Surgery, Medical Faculty, University of Pecs, Pecs, Hungary*

DAVID A. SAINT • *Cellular Biophysics Laboratory, Department of Physiology, University of Adelaide, Adelaide, Australia*

MICHAEL SIMONS • *Section of Cardiology, Dartmouth Medical School, Dartmouth Hitchcock Medical Center, Hanover, NH*

MELANIE B. SMITH • *Department of Molecular and Cellular Physiology, Louisiana State University Health Sciences Center, Shreveport, LA*

MONIKA STRNISKOVA • *Department of Cardiovascular Physiology, Institute for Heart Research, Slovak Academy of Sciences, Slovak Republic*

MARK A. SUSSMAN • *Division of Molecular Cardiovascular Biology, The Children's Hospital and Research Foundation, Cincinnati, OH*

LÁSZLÓ SZEKERES • *Department of Pharmacology and Pharmacotherapy, University of Szeged, Szeged, Hungary*

MAURIZIO TAGLIALATELA • *Section of Pharmacology, Department of Neuroscience, School of Medicine, University of Naples Federico II, Naples, Italy*

HENDRICK T. TEVAEARAI • *Department of Surgery, Duke University Medical Center, Durham, NC*

JEFFREY A. TOWBIN • *Department of Pediatrics, Cardiovascular Sciences and Molecular Human Genetics, Baylor College of Medicine, Houston, TX*

MATTEO VATTA • *Department of Pediatrics, Baylor College of Medicine, Houston, TX*

MICHAEL J. A. WALKER • *Department of Pharmacology and Therapeutics, University of British Columbia, Vancouver, Canada*

PAUL J. WILLIAMS • *Department of Pharmacy Practice, School of Pharmacy, University of the Pacific, Stockton, CA*

I

INTRODUCTION

1

Cardiac Drug Development

From Animal Models to Clinical Trials

Michael K. Pugsley

1. CARDIAC DRUGS: THE MARKET POTENTIAL FOR ANTIARRHYTHMIC DRUG DEVELOPMENT

Statistics from the American Heart Association show that the total number of arrhythmia-related mortalities is approx 500,000 of an estimated 2,000,000 US deaths per year, or nearly one-quarter of all cardiovascular-related deaths *(1)*. The majority of such deaths, which have remained at a nearly constant ratio since the 1970s when cardiac drug development programs were formally being established within the pharmaceutical industry, are caused by ventricular fibrillation (VF; Fig. 1).

The development of novel, effective cardiac (antiarrhythmic) drugs was fueled by the need for agents that would possess the so-called ideal pharmacological properties, including high oral bioavailability, marked efficacy and selectively for the abolition of ectopic ventricular arrhythmias, and a reduced adverse events profile (e.g., reduced hypotensive actions and lack of proarrhythmic tendencies). The majority of drugs developed at that time were analogs of lidocaine; however, structurally distinct classes of drugs were developed, including the trifluoroethoxybenzamides (flecainide). These compounds, according to the Vaughan Williams classification scheme *(2)*, were class I antiarrhythmic agents, that is, those that reduce the influx of sodium (Na^+) ions during phase 0 of the action potential (AP). In the mid-1980s, the development of this abundant group of diverse new chemical entities with activity in animal models of

From: *Cardiac Drug Development Guide*
Edited by: M. K. Pugsley © Humana Press Inc., Totowa, NJ

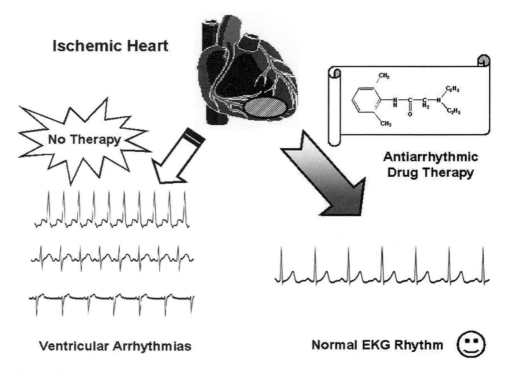

Fig. 1. The ischemic heart produces a broad spectrum of arrhythmias that precipitate sudden cardiac death. Antiarrhythmic drug therapy (ion channel-blocking drugs) can suppress fatal arrhythmias and produce a normal EKG rhythm. Unfortunately, although these drugs are beneficial, many possess side effects, including myocardial depression and proarrhythmic tendencies.

arrhythmias and efficacy in the clinic (phase 1 and 2 studies) resulted in their evaluation in larger phase 3 clinical trials. The Cardiac Arrhythmia Suppression Trial (CAST-I) study was undertaken to examine whether the incidence of cardiac death in patients with asymptomatic or mild ventricular arrhythmias, post-myocardial infarction (MI), could be reduced with class I antiarrhythmic drugs *(3)*. The CAST-I clinical trial with flecainide, encainide, and later moricizine in CAST-II *(4)* and mexiletine in the International Mexiletine and Placebo Antiarrhythmic Coronary Trial (IMPACT) trial showed an abnormally high incidence of death in drug-treated groups when compared with placebo controls *(5)*. Thus, these clinical trials, albeit not showing marked efficacy of these drugs, provided a valuable lesson as to the complex interrelationship that exists among the antiarrhythmic drug used, the arrhythmogenic substrate, and resulting drug efficacy.

Thus, despite the large number of experiments and clinical trials that have been conducted, remarkably few Na^+ channel-blocking drugs are used clinically to suppress arrhythmias. This low number of drugs accentuates the findings from the CAST-I and CAST-II trial as well as others *(3,4)*. Many studies with a variety of Na^+ channel-blocking antiarrhythmic agents suggest that these drugs can effectively suppress arrhythmias; however, this does not necessarily result in an improved survival rate after a myocardial infarction in patients *(6)*. Quinidine, for example, was shown clinically to increase the incidence of mortality as compared with mexiletine *(7)*, and lidocaine, although abolishing fatal VF, does not significantly improve survival in post-MI patients *(8)*.

The class II (beta-blocking) antiarrhythmic agents, typified by propranolol, atenolol, and esmolol, are the only drugs that have been consistently shown to produce an increased time to onset of ventricular tachycardia (VT; ref. *9*), a reduction in arrhythmia incidence *(10)*, and to improve survival post-MI *(11)*. A true appreciation for these actions seems to have been overlooked despite the overwhelming abundance of data describing the efficacy of this class of antiarrhythmic drug *(12)*. Both the class III K^+ channel-blocking and class IV Ca^{2+} channel-blocking agents have, in contrast, exhibited poor results in post-MI clinical trials *(13)*.

An examination of the developmental patterns for antiarrhythmic drugs suggests that because of the poor performance of antiarrhythmics in the past, there must be continued research in this area. Therefore, novel molecular targets must be determined and drugs for these targets developed. Some novel cardiac targets include a pathologically targeted approach whereby drugs have been developed that show marked selectivity for myocardial ischemia and have a greater therapeutic index when compared with prevous antiarrhythmic drugs *(14)*. Sodium-hydrogen exchange inhibitor drugs, such as cariporide, which target the cardiac-specific isoform of this membrane pump, may also have activity against arrhythmias and efficacy in congestive heart failure *(15)*. Thus, because of the large number of mortalities each year from cardiac disease, there is a very large unmet medical need for more efficacious antiarrhythmic drugs. Current medical expenditures in the United States for arrhythmias and arrhythmia-related conditions are over $1 billion, and the unmet medical market is estimated to be well over $3 billion.

2. GENESIS OF THE CARDIAC ACTION POTENTIAL (CAP)

To develop effective cardiac drugs, it is necessary to understand the basic tenets of heart function. The coordinated electrical activity of cardiac muscle results from the establishment of transmembrane potentials that culminate from an integration of many different ion channels. The corresponding changes in ionic permeability results in the flow of current producing contraction of heart muscle. APs in excitable cells result from the presence of voltage-gated ion channels *(16)* that open and close depending on the voltage across the membrane. Depolarization of the resting membrane potential causes the opening of voltage-gated Na^+ channels. This increase in Na^+ permeability results in the development of an inward current that enhances depolarization. Membrane potential is re-established by the rapid inactivation of voltage-gated Na^+ channels and opening of voltage-gated K^+ channels. In the heart membrane, potential is complicated by the presence of voltage-gated Ca^{2+} channels. These channels mediate the slow inward current (Isi) that is responsible for the plateau phase of the AP. In some tissues, such as the sinoatrial and atrioventricular nodes, voltage-gated Ca^{2+} channels predominate and produce the AP.

The CAP (Fig. 2A) for a ventricular myoctye consists of 4 phases. A rapid upstroke (phase 0) is followed by a brief peak (phase 1) followed by a sustained plateau (phase 2). A rapid repolarization (phase 3) begins after several hundred milliseconds, and this is followed by phase 4 that persists until the next rapid upstroke event. Thus, the shape of the AP is governed by ionic current flux via gated channels in the membrane for Na^+,

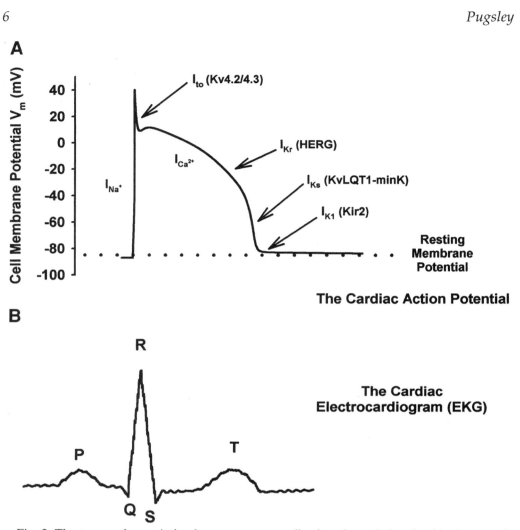

Fig. 2. The temporal association between some cardiac ion channels involved in the genesis of the AP and the EKG. (**A**), a ventricular AP is depicted with ion currents involved in its genesis. Although ion channels vary in species the fast upward spike generated by Na⁺ (I_{Na}) represents the QRS complex of the EKG (**B**). Ventricular repolarization results from the combined actions of many K⁺ currents and is delineated in the EKG by the upward deflection of the T-wave (**B**).

Ca^{2+} and K^+ (Fig. 2A). Membrane pumps and exchangers are involved as well. The properties of the AP change moderately among tissue types. In pacemaker cells of the nodal tissues phase 4 is characterized by a slow, steady depolarization from the resting membrane potential (V_m) that leads to a threshold potential. When this potential is met, a rapid upstroke (phase 0) results and a nodal AP develops that is composed of similar phases as in ventricular or other cardiac cells. Although there may be some differences regarding phase 4 development in various cardiac tissue, the fundamentals of AP generation are unchanged. The pacemaker current shapes the periodicity of oscillations in the heart because this current is activated by the hyperpolarized cell membrane at the conclusion of the AP.

The inward voltage-gated Na^+ channel is responsible for producing phase 0 and the rapid upstroke of the cardiac AP. Although Na^+ channels rapidly inactivate as V_m approaches the equilibrium potential (0 mV), a second voltage-gated ion channel is activated that is carried by Ca^{2+} ions. Calcium channels carry Isi that is responsible for the plateau phase of the AP (Fig. 2A). Although many Ca^{2+} channel subtypes occur, there are at least two isoforms found in the heart: the L and T types.

Within a short period of time (125 ms), cardiac Ca^{2+} channels inactivate and K^+ channels activate. Repolarization is rapid when the total outward K^+ current becomes appreciably greater than inward Ca^{2+} current. A large number of voltage- and nonvoltage-gated K^+ currents are involved in repolarization of the cardiac AP. The voltage-gated K^+ currents include the transient outward K^+ current (I_{to}), one of the earliest channels to open; the outward or delayed rectifier current (I_K), which opens at the end of phase 2 and is the main K^+ current responsible for ventricular repolarization. The last to open is the inward rectifier K^+ current (I_{K1}) which, unlike other K^+ currents, closes during depolarization and is responsible for maintenance of the resting membrane potential (Fig. 2A).

2.1. The Cardiac Na+ Channel

Depolarization of the cell membrane opens Na^+ channels. Molecular studies have revealed characteristics of the Na^+ channel. All voltage-gated Na^+ channels are comprised of ~2000 amino acids and contain four homologous internal repeats (DI–DIV), each of which has six putative transmembrane (SI–S6) segments (17). The subunit is the protein that forms the ion channel pore (17). Recently, Sato et al. (18) determined the crystal structure of the Na^+ channel and suggests that the Na^+ channel α-subunit is a bell-shaped membrane protein (18).

Most Na^+ channels are heterotrimeric complexes in the membrane. The α-subunit (~260 kDa) interacts with at least two small auxiliary β subunit proteins. The $β_1$ subunit (~36 kDa) regulates current amplitude and refines channel kinetics for neuronal isoforms but not the cardiac isoform of the channel (19). The $β_2$ subunit (~33 kDa) modulates Na^+ channel localization in tissue (20). Many subtypes of cardiac voltage-gated Na^+ channels have been described.

Despite many isoforms, ionic conductance of the Na^+ channel is transient. Activation occurs rapidly, and prolonged depolarization produces Na^+ channel inactivation, preventing the continued influx of Na^+ into the myocyte. Molecular studies reveal that the α-helical intracellular linker between domains III and IV (DIII–DIV) of the Na^+ channel is responsible for inactivation and channel closure (21).

Local anesthetics and antiarrhythmic drugs interact with the inactivation gate (22). The inactivation produced by a change in membrane potential and drug block of the channel are interacting processes. These occur as a result of drug binding to a site on or near the inactivation gate in a voltage-, time-, and channel state-dependent manner according to the modulated receptor hypothesis. This model suggests that as Na^+ channels change states antiarrhythmic drugs can associate or dissociate from these states (23,24). Evidence exists for a specific binding site on the Na^+ channel for drugs. Ragsdale et al. (25) identified a putative antiarrhythmic drug binding site on the S6 transmembrane spanning region of domain IV (DIVS6) that lines the pore of the Na^+ channel. Thus there exists a greater promise for cardiac drug development as a result of the molecular localization of drug action in the heart. A return of the membrane potential to its predepolarizing (resting) level begins with activation of Ca^{2+} current and repolarizing K^+ currents.

2.2. Cardiac Ca^{2+} Channels

Voltage-gated Ca^{2+} channels are important regulators of electrical signaling and mechanical function in the heart. In the myocyte, Ca^{2+} is highly regulated by voltage-gated Ca^{2+} channels, Ca^{2+} pumps and by the Na^+/Ca^{2+} exchanger.

Calcium channels are responsible for the genesis of APs in cardiac pacemaker cells, the propagation of APs in sinoatrial and atrioventricular node cells and in the control of depolarization-induced Ca^{2+} entry responsible for the plateau (phase 2) of the CAP (Fig. 2A).

Voltage-gated Ca^{2+} channels are hetero-oligomeric protein complexes that are comprised of a α_1 (~240 kDa) subunit, a β subunit (~60 kDa), and an accessory α_2-δ (~175 kDa) subunit *(26)*. Currently, six classes of voltage-gated Ca^{2+} channel have been characterized. In the heart, there is a single L- and T-type Ca^{2+} channel and each mediate an important action in the genesis of the AP.

The α_1 subunit of the Ca^{2+} channel (~1800 amino acid residues) is the major protein constituent that contains the ionic pore, selectivity filter, and gating machinery. In cardiac ventricular muscle the α_{1C} subunit encoding the L-type Ca^{2+} channel is found at appreciably high levels (>80%) whereas α_{1D} subunit expression dominates atrial muscle *(26)*. Of the three isoforms of the α_1 subunit that encode for the T-type channel only α_{1G} and α_{1H} are found in cardiac tissue *(26,27)*.

The α_1 subunit also contains the binding domain for Ca^{2+} channel-blocking drugs. The L-type channel is blocked by three groups of drugs. The phenylalkylamine (e.g., verapamil) and benzothiazepine (e.g., diltiazem) blockers are effective clinically used antiarrhythmics whereas the 1,4-dihydropyridines (e.g., nifedipine) are useful antihypertensive agents. Chemically, Ca^{2+} channels show a marked structural homology to each other and to voltage-gated Na^+ channels. This subunit is composed of four homologous domains (DI–DIV) each of which is composed of six transmembrane spanning α-helical proteins that form a pore in the membrane.

Calcium channels also require auxiliary subunits for functional expression. Currently, four mammalian isoforms of the β subunit exist but the cardiac L- and T-type Ca^{2+} channels are only co-expressed with the β_2-subunit isoform *(28)*. Of the three α_2-δsubunit isoforms that have been detected in various tissues, only the α_2-δ_1 and α_2-δ_2 types are expressed in the heart *(28,29)*. The cardiac L-type Ca^{2+} channels possess the high affinity, stereoselective-binding sites for channel block. Inhibition produces antiarrhythmic activity against supraventricular arrhythmias. The S6 regions of DIII and DIV may contain the actual high affinity binding sites for channel blocking drugs *(26)*.

2.3. Cardiac K^+ Channels

Interest in the development of drugs that prolong refractoriness, that is, possess class III antiarrhythmic action, increased markedly after the negative results of the CAST trials. Repolarization and the configuration of phase 3 of the AP in cardiac tissue seemed the next likely target for antiarrhythmic drug development. This was especially tantalizing because repolarization resulted from the complex interaction of multiple K^+ channels providing numerous targets for drug development *(30)*.

However, whereas individual K^+ currents overlap in contribution to the total membrane current during the AP, the relative importance of each may vary under different physiological conditions. During ischaemia, changes in cell properties may alter the degree to which different channels contribute to the CAP. Despite these short-comings, intensive development has continued for selective K^+ channel-blocking antiarrhyhmic drugs.

Mammalian K^+ channels have been categorized into three main families: the voltage-gated K^+ channels (Kv), the inward rectifying K^+ channels (K1), and the two pore domain channels (K2P). All K^+ currents have a similar primary amino acid sequence with highly conserved structural regions. The molecular structures of K^+ channels are described as having one or two pore-forming domains and two, four, or six transmembrane-spanning domains. The molecular diversity of K^+ channels is largely to the result of variability in the heteromeric association of pore-forming α subunits and accessory or β-subunits *(31)*. Voltage-dependent K^+ channel α subunits have six transmembrane spanning sequences and a pore-forming region. The inwardly rectifying K^+ channel α subunit is composed of two transmembrane spanning sequences and one pore-forming region.

The voltage-dependent activation of K^+ currents plays a considerable role in the repolarization of the cardiac cell membrane. Voltage-dependent inactivation may proceed either rapidly or slowly by N- and C-type inactivation, respectively *(32)*. The differential distribution of currents carried by K^+ channels is extremely important in the regulation of myocardial cell resting potential and repolarization and thus to the configuration of the cardiac AP within different cells of the heart and electrocardiogram (EKG) morphology between species.

Thus, the heterogeneity of K^+ channels provides a large potential for the development of K^+ channel-blocking drugs *(33)*. However, class III agents are bradycardic and prolong the action potential duration (APD) at low heart rates more effectively than high heart rates, reducing their efficacy.

This reverse-use dependence limits their beneficial actions in the arrhythmic condition *(34)*. The resulting bradycardia associated with new potent K^+ channel blockers, such as dofetilide and sematilide, is associated with torsade des pointes arrhythmias *(35)*. Note, however, that some drugs, such as amiodarone, lack this effect *(34)*.

Thus, although many K^+ channels exist in cardiac muscle, a complete overview of only those K^+ conductances, which carry most of the outward repolarizing current, is beyond the scope of this article. Note, however, that the K^+ currents that do contribute include the transient outward K^+ current, the delayed rectifier K^+ (I_K) current (and its components, I_{Kr} and I_{Ks}), and the inward rectifier (I_{KIR}) current.

3. ISCHEMIA-INDUCED CHANGES IN MYOCYTES PRODUCE CHANGES IN THE EKG

Electrical activity in excitable cells results from the opening and closing of ion channels in a voltage- and time-dependent manner. The depolarization of a single cardiac cell results in the electrotonic spread of electrical activity to adjacent cells and the production of current that flows in the direction of depolarization. A second, repolarizing current, is established to restore electrical excitability to cells. If these currents are recorded in individual cells, an AP is observed (Fig. 2A); if they are recorded on the surface of the body, an EKG is observed (Fig. 2B).

Thus, the EKG is defined as the global summation of all the electrical activity that is generated by cells within the heart. It is the rate of change of voltage across the cell membrane as a function of time ($\Delta dV/dt$). The intervals that are defined by the EKG present the clinician and basic researcher with a fundamental tool to diagnose disease and investigate drug activity.

Whereas electrical activity generated by atrial depolarization is recorded by the EKG as the P-wave (Fig. 2B), ventricular depolarization produces a QRS complex. Repolarization of the ventricles is recorded by the EKG as the T-wave. The QT interval represents the ventricular refractory period and includes depolarization and repolarization of ventricular muscle. In contrast to the atria, the AP in ventricular tissue is long (~300 ms) and similar to the duration of the QT interval. Thus, the QT interval is an approximate measure of ventricular repolarization and thus K^+ channel function.

The ST segment is an important measure of the EKG because it represents the early phase of ventricular repolarization. Clinically, depression in this segment can be used to diagnose conditions, such as angina. Elevation in this segment occurs in a damaged area of the ventricular wall that may be associated with myocardial ischemia or infarction. However, any abnormality in these measures may be indicative of some underlying pathophysiological process that alters the AP in cardiac cells that are a consequence of changes in voltage-gated ion channel(s) in tissue *(36)*.

Because the EKG is a composite of voltage-gated ion channels, it is not consistent between various animal species. The variability is quantitative, that is, measureable differences in current densities can be recorded and qualitative, that is, EKG shape varies because of expression of ion channel(s) distinct from that found in the human heart (Fig. 3). Although little disparity exists regarding the role of both Na^+ and Ca^{2+} channels in the hearts of various species, important species and regional differences exist in the contribution K^+ channels make to repolarization of the cardiac AP. This disparity is of particular importance when determining which species to use in establishing relevant in vivo and in vitro animal models to assess the activity of novel cardiac drugs.

4. THE ROLE OF CARDIAC ION CHANNELS IN HEART DISEASE

Implicit in the development of novel cardiac drugs is an understanding of the molecular mechanism(s) responsible for arrhythmogenesis and the proarrhythmic propensity observed for many antiarrhythmic drugs. The blockade of Na^+ channels in the heart by antiarrhythmic drugs reflects limited selectivity to ischemic tissue. Therefore, drug blockade produces an increase in the rate of delayed conduction in ischemic-damaged muscle without either the abolition of excitability or the production of complete conduction block *(37)*. This disparity increases the probability for the development of re-entrant arrhythmias. Therefore, slowed conduction in injured heart tissue along with a reduction in electrical conduction in normal tissue surrounding the damaged area may be an important factor in arrhythmogenesis.

Mutations in the cardiac Na^+ channel has directly implicated it in inherited cardiac disease. In the heart, mutations in NaV1.5 produce dramatic changes in the Na^+ channel. Usually inherited as autosomal-dominant mutations, these changes prolong the QT interval. Mutations result from an amino acid deficit in the DIII–IV linker responsible for normal channel inactivation *(38)*. The predominant intragenic mutation, a deletion of the amino acids $K_{1505}P_{1506}Q_{1507}$ (ΔKPQ) and two missense mutations (R1644H and N1325S) produce channels, but with altered inactivation properties *(38,39)*.

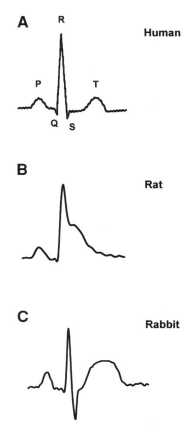

Fig. 3. A comparison of some EKG recordings from various species. (**A**) depicts a human EKG, (**B**) from a rat, and (**C**) from a rabbit. Note that the EKG tracings are not to scale.

As with many diseases, there is a prominent genetic component to the etiology of cardiac arrhythmias that relates to alterations in ion channel function. Because many ion channels mediate a basis for electrical activity in myocytes, it is of no surprise that, in a manner similar to that for Na^+ channels, altered Ca^{2+} and K^+ ion channel properties produce disease. The search is now on to determine the functional consequences associated with aberrant ion channel proteins for which novel antiarrhythmic drugs may be developed. Mechanistically, these findings will provide crucial information as to whether these disorders result from faulty voltage-gated ion channels themselves or from mutations in the regulatory protein components of the electrical-excitation coupling system in the heart.

The best characterized of the cardiac disorders involving a K^+ channel is the long-QT syndrome (LQTS). It is a specific cardiac disorder related to acquired or inherited alterations in I_K channel function and displays a torsade des pointes phenotype. The majority of genetic loci (11p15 in humans) that have been identified contain the genes responsible for LQTS and encode those subunits for the I_K channel *(39,40)*. In mammals a gene from the KCNQ (K_vLQT) subfamily, KCNQ1, when co-expressed with the auxiliary subunit, minK (or KCNE1), produces functional K^+ channels (LQTS1) similar to the slowly activating component of the I_K current (I_{Ks}; ref. *40*).

However, the association of human ether-a-go-go (HERG; or KCNH2) with KCNE1 (minK) or KCNE2 (MiRP, a minK homolog) produces the molecular equivalent of the rapidly activating I_k (I_{Kr}) *(41)*. Many mutations within the HERG α subunit suggest it is a mediator of LQTS2 *(42)*.

Before the delineation of the molecular correlates for LQTS, the development of potent and selective K^+ channel blockers resulted in QT prolongation and induction of torsade arrhythmias *(42)*. Studies indicated that methanesulfonamide drugs were potent blockers of native I_{Kr} channels in cardiac tissue and the molecular correlates of I_{Kr}, the HERG K^+ channels. Thus these drugs produce heterogeneity of refractoriness and predispose one to arrhythmia incidence. This is now a concern for the pharmaceutical and biotechnology industries, as well as government agencies (e.g., Food and Drug Administration [FDA]) because many cardiac (and noncardiac) drugs exhibit QT interval prolongation and may also block HERG K^+ channels. Thus, the potential for these adverse actions of a drug, unrelated to their primary pharmacological actions, has prompted the establishment of regulatory requirements for safety pharmacology studies that outline, using good laboratory practice methods to investigate novel cardiovascular (and noncardiovascular) drugs.

5. SAFETY PHARMACOLOGY

In the simplest sense, pharmacological studies can be separated essentially into three main categories that characterize (1) the primary pharmacodynamic, (2) the secondary pharmacodynamic actions of a new drug, which determines the mechanism of drug action, and (3) the safety pharmacology of the new drug.

Safety pharmacology is defined as those studies that investigate any potential undesirable pharmacological effects of a drug on normal physiological function *(43)*. These studies are not toxicological in nature but rather are an attempt to characterize whether or not a dose–response relationship exists between a drug and the observed response. These studies are conducted before drug administration to humans (phase 1 clinical trials) to reduce the likelihood of adverse events from occurring in the clinical setting. The information excogitated from such studies provides supplemental knowledge relating to the mechanism of action responsible for the observed beneficial, as well as any potential adverse, pharmacological effects. Safety pharmacology studies primarily examine the effects of a drug on three main vital organ systems using a core battery of in vitro and in vivo test systems. These vital organ systems are the central nervous system, respiratory system, and the cardiovascular system. All studies are conducted, optimized, and validated according to International Conference on Harmonization (ICH) ethics and scientific quality standards that reflect proper study design, conduct of experiments, data-recording methods, and data-reporting practices.

Studies are conducted according to good laboratory practice regulations set forth by global regulatory agencies *(43,44)*. Thus, safety pharmacology is a unique new discipline that bridges the gap that currently exists between pharmacology and toxicology. Thus, it is an important consequential means by which to ensure the safety of drugs, especially those being developed for cardiac disease, before their use in human studies. Thus, all new drugs must undergo rigorous safety pharmacology screening methods.

6. METHODS USED TO INVESTIGATE THE ROLE OF ION CHANNELS IN CARDIAC DRUG DEVELOPMENT

6.1. In Vivo Methods

The following describes some of the methods that can used to characterize the pharmacological actions of novel drugs on the heart. These methods are not defined according to specific use in either general or safety pharmacology studies, but are simply divided into in vivo and in vitro methods. In vivo methods require the use of whole animals (mice to primates) where the heart is functionally connected to the circulation. Selection of animal species may vary with the proposed candidate molecule, thus, a thorough understanding of the physiology and functional ion channel status of the species selected should be known. These methods are concerned with measuring the effect of the drug on electrical and mechanical heart performance. The effect on the mechanical performance of the heart in vivo can be evaluated in terms of cardiac output and ventricular pressure whereas actions on electrical properties are characterized using the EKG.

Many direct and indirect methods exist to determine drug activity on cardiac output. Direct measurement of cardiac output is best accomplished using flow probes. Flow probes can be surgically implanted around blood vessels and the volume of blood flowing through the vessel measured. Although many different types of flow probes are available for use, the most common are ultrasonic and electromagnetic *(45)*.

Electromagnetic flow probes provide a greater accuracy for absolute measures of blood flow in a vessel than do ultrasonic flow probes. Ultrasonic flow probes, however, are useful for measuring patterns of changes in flow because they use the Doppler principle of signals reflected from moving blood in the vessel rather than the distortion created by moving red blood cells in the magnetic field of the electromagnetic flow probe. This should be considered when investigating the hemodynamic actions of a drug.

Rather than the direct measurement of cardiac output by flow probes, it is possible to use indirect dye dilution techniques that use tracer materials, such as indocyanine green or Evan's blue dye *(46)*. The introduction of thermodilution methods has allowed for the precise measurement of cardiac output. This clinically used technique has been adapted for use in animal experiments; however, validation and optimization of the method is critical for accurate determination of the effects of novel cardiac drugs.

Cardiac output measurement is the preeminent method for evaluation of the effects of a drug on heart function. However, there are other physical indices of cardiac function that can complement cardiac output studies. Cardiac contractility (performance) depends upon filling pressure in the ventricle and the initial or diastolic fiber length. Therefore, drug effects on such parameters should be assessed. End diastolic pressures are easily measured in the right ventricle in vivo by the direct positioning of a catheter into the right ventricle. Left ventricular pressure recording is best accomplished by measuring pulmonary wedge pressures.

The methods described above provide the best indices of the functional state of the heart. Effective cardiac contraction, in the absence and presence of the candidate drug molecule, can only occur in vivo if adequate delivery of oxygen is supplied to the myocardium and metabolic waste products removed. Thus, coronary blood flow should be measured globally and regionally in these studies. Coronary blood flow can be measured using flow probes placed around a coronary artery or by using microspheres *(47)*.

Electrical activity in the heart can be examined at many levels providing the researcher with the ability to quantitate the effects of novel cardiac drugs at all levels. Global electrical activity is most easily quantified using the EKG. The electrical activity can be examined in different chambers and in various anatomical locations within the heart by insertion of recording electrodes into those areas (or chambers) of the heart *(48)*. With the placement of stimulating electrodes into any of these areas, it is possible to electrically challenge the heart. The electrical stimulation method allows for an assessment of the ion channel status (Na^+ and K^+) within cardiac tissue in the absence and presence of cardiac drug *(48)*. This method also permits for an evaluation of the vulnerability of the ventricle to arrhythmia (premature ventricular contraction [PVC] or VF) induction, thus, is an excellent method with which to rapidly screen novel drugs for cardiac activity.

Extracellular monophasic action potentials (MAPs) can be recorded from the endocardium or epicardium of atria, ventricles, or the whole heart *(49)*. The MAP is an extracellularly recorded potential that approximates the time course of the intracellular AP. The MAP is generated by the application of pressure to the contact electrode against the cardiac muscle wall. The MAP can be used to record myocardial activation time, repolarization (phases 1–3) of the CAP, dispersion of APD, postrepolarization refractoriness, early after-depolarization development, ischemia-induced changes in the APD, and the actions of cardiac drugs *(49)*.

Arrhythmias can seriously impair mechanical function of the heart. Thus, although VT limits or impairs cardiac output, VF terminates cardiac output. Arrhythmias can be detected experimentally by changes in both blood pressure and the EKG. The experimental methods used to induce arrhythmias are both numerous and complex. Arrhythmias may be produced electrically (as discussed previously), chemically or by ischemia *(50)*.

The induction of arrhythmias by chemical methods is usually performed in small animal species. Standard chemical methods for the induction of arrhythmias include the use of cardiac glycosides in guinea pigs, chloroform in mice, aconitine in rats and catecholamines to dogs *(48,50)*. Note that the types of arrhythmias that result are specific to the chemical agent used and are species dependent. Although the arrhythmias that result are reproducible and exhibit characteristic sensitivity to historical or control antiarrhythmic drugs, the mechanism(s) responsible for the development of the arrhythmia are not well defined. However, the use of these proarrhythmic models provide a rapid in vivo screening system with which to investigate the potential efficacy of novel cardiac drugs that can be compared with current, clinically used drugs.

Appropriate electrical stimulation, applied though the implantation of electrodes into any part of the heart, can result in the induction of arrhythmia *(48)*. A large variety of defined stimulation protocols can be used and can be chosen for either the induction of arrhythmias or for indirectly probing the functional status of either Na^+ or K^+ channels. For example, electrical currents and pulse widths required to induce single extra beats in the myocardium reflect Na^+ channel availability and excitability (or i-t curves) whereas refractory periods or effective refractory period (ERP) reflect Na^+ channel status but are highly dependent on K^+ channels which control repolarization *(46)*.

The types of arrhythmias induced by electrical stimulation include single extra beats, VT, or VF. These studies can be conducted in normal intact hearts or in previously ischemic or infarcted hearts. Thus, the flexibility that results from the availability of the numerous stimulation protocols to probe arrhythmia propensity and ion channel activity also makes this a very useful method with which to investigate novel cardiac drugs.

However, the most clinically relevant method for arrhythmia induction results from the occlusion of a coronary artery. This deprives blood flow to the cardiac region subserved by the artery, results in ischemia, and produces changes representative of a heart attack. The continued occlusion of the coronary artery results in MI. Both the duration of coronary artery occlusion and the size of the developed ischemic area determine the extent of infarction. These factors then determine the severity of arrhythmias that develop *(51)*. Reperfusion, which results from the release of the coronary artery from occlusion, produces arrhythmias that appear similar in morphology to those that result from ischemia alone but vary markedly in their development characteristic *(51)*.

VT and VF in these animal models occur at critical times after coronary artery occlusion or reperfusion subsequent to a preceding ischemic period. These methods can be used in all species but care should be taken when selecting the species with which to conduct arrhythmia studies because coronary collateralization in the heart is critical to the size of the developing ischemic area or infarct *(52)*.

Collateralization varies to a large degree among the hearts of different animal species. The hearts of guinea pigs have an abundance of coronary collateral vessels, which prevents its use in the study of regional myocardial ischemia *(46)*. Arrhythmic responses are also not uniform in dogs because of the extent of pre-existing coronary collateralization *(50)*. Coronary collaterals are not present to any significant degree in the hearts of species such as rats, pigs, rabbits, and primates; this makes them better candidates as models with which to investigate responses to ischemia and reperfusion in the heart *(50)*.

To accurately assess the efficacy of a novel cardiac drug, it is necessary to quantitate the area of ischemia or infarction that is produced by the most physiologically relevant animal model. Many diverse experimental methods can be used to quantitate the size of the infarction produced in the heart. The most accurate methods are those that directly quantitate the anatomical size of the infarct. Such gross anatomical methods include cross-sectioning the ventricle into slices and estimating the area of infarction found in each slice. Demarcation between infarcted, ischemic, and normal myocardial tissue can be resolved using stains that chemically interact with normal tissue and not necrotic tissue *(46)*. These provide an accurate estimate of infarct size that is easily determined by visual examination providing reliable results in drug assessment.

6.2. In Vitro Methods

Many types of in vitro cardiac preparations are used to study cardiac function and the electrophysiological effects of drugs on myocardial cells. Methods include single myocardial cells, isolated cardiac tissue preparations, the Langendorff isolated rat heart, and heterologous expression systems.

Although single adult myocardial cells are isolated from many different animal species, including humans, the rat and guinea pig remain the principle species used. Enzymes are perfused into isolated hearts and the dissociated cells harvested for use in electrophysiological and biochemical study. The main advantage of the use of single isolated myocytes is that the unknown electrophysiological actions of a newly developed cardiac drug can be investigated independent of other cells in the heart.

The patch clamp technique revolutionized cardiac drug discovery because it was possible to record current flow through ion channels in the many cells that comprise the CAP. The electrophysiological actions of a drug are investigated using many configurations of the patch clamp. Whole-cell recording, in which the total ionic current that flows across the cell membrane is recorded, and patch clamp recording, in which the current that only flows across a small membrane patch is recorded, are the most commonly used (53). However, for drug study, the whole-cell configuration is preferred. This method allows the investigator to determine the effects of the drug on many different ion channels using electrophysiological protocols that probe the functional properties of the channel. Many properties of the channel can be examined in the absence and presence of various concentrations of the investigational drug. The goal of these studies is to characterize the molecular actions of the drug in an attempt to elucidate both its site of action and putative mechanism.

Isolated tissue preparations have become a cornerstone of the physiological and pharmacological evaluation of natural and synthetic drugs. Note, however, that the extrapolation of drug effects on isolated tissue preparations to the whole animal is limited by the complexity of mechanisms present in intact animals. Nevertheless, the assessment of the pharmacological action of antiarrhythmic drugs in isolated tissues is an essential step in clarifying the actions of a novel drug and in determining further studies in intact animals.

The cardiovascular system is a rich source of tissues for in vitro studies. Therefore, to investigate drug action some of the most widely used cardiac preparations include isolated atrial or ventricular tissue, papillary muscles and the isolated, coronary-perfused right ventricular wall (54). The use of these tissue preparations in drug investigations is numerous. The small size of most cardiac tissues allows for the rapid and continuous diffusion of oxygen and nutrients to subcellular layers, resulting in viable, stable preparations. These preparations from different animal species are extensively used to represent the heart; therefore, the type of isolated tissue preparation used when attempting to study problems concerning drug actions or cardiac function must be carefully considered.

The isolated perfused whole heart is the most physiologically relevant isolated cardiac tissue. This preparation has many advantages compared with either isolated myocytes or isolated tissues because it lends itself to the study of the actions of cardiac drugs on mechanical, electrical, and biochemical properties of the heart. The isolated Langendorff heart is a simple preparation with which to screen for the cardiac actions of drugs because it uses physiological buffers to maintain normal heart function (55).

The greatest function of the isolated perfused heart is its usefulness in assessing drug actions on the rate of generation of ventricular pressure. It is also a sensitive indicator of the chronotropic and inotropic actions of drugs on the heart. Coronary flow and a surface EKG can also be recorded as supplementary indices of drug action on coronary vasculature resistance and ion channels. Drug activity can also be assessed in diseased hearts.

Equally, ischemia and reperfusion arrhythmias can be investigated in isolated perfused hearts. Occlusion of a coronary artery in an isolated perfused heart produces arrhythmias. The antiarrhythmic efficacy of the drug under investigation can readily be compared with that observed in vivo in the absence of blood. Isolated hearts can also be rendered globally or regionally ischemic and the effect of the drug can be investigated on measures, such as oxygen consumption and other markers of cardiac metabolism associated with these pathological states. Thus, the extensive variety of convincing applications for use of this method in normal and diseases hearts will ensure its continued use in the preclinical assessment of novel cardiac and antiarrhythmic drugs.

The use of heterologous expression systems allows for the electrophysiological measurement of the properties of cardiac drugs on isolated ion channels from the heart using voltage and patch clamp techniques. These systems are used to express high levels of the desired functional protein that is not endogenous to the system. Some available expression systems include *Xenopus* oocytes, transfected mammalian cells, such as human embryonic kidney (and Chinese hamster ovary cells, and baculovirus-infected insect cell lines, such as Sf9 and Hi5. The expression system selected should be chosen (as with isolated tissues described above) appropriately based on the questions addressed because each system has certain advantages and disadvantages. For example, one system may be appropriate for the study of drugs on ion channel function (e.g., *Xenopus* oocytes) whereas another may be more useful to synthesize large amounts of protein for biochemical analysis (e.g., baculovirus-insect cell lines).

Xenopus laevis oocytes are one of the most commonly used expression systems with which to examine cDNA (or mRNA) encoding cardiac ion channels. Their usefulness resides in the fact that oocytes do not express significant levels of endogenous Na^+, K^+, or Ca^{2+} currents. RNA that is injected into oocytes is efficiently transcribed so that the effects of cardiac and antiarrhythmic drugs on exogenous channels can be studied. One disadvantage of the oocyte system is that proteins are modified by the oocyte. In mammalian cells, protein synthesis involves many sequential processing steps that result in a unique structural or functional protein. Studies of translational mRNA processes in oocytes suggest that although similar to mammalian cells, some post-translational processing differences exist. Glycosylation of the protein in oocytes may be different from mammalian glycosylation possibly resulting in altered functional properties. However, despite this caveat, oocytes have become a gold standard for functional expression of ion channels. Today, many distinct mammalian cell lines can be used to express cloned human cardiac ion channels. The most relevant to the examination of cardiac or antiarrhythmic drugs are those cell lines that stably express the HERG K^+ ion channel that is implicated in torsade des pointes arrhythmias or the LQTS.

7. HIGH THROUGHPUT SCREENING (HTS) METHODS IN CARDIAC DRUG DEVELOPMENT

HTS defines a series of usually in vitro methodologies that can be used to rapidly screen many (thousands) potential cardiac drug candidates for activity against ion channels that eventually may exhibit efficacy in humans. Recently, the defined involvement of ion channels in multiple disease conditions (i.e., channelopathies) have re-invigorated drug development for arrhythmias. The implication of ion channels, such as I_{Kr} in torsade des pointes and the LQTS, are such an example. Thus, although the voltage-gated ion channel so-called flavor of the day may vary, ion channels in the heart remain viable targets for drug development. However, as is inherent to pharmacology, there remains a continued lag in available HTS processes that accurately quantitate the cardiac efficacy of a potentially novel molecule. Thus, the pharmacologist cannot hope to compete with chemists that develop structure–activity relationships for novel drugs. It is understood that using in vivo screens, isolated tissues, dissociated myocytes, isolated hearts, or heterologous expression systems to evaluate new drug candidates is a gravely slower, and more tedious process, than drug synthesis.

However, attempts to improve upon early screening procedures using in vitro or biochemical methods may begin to close the Grand Canyon-size gap that currently exists between chemical synthesis and determining drug efficacy and safety. Because ion channels really do not contain functionally defined binding sites and are not a receptor this further complicates the development of HTS methods.

Sodium and other ion channels characteristically contain binding sites for neurotoxins and other drugs that activate, block, or modulate channel response to drugs through known mechanisms. Thus, attempts have been made to use radioligand-binding methods to develop HTS assays for ion channels. However, complications arise because the activity of many neurotoxins involves a state-dependent binding to the Na^+ channel *(56)*. The utility of such a preliminary assay as a screen is attenuated because drugs that do not interact with the state of the channel produced by the neurotoxin would not be detected.

Fluorescence-based cellular methods may more appropriately reflect the selectivity and sensitivity that is required for HTS assays *(56)*. Briefly, the fluorescence methods use a heterocycle fluorophore or fluorescence dye molecule that localizes in a region of the cell (such as the cytoplasm) and responds to a stimulus. Fluorophores for Ca^{2+} ions include dyes, such as fura-2 and fluo-4 (Molecular Probes, Eugene, OR), whereas others are available for Na^+ and K^+ ions.

Probes such as these are measured using technologies, such as the Fluorometric Imaging Plate Recorder or FLIPR[384] (Molecular Devices, Sunnyvale, CA). Because these systems contain enhanced automation features, including potential robot integration, assays that quantitate intracellular constituents, such as Ca^{2+}, pH and Na^+ and V_m, they may be modified to conduct HTS assay development. Cell responses can be monitored in real time, kinetic data for drugs can be derived, relative drug potencies can be determined, and drug-ion channel interaction kinetics can be determined.

Radiotracers can also be used in HTS assays. Denyer et al. *(56)* describe a novel cell-based Na^+ channel assay using Cytostar-T scintillating microplates (Amersham Life Science, Piscataway, NJ). These plates have a transparent scintillant base that emits light as it is excited by the decay of the radioisotope in close proximity. Cells are grown to confluence on the microplates and various neurotoxins are used to maintain open Na^+ channels. Permeant ^{14}C-labeled guanidinium is added to the cells. Once sufficient radiotracer incorporation into the cells occurs, tetrodotoxin is used to block the channels. Blockade or inhibition of channel opening by the test drug alters the signal emitted from the scintillation base of the microplate and provides an index of activity on the Na^+ channel. Complex assays such as this may provide the necessary steps in the development of HTS screening methods for ion channels.

Coronary artery occlusion and MI development results in progressive changes in the cellular architecture of both infarcted and noninfarcted ventricular muscle. These changes are caused by remodeling within the heart. Remodeling involves changes in cellular events that modulate adaptation and include hypertrophy of myocytes, deposition of extracellular matrix components, and proliferation of fibroblasts *(57)*. These processes ultimately are responsible for ensuing dysfunction that transpires post-MI. Diminution in cardiac contractility derives from muscle dystrophy and fibrosis, events subsequent to scar formation within the damaged ventricular muscle. For this to occur within the heart, there must be an altered response and downregulation of many homeostatic mechanisms responsible for normal contractility. Ultimately such changes derive from altered gene expression, and this can be studied at the subcellular level using microarray technology.

DNA microarrays are a powerful new method by which to determine the pattern of gene expression in both normal and diseased tissues. Microarrays currently provide an initial central point for use in drug target and validation. These methods allow for the identification of those genes, whether up- or downregulated in expression that may be involved in disease. It is now recognized that many cardiac disease processes involve multiple modifications in genes. These concurrent changes may then culminate in the disease process. Thus, therapy can now ideally be directed at the cause of the disease and not simply at the symptoms.

Microarray technology may have an application in cardiac disease because it provides researchers with the ability to characterize the gene expression levels of thousands of genes in parallel *(58)*. The development of DNA microarrays for application to disease is a multistep process. Genes to be arrayed are identified and obtained from private or public genebanks. Both normal and diseased tissues are used and usually ~15,000 genes are identified that may characterize the cardiac disease under investigation. Selected genes are usually maintained in bacterial plasmids and subject to polymerase chain reaction amplification procedures before hybridization on microarray plates. The polymerase chain reaction amplification product is arrayed at a high density to either glass slides radiolabeled with a fluorescent dye (such as C4S) or nylon membranes radiolabeled with phosphorus (^{33}P). The signal intensity of the hybridized genetic sample determines the expression level of the corresponding gene and the profile is then processed using bioinformatic methods.

Although the potential impact of microarray use in many cardiac diseases is substantial, its application remains at an elementary stage. Several studies have been conducted in models of heart failure, MI, and ventricular hypertrophy *(57,59)*. In these studies, no fewer than 55 known (and unknown) genes were detected that could be involved in these cardiac diseases. Functional relevance remains inconclusive and many caveats exist that relate to the use of this methodology.Microarrays, although high throughput in nature, have a low sensitivity, and genes that exhibit ~70% homology are indistinguishable *(60)*. Quality control issues, computational resources, and a requirement that a large number of diseased and nondiseased tissues must be profiled to derive conclusions concerning the reproducibility of gene expression patterns are issues that require resolution. Owing to the ingenuity of researchers in this field, resolution is only time dependent.

8. CLINICAL DRUG TRIALS

Clinical drug trials test the activity of the drug on the disease or symptom. The extensive general and safety pharmacology studies that are conducted prior to the initiation of the testing of the drug in humans require years. However, it is critical that these studies define the pharmacological effects and the potential for serious drug toxicity before use in humans and are the sum of in vitro and in vivo studies conducted in both animal and human preparations (as described above). If these preclinical studies

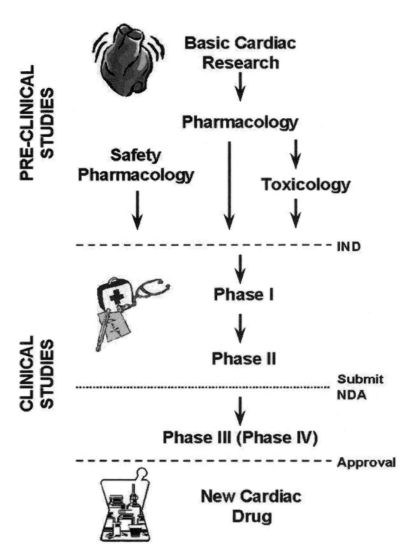

Fig. 4. The preclinical and clinical relationships for new drug development and the approval process.

are successful, then the pharmaceutical or biotechnology company provides the data in the form of an Investivational New Drug application to governmental agencies such as the FDA in the United States or to the European Agency for the Evaluation of Medicinal Products (EMEA) in Europe.

Clinical drug trials of novel antiarrhythmic or cardiovascular experimental drugs (as for all drugs) are conducted in four phases (Fig. 4). The early phases of drug testing in humans are usually broad in perspective and provide information regarding dose, drug kinetics, and tolerance. Thus these early phases concern the testing of the safety of the drug (phase 1) and the efficacy of the drug (phase 2). The attrition rate for new drugs reaches approx 60% by the end of this phase of clinical trial testing. In later trials, large controlled studies that delineate the range of the drug's effectiveness; incidence of adverse events and the benefit to potential patient population (phase 3) are conducted. The attrition rate for drugs is reduced to approx 10–20%. Successful completion allows the drug company to file a New Drug Application with the FDA or EMEA. If granted, the drug is then conditionally approved for marketing.

This conditional approval is given before phase 4 studies. However, these phase 4 (or late phase 3) studies are intended to provide for postmarketing surveillance and allow for the monitored release of the drug, whereby patients may be given the drug under specified supervision by physicians at selected medical centers.

These studies are an indispensable part of medical research and offer the only means by which to provide new therapies for cardiovascular diseases that afflict humans. However, as many clinical cardiovascular trials have taught (and cost!) the drug industry, this is a very arduous process and many cardiovascular clinical drug trials have failed. However, despite these failures, a re-evaluation of clinical trial data provides for suggestions as to how to improve clinical trials involving cardiac drugs. These suggestions include the regular requirement of phase 4 trials with surrogate endpoints, a clear definition of phase 3 study endpoints, and also by possibly reassessment of thestructure of the clinical trial hierarchy itself *(61,62)*. Recently, Lipicky *(61)* suggested that the traditional distinctions between study phases for clinical trials not be used. It is reasoned that conforming to the rigid phases currently used to conduct clinical trials with cardiac (particulary antiarrhythmic) drugs may be detrimental to drug development *(61)*. Rather, it is suggested that combining phase 2 with phase 3 trials may reduce unnecessary delays associated with independent, consecutive trials and be of a clear benefit to drug development. Additionally, it is suggested that multiple drug doses should be studied, the type of arrhythmia be defined and the doses be related to some measure of cardiac activity *(61)*. Consideration of suggestions such as these may reduce the attrition rate associated with drug development for cardiac disease, improve the safety profile for these drugs in patients, and ultimately provide novel drugs that improve symptoms associated with the disease or prevent the disease itself.

REFERENCES

1. American Heart Association. (2002) *Heart and Stroke Statistical Update*. American Heart Association, Dallas, TX.
2. Vaughan Williams, E. M. (1984). A classification of antiarrhythmic actions reassessed after a decade of new drugs. *J. Clin. Pharmacol.* **24,** 129–147.
3. The Cardiac Arrhythmia Suppression Trial (CAST) Investigators. (1989) Preliminary Report: Effect of encainide and flecainide on mortality in a randomized trial of arrhythmia suppression after myocardial infarction. *N. Eng. J. Med.* **321,** 406–412.
4. The Cardiac Arrhythmia Suppression Trial II (CAST–II) Investigators. (1992) Effect of the antiarrhythmic agent moricizine on survival after myocardial infarction. *N. Eng. J. Med.* **327,** 227–233.
5. IMPACT Research Group. (1984) International mexiletine and placebo antiarrhythmic coronary trial: I. Report on arrhythmia and other findings. *J. Am. Coll. Cardiol.* **4,** 1148–1163.
6. Myerburg, R. J., Kessler, K. M., Chakko, S., Cox, M. M., Fernando, P., Interian, A., and Castellanos, A. (1994) Future evaluation of antiarrhythmic therapy. *Am. Heart J.* **127,** 1111–1118.
7. Morganroth, J. and Goin, J. E. (1991) Quinidine-related mortality in the short- to medium-term treatment of ventricular arrhythmias: A meta analysis. *Circulation* **84,** 1977–1983.

8. Hine, L. K., Laird, N., Hewitt, P., and Chalmers, T. C. (1989) Meta-analytic evidence against prophylactic use of lidocaine in acute myocardial infarction. *Arch. Int. Med.* **149,** 2694–2698.

9. Rosenfeld, J., Rosen, M. R., and Hoffman, B. F. (1978) Pharmacologic and behavioral effects on arrhythmias that immediately follow abrupt coronary occlusion: A canine model of sudden coronary death. *Am. J. Cardiol.* **41,** 1075–1084.

10. Kam, R. M., Teo, W. S., Koh, T. H., and Lim, Y. L. (1999) Treatment and prevention of sudden cardiac death{\}what have we learnt from randomised clinical trials? *Singapore Med. J.* **40,** 707–710.

11. Ogunyankin, K. O. and Singh, B. N. (1999) Mortality reduction by antiadrenergic modulation of arrhythmogenic substrate: Significance of combining beta blockers and amiodarone. *Am. J. Cardiol.* **84,** 76R–82R.

12. Singh, B. N. (1999) The relevance of sympathetic activity in the pharmacological treatment of chronic stable angina. *Can. J. Cardiol.* **15(Suppl A),** 15A–21A.

13. Nattel, S. (1991) Antiarrhythmic drug classifications. A critical appraisal of their history, present status, and clinical relevance. *Drugs* **41,** 672–701.

14. Beatch, G. N., Barrett, T. D., Plouvier, B., Jung, G., Wall, R. A., Zolotoy, A., and Walker, M. J. A. (2002) Ventricular fibrillation, an uncontrolled arrhythmia seeking new targets. *Drug Dev. Res.* **55,** 45–52.

15. Karmazyn, M. (2000) Pharmacology and clinical assessment of cariporide for the treatment of coronary artery diseases. *Expert. Opin. Invest. Drugs* **9,** 1099–1108.

16. Hodgkin, A. L. and Huxley, A. F. (1952) A quantitative description of membrane current and its application to conduction and excitation in nerve. *J. Physiol. (Lond)* **116,** 500–544.

17. Denac, H., Mevissen, M., and Scholtysik, G. (2000) Structure, function and pharmacology of voltage-gated sodium channels. *Naunyn-Schmied. Arch. Pharmacol.* **362,** 453–479.

18. Sato, C., Ueno, Y., Asai, K., Takahashi, K., Sato, M., Engel, A., and Fujiyoshi, Y. (2001) The voltage-sensitive sodium channel is a bell-shaped molecule with several cavities. *Nature* **409,** 1047–1051.

19. Isom, L. L., DeJongh, K. S., Patton, D. E., Reber, B. F. X., Offord, J., Charbonneau, H., et al. (1992) Primary structure and functional expression of the β_1 subunit of the rat brain sodium channel. *Science* **256,** 839–842.

20. Isom, L. L., Ragsdale, D. S., De Jongh, K. S., Westenbroek, R. E., Reber, B. F. X., Scheuer, T., et al. (1995) Structure and function of the β_2 subunit of brain sodium channels, a transmembrane glycoprotein with a CAM motif. *Cell* **83,** 433–442.

21. West, J. W., Patton, D. E., Scheuer, T., Wang, Y., Goldin, A. L., and Catterall, W. A. (1992) A cluster of hydrophobic amino acid residues required for fast Na^+ channel inactivation. *Proc. Natl. Acad. Sci. USA* **89,** 10910–10914.

22. Hille, B. (1984) Mechanisms of Block, in *Ionic Channels of Excitable Membranes* (Hille, B., ed.), Sinauer, Sunderland, UK, pp. 390–422.

23. Hille, B. (1977) Local anesthetics: Hydrophilic and hydrophobic pathways for the drug–receptor reaction. *J. Gen. Physiol.* **69,** 497–515.

24. Hondeghem, L. M. and Katzung, B. G. (1977) Time- and voltage-dependent interactions of antiarrhythmic drugs with cardiac sodium channels. *Biochim. Biophys. Acta.* **472,** 373–398.

25. Ragsdale, D. S., McPhee, J. C., Scheuer, T., and Catterall, W. A. (1996) Common molecular determinants of local anesthetic, antiarrhythmic, and anticonvulsant block of voltage-gated Na+ channels. *Proc. Natl. Acad. Sci. USA* **93,** 9270–9275.

26. Streissnig, J. (1999) Pharmacology, structure and function of cardiac L-type calcium channels. *Cell. Physiol. Biochem.* **9,** 242–269.

27. Bean, B. P. and McDonough, S. I. (1998) Two for T. *Neuron* **20,** 825–828.

28. Gao, T., Puri, T. S., Gerhardstein, B. L., Chien, A. J., Green, R. D., and Hosey, M. M. (1997) Identification and subcellular localization of the subunits of L-type calcium channels and adenylyl cyclase in cardiac myocytes. *J. Biol. Chem.* **272,** 19,401–19,407.

29. Klugbauer, N., Lacinova, L., Marais, E., Hobom, M., and Hofmann, F. (1999) Molecular diversity of the calcium channel alpha2delta subunit. *J. Neurosci.* **19,** 684–691.
30. Snyders, D. J. (1999) Structure and function of cardiac potassium channels. *Cardiovasc. Res.* **42,** 377–390.
31. Nerbonne, J. M. (2000) Molecular basis of functional voltage-gated K$^+$ channel diversity in the mammalian myocardium. *J. Physiol.* **525,** 285–298.
32. Rasmusson, R. L., Morales, M. J., Wang, S., Liu, S., Campbell, D. L., Brahmajothi, M. V., and Strauss, H. C. (1998) Inactivation of voltage-gated cardiac K$^+$ channels. *Circ. Res.* **82,** 739–750.
33. Colatsky, T. J. and Follmer, C. H. (1989) K$^+$ channel blockers and activatorrs in cardiac arrhythmias. *Cardiovasc. Drug Rev.* **7,** 199–209.
34. Hondeghem, L. M. and Snyders, D. J. (1990) Class III antiarrhythmic agents have a lot of potential but a long way to go. *Circulation* **81,** 686–690.
35. Katritsis, D., and Camm, A. J. (1993) New class III antiarrhythmic drugs. *Eur. Heart J.* **14,** 93–99.
36. Janse, M. J. and Kleber, A. G. (1981) Electrophysiological changes and ventricular arrhythmias in the early phase of regional myocardial ischemia. *Circ. Res.* **49,** 1069–1081.
37. Patterson, E., Szabo, B., Scherlag, B. J., and Lazzara, R. (1995) Arrhythmogenic effects of antiarrhythmic drugs, in *Cardiac Electrophysiology, From Cell to Bedside* (Zipes, D. P., Jalife, J. eds.), W. B. Saunders, New York, NY, pp. 496–511.
38. Towbin, J. A., Wang, Z., and Li, H. (2001) Genotype and severity of long QT syndrome. *Drug Metab Dispos.* **29,** 574–579.
39. Albrecht, B., Weber, K., and Pongs, O. (1995) Characterization of a voltage-activated K-channel gene cluster on human chromosome 12p13. *Receptors Channels* **3,** 213–220.
40. Martens, J. R., Kwak, Y. G., and Tamkun, M. M. (1999) Modulation of K$_v$ channel alpha/beta subunit interactions. *Trends Cardiovasc. Med.* **9,** 253–258.
41. Roden, D. M. and Balser, J. R. (1999) A plethora of mechanisms in the HERG-related long QT syndrome. Genetics meets electrophysiology. *Cardiovasc. Res.* **44,** 242–246.
42. Mounsey, J. P., and DiMarco, J. P. (2000) Cardiovascular drugs. Dofetilide. *Circulation* **102,** 2665–2670.
43. ICH S7A. Safety pharmacology studies for human pharmaceuticals (CHMP/ICH/539/00).
44. ICH S7B (2002) Safety pharmacology studies for assessing the potential for delayed ventricular repolarization (QT interval prolongation) by human pharmaceuticals: Draft ICH Consensus Guidelines.
45. Pugsley, M. K. and Tabrizchi, R. (2000) The vascular system: An overview of structure and function. *J. Pharmacol. Toxicol. Meth.* **44,** 333–340.
46. Pugsley, M. K. and Walker, M. J.A. (1992) Methods for evaluating heart function, in *Immunopharmacology of the Heart* (Curtis, M. J., ed.), Academic Press, London, UK, pp. 7–28.
47. Pang, C. C. Y. (2000) Measurement of body venous tone. *J. Pharmacol. Toxicol. Meth.* **44,** 341–360.
48. Winslow, E. (1984) Methods in the detection and assessment of antiarrhythmic activity. *Pharmacol. Ther.* **24,** 401–433.
49. Beatch, G. N. and Barrett, T. D. (1998) Monophasic action potential recording, in *Methods in Cardiac Electrophysiology* (Walker, M. J. A., and Pugsley, M. K., eds.), CRC Press, Boca Raton, FL, pp. 117–132.
50. Cheung, P. H., Pugsley, M. K., and Walker, M. J.A. (1993) Arrhythmia models in the rat. *J. Pharmacol. Toxicol. Meth.* **29,** 179–184.
51. Botting, J. H., Curtis, M. J., and Walker, M. J.A. (1985) Arrhythmias associated with myocardial ischaemia and infarction. *Mol. Aspects Med.* **8,** 311–422.
52. Johnston, K. M., Macleod, B. A., and Walker, M. J. A. (1983) Responses to ligation of a coronary artery in conscious rats and the actions of antiarrhythmics. *Can. J. Physiol. Pharmacol.* **61,** 1340–1353.

53. Saint, D. A. (1998) Single channel recording and mathematical analysis of currents in cardiac myocytes, in *Methods in Cardiac Electrophysiology* (Walker, M. J. A., and Pugsley, M. K., eds.), CRC Press, Boca Raton, FL, pp. 63–88.

54. Walker, M. J. A. and Pugsley, M. K. (eds.) (1998) *Methods in Cardiac Electrophysiology*, CRC Press, Boca Raton, FL.

55. Doring, H. J., and Dehnert, H. (eds.) (1988) *Methods in Experimental Physiology and Pharmacology: Biological Measurement Techniques V*, Biomesstechnik-Verlag, Germany.

56. Denyer, J., Worley, J., Cox, B., Allenby, G., and Banks, M. (1998) HTS approaches to voltage-gated ion channel drug discovery. *Drug Dis. Today* **3,** 323–332.

57. Stanton L. W., Garrard, L. J., Damm, D., Garrick, B. L., Lam, A., Kapoun, A. M., et al. (2000) Altered patterns of gene expression in response to myocardial infarction. *Circ. Res.* **86,** 939–945.

58. Duggan, D. J., Bittner, M., Chen, Y., Meltzer, P., and Trent, J. M. (1999) Expression profiling using cDNA microarrays. *Nat. Genet.* **21(1 Suppl),** 10–14.

59. Remme, C. A., Lombardi, M. P., van den Hoff, M. J. B., and Lekanne dit Deprez, R. H. (2000) CDNA arrays: The ups and downs. *Cardiovasc. Drugs Ther.* **15,** 99–101.

60. Boguslavsky, J. (2000) In–house microarrays put researchers in control. *Drug Dis. Dev.* **10,** 30–36.

61. Lipicky, R. (2000) An FDA perspective on antiarrhythmic drugs in phase II trials. *Am. Heart J.* **139,** S197–S199.

62. Temple, R. (1999) Are surrogate markers adequate to assess cardiovascular disease drugs? *JAMA* **282,** 790–795.

II

Novel Molecular Targets
for Cardiac Drug Development

2

The Role of Cardiac Pacemaker Currents in Antiarrhythmic Drug Discovery

David A. Saint

1. THE PACEMAKER CURRENT AS A TARGET FOR THERAPY

From even the most basic physiological observations, it is obvious that parts of the heart can generate their own intrinsic contractile rhythm. With the development of techniques to record electrical activity from tissues, it became clear that contraction of the heart is triggered by an action potential and that most areas of the heart can, under some circumstances, generate rhythmic action potentials, although it is cells in the sinoatrial node (SAN) that have the highest intrinsic frequency, and hence it is these cells that normally provide the drive for the rest of the heart. Even a single, isolated SAN cell will generate rhythmic action potentials separated by a period of slow diastolic depolarization. It is the diastolic depolarization that repeatedly drives the membrane potential towards threshold for action potential firing. The mechanism underlying this diastolic depolarization has been a subject of much puzzlement. By the 1970s, it was clear that to provide a slow depolarization, there must be a slow increase in net inward current, although it was not clear whether this came about as a consequence of the slow inactivation of an outward current (presumed to be a carried by potassium) or the slow activation of an inward current *(1)*. Using the intracellular recording and voltage clamp techniques available at the time, it was difficult to resolve the different components of the current flowing during the diastolic depolarization *(2–4)*. With the advent of patch-clamp techniques, coupled with techniques for preparation of isolated cells

From: *Cardiac Drug Development Guide*
Edited by: M. K. Pugsley © Humana Press Inc., Totowa, NJ

from various parts of the heart, resolution of individual currents became possible. The mechanism of the diastolic depolarization was greatly clarified by the discovery in pacemaker cells of an inward current that was activated by hyperpolarization *(5–8)*. The current was shown to activate relatively slowly on hyperpolarization and to have low selectivity among cations. These properties are just what one would expect for a pacemaking current

Around the same time as it was discovered in cardiac myocytes, a similar current was identified in photoreceptors *(9)*. Subsequently, similar currents were discovered in other tissues, particularly in parts of the central nervous system (CNS). The current in cardiac tissue was christened I(f) (f for funny, because of its funny properties) and in most other tissues it was called I(h) (h, because of the activation on hyperpolarization). The terms are often used interchangeably.

I(f) or I(h) has been implicated in cardiac *(10)* and neuronal *(11–13)* rhythmogenesis, sensory adaptation *(14,15)*, shaping of synaptic potentials *(16)*, and control of synaptic transmitter release *(17,18)*.

2. THE CHARACTERISTICS OF I(F)

As noted above, the critical and unusual feature of I(f) is its voltage dependence. I(f) is activated by hyperpolarizations with a threshold of approx −40 to −50 mV in the SAN. Figure 1 shows a typical activation curve, which depicts the relative fraction of channels open at steady state as a function of membrane voltage. This relation indicates that the current is activated at voltages near the range of the diastolic depolarization in SAN cells. The fully activated current/voltage (I–V) relation reverses near +10 to +20 mV in physiological solutions as a consequence of the channel having a mixed permeability to Na^+ and K^+. The activation by hyperpolarization and permeability to Na^+ and K^+ are critical properties with respect to the role of I(f) in the generation of diastolic depolarization and hence of spontaneous activity. Hence, membrane potentials around the maximum diastolic potential in SAN cells activate the current, which, because it is a nonspecific cation current, produces an inward, depolarizing current at these potentials. To a large extent, it is this slow activation of I(f) that tends to drive the slow diastolic depolarization until the membrane potential reaches threshold for the triggering of a new action potential.

However, when it was first described, there was initially some skepticism regarding the role of I(f) in pacemaking and, indeed, there is still some degree of controversy as to just how important I(f) is to pacemaking *(19,20)*. Although I(f) seems to be a good candidate for the role of a pacemaker current, the real situation is somewhat more complex. An important caveat is that, rather than being driven by one current, the pacemaking activity of SAN cells is a product of the interplay of many currents *(21)*. This assertion is reinforced by the observation that pacemaking continues (albeit at a slowed rate) when I(f) is blocked *(22)* and from the observation that the *smo* mutant of zebra fish (which has a mutation in pacemaking channels carrying the fast kinetic component of the current which renders them nonfunctional) still has an operational pacemaker, albeit once again at a greatly slowed rate *(23)*. Hence, it seems that the autorhythmicity of SAN cells is driven and stabilized by an interplay of several currents, none of which is crucial, but all of which influence rhythm. This situation provides redundancy and pleiotropism in the regulation of rhythm *(21)*. Nevertheless, it is certainly true that one

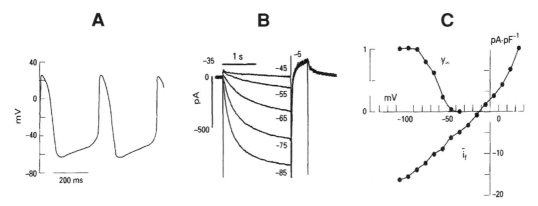

Fig. 1. The biophysical properties of I(f). (**A**) Spontaneous activity of a single SAN cell. Note that the maximum diastolic potential is about –65 mV. (**B**) I(f) current induced in a single SAN cell by a hyperpolarising pulse to the voltages indicated from a holding potential of –35 mV. (**C**) Voltage dependence of activation of I(f), (Y_∞) and fully activated I/V relationship. Reprinted from DiFrancesco, D. (1995), The onset and autonomic regulation of cardiac pacemaker activity: relevance of the f current. *Cardiovasc. Res.* **29,** 4493–4556, with permission from Elsevier Science.

of the major influences on auto rhythmicity is I(f) and, hence, it is sensible to use I(f) as a target in attempts to modulate rhythmicity.

If I(f) is indeed responsible for driving the diastolic depolarization, one would imagine that it should be modulated by sympathetic and parasympathetic stimulation in a way consistent with their chronotropic effects. I(f) is indeed modulated by adrenergic agonists in a way consistent with an increase in heart rate *(24)*.

In 1986, DiFrancesco *(25)* showed that I(f) was carried by channels having a single channel conductance of about 1 pS, and that modulation of I(f) by adrenaline at the single channel level consists of an increase in the open probability without a change in single channel conductance. This effect of adrenaline is mediated via the G-protein/ adenyl cyclase/cAMP pathway. Using patch clamp techniques, it has been shown that I(f) channels are modulated by a direct effect of intracellular cAMP at the intracellular side of the channel, independent of any phosphorylation effects *(26)*. The effect of cAMP consists of a facilitation of the opening of single I(f) channels in response to hyperpolarization. Measurement of the voltage dependence of the channel open probability shows that cAMP shifts the probability curve to more positive voltages without modifying its shape *(27)*.

Interestingly, the modulation itself seems to be subject to other influences, notably the action of phosphorylation. Hence, the phosphatase inhibitor calyculin A increases I(f) and potentates the beta-adrenergic mediated response *(28)*, suggesting that there is a so-called tonic level of phosphorylation of the channels that regulates their activity *(29)*. The channels carrying I(f) have also been reported to be modulated by various hormones and growth factors. Epidermal growth factor increases maximal I(f) conductance, apparently acting through tyrosine kinase *(30)*. Vasoactive intestinal peptide produces a slight shift in the voltage dependence of activation of I(f) *(28)*, an effect that may be related to the role of vasoactive intestinal peptide as a cotransmitter with acetylcholine released from vagal nerve endings. The thyroid hormone T3 increases the current density of I(f) in rabbit SAN cells without changing the voltage dependence, an effect that may underlie the sinus tachycardia commonly seen in hyperthyroidism *(31)*. Similar results have been reported with parathyroid hormones *(32)*. In addition, I(f) is modulated by muscarinic agonists in a way consistent with the decrease in heart rate seen with these agents *(33)*.

3. VARIABILITY OF CHARACTERISTICS OF I(F) IN DIFFERENT TISSUES

Reflecting this wide range of tissues in which it is found and the differing physiological functions with which it is therefore involved, the properties of I(f) (or I[h]) differ significantly in their voltage dependence, activation kinetics, and sensitivity to cAMP in different tissues *(12,34)*. This heterogeneity of properties of I(f) is found not only between tissues but also within organs or tissue types themselves. Hence, biophysical studies have demonstrated that I(f) has a dramatically different voltage dependence of activation in different cardiac regions, with the threshold for activation being –50 mV in SA node, –85 mV in Purkinje myocytes, and –120 mV in adult ventricular myocytes *(35)*. This difference in the voltage-dependent properties of I(f) is highly correlated with the intrinsic pacemaker activity of these tissues; the I(f) current having the most positive activation is found in the tissue with the highest pacing rate (in SA node), whereas the current having the most negative activation is found in tissue that normally exhibits no diastolic depolarization at all (ventricular myocytes). Although some of these differences in current properties may be the result of post-translational modification of the channels or functional modulation by phosphorylation, the most likely explanation is that I(f) currents are carried by different isoforms of the channel in different tissues. Current density is also an important factor, presumably controlled by the level of gene expression; as well as different voltage dependence, I(f) in ventricular cells is present at a very low current density (Fig. 2). With the recent cloning of the channels responsible for I(f), the factors controlling the level of gene expression, and which isoform of the channel is expressed, have become amenable to investigation.

4. MOLECULAR BIOLOGY OF I(F) AND I(H)

Although the properties of I(f) and the single channels underlying the current have been investigated for nearly three decades, particularly because of its importance to cardiac pacemaking *(10)*, cloning of the gene coding for I(f) was only achieved nearly three decades after the original description of I(f), and even then the clone was discovered serendipitously. While searching for proteins interacting with the SH3 binding domain of neural Src, Santoro et al. *(36)* identified a putative member of a new family of channels cloned from mouse brain. Using BLAST searches of expressed sequence tag databases, along with reverse-transcription polymerase chain reaction and screening of cDNA libraries, four isoforms of the channel were subsequently cloned in mammals *(37–40)*. Functional expression of these channels resulted in currents with the hallmarks of the cardiac I(f) or its neuronal equivalent I(h). Although the properties of different isoforms differ quantitatively, all isoforms except one yield currents that are activated by hyperpolarization, are permeable to both K^+ and Na^+, are blocked by

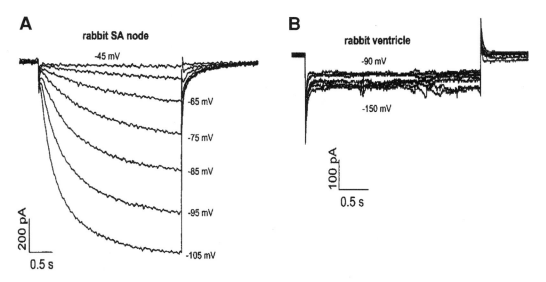

Fig. 2. The relative magnitudes of I(f) in rabbit ventricle and SAN cells. I(f) was evoked by hyperpolarizing voltage steps to the voltages indicated from a holding potential of –35 mV in either a single rabbit SAN cell (**A**) or ventricle cell (**B**). Note the different current scales. Reprinted from Shi, W., Wymore, R., Yu, H., Wu, J., Wymore, R. T., Pan, Z., Robinsin, R., Dixon, J. E., McKinnon, D., and Cohen, I. S. (1999), Distribution and prevalence of hyperpolarization-activated cation channel (HCN) mRNA expression in cardiac tissues. *Circ. Res.* **85,** e1–e6, with permission from Lippincott, Williams & Wilkins Publishers.

cesium (Cs^+) in a voltage-dependent way, and are modulated by a direct action of cAMP on the cytoplasmic side of the channel *(38,39,41)*.

Because of the serendipitous nature of their discovery, the early nomenclature of the gene and its isoforms for pacemaker channels is somewhat inconsistent. Some investigators referred to the isoforms as *HAC1* or *HAC2*, denoting hyperpolarizing activated channel. However, because of the direct action of cAMP and gating by hyperpolarization, the nomenclature suggested by Clapham *(42)* and Biel et al. *(43)* has been generally adopted; that is, of referring to the clones as *HCN* (hyperpolarization-activated, cyclic nucleotide-gated) channels. Compared with the previous nomenclature, *HCN1* corresponds to *HAC2* (*mBCNG-1*); *HCN2* corresponds to *HAC1* (*mBCNG-2*); and *HCN3* corresponds to *HAC3* (*mBCHG-4*).

Cloning of the gene for HCN channels and the consequent ability to perform site-directed mutagenesis and functional studies of channels expressed in heterologous systems has enabled rapid progress in defining the structure and function of the channel protein. The gene transcripts code for a protein of between 800 and 1200 amino acids, with the different protein isoforms having an overall sequence identity of 60%. They are members of the voltage-gated cation-channel superfamily, members of which are characterized by six membrane-spanning segments (S1–S6), including a voltage-sensing S4 segment, and an ion-conducting pore between S5 and S6. It seems safe to assume, by analogy with the voltage-gated family of potassium channels, that functional HCN channels are formed as tetramers of subunits, with each of the four subunits contributing to the pore region. In a structure analogous to the S4 voltage-sensing region of voltage-gated K^+ channels, the S4 region of HCN channels has two regions each containing five positively charged amino acids (10 positive charges compared with 5–7 in potassium channels). This raises some intriguing questions because the two families of channels are gated in opposite ways, the Kv family of potassium channels being opened by depolarization and HCN channels by hyperpolarization. This conundrum of the biophysics of gating of HCN channels has yet to be resolved *(44)*.

The pore region of HCN channels is also related to that of K^+ channels, having a signature GYG triplet *(45)*. However, the aspartate that follows the GYG signature sequence in most K^+ channels is replaced in HCN channels by arginine, alanine, or glutamine. This presumably underlies the high relative permeability to Na^+ of HCN channels compared to classic K^+ channels *(46)*; values of P_{Na}/P_K for cloned HCN channels are between 0.25 to 0.41 *(37,38,41)*.

In the carboxy terminus, HCN channels contain a sequence with a high degree of homology to the cyclic-nucleotide-binding proteins, such as cyclic nucleotide gated (CNG) channels of photoreceptors and olfactory neurons *(47)*, cAMP-dependent protein kinases, and the catabolic-activator protein of *Escherichia coli*. The mechanism of modulation of the channel by cAMP is thought to consist of a COOH-terminus mediated inhibition of opening, which is partially relieved by cAMP binding, as revealed by site directed mutagenesis of the COOH linker in *HCN1* and *HCN2* isoforms *(48)*.

When expressed in heterologous systems, three of the four *HCN* genes have been shown to generate hyperpolarization-activated currents with distinct biophysical properties. *HCN1* channels activate most quickly and require the least amount of hyperpolarization to open, with a half-maximal voltage, $V_{1/2}$, of about –73 mV *(40)*. *HCN2* channels activate more slowly, require stronger hyperpolarizations ($V_{1/2}$ of –92 mV), but are strongly modulated by cAMP *(38,49,50)*. *HCN4* may activate at even more negative potentials and with the slowest kinetics *(37,49,51)*, although $V_{1/2}$ values reported in the literature are variable. To date, *HCN3* channels have not been found to form functional homomultimers. It is possible that this is caused by the lack of a subunit necessary for full functionality because HCN channels have been shown to be modulated by co-expression of a MinK-related peptide *(52)*.

The existence of different isoforms of the HCN channel provides a convincing molecular basis for the heterogeneity in I(f) among different cells, with SAN cells expressing one isoform and ventricular cells another, consistent with the macroscopic properties of I(f), and hence meeting the physiological requirements of the cell. However, more complicated scenarios are possible. A given cell, for example, could express a mixture of HCN channel isoforms with different properties, a supposition reinforced by the finding that the I(f) current displays fast and slow components in heart *(24,53)* and in neurons *(54)*. Consistent with idea of several different components of I(f) being present simultaneously, a recent zebra fish mutant that displays a slow heart rate was found to be deficient in the fast kinetic component of I(f), whereas the slow component was unchanged *(23)*. As a further intriguing possibility because functional HCN channels are likely tetrameric assemblies of subunits, hybrid channels, or heterotetrameric assemblies of subunits, may also be synthesized in some cells. Although most investigations have been performed to date on homomeric channels, there is evidence that channels can be formed as heteromeric assemblies, which display properties intermediate between the two isoforms *(55)*. This additional complexity may be important in the fine control of pacemaking and may underlie the heterogeneity of cardiac tissue *(56)*.

5. DISTRIBUTION OF HCN CHANNELS

As a logical development of earlier studies demonstrating the presence and properties of I(f) in a variety of tissues, efforts have now been directed to studies defining the relative expression levels of the different isoforms of the *HCN* gene.

The relative expression levels of the different isoforms varies considerably throughout the heart, consistent with the different properties of I(f) and the different intrinsic pacemaker activity of the tissues. Hence, in SAN, the dominant isoform of the channel appears to be *HCN4*, with lesser amounts of *HCN1*, whereas in Purkinje fibers, there are equal amounts of *HCN1* and *HCN4* with a smaller amount of *HCN2*. In ventricle, the dominant isoform appears to be primarily *HCN2 (57)*. It should be noted that heterogeneity of cellular properties in the heart is found not only at the "gross" level (i.e., between SAN, atria, and ventricles), but that this heterogeneity can be traced down almost to a single cell level. For instance, the SAN shows a gradation of properties throughout its structure, in terms of the electrophysiology of the tissue and the ion channels expressed *(58,59)*. It may be that this phenotypic heterogeneity is a reflection of the different mix of *HCN4* and *HCN1* expressed in these cells, giving central pacemaker cells a higher intrinsic rate than peripheral cells.

As well as a high level of expression in heart, *HCN* isoforms are also expressed in various parts of the CNS, where *HCN1-4* show distinct but overlapping patterns of mRNA expression *(14,39,50,60,61)*. *HCN1* is expressed selectively in specific brain regions, including the hippocampus, layer 5 cells of the neocortex, and Purkinje cells of the cerebellum. *HCN2* is widely expressed throughout brain, including neocortex, hippocampus, and thalamus. Finally, *HCN4* is expressed in a restricted manner in subcortical and lower brain regions.

HCN expression can also be found in the periphery, notably in smooth muscle *(62)*. Indeed, it seems likely that HCN channels are expressed in any tissue that displays intrinsic rhythmic activity. Note also that HCN may be involved in some unexpected functions, for example, sour taste perception *(63)*. Importantly, in the context of side effects of specific bradycardic agents, *HCN1* channels are highly expressed in the retina *(60)*.

6. RELEVANCE OF I(F) TO CLINICAL CONDITIONS

An increased heart rate increases myocardial oxygen demand and decreases time for myocardial relaxation and diastolic ventricular filling. Because of the increased transmural pressure on the coronary perfusion vessels during systole, perfusion is greatly limited, or prevented entirely, during much of the cardiac cycle and perfusion occurs mostly during diastole. Hence, for example, in the presence of a compromised coronary flow because of coronary artery stenosis, a decrease in diastolic perfusion time secondary to an increase in heart rate may further reduce overall coronary perfusion, to the point where the myocardium can become ischemic. Generally, the subendocardium is most vulnerable to ischemia, and tachycardia has indeed been shown to exacerbate this vulnerability *(64,65)*. Under these circumstances, drugs that block sinus tachycardia, reduce heart rate at rest, or both could be expected to increase the diastolic coronary perfusion time and hence improve overall perfusion and function of the ischemic subendocardium *(66,67)*. This, at least partly, is the rationale behind the use of beta-blocking agents and the rate-lowering Ca^{2+} channel-blocking agents, such as diltiazem and verapamil. However, interpretation of the action of these agents, particularly the calcium channel blockers, is complicated by their tendency to reduce blood pressure and myocardial contractility, both of which reduce myocardial oxygen demand and, indirectly, affect coronary perfusion. One would nevertheless predict that a pure bradycardic agent without these attendant pressor effects should be beneficial in improving coronary perfusion and resistance of the myocardium to ischemia. This prediction is born out in practice: slowing heart rate with ZD 7288 in dogs reduces the severity of myocardial ischemia produced by left anterior descending coronary artery (LAD) occlusion *(68)*, with similar results having been shown in pigs *(69)*. Because I(f) is the primary determinant of heart rate, I(f) blockers therefore have a promising role as anti-ischemic agents.

In addition, blockers of I(f) may be useful in contexts other than when the myocardium is vulnerable to ischemia. I(f) appears to be upregulated in the ventricle during cardiac failure, leading to enhanced autorhythmicity *(70)*; however, note the results from a previous study *(71)*. It seems possible that this enhanced autorhythmicity may be responsible for the greater propensity to arrhythmia in cardiac failure, and hence blockers of I(f) may also be useful as antiarrhythmic agents in this situation. This would constitute an action separate from their bradycardic effects, although the bradycardic effect would still be present, and perhaps provide an additional benefit.

7. TYPES OF DRUGS UNDER CURRENT DEVELOPMENT

One of the earliest blockers of I(f) described was Cs^+ *(72)*, which is moderately specific for I(f), although it does block other ionic currents in addition, especially at higher doses *(73)*. Difficulties with using Cs^+ in physiological solutions and its lack of specificity sparked the search for organic blockers of I(f) in the hope of generating a more specific and more potent compounds. The following two broad lineages of compounds have emerged from these efforts:

1. A series of compounds related to phentolamine and clonidine, the prototype being alinidine (*N*-allyl-clonidine), with the latest compound being ZD-7288 *(74)*.
2. A series of compounds based on modifications of verapamil, the prototype being falipamil (or AQ-A 39), from which zatebradine *(75)* and ivabradine (S-16257-2) have been developed.

7.1. Alinidine and Congeners

Alinidine (or ST567) was shown to be bradycardic as long as 20 yr ago in dogs *(76)* and in humans *(77)*. Although it blocks I(f), alinidine is not very specific in its action, also blocking the slow inward current and outward currents in rabbit SAN cells *(78)*. There also have been suggestions that alinidine can block anion channels *(79)*, an action that may underlie its sometimes reported negative inotropic effect *(80)*. In addition, alinidine displays a variety of pharmacological properties, for example, it antagonizes cromakalim and hence inhibits K_{ATP} channel opening *(81)*. It has been shown that alinidine exhibits rate-independent cardioprotective effects, perhaps as a consequence of adenosine antagonist properties *(82,83)*. Alinidine has also been shown to be antimuscarinic—in paced left rat atria, alinidine acted as competitive antagonist against oxotremorine with a pA_2 of 5.82, and in guinea pig papillary muscle it antagonized carbachol with a pA_2 value of 5.58 *(84)*. Early reports that alinidine slows conduction through the atrioventricular (AV) node *(76)* have not been confirmed in later studies

(85). Although alinidine has been shown to prolong the effective refractory period in the AV node of dogs subject to coronary artery occlusion *(86,87),* an effect on refractory period was not noted in humans at a dose of 40 mg *(88).*

Despite the potential difficulties with nonspecific actions, alinidine has been shown to have very few acute side effects in humans *(89,90).* Note, however, that the latter study (albeit with a limited numbers of subjects) reported that alinidine did not appear to enhance myocardial salvage or preservation of left ventricular function or to reduce the incidence of major arrhythmias in the early phase of myocardial infarction. Nevertheless, interest in alinidine congeners continues with a number of compounds still under investigation *(91).* Many of these exhibit most of the nonspecific effects of alinidine and so are unlikely to be any more useful than alinidine as bradycardic agents. However, one compound, ZD7288, has been developed that shows some promise as a therapeutic agent.

7.1.1. ZD 7288

ZD 7288 (Fig.3A) has been shown to be bradycardic in rabbits and guinea pig *(92)* and to block I(f) in dissociated guinea pig SAN cells *(93).* The block is not use dependent (in contrast to that produced by zatebradine) and has been suggested to be caused by an action of the very hydrophobic ZD 7288 molecule at an intracellular site on the HCN channel *(94).* In sheep Purkinje fibers, the blocking of I(f) by ZD 7288 appears to show so-called reverse use-dependence, and it has been suggested that this may limit its efficacy under physiological conditions *(95).* ZD 7288 is more selective than alinidine or UL-FS 49, producing less prolongation of the action potential in SAN cells at bradycardic concentrations *(96).*

As noted previously, HCN channels are widely expressed in CNS and some peripheral tissues, and one could expect that blockers of HCN channels will have effects in these tissues as well as in the heart. In this context, most interest in ZD 7288 at present seems to be centered on its actions in neurons *(97,98).* ZD 7288 inhibits I(h) in rod photoreceptors *(99),* a finding that has relevance to one of the side effects of HCN channel blockers, which is that they produce visual disturbances.

As well as side effects produced by blockade of HCN channels in extracardiac tissues, which will be a common effect to all specific bradycardic agents, a difficulty with the clinical use of ZD 7288 may arise as a consequence of its kinetics; in in vitro preparations, the action appears to be essentially irreversible *(95).*

7.2. Falipamil (AQ-A 39) and Congeners

An alternative development track for blockers of I(f) has been made through modifications to the benzenacetonitrile Ca^{2+} channel antagonist verapamil. Structural modification by replacement of the lipophilic alpha-isopropylacetonitrile moiety by various heterocyclic ring systems has led to a new range of molecules with specific bradycardic activity, the prototype being falipamil (AQ-A 39). Falipamil has been shown to be bradycardic in many isolated tissue preparations, including guinea pig *(100);* rabbit *(101);* dog *(102);* anesthetized cats, dogs *(103),* and pigs *(104);* and in humans *(105).*

Despite the production of similar effects on heart rate, AQ-A 39 differs from alinidine and mixidine in that it does not depress cardiac contractility in anesthetized dogs with spontaneous heart rates *(106).* A similar observation has been made in anesthetized pigs, at least for arterial plasma concentrations lower than 1500 ng/mL *(104).*

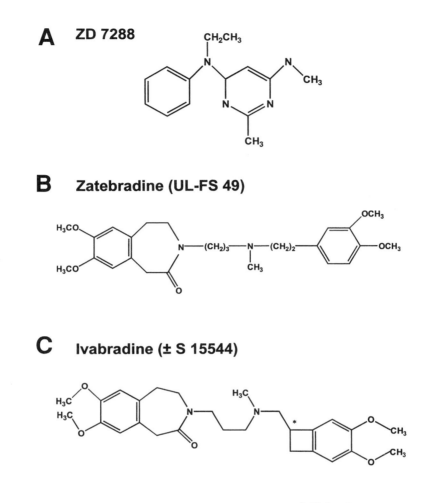

A   ZD 7288

B   Zatebradine (UL-FS 49)

C   Ivabradine (± S 15544)

* chiral centre

Fig. 3. Depicts the chemical structures of several novel I(f) blockers in development. (**A**) shows ZD 7288 (4-[*N*-ethyl-*N*-phenylamino]-1,2-dimethyl-6-[methylamino] pyridinium chloride), (**B**) shows Zatebradine (UL-FS 49 or 1,3,4,5-tetrahydro-7,8-dimethoxy-3-[3-][2-(3,4-dimethoxyphenyl)-ethyl) methylimino]propyl]-2*H*-3-benzazepin-2-on-hydrochloride), and (**C**) shows (±) S 15544 (the racemic parent of Ivabradine; (±) *S* 15544 or 7,8-dimethoxy3-[3-][(4,5-dimethoxybenzocyclobutan-1-yl) methyl] methyl-amino] propyl}1,3,4,5-tetrahydro-2*H*-3-benzazepin-2-one). Note that ivabradine has a chiral carbon center.

Consistent with these bradycardic actions, falipamil shows protective effects against ischemia in anesthetized dogs subjected to 15 min of coronary artery occlusion, followed by 3 h of reperfusion. In this study, both AQ-AH 208 and AQ-A 39 (falipamil) produced similar decreases in heart rate (24%) and increases in the endocardial/epicardial distribution of collateral blood flow. During occlusion and throughout reperfusion, both compounds also produced a significant improvement in the percentage of shortening of the ventricle in the ischemic-reperfused region *(107)*. A similar result has been reported in humans; in a randomized, controlled study 10 male patients with angiographically confirmed ischemic heart disease received AQ-A 39 (falipamil) in a single intravenous dose (2 mg/kg). After submaximal exercise, heart rate during placebo was 129 ± 3, and during AQ-A 39, it was 113 ± 3 beats min⁻¹. AQ-A 39 did not affect systolic arterial pressure and improved exercise tolerance *(108)*.

Some problems in the clinical use of falipamil may arise because of its pharmacokinetic properties, such as its terminal half-life ($t_{1/2}$). In human plasma, the $t_{1/2}$ was determined to be 1.8 ± 0.6 h *(109)*. In addition, falipamil has been reported to have anticholinergic effects in isolated SAN preparations in addition to its rate-dependent block of I(f) *(110)*. In intact animals, this anticholinergic effect can be manifest in vagolytic effects, and these can result in a paradoxical increase in heart rate in some circumstances *(111)*.

As further development has proceeded, falipamil has been submitted to further optimization mainly by manipulation of the phthalmidine moiety, resulting in a second generation of specific bradycardic agents with increased potency and selectively and a prolonged duration of action, represented by the benzazepinone-derivative UL-FS 49 (zatebradine; ref. *112*).

7.2.1. Zatebradine (UL-FS 49)

Zatebradine (Fig. 3B) blocks sinus tachycardia; it has been shown to markedly attenuate exercise-induced heart rate both in animal models *(113–116)* and in humans *(117–120)* at concentrations that do not affect the inotropic or lusitropic state or vascular tone. Zatebradine exhibits a less anticholinergic effect than falipamil *(121)*. In rabbit SAN cells *(75)* and sheep Purkinje fibers *(122)*, the bradycardic effect of zatebradine has been attributed to a use-dependent inhibition of I(f), caused by interaction with the open state of the channel that reduces open probability *(123)*. This is in contrast to the mode of action of ZD 7288 (and other alinidine-related compounds) that interact with the HCN channel in a way that reduces the single-channel conductance and that do not show the same use dependence. At concentrations that block I(f), zatebradine has minimal effects on the L-type Ca^{2+} current (ICa) or the delayed rectifier K^+ current (IKr) in rabbit sinoatrial cells *(75)*, although in spontaneously beating rabbit SAN cells zatebradine prolonged the duration of the action potential, suggesting a K^+ channel block *(75,124)*. More recent electrophysiological studies demonstrate that zatebradine also prolongs action potential duration in guinea pig papillary muscles and rabbit Purkinje fibers *(125,126)*, an effect that was more prominent in Purkinje fibers than in papillary muscles. Consistent with its bradycardic effects, zatebradine has been shown to confer protection against exercise-induced regional contractile dysfunction in dogs *(66,67,127)* and in anesthetized pigs *(69)*.

In 1999, zatebradine was in Phase III clinical trials. However, the Zatebradine Study Group, from a randomized double-blind, placebo-controlled, multicenter study in patients with chronic stable angina pectoris taking extended-release nifedipine, concluded that zatebradine seemed to provide no additional antianginal benefit. This group raised questions regarding the benefit of heart rate reduction alone as an antianginal approach to patients with chronic stable angina *(128)*. This conclusion was later reinforced by Glasser et al. *(129)*, who noted that "despite significant reductions in resting and exercise heart rate, there were no clinically significant effects on myocardial ischemia, suggesting that the anti-ischemic effect of heart rate reduction should be re-evaluated."

These studies raise some questions about the likely usefulness of specific bradycardic agents in cardiac disease, although it may be that their conclusions can only be interpreted as being relevant to zatebradine. In addition to these doubts about efficacy, the class III actions of zatebradine *(130)* have spurred efforts to improve the specificity of its I(f)-blocking actions. This has resulted in development of the compound ivabradine.

7.2.2. Ivabradine (S-16257-2)

Ivabradine is the (+)-enantiomer of the racemic compound S15544 (note that zatebradine is nonchiral). It is similarly bradycardic as zatebradine in isolated tissues *(125)*, by the same mechanism, that is, a block of I(f) *(131)*. The major improvement of ivabradine over zatebradine is that it produces much less prolongation of the action potential in the bradycardic concentration range *(125)*. Because the prototype compound for ivabradine, S15544, is a racemate, it is possible to compare the isomers and to "dissect out" the action potential prolonging action (*see* Fig. 3B for chemical structure). Most of the action potential prolonging effect resides in the (–)-enantiomer (S16260), with the (+)-enantiomer (S16257, ivabradine) having a much smaller effect *(132)*.

Ivabradine is bradycardic and alters neither myocardial contractility nor coronary vasomotion at rest and during exercise in normal dogs *(133)*. It has been shown to be effective against exercise-induced myocardial ischemia in dogs *(134)*. In humans, iv ivabradine in the first Phase I study was shown to produce a decrease of maximal heart rate during exercise *(135)*. In later Phase I trials, pharmacokinetic studies have been conducted in humans *(136)*. Ivabradine is currently in later stage clinical trials. It remains to be seen whether it will prove to be a more effective anti-ischemic agent than zatebradine, thus proving the concept that pure bradycardic agents can be useful as therapeutic agents for angina and other conditions producing myocardial ischemia.

8. CONCLUSIONS

There are a range of side effects typical for specific bradycardic agents, such as effects on the lungs. Animal studies show that relatively high iv doses of zatebradine contract guinea pig airways by a histamine-like mechanism, and zatebradine can reduce FEV1 in humans *(137)*. Besides these generalized extraneous effects of specific bradycardic agents and the usual problems of pharmacokinetics and metabolism that must be overcome, a range of side effects is possible that are related to the fundamental pharmacodynamics of these agents. Because HCN channels are found in a variety of extracardiac tissues, notably the CNS, it may be unavoidable that these agents will produce CNS actions and these may limit their usefulness as antianginal agents. Indeed, one of the common side effects already documented for these agents is a disturbance of vision, a consequence of the presence of HCN channels in the photoreceptors. However, this problem of a diffuse target for therapeutic intervention has not inhibited the development of other drugs, such as class I or class III antiarrhythmic agents. The target for these agents, sodium channels, or potassium channels, respectively, are widespread in extracardiac tissues, but this does not necessarily impede the clinical use of these agents. There is no reason to suppose that the presence of HCN channels in extracardiac tissues will be more of an impediment to the usefulness of specific bradycardic agents, although side effects may inevitably occur. In fact, the situation with specific bradycardic agents may offer more scope for drug development than has currently been exploited. Because HCN channels exist in at least four isoforms, one can speculate that it may be possible to develop blockers specific for a given isoform, in the same way that blockers of specific voltage-dependent potassium channels have been developed. If this can be done, tissue-specific blockers of HCN channels would enable the development of agents that specifically target the SAN or CNS to tailor their therapeutic actions.

REFERENCES

1. DiFrancesco, D. (1995) The onset and autonomic regulation of cardiac pacemaker activity: Relevance of the f current. *Cardiovasc Res.* **29,** 449–456.
2. Yanagihara, K. and Irisawa, H. (1980) Inward current activated during hyperpolarization in the rabbit sinoatrial node cell. *Pflugers Arch.* **385,** 11–19.
3. Brown, H. F., Giles, W., and Noble, S. J. (1977) Membrane currents underlying activity in frog sinus venosus. *J. Physiol.* **271,** 783–816.
4. DiFrancesco, D. (1981) A new interpretation of the pace-maker current in calf Purkinje fibres. *J. Physiol.* **314,** 359–376.
5. Brown, H. and DiFrancesco, D. (1980) Voltage-clamp investigations of membrane currents underlying pace-maker activity in rabbit sino-atrial node. *J. Physiol.* **308,** 331–351.
6. DiFrancesco, D. and Ojeda, C. (1980) Properties of the current if in the sino-atrial node of the rabbit compared with those of the current iK, in Purkinje fibres. *J. Physiol.* **308,** 353–367.
7. Irisawa, H. and Noma, A. (1984) Pacemaker currents in mammalian nodal cells. *J. Mol. Cell Cardiol.* **16,** 777–781.
8. Maylie, J. and Morad, M. (1984) Ionic currents responsible for the generation of pacemaker current in the rabbit sino-atrial node. *J. Physiol.* **355,** 215–235.
9. Bader, C. R., Macleish, P. R., and Schwartz, E. A. (1979) A voltage-clamp study of the light response in solitary rods of the tiger salamander. *J. Physiol.* **296,** 1–26.
10. DiFrancesco, D. (1993). Pacemaker mechanisms in cardiac tissue. *Annu. Rev. Physiol.* **55,** 455–472.
11. McCormick, D. A. and Pape, H. C. (1990) Properties of a hyperpolarization-activated cation current and its role in rhythmic oscillation in thalamic relay neurones. *J. Physiol.* **431,** 291–318.
12. Pape, H. C. (1996) Queer current and pacemaker: The hyperpolarization-activated cation current in neurons. *Annu. Rev. Physiol.* **58,** 299–327.
13. Maccaferri, G. and McBain, C. J. (1996) The hyperpolarization-activated current (Ih) and its contribution to pacemaker activity in rat CA1 hippocampal stratum oriens-alveus interneurones. *J. Physiol.* **497,** 119–130.
14. Luthi, A. and McCormick, D.A. (1998) H-current: Properties of a neuronal and network pacemaker. *Neuron* **21,** 9–12.
15. Demontis, G. C., Longoni, B., Barcaro, U., and Cervetto, L. (1999) Properties and functional roles of hyperpolarization-gated currents in guinea-pig retinal rods. *J. Physiol.* **515,** 813–828.
16. Magee, J. C. (1999) Dendritic Ih normalizes temporal summation in hippocampal CA1 neurons. *Nat. Neurosci.* **2,** 848.
17. Beaumont, V. and Zucker, R. S. (2000) Enhancement of synaptic transmission by cyclic AMP modulation of presynaptic Ih channels. *Nat. Neurosci.* **3,** 133–141.
18. Southan, A. P., Morris, N. P., Stephens, G. J., and Robertson, B. (2000) Hyperpolarization activated currents in presynaptic terminals of mouse cerebellar basket cells. *J. Physiol.* **526,** 91–97.
19. DiFrancesco, D. (1995) The pacemaker current (I(f)) plays an important role in regulating SA node pacemaker activity. *Cardiovasc. Res.* **30,** 307–308.

20. Vassalle, M. (1995) The pacemaker current (I(f)) does not play an important role in regulating SA node pacemaker activity. *Cardiovasc. Res.* **30,** 309–310.

21. Noble, D., Denyer, J. C., Brown, H. F., and DiFrancesco, D. (1992) Reciprocal role of the inward currents ib, Na and i(f) in controlling and stabilizing pacemaker frequency of rabbit sino-atrial node cells. *Proc. R Soc. Lond. B Biol. Sci.* **250,** 199–207.

22. Liu, Y. M., Yu, H., Li, C. Z., Cohen, I. S., and Vassalle, M. (1998) Cesium effects on If and IK in rabbit sinoatrial node myocytes. Implications for SA node automaticity. *J. Cardiovasc. Pharmacol.* **32,** 783–790.

23. Baker, K., Warren, K. S., Yellen, G., and Fishman, M. C. (1997) Defective "pacemaker" current (Ih) in a zebrafish mutant with a slow heart rate. *Proc. Natl. Acad. Sci. USA* **94,** 4554–4559.

24. DiFrancesco, D., Ferroni, A., Mazzanti, M., and Tromba, C. (1986) Properties of the hyperpolarizing-activated current (if) in cells isolated from the rabbit sino-atrial node. *J. Physiol.* **377,** 61–68.

25. DiFrancesco, D. (1986) Characterization of single pacemaker channels in cardiac sino-atrial node cells. *Nature* **324,** 470–473.

26. DiFrancesco, D. and Tortora, P. (1991) Direct activation of cardiac pacemaker channels by intracellular cyclic AMP. *Nature* **351,** 145–147.

27. DiFrancesco, D. and Mangoni, M. (1994) Modulation of single hyperpolarization-activated channels (i(f)) by cAMP in the rabbit sino-atrial node. *J. Physiol.* **474,** 473–482.

28. Accili, E. A., Redaelli, G., and DiFrancesco, D. (1997) Differential control of the hyperpolarization-activated current (i(f)) by cAMP gating and phosphatase inhibition in rabbit sino-atrial node myocytes. *J. Physiol.* **500,** 643–651.

29. Chang, F., Cohen, I. S., DiFrancesco, D., Rosen, M. R., and Tromba, C. (1991) Effects of protein kinase inhibitors on canine Purkinje fibre pacemaker depolarization and the pacemaker current i(f). *J. Physiol.* **440,** 367–384.

30. Wu, J. Y., Yu, H., and Cohen, I. S. (2000) Epidermal growth factor increases i(f) in rabbit SA node cells by activating a tyrosine kinase. *Biochim. Biophys. Acta.* **1463,** 1–19.

31. Renaudon, B., Lenfant, J., Decressac, S., and Bois, P. (2000) Thyroid hormone increases the conductance density of f-channels in rabbit sino-atrial node cells. *Receptors Channels* **7,** 1–8.

32. Hara, M., Liu, Y. M., Zhen, L., Cohen, I. S., Yu, H., Danilo P, Jr., et al. (1997) Positive chronotropic actions of parathyroid hormone and parathyroid hormone-related peptide are associated with increases in the current, I(f), and the slope of the pacemaker potential. *Circulation* **96,** 3704–3709.

33. DiFrancesco, D. and Tromba, C. (1988) Inhibition of the hyperpolarization-activated current (if) induced by acetylcholine in rabbit sino-atrial node myocytes. *J. Physiol.* **405,** 477–491.

34. Santoro, B. and Tibbs, G. R. (1999) The HCN gene family: Molecular basis of the hyperpolarization-activated pacemaker channels. *Ann. NY Acad. Sci.* **868,** 741–764.

35. Yu, H., Chang, F., and Cohen, I. S. (1995) Pacemaker current If in adult canine cardiac ventricular myocytes. *J. Physiol.* **485,** 469–483.

36. Santoro, B., Grant, S. G., Bartsch, D., and Kandel, E. R. (1997) Interactive cloning with the SH3 domain of N-src identifies a new brain specific ion channel protein, with homology to eag and cyclic nucleotide-gated channels. *Proc. Natl. Acad. Sci. USA* **94,** 14,815–14,820.

37. Ishii, T. M., Takano, M., Xie, L. H., Noma, A., and Ohmori, H. (1999) Molecular characterization of the hyperpolarization-activated cation channel in rabbit heart sinoatrial node. *J. Biol. Chem.* **274,** 12,835–12,839.

38. Ludwig, A., Zong, X., Jeglitsch, M., Hofmann, F., and Biel, M. (1998) A family of hyperpolarization-activated mammalian cation channels. *Nature* **393,** 587–591.

39. Santoro, B., Liu, D. T., Yao, H., Bartsch, D., Kandel, E. R., Siegelbaum, S. A., and Tibbs, G. R. (1998). Identification of a gene encoding a hyperpolarization-activated pacemaker channel of brain. *Cell* **93,** 717–729.

40. Vaccari, T., Moroni, A., Rocchi, M., Gorza, L., Bianchi, M. E., Beltrame, M., and DiFrancesco, D. (1999) The human gene coding for HCN2, the pacemaker channel of the heart. *Biochim. Biophys. Acta.* **1446**, 419–425.

41. Moroni, A., Barbuti, A., Altomare, C., Viscomi, C., Morgan, J., Baruscotti, M., and DiFrancesco, D. (2000) Kinetic and ionic properties of the human HCN2 pacemaker channel. *Pflügers Arch.* **439**, 618–626.

42. Clapham, D. E. (1998) Not so funny anymore: Pacing channels are cloned. *Neuron* **21**, 5–7.

43. Biel, M., Ludwig, A., Zong, X., and Hofmann, F. (1999) Hyperpolarization-activated cation channels: A multi-gene family. *Rev. Physiol. Biochem. Pharmacol.* **136**, 165–181.

44. Vaca, L., Stieber, J., Zong, X., Ludwig, A., Hofmann, F., and Biel, M. (2000) Mutations in the S4 domain of a pacemaker channel alter its voltage dependence. *FEBS Lett.* **479**, 35–40.

45. Doyle, D. A., Morais Cabral, J., Pfuetzner, R. A., Kuo, A., Gulbis, J. M., Cohen, S. L., et al. (1998) The structure of the potassium channel: molecular basis of K$^+$ conduction and selectivity. *Science* **280**, 69–77.

46. Heginbotham, L., Lu, Z., Abramson, T., and MacKinnon, R. (1994) Mutations in the K$^+$ channel signature sequence. *Biophys. J.* **66**, 1061–1067.

47. Zagotta, W. N. and Siegelbaum, S. A. (1996) Structure and function of cyclic nucleotide-gated channels. *Annu. Rev. Neurosci.* **19**, 235–263.

48. Wainger, B. J., DeGennaro, M., Santoro, B., Siegelbaum, S. A., and Tibbs, G. R. (2001) Molecular mechanism of cAMP modulation of HCN pacemaker channels. *Nature* **411**, 805–810.

49. Ludwig, A., Zong, X., Stieber, J., Hullin, R., Hofmann, F., and Biel, M. (1999) Two pacemaker channels from human heart with profoundly different activation kinetics. *EMBO J.* **18**, 2323–2329.

50. Santoro, B., Chen, S., Luthi, A., Pavlidis, P., Shumyatsky, G. P., Tibbs, G. R., et al. (2000) Molecular and functional heterogeneity of hyperpolarization-activated pacemaker channels in the mouse CNS. *J. Neurosci.* **20**, 5264–5275.

51. Seifert, R., Scholten, A., Gauss, R., Mincheva, A., Lichter, P., and Kaupp, U. B. (1999) Molecular characterization of a slowly gating human hyperpolarization-activated channel predominantly expressed in thalamus, heart, and testis. *Proc. Natl. Acad. Sci. USA* **96**, 9391–9396.

52. Yu, H., Wu, J., Potapova, I., Wymore, R. T., Holmes, B., Zuckerman, J., et al. (2001) MinK-related peptide 1: A beta subunit for the HCN ion channel subunit family enhances expression and speeds activation. *Circ. Res.* **88**, E847–E87.

53. Maruoka, F., Nakashima, Y., Takano, M., Ono, K., and Noma, A. (1994) Cation-dependent gating of the hyperpolarization-activated cation current in the rabbit sino-atrial node cells. *J. Physiol.* **477**, 423–435.

54. Solomon, J. S. and Nerbonne, J. M. (1993) Two kinetically distinct components of hyperpolarization-activated current in rat superior colliculus-projecting neurons. *J. Physiol.* **469**, 291–313.

55. Chen, S., Wang, J., and Siegelbaum, S. A. (2001) Properties of hyperpolarization-activated pacemaker current defined by coassembly of HCN1 and HCN2 subunits and basal modulation by cyclic nucleotide. *J. Gen. Physiol.* **117**, 491–504.

56. Boyett, M. R., Honjo, H., and Kodama, I. (2000) The sinoatrial node, a heterogeneous pacemaker structure. *Cardiovasc. Res.* **47**, 658–687.

57. Shi, W., Wymore, R., Yu, H., Wu, J., Wymore, R. T., Pan, Z., et al. (1999) Distribution and prevalence of hyperpolarization-activated cation channel (HCN) mRNA expression in cardiac tissues. *Circ. Res.* **85**, e1–e6.

58. Zhang, H., Holden, A. V., and Boyett, M. R. (2000) Gradient model versus mosaic model of the sinoatrial node. *Circulation* **103**, 584–588.

59. Nikmaram, M. R., Boyett, M. R., Kodama, I., Suzuki, R., and Honjo, H. (1997) Variation in effects of Cs$^+$, UL-FS-49, and ZD-7288 within sinoatrial node. *Am. J. Physiol.* **272,** H2782–H2792.

60. Moosmang, S., Stieber, J., Zong, X., Biel, M., Hofmann, F., and Ludwig, A. (2001) Cellular expression and functional characterization of four hyperpolarization-activated pacemaker channels in cardiac and neuronal tissues. *Eur. J. Biochem.* **268,** 1646–1652.

61. Monteggia, L. M., Eisch, A. J., Tang, M. D., Kaczmarek, L. K., and Nestler, E. J. (2000) Cloning and localization of the hyperpolarization-activated cyclic nucleotide-gated channel family in rat brain. *Brain Res. Mol. Brain Res.* **81,** 129–139.

62. Greenwood, I. A. and Prestwich, S. A. (2002) Characteristics of hyperpolarization-activated cation currents in portal vein smooth muscle cells. *Am. J. Physiol. Cell Physiol.* **282,** C744–C753.

63. Stevens, D. R., Seifert, R., Bufe, B., Muller, F., Kremmer, E., Gauss, R., et al. (2001) Hyperpolarization-activated channels HCN1 and HCN4 mediate responses to sour stimuli. *Nature* **413,** 631–635.

64. Boudoulas, H., Rittgers, S., Lewis, R., Leier, C., and Weissler, A. (1979) Changes in diastolic time with various pharmacologic agents: Implications for myocardial perfusion. *Circulation* **60,** 164–169.

65. Hoffman, J. (1990) Autoregulation and heart rate. *Circulation* **82,** 1880–1881.

66. Guth, B., Heusch, G., Seitelberger, R., and Ross, J. (1987) Elimination of exercise-induced regional myocardial dysfunction by a bradycardic agent in dogs with chronic coronary stenosis. *Circulation* **75,** 661–669.

67. O'Brien, P., Drage, D., Saeian, K., Brooks, H., and Warltier, D. (1992) Regional redistribution of myocardial perfusion by UL-FS49, a selective bradycardic agent. *Am. Heart J.* **123,** 5665–5674.

68. Schlack, W., Ebel, D., Grunert, S., Halilovic, S., Meyer, O., and Thamer, V. (1998) Effect of heart rate reduction by 4-(N-ethyl-N-phenyl-amino)-1,2-dimethyl-6-(methyl-amino)pyrimidinium chloride on infarct size in dog. *Arzneimittelforschung* **48,** 26–33.

69. Indolfi, C., Guth, B. D., Miura, T., Miyazaki, S., Schulz, R., and Ross J. Jr. (1989) Mechanisms of improved ischemic regional dysfunction by bradycardia. Studies on UL-FS 49 in swine. *Circulation* **80,** 983–993.

70. Cerbai, E., Sartiani, L., DePaoli, P., Pino, R., Maccherini, M., Bizzarri, F., et al. (2001) The properties of the pacemaker current I(F)in human ventricular myocytes are modulated by cardiac disease. *J. Mol. Cell Cardiol.* **33,** 441–448.

71. Hoppe, U. C., Jansen, E., Sudkamp, M., and Beuckelmann, D. J. (1998) Hyperpolarization-activated inward current in ventricular myocytes from normal and failing human hearts. *Circulation* **97,** 55–65.

72. DiFrancesco, D. (1982) Block and activation of the pace-maker channel in calf purkinje fibres: effects of potassium, caesium and rubidium. *J. Physiol.* **329,** 485–507.

73. Zhou, Z. and Lipsius, S. L. (1992) Properties of the pacemaker current (If) in latent pacemaker cells isolated from cat right atrium. *J. Physiol.* **453,** 503–523.

74. BoSmith, R. E., Briggs, I., and Sturgess, N. C. (1993) Inhibitory actions of ZENECA ZD7288 on whole-cell hyperpolarization activated inward current (If) in guinea-pig dissociated sinoatrial node cells. *Br. J. Pharmacol.* **110,** 343–349.

75. Goethals, M., Raes A., and Van Bogaert, P. P. (1993) Use-dependent block of the pacemaker current I(f) in rabbit sinoatrial node cells by zatebradine (UL-FS 49). On the mode of action of sinus node inhibitors. *Circulation* **88,** 2389–2401.

76. Traunecker, W. and Walland, A. (1980) Haemodynamic and electrophysiologic actions of alinidine in the dog. *Arch. Int. Pharmacodyn. Ther.* **244,** 58–72.

77. Harron, D. W., Jady, K., Riddell, J. G., and Shanks, R. G. (1982) Effects of alinidine, a novel bradycardic agent, on heart rate and blood pressure in man. *J. Cardiovasc. Pharmacol.* **4,** 213–220.

78. Satoh, H. and Hashimoto, K. (1986) Electrophysiological study of alinidine in voltage clamped rabbit sino-atrial node cells. *Eur. J. Pharmacol.* **121,** 211–219.
79. Millar, J. S. and Williams, E. M. (1981) Pacemaker selectivity: Influence on rabbit atria of ionic environment and of alinidine, a possible anion antagonist. *Cardiovasc. Res.* **15,** 335–350.
80. Jaski, B. E. and Serruys, P. W. (1985) Anion-channel blockade with alinidine: A specific bradycardic drug for coronary heart disease without negative inotropic activity? *Am. J. Cardiol.* **56,** 270–275.
81. McPherson, G. A. and Angus, J. A. (1989) Phentolamine and structurally related compounds selectively antagonize the vascular actions of the K^+ channel opener, cromromakalim. *Br. J. Pharmacol.* **97,** 941–949.
82. Streller, I. and Walland, A. (1990) Antiischemic effects of alinidine in paced isolated rat hearts. *Basic Res Cardiol.* **85,** 71–77.
83. Lang, U., Streller, I., and Walland, A. (1989) Alinidine antagonizes the myocardial effects of adenosine. *Eur. J. Pharmacol.* **164,** 13–22.
84. Lang, U. and Walland, A. (1989) Alinidine reverses the descending staircase of isolated rat atria by an antimuscarinic action. *Naunyn Schmiedebergs Arch. Pharmacol.* **339,** 456–463.
85. Takeda, M., Furukawa, Y., Ogiwara, Y., Saegusa, K., Haniuda, M., Akahane, K., et al. (1989) Effects on atrio-ventricular conduction of alinidine and falipamil injected into the AV node artery of the anesthetized dog. *Arch. Int. Pharmacodyn Ther.* **297,** 39–48.
86. Aidonidis, I., Brachmann, J., Rizos, I., Zacharoulis, A., Stavridis, I., Toutouzas, P., et al. (1995) Electropharmacology of the bradycardic agents alinidine and zatebradine (UL-FS 49) in a conscious canine ventricular arrhythmia model of permanent coronary artery occlusion. *Cardiovasc. Drugs Ther.* **9,** 555–563.
87. Boucher, M., Chassaing, C., and Chapuy, E. (1995) Cardiac electrophysiologic effects of alinidine, a specific bradycardic agent, in the conscious dog: Plasma concentration-response relations. *J. Cardiovasc. Pharmacol.* **25,** 229–233.
88. Meinertz, T., Kasper, W., and Jahnchen, E. (1987) Alinidine in heart patients: Electrophysiologic and antianginal actions. *Eur. Heart J.* **8 ,** 109–114.
89. Koenig, W., Stauch, M., Sund, M., Wanjura, D., and Henze, E. (1990) Hemodynamic effects of alinidine (ST 567) at rest and during exercise in patients with chronic congestive heart failure. *Am. Heart J.* **119,** 1348–1354.
90. Van de Werf, F., Janssens, L., Brzostek, T., Mortelmans, L., Wackers, F. J., Willems, G. M., et al. (1993) Short-term effects of early intravenous treatment with a beta-adrenergic blocking agent or a specific bradycardiac agent in patients with acute myocardial infarction receiving thrombolytic therapy. *J. Am. Coll. Cardiol.* **22,** 407–416.
91. C hallinor-Rogers, J. L., Rosenfeldt, F. L., Du, X. J., and McPherson, G. A. (1997) Antiischemic and antiarrhythmic activities of some novel alinidine analogs in the rat heart. *J. Cardiovasc. Pharmacol.* **29,** 499–507.
92. Leitch, S. P., Sears, C. E., Brown, H. F., and Paterson, D. J. (1995) Effects of high potassium and the bradycardic agents ZD7288 and cesium on heart rate of rabbits and guinea pigs. *J. Cardiovasc. Pharmacol.* **25,** 300–306.
93. BoSmith, R. E., Briggs, I., and Sturgess, N. C. (1993) Inhibitory actions of Zeneca ZD7288 on whole-cell hyperpolarization activated inward current (If) in guinea-pig dissociated sinoatrial node cells. *Br. J. Pharmacol.* **110,** 343–349.
94. Rothberg, B. S., Shin, K. S., Phale, P. S., and Yellen, G. (2002) Voltage-controlled gating at the intracellular entrance to a hyperpolarization-activated cation channel. *J. Gen. Physiol.* **119,** 83–91.
95. Berger, F., Borchard, U., Gelhaar, R., Hafner, D., and Weis, T. (1994) Effects of the bradycardic agent ZD 7288 on membrane voltage and pacemaker current in sheep cardiac Purkinje fibres. *Naunyn Schmiedebergs Arch Pharmacol.* **350,** 677–684.

96. Briggs, I., BoSmith, R. E., and Heapy, C. G. (1994) Effects of Zeneca ZD7288 in comparison with alinidine and UL-FS 49 on guinea pig sinoatrial node and ventricular action potentials. *J. Cardiovasc. Pharmacol.* **24**, 380–387.

97. Harris, N. C. and Constanti, A. (1995) Mechanism of block by ZD 7288 of the hyperpolarization-activated inward rectifying current in guinea pig substantia nigra neurons in vitro. *J. Neurophysiol.* **7**, 2366–2378.

98. Gasparini, S.and DiFrancesco, D. (1997) Action of the hyperpolarization-activated current (Ih) blocker ZD 7288 in hippocampal CA1 neurons. *Pflugers Arch.* **435**, 99–106.

99. Satoh, T. O. and Yamada, M. (2000) A bradycardiac agent ZD7288 blocks the hyperpolarization-activated current (I(h)) in retinal rod photoreceptors. *Neuropharmacology* **39**, 1289–1291.

100. Hohnloser, S., Weirich, J., Homburger, H., and Antoni, H. (1982) Electrophysiological studies on effects of AQ-A 39 in the isolated guinea pig heart and myocardial preparations. *Arzneimittelforschung* **32**, 730–734.

101. Senges, J., Rizos, I., Brachmann, J., Anders, G., Jauernig, R., Hamman, H. D., et al. (1983) Effect of nifedipine and AQ-A 39 on the sinoatrial and atrioventricular nodes of the rabbit and their antiarrhythmic action on atrioventricular nodal reentrant tachycardia. *Cardiovasc. Res.* **17**, 132–134.

102. Kawada, M., Satoh, K., and Taira, N. (1984) Analyses of the cardiac action of the bradycardic agent, AQ-A 39, by use of isolated, blood-perfused dog-heart preparations. *J. Pharmacol. Exp. Ther.* **228**, 484–490.

103. Dammgen, J., Kadatz, R., and Diederen, W. (1981) Cardiovascular actions of 5,6-dimethoxy-2-(3-[(alpha-(3,4-dimethoxy) phenylethyl)-methylamino] propyl) phthalimidine (AQ-A 39), a specific bradycardic agent. *Arzneimittelforschung* **31**, 666–670.

104. Verdouw, P. D., Bom, H. P., and Bijleveld, R. E. (1983) Cardiovascular responses to increasing plasma concentrations of AQ-A 39 Cl, a new compound with negative chronotropic effects. *Arzneimittelforschung* **33**, 702–706.

105. Hilaire, J., Broustet, J. P., Colle, J. P., and Theron, M. (1983) Cardiovascular effects of AQ-A 39 in healthy volunteers. *Br. J. Clin. Pharmacol.* **16**, 627–631.

106. Siegl, P. K., Wenger, H. C., and Sweet, C. S. (1984) Comparison of cardiovascular responses to the bradycardic drugs, alinidine, AQ-A 39, and mixidine, in the anesthetized dog. *J. Cardiovasc. Pharmacol.* **6**, 565–574.

107. Gross, G. J., Daemmgen, J. W. (1986) Beneficial effects of two specific bradycardic agents AQ-A39 (falipamil) and AQ-AH 208 on reversible myocardial reperfusion damage in anesthetized dogs. *J. Pharmacol. Exp. Ther.* **238**, 422–428.

108. Gilfrich, H. J., Oberhoffer, M., and Witzke, J. (1987) Comparison of AQ-A 39 with propanolol and placebo in ischaemic heart disease. *Eur. Heart J.* **8(Suppl L)**, 147–151.

109. Roth, W., Koss, F. W., Hallinan, D., Lambe, R., and Darragh, A. (1990) Pharmacokinetics of falipamil after intravenous administration to humans. *J. Pharm. Sci.* **79**, 415–419.

110. Osterrieder, W., Pelzer, D., Yang, Q. F., and Trautwein, W. (1981) The electrophysiological basis of the bradycardic action of AQA 39 on the sinoatrial node. *Naunyn Schmiedebergs Arch Pharmacol.* **317**, 233–237.

111. Boucher, M., Chassaing, C., Chapuy, E., and Duchene-Marullaz, P. (1994) Chronotropic cardiac effects of falipamil in conscious dogs: Interactions with the autonomic nervous system and various ionic conductances. *J. Cardiovasc. Pharmacol.* **23**, 569–575.

112. Lillie, C. and Kobinger, W. (1986) Investigations into the bradycardic effects of UL-FS 49 (1,3,4,5-tetrahydro-7,8-dimethoxy-3-[3-[[2-(3,4-dimethoxy-phenyl)ethyl]methylimino]propyl]-2H-3-benzazepin-2-on hydrochloride) in isolated guinea pig atria. *J. Cardiovasc. Pharmacol.* **8**, 791–797.

113. Johnston, W., Vinten-Johansen, J., Tommasi, E., and Little, W. (1991) ULFS-49 causes bradycardia without decreasing right ventricular systolic and diastolic performance. *J. Cardiovasc. Pharmacol.* **18**, 528–534.

114. Chen, Z. and Slinker, B. (1992) The sinus node inhibitor UL-FS 49 lacks significant inotropic effect. *J. Cardiovasc. Pharmacol.* **19,** 264–271.

115. Van Woerkens, L., van der Giessen, W., and Verdouw, P. (1992) The selective bradycardic effects of zatebradine (UL-FS 49) do not adversely affect left ventricular function in conscious pigs with chronic coronary artery occlusion. *Cardiovasc. Drugs Ther.* **6,** 59–65.

116. Breall, J., Watanabe, J., and Grossman, W. (1993) Effect of zatebradine on contractility, relaxation and coronary blood flow. *J. Am. Coll. Cardiol.* **21,** 471–477.

117. Pistchner, H., Muno, E., Vens-Cappel, F., Schulte, B., Schlepper, M., de Moura-Sieber, V., et al. Antiischemic, antianginal, and hemodynamic effects of ULFS 49 Cl (a new heart-rate-reducing agent) in patients with angiographically proven CAD, in *Sinus Node Inhibitors: A New Concept in Angina Pectoris* (Hjalmarson, Å., Remme, W., eds.), Springer, New York, 1991, pp. 45–53.

118. Baiker, W., Czako, E., Keck, M., and Nehmiz, G. Efficacy and duration of action of three doses of zatebradine (ULFS 49 Cl) in patients with chronic angina pectoris compared to placebo, in *Sinus Node Inhibitors: A New Concept in Angina Pectoris* (Hjalmarson, Å., Remme, W., eds.), Springer, New York, 1991, pp. 55–63.

119. Franke, H., Su CAPF, Schumacher, K., and Seiberling, M. (1987) Clinical pharmacology of two specific bradycardic agents. *Eur. Heart J.* **8(Suppl L),** 91–98.

120. Roth, W., Bauer, E., Heinzel, G., Cornelissen, P., van Tol, R., Jonkman, J., and Zuiderwijk, P. (1993) Zatebradine: pharmacokinetics of a novel heart-rate-lowering agent after intravenous infusion and oral administration to healthy subjects. *J. Pharm. Sci.* **82,** 99–106.

121. Kobinger, W. and Lillie, C. (1984) Cardiovascular characterization of UL-FS 49, 1,3,4,5-tetrahydro-7,8-dimethoxy-3-[3-][2-(3,4-dimethoxyphenyl)ethyl] methylimino]propyl]-2H-3-benzazepin-2-on hydrochloride, a new "specific bradycardic agent." *Eur. J. Pharmacol.* **104,** 9–18.

122. Van Bogaert, P. P., Goethals, M., and Simoens, C. (1990) Use- and frequency-dependent blockade by UL-FS 49 of the if pacemaker current in sheep cardiac Purkinje fibres. *Eur. J. Pharmacol.* **187,** 241–256.

123. DiFrancesco, D. (1994) Some properties of the UL-FS 49 block of the hyperpolarization-activated current (i(f)) in sino-atrial node myocytes. *Pflugers Arch.* **427,** 64–70.

124. Doerr, T. and Trautwein, W. (1990) On the mechanism of the "specific bradycardic action" of the verapamil derivative UL-FS 49. *Naunyn Schmiedebergs Arch Pharmacol.* **341,** 331–340.

125. Thollon, C., Cambarrat, C., Vian, J., Prost, J. F., Peglion, J. L., and Vilaine, J. P. (1994) Electrophysiological effects of S 16257, a novel sino-atrial node modulator, on rabbit and guinea-pig cardiac preparations: Comparison with UL-FS 49. *Br. J. Pharmacol.* **112,** 37–42.

126. Perez, O., Gay, P., Franqueza, L., Carron, R., Valenzuela, C., Delpon, E., et al. (1995) Electromechanical effects of zatebradine on isolated guinea pig cardiac preparations. *J. Cardiovasc. Pharmacol.* **26,** 46–54.

127. Raberger, G., Krumpl, G., and Schneider, W. (1987) Effects of the bradycardic agent UL-FS 49 on exercise-induced regional contractile dysfunction in dogs. *Int. J. Cardiol.* **14,** 343–354.

128. Frishman, W. H., Pepine, C. J., Weiss, R. J., and Baiker, W. M. (1995) Addition of zatebradine, a direct sinus node inhibitor, provides no greater exercise tolerance benefit in patients with angina taking extended-release nifedipine: Results of a multicenter, randomized, double-blind, placebo-controlled, parallel-group study. The Zatebradine Study Group. *J. Am. Coll. Cardiol.* **26,** 305–312.

129. Glasser, S. P., Michie, D. D., Thadani, U., and Baiker, W. M. (1997) Effects of zatebradine (ULFS 49 CL), a sinus node inhibitor, on heart rate and exercise duration in chronic stable angina pectoris. Zatebradine Investigators. *Am. J. Cardiol.* **79,** 1401–1405.

130. Valenzuela, C., Delpon, E., Franqueza, L., Gay, P., Perez, O., Tamargo, J., and Snyders, D. J. (1996) Class III antiarrhythmic effects of zatebradine. Time-, state-, use-, and voltage-dependent block of hKv1.5 channels. *Circulation* **94,** 562–570.

131. Bois, P., Bescond, J., Renaudon, B., and Lenfant, J. (1996) Mode of action of bradycardic agent, S 16257, on ionic currents of rabbit sinoatrial node cells. *Br. J. Pharmacol.* **118,** 1051–1057.

132. Thollon, C., Bidouard, J. P., Cambarrat, C., Lesage, L., Reure, H., Delescluse, I., et al. (1997) Stereospecific in vitro and in vivo effects of the new sinus node inhibitor (+)-S 16257. *Eur. J. Pharmacol.* **339,** 43–51.

133. Simon, L., Ghaleh, B., Puybasset, L., Giudicelli, J. F., and Berdeaux, A. (1995) Coronary and hemodynamic effects of S 16257, a new bradycardic agent, in resting and exercising conscious dogs. *J. Pharmacol. Exp. Ther.* **275,** 659–666.

134. Monnet, X., Ghaleh, B., Colin, P., de Curzon, O. P., Giudicelli, J. F., and Berdeaux, A. (2001) Effects of heart rate reduction with ivabradine on exercise-induced myocardial ischemia and stunning. *J. Pharmacol. Exp. Ther.* **299,** 1133–1139.

135. Carre, F., Denolle, T., Lecoz, F., Violet, I., Lerebours, G., and Gandon, J. M. (1995). First intravenous phase I of S 16257, a new bradycardic agent: Effects on the maximal exercise parameters. *Thérapie* **50,** 377.

136. Duffull, S. B., Chabaud, S., Nony, P., Laveille, C., Girard, P., and Aarons, L. (2000) A pharmacokinetic simulation model for ivabradine in healthy volunteers. *Eur. J. Pharm. Sci.* **10,** 285–294.

137. Maesen, F. P., Smeets, J. J., van Noord, J. A., Nehmiz, G., Wald, F. D., and Cornelissen, P. J. (1994) Effect of zatebradine, a novel 'sinus node inhibitor,' on pulmonary function compared to placebo. *Pulm. Pharmacol.* **7,** 349–355.

3

Oxygen Free Radicals in Heart Disease

Novel Therapies

Elizabeth Roth and Laszlo Hejjel

CONTENTS

1. ABOUT REACTIVE OXYGEN SPECIES

During evolutionary processes, the development of aerobic metabolism has led to the liberation of reactive oxygen species (ROS) in living creatures by leakage from terminal oxidation and other enzymatic processes even under physiological conditions. Free radicals have unpaired electrons on their outer orbit, which makes these short-lived molecular fragments highly reactive with biomolecules, such as lipids, proteins, nucleic acids, and carbohydrates. These reactions are self-perpetuating chain reactions, further increasing their destructive potential. Excessive amounts of free radicals can significantly impair cellular structure and function and even can induce different forms of cell death. The development of inheritable adaptation mechanisms against oxidative stress improved the survival of the individual and the species in general as a benefit of selection *(1,2)*. The comprehensive role of ROS in intracellular signaling mechanisms during physiological circumstances has later been recognized *(3)*. The formation, actions and inactivation of free radicals are summarized in Fig. 1.

1.1. ROS in Diseases

Oxygen free radicals have an impact in aging, reperfusion injury of different organs, including the heart, and play an important role in the pathogenesis of several chronic diseases, including atherosclerosis, heart failure, hypertension, cancer, diabetes,

From: *Cardiac Drug Development Guide*
Edited by: M. K. Pugsley © Humana Press Inc., Totowa, NJ

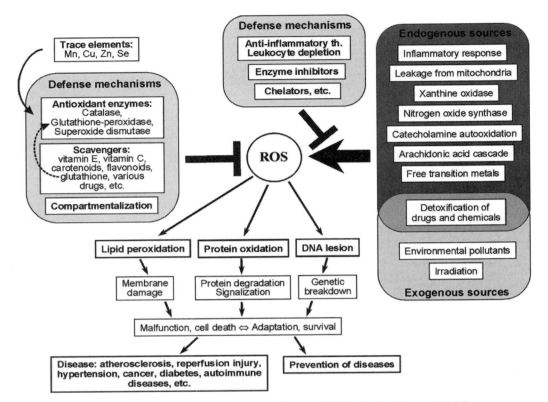

Fig. 1. The generation, detoxification, and biological effects of ROS.

autoimmune diseases, and various neurodegenerative syndromes among others *(4–6)*. Supporting and/or augmenting the natural defensive mechanisms against ROS have been expected to be an effective therapeutic option in the area of many clinical subspecialties.

1.2. The Chemistry of ROS

The sequential univalent (one electron) reduction of molecular oxygen generates a superoxide anion ($O_2^{-\bullet}$), hydrogen-peroxide (H_2O_2), a hydroxyl radical ($HO^\bullet$), and finally water (H_2O). The mitochondrial oxidative chain catalyses this same tetravalent reduction during the terminal oxidation with just a minimal escape of ROS. The super-oxide radical is less harmful directly; and the hydrogen peroxide is not a true free radical. However, they are the precursors of the extremely aggressive hydroxyl radical generated in the Haber–Weiss reaction (Eq. 1), or in the presence of a transition metal ion (such as Fe or Cu) during the much more rapidly acting Fenton-reaction (Eq. 2/a, b; refs. *1,7*):

$$O_2^{-\bullet} + H_2O_2 \rightarrow {}^1O_2 + OH^- + HO^{-\bullet} \tag{1}$$

$$O_2^{-\bullet} + Me^{(n+1)+} \rightarrow Me^{n+} + O_2 \tag{2a}$$

$$Me^{n+} + H_2O_2 \rightarrow Me^{(n+1)+} + OH^- + HO^{-\bullet} \tag{2b}$$

The pathophysiologic role of another nonradical ROS, singlet oxygen ($^1O_2$), has later been recognized in myocardial reperfusion injury. Singlet oxygen can be generated in the Haber–Weiss reaction (Eq. 1), during spontaneous disproportionation of H_2O_2 (Eq. 3), or in several enzymatic processes *(8)*:

$$2H_2O_2 \rightarrow 2H_2O + {}^1O_2 \tag{3}$$

Other nonradical ROS include peroxynitrite ($ONOO^-$), which results from the interaction of nitric oxide (NO) and the superoxide anion, and hypochlorous acid (HOCl), a neutrophil myeloperoxidase product. The enumerated ROS are or can be converted to extremely aggressive substances that can oxidize practically all cellular components. Polyunsaturated fatty acid constituents in lipids are highly vulnerable to oxidation resulting in lipid radicals (alkyl radical), subsequently lipid peroxides (peroxiradical), as well as lipid–lipid, lipid–protein, or lipid–carbohydrate crossbinding and lipid fragmentation. These self-perpetuating reactions, termed uniformly as lipid peroxidation, can damage membrane integrity and consequently impair cellular compartmentalization.

In the proteins potentially all amino acid residues (but principally the sulfhydryl (–SH) groups) are the target of oxidation, producing reversible protein–protein or protein-free amino acid disulfide bridges, causing conformational changes and/or protein–protein crosslinks. These modifications are related to protein activity and selective degradation *(3)*. Thus, free radicals can directly act on structural, regulatory, and other proteins *(9–12)*. In the control of gene expression, several transcriptional factors, such as nuclear factor kappa B (NF-κB), the glucocorticoid receptor, and activator protein 1 have zinc-coordinated cysteine SH groups. These systems are termed the zinc finger, which acts as a molecular redox-sensor *(12)*. ROS can directly depress myocardial enzymes, such as Na^+-K^+ ATP-ase and the Na^+-Ca^{2+} exchanger, and affect other Ca^{2+}-transporters *(13)* as well as cytochrome oxidase, glucose-6-phosphatase, and further enzymes required in energy metabolism in the heart *(8)*. Excitation-contraction coupling can also be disturbed by ROS *(14)*.

Malondialdehyde or other unsaturated aldehydes, the end-products of lipid peroxidation, can intercalate into cellular DNA, causing strand scission and irreversible changes in the genome leading to a genetic breakdown. Thus, ROS can both regulate and damage cellular function via modification of the redox state of subcellular constituents and, in extreme cases, they can destroy the cell *(1,6,7)*.

1.3. Potential Sources of ROS

ROS are endogenously formed during normal cellular metabolism and remain sequestrated with negligible escape; however, in certain pathologic conditions, their levels can increase enormously. Such uncontrolled increases in cellular levels allow their destructive oxidative effects to come into the forefront. Exogenous ROS sources include tobacco smoke and air pollutants, whereas other indirect sources include many drugs and different chemicals via their metabolism by the organism. High-energy radiation also acts, in part, through oxygen free radicals in biological systems *(3,15)*.

The inflammatory components of reperfusion injury are well known *(16)*. To destroy pathogens, foreign or damaged tissues, activated neutrophil cells produce superoxide anion by the membrane-associated NAD(P)H oxidase (Eq. 4) and hypochlorous acid by the secreted myeloperoxidase in the presence of chloride (Eq. 5; refs. *8,17*).

$$NAD(P)H + 2O_2 \rightarrow NAD(P)^+ + H^+ + 2O_2^{-\bullet} \tag{4}$$

$$H_2O_2 + H^+ + Cl^- \rightarrow H_2O + HOCl \qquad (5)$$

Different isoforms of NAD(P)H oxidase can be found in the endothelium, fibroblasts, vascular smooth muscle cells, and myocardial cells. They are the major intrinsic sources of ROS both in the heart and in vascular tissues. The cardiovascular forms are slow-release, low-output enzymes compared with those in neutrophils. The activity and expression of vascular NAD(P)H oxidase and thus the production of ROS are under the control of cytokines, hormones, and mechanical shear stress. The most important regulators are thrombin, platelet-derived growth factor, tumor necrosis factor-alpha, interleukin 1, and angiotensin II. The vascular NAD(P)H oxydases are strongly associated with atherosclerosis and hypertension *(8,17,18)*.

The leak of partially reduced oxygen species from the mitochondrial electron transport chain can be augmented during increased oxygen supply or during ischemia, when the respiratory chain is highly reduced and the mitochondria are overloaded with calcium *(2)*.

The dehydrogenase form of the interconvertible xanthine oxidase/dehydrogenase catalyzes the oxidation of hypoxanthine and xanthine during purine catabolism using NAD^+ as electron acceptor. The oxidase form consumes molecular oxygen (O_2) instead of NAD^+ and produces the superoxide radical. Ischemia in myocardial tissue enhances the unfavorable conversion of the enzyme. The accumulation of adenosine monophosphate facilitates its own breakdown to adenosine, inosine, hypoxanthine, and xanthine, respectively, promoting the formation of superoxide radical by xanthine oxidation. The main location of xanthine oxidase/dehydrogenase is the endothelium, whereas the myocardium contains only a limited amount of this enzyme, probably as a part of natural protection *(2,18)*.

The most important source of the short-lived but rapidly diffusible NO is the endothelium in the cardiovascular system. NO has several effects on other tissues, including relaxation of vascular smooth muscle or modulating mitochondrial respiration within the myocardium. NO synthase (NOS) uses L-arginine and NADPH to produce NO in the presence of tetrahydrobiopterin as an electron carrier. However, in the absence of either L-arginine or tetrahydrobiopterin, the enzyme generates superoxide radical and hydrogen peroxide *(18,19)*.

Catecholamine auto-oxidation can also produce ROS; however, its native role in reperfusion injury is uncertain. Free iron and other transition metal ions can amplify the conversion of superoxide to the much more aggressive hydroxyl radical through the Fenton-reaction (*see* Eq. 2a and 2b).

The formation of prostaglandins, thromboxanes, and leukotrienes from arachidonic acid also generates reactive oxygen species by products through cyclooxygenase, lipoxygenase, and cytochrome P450 enzymes *(2)*.

1.4. Endogenous Defense Mechanisms Against ROS

The earliest protective attempt against ROS must have been the compartmentalization of different cellular components by lipid membranes resulting in a moderately effective physical barrier. Recyclable or replaceable sacrificial molecules can scavenge ROS in order to prevent the damage of vital biomolecules by buffering the oxidants. Ascorbic acid, tocopherols, carotenoids, uric acid, ubiquinone, bilirubin, glutathione, metallothioneins and albumin are mentioned as natural scavengers or nonenzymatic antioxidants *(1,20)*. The most aggressive hydroxyl radical oxidizes everything it contacts, and thus there is no specific enzymatic defense mechanism neutralizing it, but there are several ways to prevent the formation of the hydroxyl radical. The Fenton reaction can be avoided with binding and inactivation of the transition metal ions by specific or nonspecific proteins including ferritin, transferrin, ceruloplasmin, metallothioneins, and albumin. The precursors of hydroxyl radicals can be enzymatically converted to less harmful substrates by superoxide dismutase (SOD; Eq. 6), catalase (CAT; Eq. 7), and glutathione peroxidase (Eq. 8). The oxidized glutathione is recycled by the NADPH-consuming glutathione reductase (Eq. 9; refs. *1,3,9,20*):

$$2O_2^{-\cdot} + 2H^+ \rightarrow H_2O_2 + O_2 \tag{6}$$

$$2H_2O_2 \rightarrow 2H_2O + O_2 \tag{7}$$

$$H_2O_2 + 2GSH \rightarrow 2H_2O + GSSG \tag{8}$$

$$GSSG + NADPH + H^+ \rightarrow 2GSH + NADP^+ \tag{9}$$

SOD has Mn, Cu, or Zn in its catalytic site. Mn-SOD is present in mitochondria, whereas Cu-SOD and Zn-SOD can be found in the cytoplasm and in an immunologically distinct form (extracellular type) on the endothelial cell surface and in the extracellular space. Catalase is a membrane-bound enzyme in peroxisomes and mitochondria. The selenium-containing glutathione peroxidase is the most significant antioxidant enzyme in the myocardium. This enzyme is located in the cytoplasm and uses reduced glutathione as a reducing substrate. The ratio of oxidized vs reduced glutathione is recognized as a marker of the cellular redox state. The glutathione peroxidase can also recycle the oxidized thiol groups of proteins; thus, it plays an important role in the determination of the redox state of proteins. Thioredoxin and peroxiredoxins are evolutionary conserved SH oxidoreductases, which can oxidize or reduce protein thiol groups regulating intracellular redox conditions. Metallothioneins are small (6000–7000 Dalton), ubiquitous intracellular proteins that are loaded with SH groups. Metallothioneins are involved in SH-redox cycles, chelation of toxic heavy metals, and in controlling intracellular zinc levels according to cellular redox conditions *(2,3,12,20)*. The proton-rich mitochondrial surface can also facilitate nonenzymatic dismutation of extramitochondrial superoxide anions *(21,22)*. The total antioxidant capacity of the highly exposed serum mainly comes from albumin and a lesser amount (in 20–25%) from uric acid *(3)*. Plasma extracellular SOD is significantly lower in males vs females, current smokers, and in patients with a history of acute myocardial infarction as surveyed in 590 white Australian patients with coronary artery disease *(23)*.

Here it must be mentioned that many enzymes are involved in the repair or elimination of damaged biomolecules. These enzymes include heat shock proteins *(24)*, phospholipases, proteases, and redoxiendonucleases, the latter of which can restore DNA lesions *(3)*.

1.5. ROS as Intracellular Messengers

The physiopathology of reperfusion injury *(2)*, cardiomyopathies *(25)*, atherosclerosis, hypertension, and restenosis *(11,18)* are strongly related to ROS formation and their destructive effects. However, the use of free radical scavengers for these clinical conditions has produced controversial results, especially in clinical practice, which has raised the concept of both physiological and pathophysiological roles for ROS. In vascular smooth muscle cells, ROS (mainly H_2O_2) play a role as intracellular signaling molecules for proliferation, hypertrophy, survival, and apoptosis, induced by different extracellular signals. ROS messengers also control endothelial cell function and survival. Their targets include redox sensitive signaling molecules, such as NF-κB, activator protein 1, cellular oncogenes like ras/rac and c-src, stress-activated protein kinases, extracellular signal-regulated kinases, protein kinase C (PKC), tyrosine phosphatases, and caspases. Nevertheless, the regulatory effects of ROS strongly depend on their quality, amount, and the oxidative status of the cell *(9,11,17)*.

Preconditioning of the heart can increase the antioxidant capacity of the myocardium *(20)*. However, antioxidants applied simultaneously with the preconditioning stimuli can blunt the protection *(26–28)*. The antioxidant mercaptopropionyl-glycine given before heat exposure prevented both Mn-SOD and heat shock protein induction *(29)*. These results reflect the mediator role of ROS in preconditioning. Indeed, several of the above-mentioned signaling factors are also involved in preconditioning. The kinetics of the ATP-dependent K-channel, the main effector of preconditioning, is also influenced by ROS according to patch-clamp studies *(30)*. In cardiac fibroblasts, oxidative stress can decrease collagen synthesis and increase matrix metalloproteinase activity that has an important role in myocardial remodeling *(31)*.

In summary, ROS have a crucial role in the regulation of many of the most important cellular functions in the heart, such as control of enzyme or transporter protein activity, mitochondrial respiration and Ca homeostasis *(19,32)*, cell survival or apoptosis, gene transcription, and mitosis *(9,11,12,17,33)*.

1.6. Oxygen Free Radicals and NO

The interaction of NO and ROS results in the production of peroxynitrite and other reactive NO species, all of which are oxidizing agents. The NO liberated from activated macrophages or synthesized in the mitochondria of other cells can block mitochondrial respiration and further functions of the target cells. Therefore, on the one hand NO is considered harmful, but on the other hand it has a useful purpose as well. The so-called good NO is a ROS scavenger, can prevent lipid peroxidation, and has several beneficial effects against oxidative injury as a mediator. It is a vasorelaxing factor and restores blood flow, inhibits neutrophil and leukocyte adhesion and activation, limits the ROS production of NAD(P)H oxidase, induces preconditioning, and inhibits platelet aggregation. NO can decrease low-density lipoprotein (LDL) oxidation, thus, entirely it is antiatherosclerotic as well. In a different view, the actions of NO can be prevented by its consumption by reactive NO species formation. The actions of the NO molecule probably depend on its concentration, the dynamics of release, and the actual cellular redox state *(19,32,34,35)*.

2. LOW-MOLECULAR-WEIGHT ANTIOXIDANTS

A variety of low-molecular-weight organic compounds can directly quench and/or scavenge ROS before they damage biomolecules in the cells. Some can even restore oxidized constituents, thus preventing or reducing oxidative cell injury. These substances are typically crucial elements of intermediary metabolism and therefore are naturally occurring molecules. The popular word nutriceutical derives from nutrient and pharmaceutical and stands for nonprescription products used to enhance health.

They are natural substances or formulations, and their activity is primarily based on a scientific paradigm that has been verified by clinical trials. The most important nutriceuticals are vitamin E, vitamin C, coenzyme Q_{10}, carotenoids, flavonoids, and L-arginine *(36)*. A number of drugs have a significant antioxidant activity as well in addition to their primary effects.

2.1. Nutriceuticals

Vitamin E is the collective name of tocols and tocotrienol derivatives that represent α-tocopherol activity. The latter is considered the most important lipid soluble chain-breaking (i.e., in the lipid peroxidation chain-reaction) antioxidant. It can be recycled by vitamin C or glutathione. Each LDL particle contains 5–9 vitamin E molecules that are effective in preventing lipid peroxidation. Oxidized LDL plays a crucial role in the pathogenesis of atherosclerosis. Other beneficial cardiovascular effects of vitamin E include the decrease of platelet aggregation and adhesion, reduction in the expression of adhesion molecules that organize neutrophil–endothelium interaction, inhibition of vascular smooth muscle cell proliferation, protection of NO from inactivation, and the preservation of vasorelaxation *(20,36–38)*. Vitamin E pretreatment has also been shown to have cardioprotective and antiarrhythmic effects via its ROS scavenging activity in acute myocardial infarction in rats *(39)*. Dietary vitamin E slowed the progression of atherosclerosis of the carotid artery in the Atherosclerosis Risk in Communities (ARIC) study *(40)* and of the coronary arteries in the Cholesterol Lowering Atherosclerosis Study (CLAS; ref. *41*). In the Cambridge Heart Antioxidant Study (CHAOS), 400 or 800 U/d of α-tocopherol intake significantly reduced the occurrence of nonfatal myocardial infarction in more than 2000 men with established coronary heart disease *(42)*. The Gruppo Italiano di Studio Sopravvivenza Infarto (GISSI) Prevenzione study demonstrated a statistically nonsignificant beneficial effect of vitamin E on coronary heart disease mortality in patients that survived an episode of acute myocardial infarction *(43)*. However, primary prevention studies related to vitamin E intake have shown that there is a decreased risk for nonfatal myocardial infarction, coronary revascularization, and heart disease in men in the Health Professionals Follow-up Study *(44)*. Similarly, decreased relative risk of nonfatal myocardial infarction and mortality from coronary disease were found in women in the Nurses' Health Study *(45)*. However, in the Heart Outcomes Prevention Evaluation (HOPE) study, the rate of cardiovascular mortality, myocardial infarction, and stroke were not improved by vitamin E (RRR-alpha-tocopheryl acetate, 400 IU/d) intake in cardiovascular high-risk patients *(46)*. In a HOPE substudy called the Study to Evaluate Carotid Ultrasound Changes in patients treated with Ramipril and vitamin E (SECURE), vitamin E did not influence the progression of atherosclerosis *(47)*.

Vitamin C is considered the main water-soluble antioxidant that regenerates vitamin E and directly captures peroxyl radicals. Vitamin C improves endothelium (NO)-dependent vasorelaxation in both human coronary *(48)* and peripheral *(49)* arteries. The ARIC study showed a reduced progression of atherosclerosis with supplementary vitamin C *(40)*; however, the CLAS study did not find any coronary angiographic advantage owed to the separate or additional intake of vitamin C *(41)*. The Health Professionals Follow-up Study did not show any reduction in the risk of coronary disease with increased intake of vitamin C *(44)*.

Coenzyme Q_{10} is a redox active electron carrier and a free radical scavenger in the lipid-phase. It has been shown to have a protective effect on coronary endothelial function during ischemia–reperfusion in isolated perfused rat hearts *(50)*. In a review based on publications found in the MEDLINE database *(51)*, coenzyme Q_{10} is orally administered as an adjuvant therapy and has been recommended to patients with chronic heart failure but not angina or hypertension. It is important to mention that the serum cholesterol lowering statins inhibit the synthesis of coenzyme Q_{10} *(36)*.

Carotenoids are lipid-soluble plant pigments with considerable singlet oxygen and peroxyl radical scavenging activity. In animals and in humans they are present in lipoproteins preventing lipid peroxidation in loco. The most studied carotenoid is the β-carotene or provitamin A, found in carrots, yellow–orange fruits, and leafy vegetables *(36,37)*. In the Health Professionals Follow-up Study *(44)* in men who smoke or smoked and in the Nurses' Health Study *(45)*, a reduced risk of coronary heart disease by β-carotene has been confirmed. However, the Carotene and Retinol Efficacy Trial (CARET) and the Alpha-Tocopherol, Beta-Carotene Cancer Prevention Study (ATBC) suggest that β-carotene did not provide any benefit to cardiovascular disease *(36)*. Lycopene, another carotenoid and valuable antioxidant, can be found in tomatoes. In the European Community Multicenter Study of Antioxidants, Myocardial Infarction, and Cancer of the Breast (EURAMIC), elevated tissue levels of lycopene were linked to reduced risk of myocardial infarction *(36)*.

Flavonoids are structurally polyphenols. More than 4000 natural flavonoids are known. Flavonoids, as the name suggests, give the color, texture, and taste to fruits and vegetables. The most investigated sources are red wine and grapes (quercetin), green tea (catechin, epicatechin), milk thistle (or Silybum marianum, silymarin), and Ginkgo biloba (quercetin, myricetin, kaempferol, and rutin; ref. *52*). Flavonoids are efficient free radical scavengers and they have other advantageous biological effects as well *(36,52)*. Low doses of riboflavin decreased the reperfusion injury in isolated perfused rabbit hearts *(53)*. In the Zutphen Elderly Study *(54)* and in a Finnish clinical study *(55)*, a significant reduction of coronary artery disease mortality has been found that relates to the amount of flavonoid intake. In the Health Professionals Follow-up Study, a nonsignificant inverse association was found between flavonoid intake and coronary heart disease in men *(56)*. Also, some polyphenols, called phytoestrogens because of their stilbene-like chemical structure and activity, are flavonoids. Important members of this group are genistein (soybean) and resveratrol (red wine, grape, peanut). Resveratrol seems to be very efficient in the chemoprevention of various heart diseases *(57)*.

L-arginine is a semi-essential amino acid and acts as a substrate for NOS. Administration of this amino acid can improve coronary and peripheral blood flow in patients. The relatively high dosage required for its efficacy (9 g/d) can be taken orally as an L-arginine-enriched "nutrient bar" (the HeartBar; ref. *36*).

Glutathione is a direct intracellular antioxidant and cofactor of glutathione peroxidase or other redox enzymes. Also, uric acid, urea, and bilirubin are effective antioxidants. Pyruvate, as an adjunct to cardioplegia and storage solutions, has been shown to significantly reduce reperfusion injury in a rat model of heart transplantation via its hydroxyl radical scavenging activity *(58)*. Taurine improved reperfusion arrhythmias and malondialdehyde levels by its ROS scavenger and membrane stabilizer effects in isolated perfused rat hearts *(59)*. The hormone melatonin has very efficient direct scavenger and indirect antioxidant properties that must be further investigated *(60)*. Also, the intake of folate and vitamin B6 above the recommended daily intake reduced the risk of coronary disease in the Nurses' Health Study *(61)*. Certain trace elements (Cu, Mn, Se, and Zn) are necessary for the catalytic activity of antioxidant enzymes, thus, the quantity of their dietary ingestion can influence endogen protective mechanisms *(62)*. Dietary intake and blood levels of selenium may correlate with the severity of congestive heart failure *(63)*.

2.2. Pharmaceuticals with Antioxidant Activity

Several drugs have been shown to possess antioxidant properties in addition to their basic action(s) that can assure an additional therapeutic benefit. Some of the widely used angiotensin-converting enzyme inhibitors contain a sulfhydryl group that can act as a free radical scavenging and copper-chelating arm *(64,65)*. These drugs also reduce the free radical formation of NAD(P)H oxidase as well (*see* following page; refs. *10,17,64*).

Carvedilol is a combined $\alpha1$-$\beta1,2$-blocker with confirmed efficacy in angina, hypertension, and heart failure. Furthermore, this drug has strong antioxidant and antiapoptotic actions *(66)*. Both the ultrashort-acting beta-blocker esmolol-HCl *(67)* and the antiarrhythmic drug bisaramil *(68)* reduced free radical production during ischemia–reperfusion in the dog. Esmolol-HCl inhibits the platelet aggregability as well in a dog model of acute myocardial infarction and reperfusion *(69)*. The 8-oxo derivatives of pentoxifylline and lisofylline are potent hydroxyl and peroxyl radical scavengers *(70)*. In an isolated rat heart model of either normothermic ischemia or cold cardioplegic arrest, the intravenous anesthetic propofol added to the perfusate had substantial antioxidative and cardioprotective effect *(71)*. The sugar alcohol mannitol, a highly effective hydroxyl radical scavenger, when applied as a cardioplegic adjunct significantly reduced myocardial oxidative damage in patients undergoing coronary artery bypass graft procedures *(72)*. Patients undergoing heart valve replacement and mainly anesthetized by isoflurane or sevoflurane showed significantly reduced plasma lipid peroxide levels during the operation compared to those anesthetized principally by fentanyl *(73)*.

There are an increasing number of drugs primarily indicated as antioxidants. *N*-acetylcysteine (NAC), a widely used mucolytic, is a very efficient direct antioxidant and SH donor. Its beneficial effects in reducing myocardial reperfusion injury have been proved both in a variety of animal and human studies, as well as in preventing myocardial infarction in patients with unstable angina *(74,75)*. In several human and experimental studies, NAC was shown to improve high levels of homocysteine and lipoprotein(a), both of which are associated with increased risk of various cardiovascular diseases. NAC also limits nitrate tolerance *(74)*. This drug can also improve human coronary artery and peripheral endothelium-dependent vasodilation *(76)*. The fat-soluble drug probucol, originally a lipid-lowering agent, has a significant antistunning effect in the rabbit because of its ROS-scavenging activity *(77)*. Mercaptopropionyl–glycine therapy has been shown to reduce myocardial infarct size via its hydrogen peroxide scavenging property in the dog *(78)* but not in the rabbit *(79)*. Dimethylthiourea *(80)*, T-0970 *(81)*, and tempol *(82)* are some additional examples of novel antioxidants found to show efficacy at reducing myocardial infarct size in conditions.

3. MODULATING ROS-PRODUCING ENZYMES

Endothelial xanthine oxidase is considered to be a potential source of ROS in ischemia and reperfusion of the heart *(2)*. Its competitive inhibitor, allopurinol, has been found effective both in animal *(83,84)* and in human *(85)* studies in preserving myocardial function and in reducing lower limb edema after femoropopliteal bypass surgery *(86)*. Oxypurinol, another inhibitor of xanthine oxidase, improved endothelium-dependent vasorelaxation in hypercholesterolemic but not in essential hypertensive patients *(87)*. The catechine components of tea may also decrease ROS production via xanthine oxidase inhibition *(88)*.

Angiotensin II indirectly activates vascular NAD(P)H oxidase to produce ROS, which interacts with mitogen-activated protein kinase system, resulting in disturbed vascular function and growth. This alteration in vascular function and growth has been termed remodeling. The antiremodeling effects of angiotensin-converting enzyme inhibitors can be explained, at least in part, by this mechanism *(10,17,64)*. In streptozotocin-induced diabetic rats, the coadministration of enalapril improved lipid, protein, and glutathione oxidation and consequently reduced the occurrence of heart, kidney, and liver lesions *(89)*. In the HOPE study, ramipril significantly reduced the risk of death, myocardial infarction, and stroke in high-risk patients without heart failure *(90)*. Endothelial NOS can act as a ROS source in diabetics, where PKC activation by elevated glucose levels upregulates NOS expression. According to expectations, PKC inhibition improved the endothelium-dependent vasodilation in streptozotocin-induced diabetic rats, suggesting a potential new therapeutic target with which to prevent or treat diabetic endothelial dysfunction *(91)*. Chronic nitrate treatment in rats is suggested to trigger crosstolerance to endothelial vasodilators, a phenomenon whereby the consecutive expression of dysfunctional endothelial NOS produces excessive amounts of superoxide anion. In the same experiment PKC inhibition significantly reduced superoxide production *(92)*. In diabetic patients lipoic acid and high doses of ascorbic acid reduced vascular oxidative stress and improved endothelium-mediated vasorelaxation in an experiment *(93)*.

Tetrahydrobiopterin is an essential cofactor of NOS, in the lack of which the enzyme produces ROS instead of NO. Tetrahydrobiopterin supplementation has been shown to improve endothelial dysfunction in diabetic patients *(94)* and in chronic smokers *(95)*.

4. METAL ION CHELATORS

Chelating transition metal ions preclude the Fenton reaction; thus, hydroxyl radical production may be limited. However, such a concept presents some controversy *(2,96)*. Bathocuproine, a copper chelator, and deferoxamine, an iron chelator, were both useful in limiting free radical generation in a canine study *(97)*. Deferoxamine also improved the postischemic ventricular recovery in dogs *(98)*. Deferiprone, also an effective iron chelator, had a considerable antioxidant effect on lipoproteins in vitro and significantly reduced thoracic aorta cholesterol content, LDL, very low-density lipoprotein, and total plasma cholesterol levels in rabbits in vivo *(99)*. Deferoxamine has an antiproliferative effect on vascular smooth muscle cells, thus limiting myointimal proliferation *(100)* and in an experiment in humans improved endothelium-dependent vasodilatation in coronary artery diseased patients but not in healthy volunteers *(101)*.

Through its mechanical and immunological effects, the extracorporeal circulation causes detectable hemolysis with iron liberation that can be absorbed by transferrin. However, transferrin becomes saturated in approx 13% of patients, and free iron appears in the blood promoting the Fenton reaction *(102)*. The reverse is also true: ROS-formation can increase hemolysis *(5)*. In an isolated, perfused rat heart model of cardioplegia, the addition of deferoxamine to the perfusate improved the cardioprotection observed *(103)*. These same authors showed lower neutrophil-mediated free radical production in patients treated with deferoxamine undergoing cardiopulmonary bypass *(104)*. However, in another human study, this same iron chelator did not improve the postoperative clinical outcome despite reducing free radical production during cardiopulmonary bypass *(105)*. Deferoxamine-conjugated hydroxyethyl starch solution added to the priming solution of the heart–lung machine did not improve pulmonary injury in a sheep experiment *(106)*.

5. ANTI-INFLAMMATORY THERAPY

Ischemic injury activates the immune system via convoluted interactions between the myocardium, endothelium, and different immune cells, especially neutrophils. Activated neutrophils release a variety of ROS and hydrolytic enzymes to necrotic tissue and neighboring viable tissues as well, further increasing the damage caused by ischemia. In animal experiments reperfusion injury can be diminished by neutrophil filters, antineutrophil antibodies, inhibition of the release of proinflammatory mediators, complement depletion, and by masking cellular adhesion molecules to moderate endothelial cell and neutrophil interaction and activation. On the contrary, a human anti-CD11b/CD18 (neutrophil adhesion molecule) antibody was not shown to be beneficial to patients with acute myocardial infarction *(16,107,108)*. In pediatric patients undergoing cardiac surgery, neutrophil depleted blood cardioplegia significantly reduced myocardial injury *(109)*. The recombinant human C5a (complement fragment, neutrophil chemotactic) antagonist, CGS 32359 significantly reduced neutrophil invasion and myocardial injury in a porcine model of surgical revascularization *(110)*.

BW 755 C, an anti-inflammatory drug, significantly reduced the infarct size of pigs when administered before ischemia but not during reperfusion *(111)*. 7-Oxo-prostacyclin pretreatment resulted in a better preservation of metabolic and ventricular function in isolated perfused rat hearts *(112)*. NCX-4016, an aspirin nitroderivative, reduced infarct size and reperfusion arrhythmias in anesthetized rats, an effective suggested to mainly be related to its NO moiety. Acetyl salicylic acid provided only minimal protection *(113)*. COX-2 inhibition or thromboxane synthase inhibition, but not COX-1 inhibition, preserved endothelium dependent vasorelaxation in isolated rat hearts; however, no correlation could be made to ventricular function *(114)*. Flavonoids (catechin, quercetin, silymarin) also have considerable anti-inflammatory effects *(52)*. The antiarrhythmics bisaramil *(68)* and esmolol–HCl *(69)* reduced free radical production from isolated neutrophils and can provide an additional beneficial effect in the treatment of ischemic syndromes.

6. EXOGENOUS ANTIOXIDANT ENZYMES

Exogenous SOD can improve postischemic recovery of myocardial function *(115)*, limit infarct size *(116,117)*, and apoptosis *(118)* in the dog. Exogenous SOD alone also limits infarct size in the pig *(119)* or in combination with CAT *(120)*. Myocardial contractile dysfunction and cell damage after cardiopulmonary bypass can be moderated by the application of SOD and CAT in a canine model of cardioplegic arrest *(121)*. However, there are controversial studies as well *(122–124)*, including an unsuccessful human study investigating the efficacy of human SOD in salvaging left ventricular function during PTCA for acute transmural myocardial infarction *(125)*. These results suggest that it may be warranted to review and revise the current animal models that are used in this field and also find alternative therapeutic approaches *(126)*. One novel therapeutic approach may reside in development of drugs, such as the organometallic, low-molecular SOD-mimetic, SC-52608, that has shown to be effective in preclinical studies *(126)*. Conjugation of SOD with lecithin results in a longer half life and increased affinity to cell membranes and thus in its superior affectivity *(127)*.

7. GENE THERAPY

Progress in biotechnology has made it possible for the transfer of genes encoding antioxidant enzymes both in vitro and in vivo. Their expression in the heart may be cardioprotective in oxidative stress. Studies showing the effective viral transfection into rat hearts by the intracoronary administration of the *Mn-SOD* gene *(128)*, or transfection into rabbit hearts of the extracellular *SOD* gene *(129)* have resulted in significantly improved myocardial protection against reperfusion injury. Adenoviral transfer of the *CAT* gene efficiently and redox independently complemented the antioxidant effect of glutathione–peroxidase, the main myocardial antioxidant enzyme that requires reduced glutathione for its function *(130)*. Adenoviral transfection of rat hearts by direct injection of either *Mn-SOD* or *NOS* gene resulted in smaller infarct size, but there were no additive effect when they were given in combination *(131)*.

Transgenic mice overexpressing or lacking (knockout) certain antioxidant enzymes help us in understanding the role of these enzymes in physiologic circumstances and in several pathologies *(126,132,133)*. Transgenic mice overexpressing *Mn-SOD (134)* and *CAT (129)* show improved functional and biochemical recovery in ischemia–reperfusion studies. Mice that genetically overexpress metallothionein in the heart present improved myocardial preservation in various forms of acute and chronic ischemia–reperfusion models *(135)*. Redox-modulating gene manipulation may be an effective therapeutic approach both in environmentally induced and genetically predetermined diseases related to ROS formation *(21)*.

8. CARDIAC DRUG TOXICITY

Anthracyclines are potent chemotherapeutic agents with chronic cardiotoxic side effects that can be mediated by free radical generation. Improving cardiac antioxidant capacity is addressed by several studies on anthracycline toxicity to obtain a better quality of life for cancer survivors and make possible the use of higher dosage of cytostatic agents *(136,137)*. Interestingly, another cytostatic agent, 5-fluorouracil has an antioxidant effect and thus it could be given in combination with anthracyclines to reduce their cardiotoxic effects *(138)*.

9. FUTURE DIRECTIONS

Both experimental and especially clinical results with free radical scavengers are currently ambivalent in their outcome. However, only the dosage of the antioxidant is usually standardized, ignoring the considerable interindividual differences in antioxidant status and responsiveness to the given substance. A greater understanding of the physiological roles of ROS can lead to the development of optimized antioxidant management and the development of novel therapeutic drugs. Individual-matched and chemically monitored antioxidant therapy or prophylaxis may dissolve existing controversies.

REFERENCES

1. Benzie, I. F. F. (2000) Evolution of antioxidant defence mechanisms. *Eur. J. Nutr.* **39,** 53–61.
2. Maxwell, S R. J. and Lip, G Y. H. (1997) Reperfusion injury: A review of the pathophysiology, clinical manifestations and therapeutic options. *Int. J. Cardiol.* **58,** 95–117.
3. Bourdon, E. and Blache, D. (2001) The importance of proteins in defense against oxidation. *Antiox. Redox Sign.* **3,** 293–311.
4. Bolli, R. (1998) Causative role of oxyradicals in myocardial stunning: A proven hypothesis. *Basic. Res. Cardiol.* **93,** 156–162.
5. Das, D K., Engelman, R M., Liu, X., Maity, S., Rousou, J. A., Flack, J., et al. (1992) Oxygen-derived free radicals and hemolysis during open heart surgery. *Mol. Cell. Biochem.* **111,** 77–86.
6. Singal, P K, Khaper, N., Palace, V., and Kumar, D. (1998) The role of oxidative stress in the genesis of heart disease. *Cardiovasc. Res.* **40,** 426–432.
7. Hejjel, L. and Roth, E. (2000) Molecular, cellular, and clinical aspects of myocardial ischemia. *Orv. Hetil.* **141,** 539–546.
8. Toufektsian, M C., Boucher F R., Morel, T S., and De Leiris, J G. (2001) Cardiac toxicity of singlet oxygen: Implication in reperfusion injury. *Antiox. Redox Sign.* **3,** 63–69.
9. Das, D K. (2001) Redox regulation of cardiomyocyte survival and death. *Antiox. Redox Sign.* **3,** 23–37.
10. Griendling, K K. and Ushio-Fukai, M. (2000) Reactive oxygen species as mediators of angiotensin II signaling. *Regul. Pept.* **91,** 21–27.
11. Irani, K. (2000) Oxidant signaling in vascular cell growth, death, and survival. *Circ. Res.* **87,** 179–183.
12. Webster, K A., Prentice, H., and Bishopric, N H. (2001) Oxidation of zinc finger transcription factors: Physiological consequences. *Antiox. Redox Sign.* **3,** 535–548.
13. Okabe, E., Tsujimoto, Y., and Kobayashi, Y. (2000) Calmodulin and cyclic ADP-ribose interaction in Ca signaling related to cardiac sarcoplasmic reticulum: Superoxide anion radical-triggered Ca-release. *Antiox. Redox Signal.* **2,** 47–54.
14. Goldhaber, J I. and Qayyum, M S. (2000) Oxygen free radicals and excitation-contraction coupling. *Antiox. Redox Signal.* **2,** 55–64.
15. Agrawal, A. and Kale, R K. (2001) Radiation induced peroxidative damage: Mechanism and significance. *Indian J. Exp. Biol.* **39,** 291–309.
16. Entman, M L. and Smith, C W. (1994) Postreperfusion inflammation: A model for reaction to injury in cardiovascular disease. *Cardiovasc. Res.* **28,** 1301–1311.
17. Griendling, K K., Sorescu, D., and Ushio-Fukai, M. (2000) NAD(P)H oxidase. Role in cardiovascular biology and disease. *Circ. Res.* **86,** 494–501.
18. Cai, H. and Harrison, D G. (2000) Endothelial dysfunction in cardiovascular diseases. The role of oxidant stress. *Circ. Res.* **87,** 840–844.

19. Trochu, J.-N., Bouhour, J.-B., Kaley, G., and Hintze, T H. (2000) Role of endothelium-derived nitric oxide in the regulation of cardiac oxygen metabolism. *Circ. Res.* **87,** 1108–1117.

20. Dhalla, N. S., Elmoselhi, A B., Hata, T., and Makino, N. (2000) Status of myocardial antioxidants in ischemia-reperfusion injury. *Cardiovasc. Res.* **47,** 446–456.

21. Engelhardt, J. F., Sen, C K., and Oberley, L. (2001) Redox-modulating gene therapies for human diseases. *Antiox. Redox Sign.* **3,** 341–346.

22. Guidot, D. M., Repine, J. E., Kitlowski, A. D., Flores, S. C., Nelson, S. K., Wright, R. M., et al. (1995) Mitochondrial respiration scavenges extramitochondrial superoxide via non-enzymatic mechanism. *Clin. Invest.* **96,** 1131–1136.

23. Wang, X. L., Adachi, T., Sim, A. S., and Wilcken, D. E. (1998) Plasma extracellular superoxide dismutase levels in an Australian population with coronary artery disease. *Arterioscler. Thromb. Vasc. Biol.* **18,** 1915–1921.

24. Benjamin, I. J. and McMillan, D. R. (1998) Stress (heat shock) proteins. Molecular chaperones in cardiovascular biology and disease. *Circ. Res.* **83,** 117–132.

25. Das, U. N. (2000) Free radicals, cytokines and nitric oxide in cardiac failure and myocardial infarction. *Mol. Cell. Biochem.* **215,** 145–152.

26. Chen, W., Gabel, S., Steenberger, C., and Murphy, E. (1995) A redox-based mechanism for cardioprotection induced by ischemic preconditioning in perfused rat heart. *Circ. Res.* **77,** 424–429.

27. Cohen, M. V., Yang, X-M., Liu, G. S., Heusch, G., and Downey, J. M. (2001) Acetylcholine, bradykinin, opioids, and phenylephrine, but not adenosine, trigger preconditioning by generating free radicals and opening mitochondrial KATP channels. *Circ. Res.* **89,** 273–278.

28. Tanaka, M., Fujiwara, H., Yamasaki, K., and Sasayama, S. (1994) Superoxide dismutase and N-2-mercaptopropionyl glycine attenuate infarct size limitation effect of ischemic preconditioning in the rabbit. *Cardiovasc. Res.* **28,** 980–986.

29. Yamashita, N., Hoshida, S., Taniguchi, N., Kuzuya, T., and Hori, M. (1998) Whole-body hyperthermia provides biphasic cardioprotection against ischemia/reperfusion injury in the rat. *Circulation* **98,** 1414–1421.

30. Tritto, I. and Ambrosio, G. (2001) Role of oxidants in the signaling pathway of preconditioning. *Antiox. Redox Sign.* **3,** 3–10.

31. Siwik, D. A., Pagano, P. J., and Colucci, W. S. (2001) Oxidative stress regulates collagen synthesis and matrix metalloproteinase activity in cardiac fibroblasts. *Am. J. Physiol.* **280,** C53–C60.

32. Szibor, M., Richter, C., and Ghafourifar, P. (2001) Redox control of mitochondrial functions. *Antiox. Redox Sign.* **3,** 515–523.

33. Semenza, G. L. (2000) Cellular and molecular dissection of reperfusion injury. ROS within and without. *Circ. Res.* **86,** 117–118.

34. Rakhit, R. D. and Marber, M. S. (2001) Nitric oxide: An emerging role in cardioprotection? *Heart* **86,** 368–372.

35. Wink, D. A., Miranda, K. M., Espey, M. G., Pluta, R. M., Hewett, S. J., Colton, C., et al. (2001) Mechanism of the antioxidant effects of nitric oxide. *Antiox. Redox Sign.* **3,** 203–213.

36. Cooke, J. P. (1998) Nutriceuticals for cardiovascular health. *Am. J. Cardiol.* **82,** 43S–46S.

37. Guigliano, D. (2000) Dietary antioxidants for cardiovascular prevention. *Nutr. Metab. Cardiovasc. Dis.* **10,** 38–44.

38. Pryor, W. (2000) Vitamin E and heart disease: Basic science to clinical intervention trials. *Free Rad. Biol. Med.* **28,** 141–164.

39. Sethi, R., Takeda, N., Nagano, M., and Dhalla, N. S. (2000) Beneficial effects of vitamin E treatment in acute myocardial infarction. *J. Cardiovasc. Pharmacol. Ther.* **5,** 51–58.

40. Kritchevsky, S. B., Shimakawa, T., Tell, G. S., et al. (1995) carotid artery wall thickness. The ARIC Study. Atherosclerosis Risk in Communities Study. *Circulation* **92,** 2142–2150.

41. Hodis, H. N., Mack, W. J., LaBree, L., et al. (1995) Serial coronary angiographic evidence that antioxidant vitamin intake reduces progression of coronary artery atherosclerosis. *JAMA* **273,** 1849–1854.

42. Stephens, N. G., Parsons, A., Schofield, P. M., Kelly, F., Cheeseman, K., and Mitchinson, M. J. (1996) Randomised controlled trial of vitamin E in patients with coronary disease: Cambridge Heart Antioxidant Study (CHAOS). *Lancet* **347,** 781–786.

43. GISSI (1999) Dietary supplementation with n-3 polyunsaturated fatty acids and vitamin E after myocardial infarction: Results of the GISSI-Prevenzione trial. Gruppo Italiano per lo Studio della Sopravvivenza nell'Infarto miocardico. *Lancet* **354,** 447–455.

44. Rimm, E. B., Stampfer, M. J., Ascherio, A., Giovannucci, E., Colditz, G. A., and Willett, W. C. (1993) Vitamin E consumption and the risk of coronary heart disease in men. *N. Engl. J. Med.* **328,** 1450–1456.

45. Stampfer, M. J., Hennekens, C. H., Manson, J. E., Colditz, G. A., Rosner, B., and Willett, W. C. (1993) Vitamin E consumption and the risk of coronary disease in women. *N. Engl. J. Med.* **328,** 1444–1449.

46. Yusuf, S., Dagenais, G., Pogue, J., Bosch, J., and Sleight, P. (2000) Vitamin E supplementation and cardiovascular events in high-risk patients. The Heart Outcomes Prevention Evaluation Study Investigators. *N. Engl. J. Med* **342,** 154–160.

47. Lonn, E., Yusuf, S., Dzavik, V., Doris, C., Yi, Q., Smith, S., et al., for the SECURE Investigators. (2001) Effects of ramipril and vitamin E on atherosclerosis: The study to evaluate carotid ultrasound changes in patients treated with ramipril and vitamin E (SECURE). *Circulation* **103,** 919–925.

48. Solzbach, U., Hornig, B., Jeserich, M., and Just, H. (1997) Vitamin C improves endothelial dysfunction of epicardial coronary arteries in hypertensive patients. *Circulation* **96,** 1513–1519.

49. Hornig, B., Arakawa, N., Kohler, C., and Drexler, H. (1998) Vitamin C improves endothelial function of conduit arteries in patients with chronic heart failure. *Circulation* **97,** 363–368.

50. Yokoyama, H., Lingle, D. M., Crestanello, J. A., Kamelgard, J., Kott, B. R., Momeni, R., et al. (1996) Coenzyme Q10 protects coronary endothelial function from ischemia reperfusion injury via an antioxidant effect. *Surgery* **120,** 189–196.

51. Tran, M. T., Mitchell, T. M., Kennedy, D. T., and Giles, J. T. (2001) Role of coenzyme Q10 in chronic heart failure, angina, and hypertension. *Pharmacotherapy* **21,** 797–806.

52. Miller, A. L. (1996) Antioxidant flavonoids: Structure, function and clinical usage. *Alt. Med. Rev.* **1,** 103–111.

53. Hultzquist, D. E., Xu, F., Quandt, K. S., Shlafer, M., Mack, C. P., Till, G. O., et al. (1993) Evidence that NADPH-dependent methemoglobin reductase and administered riboflavin protect tissues from oxidative injury. *Am. J. Hematol.* **42,** 13–18.

54. Herrog, M. G. L., Feskens, E. J. M., Hollman, P. C. H., Katman, M. B., and Krombout, D. (1993) Dietary antioxidant flavonoids and risk of coronary heart disease: The Zutphen elderly study. *Lancet* **342,** 1007–1011.

55. Knekt, P., Reunanen, A., Järvinen, R., Seppänen, R., Heliövaara, M., and Aromaa, A. (1994) Antioxidant vitamin intake and coronary mortality in a longitudinal population study. *Am. J. Eepidemiol.* **139,** 1180–1189.

56. Rimm, E. B., Katan, M. B., Ascherio, A., Stampfer, M. J., and Willett, W. C. (1996) Relation between intake of flavonoids and risk for coronary heart disease in male health professionals. *Ann. Intern. Med.* **125,** 384–389.

57. Lin, J. K. and Tsai, S. H. (1999) Chemoprevention of cancer and cardiovascular disease by resveratrol. *Proc. Natl. Sci. Counc. Repub. China B* **203,** 99–106.

58. Dobsak, P., Courderot-Masuyer, C., Zeller, M., Vergely, C., Laubriet, A., Assem, M., et al. (1999) Antioxidative properties of pyruvate and protection of the ischemic rat heart during cardioplegia. *J. Cardiovasc. Pharmacol.* **34,** 651–659.

59. Chahine, R. and Feng, J. (1998) Protective effects of Taurine against reperfusion-induced arrhythmias in isolated ischemic rat heart. *Arzneimittelforschung* **48,** 360–364.

60. Reiter, R. J., Tan, D. X., Qi, W., Manchester, L. C., Karbownik, M., and Calvo, J. R. (2000) Pharmacology and physiology of melatonin in the reduction of the oxidative stress in vivo. *Biol. Signals Recept.* **9,** 160–171.

61. Rimm, E. B., Willett, W. C., Hu, F. B., Sampson, L., Colditz, G. A., Manson, J. E., et al. (1998) Folate and vitamin B6 from diet and supplements in relation to risk of coronary heart disease among women. *JAMA* **279,** 359–364.

62. Barandier, C., Tanguy, S., Pucheu, S., Boucher, F., and de Leiris, J. (1999) Effect of antioxidant trace elements on the response of cardiac tissue to oxidative stress. *Ann. N. Y. Acad. Sci.* **874,** 138–155.

63. de Lorgeril, M., Salen, P., Accominotti, M., Cadau, M., Steghens, J. P., Boucher, F., et al. (2001) Dietary and blood antioxidants in patients with chronic heart failure. Insights into the potential importance of selenium in heart failure. *Eur. J. Heart. Failure* **3,** 661–669.

64. Munzel, T. and Keaney, J. F. Jr. (2001) Are ACE inhibitors a "magic bullet" against oxidative stress? *Circulation* **104,** 1571–1574.

65. Tamba, M. and Torreggiani, A. (2000) Free radical scavenging and copper chelation: a potentially beneficial action of captopril. *Free Rad. Res.* **32,** 199–211.

66. Feuerstein, G., Yue, T. L., Ma, X., and Ruffolo, R. R. (1998) Novel mechanisms in the treatment of heart failure: inhibition of oxygen radicals and apoptosis by carvedilol. *Prog. Cardiovasc. Dis.* **41,** S17–24.

67. Roth, E. and Torok, B. (1991) Effect of the ultrashort-acting beta-blocker Brevibloc on free-radical-mediated injuries during the early reperfusion state. *Basic Res. Cardiol.* **86,** 422–433.

68. Paroczai, M., Roth, E., Matos, G., Temes, G., Lantos, J., and Karpati, E. (1996) Effects of bisaramil on coronary-occlusion-reperfusion injury and free-radical-induced reactions. *Pharmacol. Res.* **33,** 327–336.

69. Roth, E., Matos, G., Guarnieri, C., Papp, B., and Varga, J. (1995) Influence of the beta-blocker therapy on neutrophil superoxide generation and platelet aggregation in experimental myocardial ischemia and reflow. *Acta Physiol. Hung.* **83,** 163–170.

70. Bhat, V. B. and Madyastha, K. M. (2001) Antioxidant and radical scavenging properties of 8-oxo derivatives of xanthine drugs pentoxifylline and lisofylline. *Biochem. Biophys. Res. Commun.* **288,** 1212–1217.

71. Javadov, S. A., Lim, K. H., Kerr, P. M., Suleiman, M. S., Angelini, G. D., and Halestrap, A. P. (2000) Protection of hearts from reperfusion injury by propofol is associated with inhibition of the mitochondrial permeability transition. *Cardiovasc. Res.* **45,** 360–369.

72. Ferreira, R., Burgos, M., Llesuy, S., Molteni, L., Milei, J., Flecha, B. G., et al. (1989) Reduction of reperfusion injury with mannitol cardioplegia. *Ann. Thorac. Surg.* **48,** 77–83.

73. Xu, J., Chang, Y., Ouyang, B., Lu, Z., and Li, L. (1998) Influence of isoflurane and sevoflurane on metabolism of oxygen free radicals in cardiac valve replacement (abstract). *Hunan. Yi. Ke. Da. Xue. Bao.* **23,** 489–491.

74. Kelly, G. S. (1998) Clinical applications of N-acetylcysteine. *Altern. Med. Rev.* **3,** 114–127.

75. Marchetti, G., Lodola, E., Licciardello, L., and Colombo, A. (1999) Use of N-acetyl-cysteine in the management of coronary artery diseases. *Cardiologia* **44,** 633–637.

76. Andrews, N. P., Prasad, A., and Quyyumi, A. A. (2001) N-acetylcysteine improves coronary and peripheral vascular function. *J. Am. Coll. Cardiol.* **37,** 117–123.

77. Dage, R. C., Anderson, B. A., Mao, S. J., and Koerner, J. E. (1991) Probucol reduces myocardial dysfunction during reperfusion after short-term ischemia in rabbit heart. *J. Cardiovasc. Pharmacol.* **17,** 158–165.

78. Horwitz, L. D., Fennessey, P. V., Shikes, R. H., and Kong, Y. (1994) Marked reduction in myocardial infarct size due to prolonged infusion of an antioxidant during reperfusion. *Circulation* **89**, 1792–1801.

79. Miki, T., Cohen, M. V., and Downey, J. M. (1999) Failure of N-2-mercaptopropionyl glycine to reduce myocardial infarction after 3 days of reperfusion in rabbits. *Basic Res. Cardiol.* **94**, 180–187.

80. Kinugawa, S., Tsutsui, H., Hayashidani, S., Ide, T., Suematsu, N., Satoh, S., et al. (2000) Treatment with dimethylthiourea prevents left ventricular remodeling and heart failure after experimental myocardial infarction in mice: Role of oxidative stress. *Circ. Res.* **87**, 392–398.

81. Hashimoto, K., Minatoguchi, S., Hashimoto, Y., Wang, N., Qiu, X., Yamashita, K., et al. (2001) role of protein kinase C, KATP channels and DNA fragmentation in the infarct size reducing effects of the free radical scavenger T-0970. *Clin. Exp. Pharmacol. Physiol.* **28**, 193–199.

82. McDonald, M. C., Zacharowski, K., Bowes, J., Cuzzocrea, S., and Thiemermann, C. (1999) Tempol reduces infarct size in rodent models of regional myocardial ischemia and reperfusion. *Free Rad. Biol. Med.* **27**, 493–503.

83. Headrick, J. P., Armiger, L. C., and Willis, R. J. (1990) Behaviour of energy metabolites and effect of allopurinol in the "stunned" isovolumic rat heart. *J. Mol. Cell. Cardiol.* **22**, 1107–1116.

84. Khatib, S. Y., Farah, H., and El-Migdadi, F. (2001) Allopurinol enhances adenine nucleotide levels and improves myocardial function in isolated hypoxic rat heart. *Biochemistry (Mosc)* **66**, 328–333.

85. Clancy, R. R., McGaurn, S. A., Goin, J. E., Hirtz, D. G., Norwood, W. I., Gaynor, J. W., et al. (2001) Allopurinol neurocardiac protection trial in infants undergoing heart surgery using deep hypothermic circulatory arrest. *Pediatrics* **108**, 61–70.

86. Soong, C. V., Young, I. S., Lightbody, J. H., Hood, J. M., Rowlands, B. J., Trimble, E. R., and BarrosD'Sa, A. A. (1994) Reduction of free radical generation minimises lower limb swelling following femoropopliteal bypass surgery. *Eur. J. Vasc. Surg.* **8**, 435–440.

87. Cardillo, C., Kilcoyne, C. M., Cannon, R. O. 3rd, Quyyumi, A. A., and Panza, J. A. (1997) Xanthine oxidase inhibition with oxypurinol improves endothelial vasodilator function in hypercholesterolemic but not in hypertensive patients. *Hypertension* **30**, 57–63.

88. Aucamp, J., Gaspar, A., Hara, Y., and Apostolides, Z. (1997) Inhibition of xanthine oxidase by catechins from tea (*Camellia sinensis*). *Anticancer Res.* **17**, 4381–4385.

89. de Cavanagh, E. M., Inserra, F., Toblli, J., Stella, I., Fraga, C. G., and Ferder, L. (2001) Enalapril attenuates oxidative stress in diabetic rats. *Hypertension* **38**, 1130–1136.

90. Yusuf, S., Sleight, P., Pogue, J., Bosch, J., Davies, R., and Dagenais, G. (2000) Effects of an angiotensin-converting-enzyme inhibitor, ramipril, on cardiovascular events in high-risk patients. The Heart Outcomes Prevention Evaluation Study Investigators. *N. Engl. J. Med.* **342**, 145–153.

91. Hink, U., Li, H., Mollnau, H., Oelze, M., Matheis, E., Hartmann, M., et al. (2001) Mechanisms underlying endothelial dysfunction in diabetes mellitus. *Circ. Res.* **88**, E14–22.

92. Munzel, T., Li, H., Mollnau, H., Hink, U., Matheis, E., Hartmann, M., et al. (2000) Effects of long-term nitroglycerin treatment on endothelial nitric oxide synthase (NOS III) gene expression, NOS III-mediated superoxide production, and vascular NO bioavailability. *Circ. Res.* **86**, E7–E12.

93. Heitzer, T., Finckh, B., Albers, S., Krohn, K., Kohlschutter, A., and Meinertz, T. (2001) Beneficial effects of alpha-lipoic acid and ascorbic acid on endothelium-dependent, nitric oxide-mediated vasodilation in diabetic patients: Relation to parameters of oxidative stress. *Free Rad. Biol. Med.* **31**, 53–61.

94. Heitzer, T., Krohn, K., Albers, S., and Meinertz, T. (2000) Tetrahydrobiopterin improves endothelium-dependent vasodilation by increasing nitric oxide activity in patients with Type II diabetes mellitus. *Diabetologia* **43**, 1435–1438.

95. Heitzer, T., Brockhoff, C., Mayer, B., Warnholtz, A., Mollnau, H., Henne, S., et al. (2000) Tetrahydrobiopterin improves endothelium-dependent vasodilation in chronic smokers: Evidence for a dysfunctional nitric oxide synthase. *Circ. Res.* **86**, E36–E41.

96. Reddy, B. R., Wynne, J., Kloner, R. A., and Przyklenk, K. (1991) Pretreatment with the iron chelator desferrioxamine fails to provide sustained protection against myocardial ischaemia-reperfusion injury. *Cardiovasc. Res.* **25**, 711–718.

97. Spencer, K. T., Lindower, P. D., Buettner, G. R., and Kerber, R. E. (1998) Transition metal chelators reduce directly measured myocardial free radical production during reperfusion. *J. Cardiovasc. Pharmacol.* **32**, 343–348.

98. Bolli, R., Patel, B. S., Zhu, W. X., O'Neill, P. G., Hartley, C. J., Charlat, M. L., et al. (1987) The iron chelator desferrioxamine attenuates postischemic ventricular dysfunction. *Am. J. Physiol.* **253**, H1372–1380.

99. Matthews, A. J., Vercellotti, G. M., Menchaca, H. J., Bloch, P. H., Michalek, V. N., Marker, P. H., et al. (1997) Iron and atherosclerosis: Inhibition by the iron chelator deferiprone (L1). *J. Surg. Res.* **73**, 35–40.

100. Porreca, E., Ucchino, S., Di Febbo, C., Di Bartolomeo, N., Angelucci, D., Napolitano, A. M., et al. (1994) Antiproliferative effect of desferrioxamine on vascular smooth muscle cells in vitro and in vivo. *Arterioscler. Thromb.* **14**, 299–304.

101. Duffy, S. J., Biegelsen, E. S., Holbrook, M., Russell, J. D., Gokce, N., Keaney, J. F. Jr., and Vita, J. A. (2001) Iron chelation improves endothelial function in patients with coronary artery disease. *Circulation* **103**, 2799–2804.

102. Pepper, J. R., Mumby, S., and Gutteridge, J. M. (1994) Transient iron-overload with bleomycin-detectable iron present during cardiopulmonary bypass surgery. *Free Rad. Res.* **21**, 53–58.

103. Menasche, P., Grousset, C., Gauduel, Y., Mouas, C., and Piwnica, A. (1988) A new concept of cardioplegic protection in cardiac surgery: iron chelation. *Arch. Mal. Coeur Vaiss.* **81**, 811–816.

104. Menasche, P., Pasquier, C., Bellucci, S., Lorente, P., Jaillon, P., and Piwnica, A. (1988) Deferoxamine reduces neutrophil-mediated free radical production during cardiopulmonary bypass in man. *J. Thorac. Cardiovasc. Surg.* **96**, 582–589.

105. Bel, A., Martinod, E., and Menasche, P. (1996) Cardioprotective effect of desferrioxamine. *Acta Haematol.* **95**, 63–65.

106. Stamler, A., Wang, S. Y., Aquirre, D. E., Sellke, F. W., and Johnson R. G. (1996) Effects of pentastarch-deferoxamine conjugate on lung injury after cardiopulmonary bypass. *Circulation* **94**, II358–II363.

107. Black, S. C. (2000) In vivo models of myocardial ischemia and reperfusion injury. Application to drug discovery and evaluation. *J. Pharm. Toxicol. Meth.* **43**, 153–167.

108. Jordan, J. E., Zhao, Z. Q., and Vinten-Johansen, J. (1999) The role of neutrophils in myocardial ischemia-reperfusion injury. *Cardiovasc. Res.* **43**, 860–878.

109. Hayashi, Y., Sawa, Y., Nishimura, M., Ichikawa, H., Kagisaki, K., Ohtake, S., et al. (2000) Clinical evaluation of leukocyte-depleted blood cardioplegia for pediatric open heart operation. *Ann. Thorac. Surg.* **69**, 1914–1919.

110. Riley, R. D., Sato, H., Zhao, Z. Q., Thourani, V. H., Jordan, J. E., Fernandez, A. X., et al. (2000) Recombinant human complement C5a receptor antagonist reduces infarct size after surgical revascularization. *J. Thorac. Cardiovasc. Surg.* **120**, 350–358.

111. Klein, H. H., Pich, S., Bohle, R. M., Lindert, S., Nebendahl, K., Buchwald, A., et al. (1988) Antiinflammatory agent BW 755 C in ischemic reperfused porcine hearts. *J. Cardiovasc. Pharmacol.* **12**, 338–344.

112. Ravingerova, T., Styk, J., Tregerova, V., Pancza, D., Slezak, J., Tribulova, N., et al. (1991) Protective effect of 7-oxo-prostacyclin on myocardial function and metabolism during postischemic reperfusion and calcium paradox. *Basic Res. Cardiol.* **86**, 245–253.

113. Rossoni, G., Manfredi, B., Colonna, V. D., Bernareggi, M., and Berti, F. (2001) The nitroderivative of aspirin, NCX 4016, reduces infarct size caused by myocardial ischemia-reperfusion in the anesthetized rat. *J. Pharmacol. Exp. Ther.* **297**, 380–387.

114. Bouchard, J. F. and Lamontagne, D. (1999) Mechanisms of protection afforded by cyclooxygenase inhibitors to endothelial function against ischemic injury in rat isolated hearts. *J. Cardiovasc. Pharmacol.* **34**, 755–763.

115. Buchwald, A., Klein, H. H., Lindert, S., Pich, S., Nebendahl, K., Wiegand, V., and Kreuzer, H. (1989) Effect of intracoronary superoxide dismutase on regional function in stunned myocardium. *J. Cardiovasc. Pharmacol.* **13**, 258–264.

116. Ambrosio, G., Becker, L. C., Hutchins, G. M., Weisman, H. F., and Weisfeldt, M. L. (1986) Reduction in experimental infarct size by recombinant human superoxide dismutase: Insights into the pathophysiology of reperfusion injury. *Circulation* **74**, 1424–1433.

117. Werns, S. W., Simpson, P. J., Mickelson, J. K., Shea, M. J., Pitt, B., and Lucchesi, B. R. (1988) Sustained limitation by superoxide dismutase of canine myocardial injury due to regional ischemia followed by reperfusion. *J. Cardiovasc. Pharmacol.* **11**, 36–44.

118. Ambrosio, G., Zweier, J. L., and Becker, L. C. (1998) Apoptosis is prevented by administration of superoxide dismutase in dogs with reperfused myocardial infarction. *Basic. Res. Cardiol.* **93**, 94–96.

119. Naslund, U., Haggmark, S., Johansson, G., Marklund, S. L., and Reiz, S. (1990) Limitation of myocardial infarct size by superoxide dismutase as an adjunct to reperfusion after different durations of coronary occlusion in the pig. *Circ. Res.* **66**, 1294–1301.

120. Naslund, U., Haggmark, S., Johansson, G., Marklund, S. L., Reiz, S., and Oberg, A. (1986) Superoxide dismutase and catalase reduce infarct size in a porcine myocardial occlusion-reperfusion model. *J. Mol. Cell. Cardiol.* **18**, 1077–1084.

121. Prasad, K., Chan, W. P., and Bharadwaj, B. (1996) Superoxide dismutase and catalase in protection of cardiopulmonary bypass-induced cardiac dysfunction and cellular injury. *Can. J. Cardiol.* **12**, 1083–1091.

122. Tanaka, M., Richard, V. J., Murry, C. E., Jennings, R. B., and Reimer, K. A. (1993) Superoxide dismutase plus catalase therapy delays neither cell death nor the loss of the TTC reaction in experimental myocardial infarction in dogs. *J. Mol. Cell. Cardiol.* **25**, 367–378.

123. Omar, B. A. and McCord, J. M. (1990) The cardioprotective effect of Mn-superoxide dismutase is lost at high doses in the postischemic isolated rabbit heart. *Free Rad. Biol. Med.* **9**, 473–478.

124. Omar, B. A., Gad, N. M., Jordan, M. C., Striplin, S. P., Russell, W. J., Downey, J. M., et al. (1990) Cardioprotection by Cu,Zn-superoxide dismutase is lost at high doses in the reoxygenated heart. *Free Rad. Biol. Med.* **9**, 465–471.

125. Flaherty, J. T., Pitt, B., Gruber, J. W., Heuser, R. R., Rothbaum, D. A., Burwell, L. R., et al. (1994) Recombinant human superoxide dismutase (h-SOD) fails to improve recovery of ventricular function in patients undergoing coronary angioplasty for acute myocardial infarction. *Circulation* **89**, 1982–1991.

126. Black, S. C., Schasteen, C. S., Weiss, R. H., Riley, D. P., Driscoll, E. M., and Lucchesi, B. R. (1994) Inhibition of in vivo myocardial ischemic and reperfusion injury by a synthetic manganese-based superoxide dismutase mimetic. *J. Pharm. Exp. Ther.* **270**, 1208–1215.

127. Hangaishi, M., Nakajima, H., Taguchi, J., Igarashi, R., Hoshino, J., Kurokawa, K., et al. (2001) Lecithinized Cu, Zn-superoxide dismutase limits the infarct size following ischemia-reperfusion injury in rat hearts in vivo. *Biochem. Biophys. Res. Commun.* **285**, 1220–1225.

128. Suzuki, K., Sawa, Y., Ichikawa, H., Kaneda, Y., and Matsuda, H. (1999) Myocardial protection with endogenous overexpression of manganese superoxide dismutase. *Ann. Thorac. Surg.* **68,** 1266–1271.

129. Li, G., Chen, Y., Saari, J. T., and Kang, Y. J. (1997) Catalase-overexpressing transgenic mouse heart is resistant to ischemia-reperfusion injury. *Am. J. Physiol.* **273,** H1090–H1095.

130. Zhu, H. L., Stewart, A. S., Taylor, M. D., Vijayasarathy, C., Gardner, T. J., and Sweeney, H. L. (2000) Blocking free radical production via adenoviral gene transfer decreases cardiac ischemia-reperfusion injury. *Mol. Ther.* **2,** 470–475.

131. Abunasra, H. J., Smolenski, R. T., Morrison, K., Yap, J., Sheppard, M. N., O'Brien, T., et al. (2001) Efficacy of adenoviral gene transfer with manganese superoxide dismutase and endothelial nitric oxide synthase in reducing ischemia and reperfusion injury. *Eur. J. Cardiothorac. Surg.* **20,** 153–158.

132. Ho, Y. S., Magnenat, J. L., Gargano, M., and Cao, J. (1998) The nature of antioxidant defense mechanisms: A lesson from transgenic studies. *Environ. Health Perspect.* **106(S5),** 1219–28.

133. Huang, T. T., Carlson, E. J., Raineri, I., Gillespie, A. M., Kozy, H., and Epstein, C., J. (1999) The use of transgenic and mutant mice to study oxygen free radical metabolism. *Ann. N. Y. Acad. Sci.* **893,** 95–112.

134. Chen, Z., Siu, B., Ho, Y.S., Vincent, R., Chua, C. C., Hamdy, R. C., et al. (1998) Overexpression of MnSOD protects against myocardial ischemia/reperfusion injury in transgenic mice. *J. Mol. Cell. Cardiol.* **30,** 2281–2289.

135. Kang, Y. J., Li, G., and Saari, J. T. (1999) Metallothionein inhibits ischemia-reperfusion injury in mouse heart. *Am. J. Physiol.* **276,** H993–H997.

136. Horenstein, M. S., Vander Heide, R. S., and L'Ecuyer, T. J. (2000) Molecular basis of anthracyclin-induced cardiotoxicity and its prevention. *Mol. Gen. Metab.* **71,** 436–444.

137. Mohamed, H. E., El-Swefy, S. E., and Hagar, H. H. (2000) The protective effect of glutathione administration on adriamycin-induced acute cardiac toxicity in rats. *Pharmacol. Res.* **42,** 115–121.

138. Stathopoulos, G. P., Malamos, N. A., Dontas, I., Deliconstantinos, G., Perrea-Kotsareli, D., and Karayannacos, P. E. (1998) Inhibition of adriamycin cardiotoxicity by 5-fluorouracil: A potential free oxygen radical scavenger. *Anticancer Res.* **18,** 4387–4392.

4

Mitogen-Activated Protein Kinases-Mediated Signaling in Cardiac Pathology

A Perspective of Novel Therapeutic Targets?

Tanya Ravingerova, Miroslav Barancik, and Monika Strniskova

CONTENTS

INTRODUCTION
REGULATORY ROLE OF MAPKs IN THE MYOCARDIUM
ROLE OF MAPKs IN CARDIAC PATHOLOGY
ROLE OF MAPKs IN CARDIOPROTECTION
PHARMACOLOGICAL MODULATION OF MAPK ACTIVITY
CONCLUSION
ACKNOWLEDGMENTS
REFERENCES

1. INTRODUCTION

It has been recognized that eucaryotic cells respond to different external stimuli by activation of mechanisms of cell signaling. One of the major systems participating in the transduction of signal from the cell membrane to nuclear and other intracellular targets is the highly conserved mitogen-activated protein kinase (MAPK) superfamily. The members of MAPK family are involved in the regulation of a large variety of cellular processes, such as cell growth, differentiation, development, cell cycle, death, and survival. Several MAPK subfamilies, each with apparently unique signaling pathway, have been identified in the mammalian myocardium. These cascades differ in their upstream activation sequence and in downstream substrate specificity. Each pathway follows the same conserved three-kinase module consisting of MAPK, MAPK kinase (MKK or MEK), and MAPK kinase kinase. The major groups of MAPKs found in cardiac tissue include the extracellular signal-regulated kinases (ERKs), the stress-activated/c-Jun NH2-terminal kinases (SAPK/JNKs), p38-MAPK, and ERK5/big MAPK 1 (BMK1). The ERKs are strongly activated by mitogenic and growth factors and by physical stress, SAPK/JNKs and p38-MAPK can be activated by various cell stresses, such as hyperosmotic shock, metabolic stress, or protein synthesis inhibitors, ultraviolet radiation, heat shock, cytokines, and ischemia. Recently it has been proposed that activation of MAPK family and their downstream effectors plays a key role

From: *Cardiac Drug Development Guide*
Edited by: M. K. Pugsley © Humana Press Inc., Totowa, NJ

in the pathogenesis of various deleterious processes in the heart, for example, myocardial hypertrophy and its transition to heart failure, in ischemic and reperfusion injury, as well in the cardioprotection induced by ischemic preconditioning or pharmacologically. The role of MAPKs in the myocardium was documented by (1) studies of the effects of myocardial processes (such as ischemia–reperfusion, preconditioning, hypertrophy, etc.) on the activation of these kinases; (2) pharmacological modulations of MAPK activity and evaluation of their impact on the (patho)physiological processes in the heart; (3) gene targeting or expression of constitutively active and dominant-negative forms of enzymes (adenovirus-mediated gene transfer).

This chapter focuses on the regulatory role of MAPKs in the myocardium, with particular regard to involvement of different MAPK pathways in pathophysiological processes, such as myocardial hypertrophy and heart failure, ischemia–reperfusion injury, as well as in mechanisms of ischemic preconditioning-induced cardioprotection. The chapter summarizes current information on pharmacological modulations aimed at the stimulation and/or inhibition of MAPK activity and their impact on the cardiac response to pathophysiological processes, as well as on potential protective actions.

2. REGULATORY ROLE OF MAPKS IN THE MYOCARDIUM

The cardiomyocyte is a terminally differentiated cell that responds to appropriate external stimuli by adaptive growth (hypertrophy) in the absence of cell division *(1)*. One of the characteristic features of this physiological response is an increased expression of proto-oncogenes c-*fos* and c-*jun*, which could be induced by low levels of stress *(1)*. Extracellular stimuli, such as growth factors, cytokines, physical, and/or chemical stress initiate signal transduction from the plasma membrane mediated by sequential phosphorylation and activation of specific components of MAPK cascades. Regulation of gene expression in response to extracellular stimuli belongs to one of the most explored roles of MAPKs in the mammalian myocardium. Although cardiac myocytes cannot respond to mitogenic stimuli with cell division, the expression of MAPKs and their activity was demonstrated in the heart cells of all animal species studied *(2–7)*. In the cardiomyocytes, these kinase systems gained a different function than in the noncardiac cells and are involved mainly in the mechanisms of response to stress and in the processes of cell survival and death (apoptosis).

The three major MAPKs cascades identified in the myocardium are the ERKs and two stress-activated MAPKs subfamilies: SAPK/JNK and p38 MAPKs. These kinases are encoded by different genes and differ in the amino acid activation motif. Each cascade consists of the same three-kinase module *(8)*. Activation of upstream-located MAPK kinase kinase is followed by phosphorylation of MAPK kinase (MKK or MEK) on serine–threonine residues. Activation of the MAPK by MKK requires phosphorylation of threonine and tyrosine residues *(9)*. The MAPKs themselves are proline-directed serine–threonine kinases, phosphorylating serine and threonine residues *(9,10)*.

Differences in upstream activation mechanisms and substrates specificity do not exclude parallel activation of different MAPK cascades and their crosstalk at various levels of pathways (upstream of the cascades, within the cascades, within the substrates). This is particularly important for the transcriptional regulation in the heart because MAPKs phosphorylate and increase transactivating/DNA-binding activity of several transcription factors in a cooperative way *(11–14)*.

2.1. ERKs

This cascade is the best studied. The activation of the ERK subfamily occurs in response to mitogenic and growth factors acting through receptor protein tyrosine kinases or G protein-coupled receptors *(9,15)*. Recently, an activation of ERK1/2 and translocation to the nucleus has been demonstrated in isolated rat heart in response to a physical stretch induced by an increase in intraventricular pressure *(16)*. In isolated rat cardiomyocytes, activation of the ERK pathway was shown to be initiated by enhanced calcium entry into the cells through L-type Ca^{2+} channels and signaling mechanisms involved phosphorylation of proline-rich tyrosine kinase 2 (Pyk2) and epidermal growth factor receptor *(17)*. An immediate upstream regulator of the ERKs is MEK 1/2. Activation of MEK involves the small G-protein (Ras), the 74-kDa protein Ser–Thr kinase, the Raf-1 kinase and some kinases that might belong to the protein kinase C (PKC) family *(18–20)*. Mechanism of MEK activation involves phosphorylation on two Ser residues within MEK subdomains VII and VIII. Activated MEKs demonstrate a high degree of specificity for the native form of their downstream substrates, the ERK 1 and ERK 2. The phosphorylation motif of ERKs is Thr–Glu–Tyr *(21)*.

2.1.1. Consequences of ERK Pathway Activation

Phosphorylation of Thr and Tyr residues is essential not only for activation of ERKs but also for their translocation to the nucleus. Activated ERKs phosphorylate a large number of regulatory proteins and thus directly control several cellular processes, including transcription, translation, and cytoskeletal rearrangement *(22)*. In addition, ERKs can transmit the signal to downstream kinases, such as the ribosomal S6 kinase (RSK) or MAPKAP kinase 1 *(23)*. RSK can phosphorylate and activate regulatory molecules, such as the transcription factor c-Fos, cAMP response element-binding protein, estrogen receptor, nuclear factor (NF)κB/IκB α, the ribosomal S6 protein, stimulate Na^+/H^+ exchanger and can also transmit the signal to a downstream kinase, glycogen synthase kinase-3, which participates in the downregulation of transcription. RSK also phosphorylates the Ras GTP/GDP-exchange factor Sos, leading to feedback inhibition of the Ras–ERK pathway *(24,25)*. Perhaps the two best-characterized ERK substrates are cytoplasmic phospholipase A_2 (cPLA$_2$) and the transcription factor Elk-1. Phosphorylation of cPLA$_2$ by ERKs causes an increase in the enzymatic activity of cPLA$_2$, resulting in an increased arachidonic acid release and formation of lysophospholipids from membrane phospholipids *(26)*. ERKs can therefore trigger the formation of multiple secondary signaling molecules. Elk-1 is also a direct target of the ERK cascade. This transcription factor binds to the promoters of many genes and its increased phosphorylation and stimulation of transcriptional activity can mediate the effects of the MAPK signal transduction pathway on gene expression *(27)*.

2.2. p38–MAPK Subfamily

These enzymes, also termed cytokine-suppressive anti-inflammatory drug-binding proteins *(28)*, are osmoregulatory protein kinases that are activated after exposure to many forms of cellular stress. They are also poorly activated by mitogens but strongly respond to endotoxin, proinflammatory cytokines, tumor necrosis factor alpha (TNF-α), interleukin-1, osmotic shock, heat stress, or metabolic inhibitors, such as sodium arsenite *(29,30)*. The p38 subfamily consists of four isoforms (α, β, γ and δ); however, only p38α and p38β have been detected in the cardiac tissue *(31)*. MKK3 and MKK6 selectively activate p38–MAPK in different cell types and exhibit isoform specificity: MKK3 activates only α and γ isoforms, whereas MKK6 can activate α, β, and γ isoforms *(31)*. The phosphorylation motif of p38–MAPK is Thr–Gly–Tyr.

With the use of a cotransfection technique, several other potential regulators of the p38–MAPK pathway have been defined. They include GTP-binding protein Ras, p21-activated kinase (PAK) *(32,33)*, and two new kinases named mixed-lineage kinase 3 (MLK 3) and dual leucine zipper-bearing kinase *(34,35)*. It is unknown, however, how these signaling molecules are coupled to receptor signals or how they mediate different extracellular signals that ultimately lead to p38–MAPK activation.

2.2.1. Consequences of p38–MAPK Pathway Activation

The primary substrate of p38–MAPK is MAPK-activated protein kinase 2 (MAPKAPK-2; *36*) that in turn phosphorylates the small heat shock protein HSP27, which promotes polymerization of actin filaments and maintains integrity of the cytoskeleton *(37)*. The activation of this pathway prevents oxygen radical- and cytochalasin D-induced fragmentation of actin filaments and cell damage *(37)*. In addition, activated MAPKAPK-2 has also been reported to phosphorylate glycogen synthase *(14)* and cAMP response element-binding protein *(38)*. It has been demonstrated that MAPKAPK-2 activity in neonatal cardiomyocytes can be increased after PKC activation by the G protein–coupled receptor agonists, endothelin-1 and phenylephrine *(39)*, suggesting a link between PKC and p38-MAPK cascades. However, intermediate processes are still not clear.

Many transcription factors have been suggested as potential substrates for p38-MAPK, such as activating transcription factor-1 (ATF-1), ATF-2, Elk-1, and serum response factor *(12,29,40)*. Activation of p38-MAPK by numerous inflammatory stimuli followed by transcription of genes encoding inflammatory molecules indicates an important role of this stress cascade in the cell inflammatory responses *(40,41)*.

2.3. SAPK/JNK Subfamily

This group of MAPKs was first identified as protein kinases that phosphorylate the transcription factor c-Jun within its N-terminal activation domain in the cells exposed to ultraviolet radiation *(42)*. Two isoforms of JNKs, the 46-kDa JNK1 and the 54-kDa JNK2, have been demonstrated, both of which are present in the heart tissue *(2,43)*. Simultaneously, a family of MAPK-related kinases with properties of JNKs has been cloned. Because these kinases were more strongly activated by stress-inducing stimuli, they were named, as mentioned in the Introduction, SAPKs. SAPKs have been found to be similar to JNKs in terms of their molecular mass and, therefore, this group of kinases has been named SAPK/JNK *(43,44)*. Direct activators of these kinases are upstream kinases MKK4 and MKK7. MKK4 is unique in its ability to activate both, p38-MAPK and JNK in vitro *(45)*, whereby MKK7 is activating JNK isoforms *(46)*. Upstream activators of MKKs are isoforms of MEKK *(45)*. Furthermore, activation of Gq-coupled receptors and PKC can mediate activation of SAPK/JNKs *(47)*.

Different from the ERK cascade, SAPK/JNKs are weakly activated by growth factor, phorbol esters or activated Ras. On the other hand, inflammatory cytokines, various cellular stresses such as ultraviolet radiation, heat shock or osmotic shock, as well as protein synthesis inhibition (anisomycin) appear to play a strong role in the mechanisms of SAPK/JNK activation *(44,48–50)*.

2.3.1. Consequences of SAPK/JNK Activation

The primary substrate for SAPK/JNKs is the transcription factor c-Jun *(31)*. The presence of binding sites for SAPK/JNKs (the δ-subdomains) on the amino-terminal activation domains of c-Jun separated from the sites of c-Jun phosphorylation has been demonstrated, and it has been suggested that strong interaction between SAPK/JNKs and the δ-subdomain of c-Jun is required for the phosphorylation of c-Jun by SAPK/JNKs *(43,48)*. In addition, further substrates for the phosphorylation by SAPK/JNKs are transcription factors ATF-2, Elk-1, and/or antiapoptotic Bcl-2 protein *(12,49,51)*.

3. ROLE OF MAPKS IN CARDIAC PATHOLOGY

Table 1 summarizes the implication of members of MAPK superfamily in various cardiovascular diseases.

Ischemic heart disease and acute myocardial infarction are major causes of morbidity and mortality and represent major therapeutic targets. Ischemic damage to the myocardium and cell death is often associated with a reactive hypertrophy of the surviving cardiomyocytes in the noninfarcted area and myocardial remodeling to maintain contractility and cardiac output. It is likely that the response of cardiomyocytes to these stress factors is mediated through the activation of different MAPK cascades. To elucidate the real biological role of MAPK signaling cascades in the mechanisms of cell death and/or survival, activation or inactivation of specific MAPKs either by pharmacological modulations or by gene targeting can be employed.

3.1. Role of MAPKs in Hypertrophic Response and Heart Failure

Cardiac hypertrophy represents a major risk factor for the development of congestive heart failure. Being a compensatory adaptive response in the early phase, a transition to decompensated hypertrophy eventually leads to the death of the patient if the pathological stimulus persists. Involvement of all three classic MAPK pathways has been implicated in the mechanisms of cardiac hypertrophy. Numerous pathological mediators of cardiac hypertrophy (neurohormones, cytokines, mechanical stretch) have been shown to activate different MAPK pathways *(57,76–80)*.

Most of the studies point to the key role of ERK cascade in the mechanisms of hypertrophic response. Hypertrophic G protein-coupled receptors agonists, such as endothelin-1 (ET-1) and phenylephrine (PE) stimulate ERK pathway in the heart *(65,81)*. It was found that in the neonatal rat cardiomyocytes, specific inhibition of ERK pathway reversed the ET-1- and PE-induced protein synthesis and increased cell size, sarcomeric reorganization, and expression of beta-myosin heavy chains *(65)*. In the adult rat ventricular myocytes, stimulation of alpha1-adrenergic receptors caused hypertrophy dependent on the MEK1/2-ERK1/2 signaling pathway *(82)*. In accordance, concentric hypertrophy without signs of cardiomyopathy or lethality was demonstrated in MEK1 transgenic mice *(66)*. In addition, the involvement of MAPKs in hypertrophic responses was also demonstrated using antisense oligodeoxynucleotide approach, when anti-MAPK oligodeoxynucleotide inhibited the development of morphological features of hypertrophy in cardiomyocytes exposed to phenylephrine *(67)*. An increase in the ERK1/2 activity was observed in rat myocardium with volume overload-induced hypertrophy *(79)* and in normal guinea pig hearts exposed to acute mechanical stretch, as well as during chronic pressure overload (as the result of aortic banding), leading to

Table 1
Summary of MAPKs Involvement in Cardiac Pathology

Cardiac pathologies	MAPKs studied	Refs.
Heart failure	p38–MAPK	*52–55*
	JNK	*53–55*
	ERK	*53,55–57*
Hypertensive cardiac hypertrophy	p38–MAPK	*58,59*
	JNK	*58*
	ERK	*58*
Hypertrophy	p38–MAPK	*58–61*
	JNK	*62–64*
	ERK	*57,65–67*
Cardiomyopathies	p38–MAPK	*61,68*
	ERK	*56*
Ischemia–reperfusion injury	p38–MAPK	*69–74*
Inflammatory diseases	p38–MAPK	*41,75*

a transition of compensated hypertrophy to decompensated congestive heart failure *(57)*. The latter study also demonstrated differential activation of members of MAPKs family (ERK1/2, p38, Src, p90RSK, and BMK1) during progression of hypertrophy and pointed to the specific role of novel pathways (p90RSK and BMK1) in the development of heart failure.

Possible role of three classic MAPK pathways in hypertrophic responses was demonstrated using adenovirus-mediated gene transfer, whereby constitutive expression of dual-specificity phosphatase MKP-1 in cultured primary myocytes blocked the activation of p38-MAPK, SAPK/JNKs, and ERKs and prevented the agonist (catecholamine)-induced hypertrophy *(83)*. Another co-transfection experiment showed that the action of constitutively active MKK3 is followed by an activation of the p38α isoform of p38-MAPK, but it is the p38β that appears to mediate the hypertrophic response independently on the MKK3 pathway *(60)*. The activation of p38-MAPK signaling pathway was associated with the development of hypertrophy also in transgenic mice with Angiotensin II (Ang II)-induced cardiac hypertrophy *(58)* and in a model of hypertensive cardiac hypertrophy in spontaneously hypertensive stroke-prone rats *(59)*. Recently, it was demonstrated that targeted activation of p38–MAPK in vivo using a gene-switch transgenic technique with activated mutants of upstream kinases MKK3 and MKK6 resulted in the development of cardiac remodeling (marked interstitial fibrosis) and the expression of fetal genes characteristic of heart failure in conjunction with systolic contractile depression and restrictive diastolic defects related to increased chamber stiffness *(61)*.

Some studies also have documented the possible role of another stress kinase pathway, SAPK/JNK, in hypertrophic responses to Gq receptor-coupled hypertrophic agonists. Wang et al *(62)* found that expression of both wild-type and constitutive mutants of MKK7 and specific activation of JNK pathway led to the induction of the hypertrophic responses. Activation of JNK pathway by ET-1 and PE was shown to contribute to the morphological response of neonatal rat cardiomyocytes and to increase the expression of hypertrophy-related genes *(63)*. Overexpression of JNK-interacting protein 1, which binds to JNK and inhibits its signaling, inhibited the changes in gene expression and cell shape induced by the above agents and attenuated reporter gene activation induced by a constitutively active mutant of MEKK1, an upstream kinase that preferentially activates JNKs *(63)*. Moreover, a dominant inhibitory mutant of SEK-1 (MKK4), an immediate upstream activator of SAPK/JNKs, completely inhibited the ET-1–induced increase of protein synthesis, sarcomeres reorganization and JNK activation *(64)*. On the contrary, the JNK activation was reported not to be involved in response to acute mechanical stress or to aortic banding-induced chronic hypertrophy in the guinea pig heart *(57)*.

A few studies were performed recently to clarify the role of MAPKs in human pathology. In the study of Takeishi *(56)*, a differential regulation of multiple MAPK kinases, p90RSK and Src, was demonstrated in patients with failing heart as the result of dilated cardiomyopathy. ERK1/2 and p90RSK were activated in failed myocardium with end stage of disease, whereas SAPK/JNKs were unchanged. On the contrary, the activities of p38–MAPK, Src, and BMK1 were significantly reduced in end-stage heart failure. In patients with ischemic and idiopathic failing hearts, the predominant isoform of p38–MAPK was found to be p38α, and its activity was markedly decreased before the end-stage heart failure that correlated with a decreased phosphorylation of its substrate MAPKAPK-2 *(52)*. Interestingly, differential regulation of MAPKs was also observed in failing human heart after its mechanical unloading with a left ventricular assist device. This intervention led to a reduction in ERK1/2 and SAPK/JNKs activities and an increase in p38 activity, and these changes were associated with attenuation of morphological signs of hypertrophy *(53)*.

3.2. Role of MAPKs in Ischemia–Reperfusion Injury

Mammalian cells respond to ischemia with activation of numerous cell-signaling cascades that lead eventually to cell death unless early onset of reperfusion salvages viable myocytes. It was found that ischemia and reperfusion induce distinct regulation of various MAPK cascades, and some differences in the intensity and time course of their activation, as well as interspecies differences (rat, rabbit, pig) were observed.

3.2.1. ERKs and Response to Ischemia–Reperfusion

The ERK cascade has been shown to be activated during ischemia in the in vivo pig *(84–86)* and rat *(87)* models, in neonatal rat cardiomyocytes *(65)*, as well as in human hearts *(3)*. ERK activation was also observed during ischemia and reperfusion in human, bovine, rat, and guinea pig heart by several *(3,65,86,88,89)* but not all investigators *(2,90)*. Results of several studies show that the activation of ERK plays an important role in prevention of myocardial necrosis and apoptosis *(6,91,92)*. Inhibition of the ERK cascade during sustained ischemia or ischemia–reperfusion significantly increased the size of myocardial infarction in pig myocardium *(6)*, exaggerated reperfusion injury in isolated rat hearts, and enhanced ischemia–reperfusion-induced apoptosis in neonatal cardiomyocytes *(65)*. Moreover, the protective effect of ERK cascade activation has been demonstrated in MEK1 transgenic mice and MEK1 adenovirus-infected cultured cardiomyocytes that exhibited an increased resistance to apoptotic stimuli *(66)*.

A positive role of the ERK cascade in the mechanisms of cell survival is also supported by the observations that several growth factors, such as insulin-like growth factors *(93–95)*, fibroblast growth factors *(96,97)*, cardiotrophin-1 *(98,99)*, which also activate ERKs *(99,100)*, exert the antiapoptotic effects *(94,101)* or limit the ischemia–reperfusion injury *(93,95–98,101,102)*.

3.2.2. *"Stress" Kinases and Response to Ischemia–Reperfusion*

p38–MAPK pathway belongs to the most investigated but also the most controversial signaling pathway in myocardial responses to ischemic injury. With a few exceptions *(103–105)* most studies (regardless of the species or model) showed the activation of p38–MAPK either by ischemia alone, or persisting throughout reperfusion, and reported a negative role of p38–MAPK during ischemia–reperfusion injury. Inhibition of p38–MAPK activation delayed the development of infarcts, increased cell survival, reduced myocardial apoptosis, and improved postischemic recovery of cardiac function, suggesting that it could be considered as an essential element of cardioprotection *(69–74,106,107)*. In contrast, others showed that the inhibition of p38–MAPK during lethal ischemia did not influence the extent of ischemia–reperfusion-induced injury or even increased it *(4,105,108,109)*, suggesting a protective role of p38–MAPK activation during ischemia.

In contrast with the p38–MAPK pathway, the SAPK/JNK signaling pathway shows a different pattern of activation. Several studies showed that this kinase pathway is moderately or not activated during ischemia; however, a stronger activation of JNKs was found during reperfusion after a brief ischemic stimulus *(84,88,90)*. The precise role of SAPK/JNK in pathophysiology of ischemic injury remains unresolved.

4. ROLE OF MAPKS IN CARDIOPROTECTION

Prolonged ischemia causes necrotic changes in the myocardium and contractile dysfunction, whereas brief ischemic episodes before sustained ischemic challenge render the heart more resistant to ischemic injury *(110)*. Numerous studies demonstrate the involvement of various MAPK cascades in the mechanisms of this adaptive phenomenon termed as ischemic preconditioning (IP; ref. *111*).

4.1. *Ischemic Preconditioning*

A positive role for ERK cascade in the mechanisms of IP-mediated cardioprotection has been demonstrated in pig myocardium, when inhibition of ERK pathway during the IP protocol inhibited both the IP-induced limitation of infarct size and the stimulation of ERK activities during IP *(6)*. Other studies also confirmed the positive role of ERKs in regulation of both the classic early *(112)* and late *(91,92)* phase of IP-mediated cardioprotection. A key role for ERK-1 was documented also in opioid-induced cardioprotection in rats *(92,112)*.

On the contrary, the role of p38–MAPK cascade in IP remains still unclear. In some studies, a downregulation of the p38–MAPK during repeated periods of short ischemia and reperfusion was observed *(5,72,84)* with a subsequent further decrease in p38–MAPK activities during sustained ischemia *(4,69,72,84)*. However, in some studies it was found that IP mediated a subsequent increase in p38–MAPK activities *(103,108,109,113)*. These discrepancies suggest that, apart from species differences, specific p38–MAPK isoforms might play a role.

Recent studies revealed a different role for p38α and β isoforms in apoptotic responses and cell survival *(60,114)*: a negative role of p38α and positive of p38β (mediating hypertrophic response). One possible explanation for these divergent functions of p38–MAPK isoforms is that they mediate phosphorylation of different downstream-located substrates that can play different roles in apoptosis. It is also possible that ischemia and IP differentially activate p38–MAPK isoforms and that this contributes to the conflicting data. p38α activation was observed in response to ischemia and reperfusion *(72,73,90)*. Also, in myocytes with ectopically expressed p38α and p38β, p38α was activated during sustained simulated ischemia, whereas the p38β isoform was deactivated *(115)*. Moreover, in rat heart cells expressing wild-type p38α injury was reduced by p38–MAPK inhibition, suggesting that the selective inhibition of the p38α isoform of the p38–MAPK pathway may underlie the mechanism responsible for anti-ischemic effects observed after p38–MAPK inhibition *(114)*. However, the p38–MAPK(β) isoform appears to play a positive role in the protection against apoptotic cell death *(60)*.

There is only little evidence about the role of SAPK/JNK pathway in IP-mediated cardioprotection. Recently, it was demonstrated in the in vivo rat model that SAPK/JNK activation is an important component of IP- or opioid receptor-mediated reduction of infarct size *(112,116)*. This is strengthened by the observation that IP increased SAPK/JNKs activities *(5)*. Moreover, pharmacological preconditioning with protein synthesis inhibitor anisomycin conferred the IP-like anti-infarct protection in pigs *(117)*, rabbits *(103, 104)*, and rats *(106)* and was found to be accompanied by an activation of SAPK/JNKs only *(117)* or both SAPK/JNK and p38–MAPK cascades *(103,104,106,118)*. Although the JNK pathway, as well as the p38–MAPK pathway, is generally implicated in apoptotic processes, its activation is not universally proapoptotic *(62)*, and the effects could be isoenzyme specific and dependent on the extent, intensity, and the timing of JNKs activation.

4.2. Delayed Cardioprotection

Apart from the classic short-lasting ischemic preconditioning, a delayed phase of protection appears several hours after the initial stimulus and lasts longer. Molecular mechanisms of this form of cardioprotection termed second window of cardioprotection involve the induction of immediate early genes (c-*myc*, c-*fos*, and c-*jun*), leading to the expression of late genes encoding various cardioprotective proteins, for example, heat shock proteins (HSP70), antioxidants, and/or inducible nitric oxide synthase (iNOS; reviewed by Yellon and Baxter in ref. *119*). Delayed protection against myocardial necrosis and contractile dysfunction in mice 48 h after heat stress has been found to be associated with an increased phosphorylation of JNK and accumulation of HSP72 protein *(7)*. Similar improvement of heart function and reduction in infarct size was observed in Langendorff-perfused rat hearts 24 h after treatment with p38 activator anisomycin. The latter induced activation of nuclear factor NFκB and increased expression of iNOS, suggesting that activation of p38 triggers delayed protection by mechanisms involving activation of NFκB and synthesis of NO by iNOS *(120)*. Although the role of ERKs activation in the delayed cardioprotection in rat myocardium induced by pretreatment with noradrenaline has not been confirmed *(121)*, more recent studies indicate that activation of ERKs cascade may be involved in the delayed protective effect in conscious rabbits *(91)* and also be a component of opioid-induced cardioprotection *(92,112)*.

5. PHARMACOLOGICAL MODULATION OF MAPK ACTIVITY

The activities of distinct MAPKs are positively or negatively modulated by several pharmacological substances. Specific inhibitors are most often used for the study of role MAPKs in the cellular processes. At present, specific inhibitors of ERK and p38–MAPK pathways are available. PD98059 [2-(2-amino-3-methoxyphenyl)-4H-1-benzopyran-4-one] and UO126 (1,4-diamino-2,3-dicyano-1,4-bis[2-aminophenyl-thio]butadiene) are known as selective and potent inhibitors of ERK1/2 pathway in vitro as well as in vivo (122,123). A recent study showed that these substances can inhibit also the epidermal-growth factor-induced and MEK5-mediated activation of other members of the ERK family, such as ERK5/BMK1 (124).

On the other hand, several pyridinyl imidazole derivatives, SB203580, SB202190, and SB242719, were found to inhibit the p38–MAPK signaling pathway *(125,126)*. The availability of these specific inhibitors helps to clarify the role of ERK and p38–MAPK pathways in the myocardium.

To resolve the question whether activation of p38–MAPK by ischemia and/or ischemia–reperfusion is only an epiphenomenon or whether it is causative for myocardial necrosis and/or apoptosis, several groups used pharmacological inhibition of p38–MAPKs. It was found that the inhibition of p38–MAPK during sustained ischemia with SB203580, SB202190, or SB242719 induced cardioprotective effects *(4,69–74,106,115)*. The application of SB substances before and during sustained ischemia delayed the development of infarcts *(69–71,73,106)* reduced myocardial apoptosis *(70, 107)* and improved postischemic recovery of cardiac function in several animal models *(69,70,106)*.

The inhibition of p38–MAPK with SB203580 also decreased ischemia-induced TNF-α production and facilitated limitation of functional impairment after ischemia–reperfusion in human myocardium. It was suggested that this may represent a potent therapeutic strategy for improving myocardial function after angioplasty, coronary bypass, or heart transplantation.

The inhibition of p38–MAPK cascade was used also for the investigation of the role of this kinase cascade in the IP-induced cardioprotection. In isolated rat *(106,109,127)*, rabbit *(108)* and mouse *(7)* hearts, rabbit cardiomyocytes *(103,105)*, the treatment with SB203550 reversed the protective effects of IP-mediated cardioprotection. However, in another group of studies, suppression of the cardioprotective effect of IP by SB203580 and/or by other SB-related p38–MAPK inhibitors was not observed.

Pharmacological inhibition of p38–MAPK suggests also the involvement of this kinase cascade in the immune and inflammatory responses and in hypertrophy. In healthy human volunteers, it was demonstrated that inhibition of p38–MAPK by pyridinyl imidazole RWJ-67657 might be a tool to intervene in the deranged immune response in sepsis and other inflammatory diseases *(75)*. The inhibition of p38–MAPK activity by SB203580 reduced also myocyte secretion of TNF-α and prevented burn-mediated cardiac dysfunction *(128)*. It was also found that long-term oral treatment of hypertensive stroke-prone rats with a selective p38–MAPK inhibitor (SB239063) significantly enhanced survival, whereby echocardiographic analysis revealed a significant reduction in left ventricular (LV) hypertrophy and dysfunction in the SB239063-treated groups *(59)*.

PD98059 and UO126 are able to specifically inhibit the ERK signaling pathway. It was found that pharmacological inhibition of the ERK cascade during ischemia–reperfusion by PD98059 injured isolated rat hearts and enhanced the ischaemia–reperfusion-induced apoptosis in neonatal cardiomyocytes *(107)*. In pig myocardium, an augmentation of infarct size after inhibition of ERKs during sustained ischaemia by both PD98059 and UO126 was observed *(6)*. Moreover, the presence of these inhibitors during the IP protocol inhibited the IP-induced cardioprotection. Also survival-promoting effects of urocortin endogenous cardiac factor were blocked by PD98059 *(129)*. Using spontaneously hypertensive and aortic-banded rats, it was found that expression of myocardial osteopontin, an extracellular matrix protein, coincides with the development of heart failure and is inhibited by captopril. Evidence that ERK cascade plays a key role in the regulation of osteopontin gene expression and is critical component of the reactive oxygen species-sensitive signaling pathways activated by angiotensin II was also obtained using PD98059 *(130)*.

It has been found that effects of numerous hypertrophic stimuli are mediated by the activation of MAPK pathways *(76–80,131)*. Ang II stimulates cardiac fibroblast growth and this effect was associated with the activation of ERK, p38–MAPK, and STAT3 pathways *(131)*. The angiotensin-converting enzyme inhibitors moexiprilat and enaprilat inhibited the Ang II-induced proliferation of cardiac fibroblasts and also completely inhibited Ang II-induced activation of ERKs, p38–MAPK, and STAT3 *(131)*. Another angiotensin-converting enzyme inhibitor, cilazapril, remarkably suppressed the arterial JNK activation after balloon injury *(132)*. The activation of both JNKs and ERKs was prevented also by E4177, an angiotensin AT1 receptor antagonist *(132)*. Carvedilol, a vasodilating beta-adrenoceptor antagonist and potent antioxidant, prevented myocardial ischemia–reperfusion-induced apoptosis in rabbit cardiomyocytes possibly by the inhibition (downregulation) of JNK signaling pathway *(133)*.

Another group of pharmacological substances that influence and possibly act through MAPK-signaling pathways is represented by alpha- and beta-adrenergic receptor agonists. Selective beta-2 adrenergic receptor stimulation markedly stimulated ERKs as well as PI-3K/Akt activities and this was connected with a protection of the rat neonatal cardiomyocytes against apoptosis *(134)*. The agonist-induced activation of the kinase pathways was blocked using specific inhibitors of these pathways (PD98059 and LY 294002). Activation of alpha-1 adrenergic receptors in the heart was shown to influence heart physiology and increase contractile activity, cardiac fetal genes re-expression, and myocyte hypertrophy. G(q)-coupled receptor agonists, such as phenylephrine, a promoter of hypertrophic responses in cardiac cells, were found to activate the ERKs, p38-MAPK, and also JNKs in perfused contracting rat hearts *(79)*. Phenylephrine was also found to stabilize the B-type natriuretic peptide mRNA. Using specific inhibitors (PD98059 for ERKs and GF 109203X for PKC) the role of PKC and ERKs in this alpha1-adrenergic receptor-mediated stabilization of the B-type natriuretic peptide mRNA was established *(135)*.

It has been also found that some protein phosphatase inhibitors (okadaic acid) and protein synthesis inhibitors (anisomycin) stimulate myocardial MAPKs activities. It was found that pharmacological inhibition of Ser–Thr protein phosphatases by okadaic acid *(117)* exerted cardioprotective effects and this was connected with the stimulation of SAPK/JNKs activities.

Also anisomycin, a potent but unspecific activator of stress kinases (SAPK/JNKs and p38–MAPK) in mammalian cells *(136)* mimicked the anti-infarct effects of IP in several animal models *(106,108,117,137)*.

6. CONCLUSION

Recent evidence suggests the involvement of MAPKs in several pathophysiological processes in the heart (hypertrophy, heart failure, ischemia–reperfusion, cardioprotective responses). Because all three major MAPK pathways were found to be activated during ischemia–reperfusion, crosstalk between the ERK, p38-MAPK, and JNK cascades in ischemia-associated processes cannot be excluded. The activation of ERKs during ischemia is linked to cell survival. In contrast, the role of the p38–MAPK pathway is not unequivocal and may be linked to the activation of different p38–MAPK isoforms by ischemia and IP: although the p38α isoform activation is believed to accelerate the death pathway, the p38β pathway may be antiapoptotic. The literature on the JNK pathway is sparse. However, there is an agreement that the apoptotic response can be mediated by sustained JNK activation, but transient and more marked JNK activation (in response to reperfusion after brief ischemia) can also cause cardioprotective responses.

The precise role of distinct MAPKs during pathophysiological processes in the myocardium will be probably resolved only by using isoenzyme-specific MAPK inhibitors and activators and elucidation of physiological (in vivo) substrates for distinct MAPKs that are phosphorylated under some specific conditions.

Pharmacological modulation of MAPKs may represent a novel therapeutic target to confer protection to the myocardium by way of either inhibition of deleterious pathways and shifting the balance toward cell survival or by activation of pathways participating in the endogenous cardioprotective cascades.

ACKNOWLEDGMENTS

Supported, in part, by grant VEGA SR 2/2063/22 and APVT 51-013802.

REFERENCES

1. Chien, K. R., Knowlton, K. U., Zhu, H., and Chien, S. (1991) Regulation of cardiac gene expression during myocardial growth and hypertrophy: Molecular studies of an adaptive physiologic response. *FASEB J.* **5,** 3037–3046.
2. Clerk, A., Fuller, S. J., Michael, A., and Sugden, P. H. (1998) Stimulation of "stress-regulated" mitogen-activated protein kinases (stress-activated protein kinases/c-Jun N-terminal kinases and p38-mitogen-activated protein kinases) in perfused rat hearts by oxidative and other stresses. *J. Biol. Chem.* **273,** 7228–7334.
3. Talmor, D., Applebaum, A., Rudich, A., Shapira, Y., and Tirosh, A. (2000) Activation of mitogen-activated protein kinases in human heart during cardiopulmonary bypass. *Circ. Res.* **86,** 1004–1007.
4. Sanada, S., Kitakaze, M., Papst, P. J., Hatanaka, K., Asanuma, H., Aki, T., et al. (2001) Role of phasic dynamism of p38 mitogen-activated protein kinase activation in ischemic preconditioning of the canine heart. *Circ. Res.* **88,** 175–180.
5. Ping, P., Zhang, J., Huang, S., Cao, X., Tang, X. L., Li, R. C., et al. (1999) PKC-dependent activation of p46/p54 JNKs during ischemic preconditioning in conscious rabbits. *Am. J. Physiol. Heart Circ. Physiol.* **277,** H1771–1785.

6. Strohm, C., Barancik, M., Bruehl, M. L., Kilian, S. A. R., and Schaper, W. (2000) Inhibition of the ER-Kinase by PD98059 and UO126 counteracts ischemic preconditioning in pig myocardium. *J. Cardiovasc. Pharmacol.* **36,** 218–229.

7. Tekin, D., Xi, L., Zhao, T., Tejero-Taldo, M. I., Atluri, S., and Kukreja, R. C. (2001) Mitogen-activated protein kinases mediate heat shock-induced delayed protection in mouse heart. *Am. J. Physiol. Heart Circ. Physiol.* **281,** H523–532.

8. Robinson, M. J. and Cobb, M. H. (1997) Mitogen-activated protein kinase pathways. *Curr. Opin. Cell Biol.* **9,** 180–186.

9. Sugden, P. H. and Bogoyevitch, M. A. (1995) Intracellular signalling through protein kinases in the heart. *Cardiovasc. Res.* **30,** 478–492.

10. Marshall, C. J. (1994) MAP kinase kinase kinase, MAP kinase kinase and MAP kinase. *Rev. Curr. Opin. Genet. Dev.* **4,** 82–89.

11. Minden, A., Lin, A., McMahon, M., Lange-Carter, C., Dérijard, B., Davis, R. J., et al. (1994) Differential activation of ERK and JNK mitogen-activated protein kinases by Raf-1 and MEKK. *Science* **266,** 1719–1723.

12. Whitmarsh, A. J., Shore, P., Sharrocks, A. D., and Davis, R. J. (1995) Integration of MAP kinase signal transduction pathways at the serum response element. *Science* **269,** 403–407.

13. Lange-Carter, C. A., Pleiman, C. E., Gardner, A. M., Blumer, K. J., and Johnson, G. L. (1993) A divergence in the MAP kinase regulatory network defined by MEK kinase and Raf. *Science* **260,** 315–319.

14. Stokoe, D., Campbell, D. G., Nakielny, S., Hidaka, H., Leevers, S. J., Marshall, C., et al. (1992) MAPKAP kinase-2: A novel protein kinase activated by mitogen-activated protein kinase. *EMBO J.* **11,** 3985–3994.

15. Sadoshima, J., Qiu, Z., Morgan, J. P., and Izumo, S. (1995) Angiotensin and other hypertrophic stimuli mediated by G protein-coupled receptors activate tyrosine kinase, mitogen-activated protein kinase, and 90 kD S6 kinase in cardiac myocytes: the critical role of Ca^{2+}-dependent signaling. *Circ. Res.* **76,** 1–15.

16. Domingos, P. P., Fonseca, P. M., Nadruz, W. Jr., and Franchini, K. G. (2002) Load-induced focal adhesion kinase activation in the myocardium: Role of stretch and contractile activity. *Am. J. Physiol.* **282,** H556–H564.

17. Tahara, S., Fukuda, K., Kodama, H., Kato, T., Miyoshi, S., and Ogawa, S. (2001) Potassium channel blocker activates extracellular signal-regulated kinases through Pyk2 and epidermal growth factor receptor in rat cardiomyocytes. *J. Am. Coll. Cardiol.* **38,** 554–563.

18. Ahn, N. G., Seger, R., Bratlien, R. L., Diltz, C. D., Tonks, N. K., and Krebs, E. G. (1991) Multiple components in an epidermal growth factor-stimulated protein kinase cascade. In vitro activation of a myelin basic protein/microtubule-associated protein 2 kinase. *J. Biol. Chem.* **266,** 4220–4227.

19. Warne, P. H., Viciana, P. R., and Downward, J. (1993) Direct interaction of Ras and the amino-terminal region of Raf-1 *in vitro. Nature* **364,** 352–355.

20. Kolch, W., Heidecker, G., Kochs, G., Hummel, R., Vahidi, H., Mischak, H., et al. (1993) Protein kinase C activates Raf-1 by direct phosphorylation. *Nature* **364,** 249–252.

21. Cano, E. and Mahadevan, L. C. (1995) Parallel signal processing among mammalian MAPKs. *Trends Biochem. Sci.* **20,** 117–122.

22. Reszka, A. A., Seger, R., Diltz, C. D., Krebs, E. G., and Fischer, E. H. (1995) Association of mitogen-activated protein kinase with the microtubule cytoskeleton. *Proc. Natl. Acad. Sci. USA* **92,** 8881–8885.

23. Erikson, R. L. (1991) Structure expression, and regulation of protein kinases involved in the phosphorylation of ribosomal protein S6. *J. Biol. Chem.* **266,** 6007–6010.

24. Eldar-Finkelman, H., Seger, R., Vandenheede, J. R., and Krebs, E. G. (1995) Inactivation of glycogen synthase kinase-3 by epidermal growth factor is mediated by mitogen-activated protein kinase/p90 ribosomal protein S6 kinase signaling pathway in NIH/3T3 cells. *J. Biol. Chem.* **270,** 987–990.

25. Frödin, M. and Gammeltoft, S. (1999) Role and regulation of 90kDa ribosomal S6 kinase (RSK) in signal transduction. *Mol. Cell Endocrinol.* **151,** 65–77.

26. Lin, L. L., Wartmann, M., Lin, A. Y., Knopf, J. L., Seth, A., and Davis, R. J. (1993) cPLA$_2$ is phosphorylated and activated by MAP kinase. *Cell* **72,** 269–278.

27. Davis, R. J. (1993) The mitogen-activated protein kinase signal transduction pathway. *J. Biol. Chem.* **268,** 14553–14556.

28. Lee, J. C., Laydon, J. T., McDonnell P. C., Gallagher, T. F., Kumar, S., Green, D., et al. (1994) A protein kinase involved in the regulation of inflammatory cytokine biosynthesis. *Nature* **372,** 739–746.

29. Han, J., Lee, J. D., Bibbs, L., and Ulevitch, R. J. (1994) A MAP kinase targeted by endotoxin and hyperosmolarity in mammalian cells. *Science* **265,** 808–811.

30. Rouse, J., Cohen, P., Trigon, S., Morange, M., Alonso-Llamazares, A., Zamanillo, D., et al. (1994) A novel kinase cascade triggered by stress and heat shock that stimulates MAPKAP kinase-2 and phosphorylation of the small heat shock proteins. *Cell* **78,** 1027–1037.

31. Sugden, P. H. and Clerk, A. (1998) "Stress-responsive" mitogen-activated protein kinases (c-Jun N-terminal kinases and p38 mitogen-activated protein kinases) in the myocardium. *Circ. Res.* **83,** 345–352.

32. Zhang, S., Han, J., Sells, M. A., Chernoff, J., Knaus, U. G., Ulevitch, R. J., et al. (1995) Rho family GTP-ases regulate p38 mitogen-activated protein kinase through the downstream mediator Pak 1. *J. Biol. Chem.* **270,** 23934–23936.

33. Bagrodia, S., Derijard, B., Davis, R. J., and Cerione, R. A. (1995) Cdc42 and PAK-mediated signaling leads to Jun kinase and p38 mitogen-activated protein kinase activation. *J. Biol. Chem.* **270,** 27995–27998.

34. Fan, G., Merrit, S. E., Kortenjann, M., Shaw, P. E., and Holzman, L. B. (1996) Dual leucine zipper-bearing kinase (DLK) activates p46SAPK and p38 MAPK but not ERK2. *J. Biol. Chem.* **271,** 24788–24793.

35. Tibbles, L. A., Ing, Y. L., Kiefer, F., Chan, J., Iscove, N., Woodgett, J. R., et al. (1996) MLK-3 activates the SAPK/JNK and p38/RK pathways via SEK1 and MKK3/6. *EMBO J.* **15,** 7026–7035.

36. Freshney, N. W., Rawlinson, L., Guesdon, F., Jones, E., Cowley, S., Hsuan, J., et al. (1994) Interleukin-1 activates a novel protein kinase cascade that results in the phosphorylation of Hsp27. *Cell* **78,** 1039–1049.

37. Guay, J., Lambert, H., Gingras-Breton, G., Lavoie, J. N., and Huot, J. (1997) Regulation of actin filament dynamics by p38 map kinase-mediated phosphorylation of heat shock protein 27. *J. Cell Sci.* **110,** 357–368.

38. Tan, Y., Rouse, J., Zhang, A., Cariati, S., Cohen, P., and Comb, M. J. (1996) FGF and stress regulate CREB and ATF-1 via a pathway involving p38 MAP kinase and MAPKAP kinase-2. *EMBO J.* **15,** 4629–4642.

39. Clerk, A., Michael, A., and Sugden, P. H. (1998) Stimulation of the p38 mitogen-activated protein kinase pathway in neonatal rat ventricular myocytes by the G protein-coupled receptor agonists, endothelin-l and phenylephrine: a role in cardiac myocyte hypertrophy? *J. Cell Biol.* **142,** 523–535.

40. Raingeaud, J., Gupta, S., Rogers, J. S., Dickens, M., Han J., Ulevitch, R. J., et al. (1995) Pro-inflammatory cytokines and enviromental stress cause p38 mitogen-activated protein kinase activation by dual phosphorylation on tyrosine and threonine. *J. Biol. Chem.* **270,** 7420–7426.

41. Han, J., Jiang, Y., Li, Z., Kravchenko, V. V., and Ulevitch, R. J. (1997) Activation of the transcription factor MEF 2C by the MAP kinase p38 in inflammation. *Nature* **386,** 296–299.

42. Pulverer, B. J., Kyriakis, J. M., Avruch, J., Nikolakaki, E., and Woodgett, J. R. (1991) Phosphorylation of c-jun mediated by MAP kinases. *Nature* **353,** 670–674.

43. Derijard, B., Hibi, M., Wu, I. H., Barrett, T., Su, B., Deng, T., et al. (1994) JNK1: A protein kinase stimulated by UV light and Ha-Ras that binds and phosphorylates the c-Jun activation domain. *Cell* **76**, 1025–1037.

44. Kyriakis, J. M., Banerjee, P., Nikolakaki, E., Dai, T., Rubie, E. A., Ahmad, M. F., et al. (1994) The stress-activated protein kinase subfamily of c-Jun kinases. *Nature* **369**, 156–160.

45. Deacon, K. and Blank, J. L. (1997) Characterization of the mitogen-activated protein kinase 4 (MKK4)/c-Jun NH2-terminal kinase 1 and MKK/p38 pathways regulated by MEK kinase 2 and 3: MEK kinase 3 activates MKK3 but does not cause activation of p38 kinase in vivo. *J. Biol. Chem.* **272**, 14,489–14,496.

46. Foltz, I. N., Gerl, R.e., Wieler, J. S., Luckach, M., Salmon, R. A., and Schrader, J. W. (1998) Human mitogen-activated protein kinase kinase 7 (MKK7) is a highly conserved c-Jun N-terminal kinase/stress-activated protein kinase (SAPK/JNK) activated by environmental stresses and physiological stimuli. *J. Biol. Chem.* **273**, 9344–9351.

47. Nagao, M., Yamauchi, J., Kaziro, Y., and Itoh, H. (1998) Involvement of protein kinase C and Src family tyrosine kinase in $G\alpha_{q/11}^-$ induced activation of c-Jun N-terminal kinase and p38 mitogen-activated protein kinase. *J. Biol. Chem.* **273**, 22,892–22,898.

48. Hibi, M., Lin, A., Smeal, T., Minden, A., and Karin, M. (1993) Identification of an oncoprotein- and UV- responsive protein kinase that binds and potentiates the c-Jun activation domain. *Genes Dev.* **7**, 2135–2148.

49. Gupta, S., Campbell, D., Derijard, B., and Davis, R. J. (1995) Transcription factor ATF2 regulation by the JNK signal transduction pathway. *Science* **267**, 389–393.

50. Bogoyevitch, M. A., Ketterman, A. J., and Sugden, P. H. (1995) Cellular stresses activate c-Jun N-terminal kinases (JNKs) in ventricular myocytes cultured from neonatal rat hearts. *J. Biol. Chem.* **270**, 29,710–29,717.

51. Gross, A., McDonnell, J. M., and Korsmeyer, S. J. (1999) BCL-2 family members and the mitochondria in apoptosis. *Genes Dev.* **13**, 1899–1911.

52. Lemke, L. E., Bloem, L. J., Fouts, R., Esterman, M., Sandusky, G., and Vlahos, C. J. (2001) Decreased p38 MAPK activity in end-stage failing human myocardium: p38 MAPK alpha is the predominant isoform expresed in human heart. *J. Mol. Cell Cardiol.* **33**, 1527–1540.

53. Flesch, M., Margulies, K. B., Mochmann, H. C., Engel, D., Sivasubramanian, N., and Mann, D. L. (2001) Diferential regulation of mitogen-activated protein kinases in the failing human heart in response to mechanical unloading. *Circulation* **104**, 2273–2276.

54. Cook, S. A., Sugden, P. H., and Clerk, A. (1999) Activation of c-Jun N-terminal kinases and p38-mitogen-activated protein kinases in human heart failure secondary to ischaemic heart disease. *J. Mol. Cell Cardiol.* **31**, 1429–1434.

55. Haq S., Choukroun G., Lim H., Tymitz K. M., del Monte F., Gwathmey J., et al. (2001) Differential activation of signal transduction pathways in human hearts with hypertrophy versus advanced heart failure. *Circulation* **103**, 670–677.

56. Takeishi, Y., Huang, Q., Abe, J., Che, W., Lee, J. D., Kawakatsu, H., et al. (2002) Activation of mitogen-activated protein kinases and p90 ribosomal S6 kinase in failing human hearts with dilated cardiomyopathy. *Cardiovasc. Res.* **53**, 131–137.

57. Takeishi, Y., Huang, Q., Abe, J., Glassman, M., Che, W., Lee, J. D., et al. (2001) Src and multiple MAP kinase activation in cardiac hypertrophy and congestive heart failure under chronic pressure-overload: Comparison with acute mechanical stretch. *J. Mol. Cell Cardiol.* **33**, 1637–1648.

58. Pellieux, C., Sauthier, T., Aubert, J. F., Brunner, H. R., and Pedrazzini, T. (2000) Angiotensin II-induced cardiac hypertrophy is associated with different mitogen-activated protein kinase activation in normotensive and hypertensive mice. *J. Hypertens* **18**, 1307–1317.

59. Behr, T. M., Nerurkar, S. S., Nelson, A. H., Coatney, R. W., Woods, T. N., Sulpizio, A., et al. (2001) Hypertensive end-organ damage and premature mortality are p38 mitogen-

activated protein kinase-dependent in a rat model of cardiac hypertrophy and dysfunction. *Circulation* **11,** 1292–1298.

60. Wang, Y., Huang, S., Sah, V. P., Ross, J., Brown, J. H., Han, J., et al. (1998) Cardiac muscle cell hypertrophy and apoptosis induced by distinct members of the p38 mitogen-activated protein kinase family. *J. Biol. Chem.* **273,** 2161–2168.

61. Liao, P., Georgakopoulos, D., Kovacs, A., Zheng, M., Lerner, D., Pu, H., et al. (2001) The in vivo role of p38 MAP kinases in cardiac remodeling and restrictive cardiomyopathy. *Proc. Natl. Acad. Sci. USA* **9,** 12,283–12,288.

62. Wang, Y., Su, B., Sah, V. P., Brown, J. H., Han, J., and Chien, K. R. (1998) Cardiac hypertrophy induced by mitogen-activated protein kinase kinase 7, a specific activator for c-Jun NH2-terminal kinase in ventricular muscle cells. *J. Biol. Chem.* **273,** 5423–5426.

63. Finn, S. G., Dickens, M., and Fuller, S. J. (2001) c-Jun N-terminal kinase/interacting protein 1 inhibits gene expression in response to hypertrophic agonists in neonatal rat ventricular myocytes. *Biochem. J.* **358,** 489–495.

64. Choukroun, G., Hajjar, R., Kyriakis, J. M., Bonventre, J. V., Rosenzweig, A., and Force, T. (1998) Role of the stress-activated protein kinases in endothelin-induced cardiomyocyte hypertrophy. *J. Clin. Invest.* **102,** 1311–1320.

65. Yue, T. L., Gu, J. L., Wang, C., Reith, A. D., Lee, J. C., Mirabile, R. C., et al. (2000) Extracellular signal-regulated kinase plays an essential role in hypertrophic agonists, endothelin-1 and phenylephrine-induced cardiomyocyte hypertrophy. *J. Biol. Chem.* **275,** 37,895–37,901.

66. Bueno, O. F., De Windt, L. J., Tymitz, K. M., Witt, S. A., Kimball, T. R., Klevitsky, R., et al. (2000) The MEK1-ERK1/2 signaling pathway promotes compensated cardiac hypertrophy in transgenic mice. *EMBO J.* **19,** 6341–6350.

67. Glennon, P. E., Kaddoura, S., Sale, E. M., Sale, G. J., Fuller, S. J., and Sugden, P. H. (1996) Depletion of mitogen-activated protein kinase using an antisense oligodeoxynucleotide approach downregulates the phenylephrine-induced hypertrophic response in rat cardiac myocytes. *Circ. Res.* **78,** 954–961.

68. Kang Y. J., Zhou Z. X., Wang G. W., Buridi A., and Klein J. B. (2000) Suppression by metallothionein of doxorubicin-induced cardiomyocyte apoptosis through inhibition of p38 mitogen-activated protein kinases. *J. Biol. Chem.* **275,** 1390–1398.

69. Schneider, S. Chen W, Hou J, Steenbergen C, and Murphy E. (2001) Inhibition of p38 MAPK alpha/beta reduces ischemic injury and does not block protective effects of preconditioning. *Am. J. Physiol. Heart Circ. Physiol.* **280,** H499–508.

70. Ma, XL., Kumar, S., Gao, F., Louden, C. S., Lopez, B. L., Christopher, T. A., et al. (1999) Inhibition of p38 mitogen-activated protein kinase decreases cardiomyocyte apoptosis and improves cardiac function after myocardial ischemia and reperfusion. *Circulation* **99,** 1685–1691.

71. Gysembergh, A., Simkhovich, B. Z., Kloner, R. A., and Przyklenk, K. (2001) p38 MAPK activity is not increased early during sustained coronary artery occlusion in preconditioned versus control rabbit heart. *J. Mol. Cell Cardiol.* **33,** 681–690.

72. Marais, E., Genade, S., Huisamen, B., Strijdom, J. G., Moolman, J. A., and Lochner, A. (2001) Activation of p38 MAPK induced by a multi-cycle ischaemic preconditioning protocol is associated with attenuated p38 MAPK activity during sustained ischaemia and reperfusion. *J. Mol. Cell Cardiol.* **33,** 769–778.

73. Barancik, M., Htun, P., Strohm, C., Kilian, S., and Schaper, W. (2000) Inhibition of the cardiac p38-MAPK pathway by SB203580 delays ischemic cell death. *J. Cardiovasc. Pharmacol.* **35,** 474–483.

74. Cain, B. S., Meldrum, D. R., Meng, X., Dinarello, C. A., Shames, B. D., Banerjee, A., et al. (1999) p38 MAPK inhibition decreases TNF-alpha production and enhances postischemic human myocardial function. *J. Surg. Res.* **83,** 7–12.

75. Fijen, J. W., Zijlstra, J. G., De Boer, P., Spanjersberg, R., Cohen Tervaert, J. W., Van Der Werf, T. S., et al. (2001) Suppression of the clinical and cytokine response to endotoxin by RWJ-67657, a p38 mitogen-activated protein-kinase inhibitor, in healthy human volunteers. *Clin. Exp. Immunol.* **124,** 16–20.

76. Yamazaki, T., Tobe, K., Hoh, E., Maemura, K., Kaida, T., Komuro, I., et al. (1993) Mechanical loading activates mitogen-activated protein kinase and S6 peptide kinase in cultured rat cardiac myocytes. *J. Biol. Chem.* **268,** 12,069–12,076.

77. Kudoh, S., Komuro, I., Hiroi, Y., Zou, Y., Harada, K., Sugaya, T., et al. (1998) Mechanical stretch induces hypertrophic responses in cardiac myocytes of angiotensin II type 1a receptor knockout mice. *J. Biol. Chem.* **273,** 24,037–24,043.

78. Hayashida, W., Kihara, Y., Yasaka, A., Inagaki, K., Iwanaga, Y., and Sasayama, S. (2001) Stage-specific differential activation of mitogen-activated protein kinases in hypertrophied and failing rat hearts. *J. Mol. Cell Cardiol.* **33,** 733–744.

79. Lazou, A., Sugden, P. H., and Clerk, A. (1998) Activation of mitogen-activated protein kinases (p38-MAPKs, SAPKs/JNKs and ERKs) by the G-protein-coupled receptor agonist phenylephrine in the perfused rat heart. *Biochem. J.* **332,** 459–465.

80. Ng, D. C., Long, C. S., and Bogoyevitch, M. A. (2001) A role for the extracellular signal-regulated kinase and p38 mitogen-activated protein kinases in interleukin-1 beta-stimulated delayed signal tranducer and activator of transcription 3 activation, atrial natriuretic factor expression, and cardiac myocyte morphology. *J. Biol. Chem.* **276,** 29,490–29,498.

81. Clerk, A., Bogoyevitch, M. A., Anderson, M. B., and Sugden, P. H. (1994) Differential activation of protein kinase C isoforms by endothelin-1 and phenylephrine, and subsequent stimulation of p42 and p44 mitogen-activated protein kinases in ventricular myocytes cultured from neonatal rat hearts. *J. Biol. Chem.* **269,** 32,848–32,857.

82. Xiao, L., Pimental, D. R., Amin, J. K., Singh, K., Sawyer, D. B., and Colucci, W. S. (2001) MEK1/2-ERK1/2 mediates alpha1-adrenergic receptor-stimulated hypertrophy in adult rat ventricular myocytes. *J. Mol. Cell Cardiol.* **33,** 779–787.

83. Bueno, O. F., De Windt, L. J., Lim, H. W., Tymitz, K. M., Witt, S. A., Kimball, T. R., et al. (2001) The dual-specificity phosphatase MKP-1 limits the cardiac hypertrophic response in vitro and in vivo. *Circ. Res.* **88,** 88–96.

84. Barancik, M., Htun, P., Maeno, Y., Zimmermann, R., and Shaper, W. (1997) Differential regulation of distinct protein kinase cascades by ischemia and ischemia/reperfusion in porcine myocardium (asbtr.). *Circulation* **96,** I–252.

85. Behrends, M., Schulz, R., Post, H., Alexandrov, A., Belosjorow, S., Michel, M. C., et al. (2000) Inconsistent relation of MAPK activation to infarct size reduction by ischemic preconditioning in pigs. *Am. J. Physiol. Heart Circ. Physiol.* **279,** H1111–1119.

86. Araujo, E. G., Bianchi, C., Faro, R., and Sellke, F. W. (2001) Oscilation in the activities of MEK/ERK1/2 during cardiopulmonary bypass in pigs. *Surgery* **130,** 182–191.

87. Yoshida, K., Yoshiyama, M., Omura, T., Nakamura, Y., Kim, S., Takeuchi, K., et al. (2001) Activation of mitogen-activated protein kinases in the non-ischemic myocardium of an acute myocardial infarction in rats. *Jpn. Circ. J.* **65,** 808–814.

88. Knight, R. J. and Buxton, D. B. (1996) Stimulation of c-Jun kinase and mitogen-activated protein kinase by ischemia and reperfusion in the perfused rat hearts. *Biochem. Biophys. Res. Commun.* **218,** 83–88.

89. Takeishi, Y., Huang, Q., Wang, T., Glassman, M., Yoshizumi, M., Baines, C. P., et al. (2001) Src family kinase and adenosine differentially regulate multiple MAP kinases in ischemic myocardium: Modulation of MAP kinases activation by ischemic preconditioning. *J. Mol. Cell Cardiol.* **33,** 1989–2005.

90. Bogoyevitch, M. A., Gillespie-Brown, J., Ketterman, A. J., Fuller, S. J., Ben-Levy, R., Ashworth, A., et al. (1996) Stimulation of the stress-activated mitogen-activated protein

kinases subfamilies in perfused heart. p38/RK mitogen-activated protein kinases and c-jun N-terminal kinases are activated by ischemia/reperfusion. *Circ. Res.* **79,** 162–173.

91. Ping, P., Zhang, J., Cao, X., Kong, D., Tang, X. L., Qiu, Y., et al. (1999) PKC-dependent activation of p44/p42 MAPKs during myocardial ischemia-reperfusion in conscious rabbits. *Am. J. Physiol. Heart Circ. Physiol.* **276,** H1468–1481.

92. Fryer, R. M., Hsu, A. K., and Gross, G. J. (2001) ERK and p38 MAP kinase activation are components of opioid-induced delayed cardioprotection. *Basic Res. Cardiol.* **96,** 136–142.

93. Buerke, M., Murohara, T., Skurk, C., Nuss, C., Tomaselli, K., and Lefer, A. (1995) Cardioprotective effect of insulin-like growth factor I in myocardial ischemia followed by reperfusion. *Proc. Natl. Acad. Sci. USA* **92,** 8031–8035.

94. Parrizas, M., Saltiel, A. R., and LeRoith, D. (1997) Insulin-like growth factor 1 inhibits apoptosis using the phosphatidylinositol 3'-kinase and mitogen-activated protein kinase pathways. *J. Biol. Chem.* **272,** 154–161.

95. Vogt, A., Htun, P., Kluge, A., Zimmermann, R., and Schaper, W. (1997) Insulin like growth factor II delays myocardial infarction in experimental coronary artery occlusion. *Cardiovasc. Res.* **33,** 469–477.

96. Htun, P., Ito, W. D., Hoefer, I. E., Schaper, J., and Schaper, W. (1998) Intramyocardial infusion of FGF-1 mimics ischemic preconditioning in pig myocardium. *J. Mol. Cell Cardiol.* **30,** 867–877.

97. Padua, R. R., Sethi, R., Dhalla, N. S., and Kardami, E. (1995) Basic fibroblast growth factor is cardioprotective in ischemia-reperfusion injury. *Mol. Cell. Biochem.* **143,** 129–135.

98. Ghosh, S., Ng, L. L., Talwar, S., Squire, I. B., and Galinanes, M. (2000) Cardiotrophin-1 protects the human myocardium from ischemic injury: Comparison with the first and second window of protection by ischemic preconditioning. *Cardiovasc. Res.* **48,** 440–447.

99. Kuwahara, K., Saito, Y., Kishimoto, I., Miyamoto, Y., Harada, M., Ogawa, E., et al. (2000) Cardiotrophin-1 phosphorylates Akt and BAD, and prolongs cell survival via a PI3K-dependent pathway in cardiac myocytes. *J. Mol. Cell Cardiol.* **32,** 1385–1394.

100. Bogoyevitch, M. A., Glennon, P. E., Andersson, M. B., Clerk, A., Lazou, A., Marshall, C. J., et al. (1994) Endothelin-1 and fibroblast growth factors stimulate the mitogen-activated protein kinase signaling cascade in cardiac myocytes. The potential role of the cascade in the integration of two signaling pathways leading to myocyte hypertrophy. *J. Biol. Chem.* **269,** 1110–1119.

101. Stephanou, A., Brar, B., Heads, R., Knight, R. D., Marber, M. S., Pennica, D., et al. (1998) Cardiotrophin-1 induces heat shock protein accumulation in cultured cardiac cells and protects them from stressful stimuli. *J. Mol. Cardiol.* **30,** 849–855.

102. Sheng, Z., Knowlton, K., Chen, J., Hoshijima, M., Brown, J. H., and Chien, K. R. (1997) Cardiotrophin 1 (CT-1) inhibition of cardiac myocyte apoptosis via a mitogen-activated protein kinase-dependent pathway. Divergence from downstream CT-1 signals for myocardial cell hypertrophy. *J. Biol. Chem.* **272,** 5783–5791.

103. Weinbrenner, C., Liu, G. S., Cohen, M. V., and Downey, J. M. (1997) Phosphorylation of tyrosine 182 of p38 mitogen-activated protein kinase correlates with the protection of preconditioning in rabbit heart. *J. Mol. Cell Cardiol.* **29,** 2383–2391.

104. Nakano, A., Baines, C. P., Kim, C. O., Pelech, S. L., Downey, J. M., Cohen, M. V., et al. (2000) Ischemic preconditioning activates MAPKAPK2 in isolated rabbit heart. Evidence for involvement of p38 MAPK. *Circ. Res.* **86,** 144–151.

105. Armstrong, S. C., Delacey, M., and Ganote, C. E. (1999) Phosphorylation state of hsp27 and p38 MAPK during preconditioning and protein phosphatase inhibitor protection of rabbit cardiomyocytes. *J. Mol. Cell Cardiol.* **31,** 555–567.

106. Sato, M., Cordis, G. A., Maulik. N., and Das, D. K. (2000) SAPKs regulation of ischemic preconditioning. *Am. J. Physiol. Heart Circ. Physiol.* **279,** H901–907.

107. Yue, T. L., Wang, C., Gu, J. L., Ma, X. L., Kumar, S., Lee, J. C., et al. (2000) Inhibition of extracellular signal-regulated kinase enhances ischemia/reoxygenation-induced apoptosis in cultured cardiac myocytes and exaggerates reperfusion injury in isolated perfused heart. *Circ. Res.* **86,** 692–699.

108. Nakano, A., Cohen, M. V., Critz, S., and Downey, J. M. (2000) SB 203580, an inhibitor of p38 MAPK, abolishes infarct-limiting effect of ischemic preconditioning in isolated rabbit hearts. *Basic Res. Cardiol.* **95,** 466–471.

109. Mocanu, M. M., Baxter, G. F., Yue, Y., Critz, S. D., and Yellon, D. M. (2000) The p38 MAPK inhibitor, SB203580, abrogates ischaemic preconditioning in rat heart but timing of administration is critical. *Basic Res. Cardiol.* **95,** 472–478.

110. Murry, C. E., Jennings, R. B., and Reimer, K. A. (1986) Preconditioning with ischemia: a delay of lethal cell injury in ischemic myocardium. *Circulation* **74,** 1124–1136.

111. Cohen, M. V., Baines, Ch. P., and Downey, J. M. (2000) Ischemic Preconditioning: From adenosine receptor to K_{ATP} Channel. *Annu. Rev. Physiol.* **62,** 79–109.

112. Fryer, R. M., Pratt, P. F., Hsu, A. K., and Gross, G. J. (2001) Differential activation of extracellular signal regulated kinase isoforms in preconditioning and opioid-induced cardioprotection. *J. Pharmacol. Exp. Ther.* **296,** 642–649.

113. Maulik, N., Watanabe, M., Zu, Y. L., Huang, C. K., Cordis, G. A., Schley, J. A., et al. (1996) Ischemic preconditioning triggers the activation of MAP kinases and MAPKAP kinase 2 in rat heart. *FEBS Lett.* **396,** 233–237.

114. Martin, J. L., Avkiran, M., Quinlan, R. A., Cohen, P., and Marber, M. S. (2001) Antiischemic effects of SB203580 are mediated through the inhibition of p38alpha mitogen-activated protein kinase: evidence from ectopic expression of an inhibition-resistant kinase. *Circ. Res.* **89,** 750–752.

115. Saurin, A. T., Martin, J. L., Heads, R. J., Foley, C., Mockridge, J. W., Wright, M. J., et al. (2000) The role of differential activation of p38-mitogen-activated protein kinase in preconditioned ventricular myocytes. *FASEB J.* **14,** 2237–2246.

116. Fryer, R. M., Patel, H. H., Hsu, A. K., and Gross, G. J. (2001) Stress-activated protein kinase phosphorylation during cardioprotection in the ischemic myocardium. *Am. J. Physiol. Heart Circ. Physiol.* **281,** H1184–1192.

117. Barancik, M., Htun, P., and Schaper, W. (1999) Okadaic acid and anisomycin are protective and stimulate the SAPK/JNK pathway. *J. Cardiovasc. Pharmacol.* **34,** 182–190.

118. Mackay, K. and Mochly-Rosen, D. (1999) An inhibitor of p38 mitogen-activated protein kinase protects neonatal rat cardiac myocytes from ischemia. *J. Biol. Chem.* **274,** 6272–6279.

119. Yellon, D. M. and Baxter, G. F. (1995) "A second window of protection" or delayed preconditioning phenomenon: Future horizons for myocardial protection. *J. Mol. Cell Cardiol.* **27,** 1023–1034.

120. Zhao, T. C., Taher, M. M., Valerie, K. C., and Kukreja, R. C. (2001) p38 triggers late preconditioning elicited by anisomycin in heart: Involvement of NF-kappaB and iNOS. *Circ. Res.* **89,** 915–922.

121. Wilson, S., Wu, S., Kaszala, K., Ravingerova, T., Vegh, A., Papp, J., et al. (1996) Delayed cardioprotection is associated with the subcellular relocalisation of ventricular protein kinase Cε, but not p42/44MAPK. *Mol. Cell Biochem.* **161,** 225–230.

122. Alessi, D. R., Cuenda, A., Cohen, P., Dudley, D. T., and Saltiel, A. R. (1995) PD 098059 is a specific inhibitor of activation of mitogen-activated protein kinase kinase *in vitro* and *in vivo*. *J. Biol. Chem.* **270,** 27,489–27,494.

123. Favata, M. F., Horiuchi, K. Y., Manos, E. J., Daulerio, A. J., Stradley, D. A., Feeser, W. S., et al. (1998) Identification of a novel inhibitor of mitogen-activated protein kinase kinase. *J. Biol. Chem.* **273,** 18623–18632.

124. Kamakura, S., Moriguchi, T., and Nishida, E. (1999) Activation of the protein kinase ERK5/BMK1 by receptor tyrosine kinases. *J. Biol. Chem.* **274,** 26,563–26,571.

125. Tong, L., Pav, S., White, D., Rogers, S., Crane, K. M., Cywin, C. L., et al. (1997) A highly specific inhibitor of human p38 MAP kinase binds in the ATP pocket. *Nat. Struct. Biol.* **4,** 311–316.

126. Kumar, S., Jiang, M. S., Adams, J. L., and Lee, J. C. (1999) Pyridinylimidazole compound SB 203580 inhibits the activity but not the activation of p38 mitogen-activated protein kinase. *Biochem. Biophys. Res. Commun.* **263,** 825–831.

127. Sakamoto, K., Urushidani, T., and Nagao, T. (2000) Translocation of HSP27 to sarcomere induced by ischemic preconditioning in isolated rat hearts. *Biochem. Biophys. Res. Commun.* **269,** 137–142.

128. Ballard-Croft, C., White, D. J., Maass, D. L., Hybki, D. P., and Horton, J. W. (2001) Role of p38 mitogen-activated protein kinase in cardiac myocyte secretion of the inflammatory cytokine TNF-alpha. *Am. J. Physiol. Heart Circ. Physiol.* **280,** H1970–1981.

129. Brar, B. K., Jonassen, A. K., Stephanou, A., Santilli, G., Railson, J., Knight, R. A., et al. (2000) Urocortin protects against ischemia and reperfusion injury via a MAPK-dependent pathway. *J. Biol. Chem.* **275,** 8508–8514.

130. Xie, Z., Pimental, D. R., Lohan, S., Vasertriger, A., Pligavko, C., Colucci, W. S., et al. (2001) Regulation of angiotensin II-stimulated osteopontin expression in cardiac microvascular endothelial cells: Role of p42/44 mitogen-activated protein kinase and reactive oxygen species. *J. Cell Physiol.* **188,** 132–138.

131. van Eickels, M., Grohe, C., Lobbert, K., Stimpel, M., and Vetter, H. (1999) Angiotensin converting enzyme inhibitors block mitogenic signalling pathways in rat cardiac fibroblasts. *Naunyn Schmiedebergs Arch. Pharmacol.* **359,** 394–399.

132. Kim, S., Izumi, Y., Yano, M., Hamaguchi, A., Miura, K., Yamanaka, S., et al. (1998) Angiotensin blockade inhibits activation of mitogen-activated protein kinases in rat balloon-injured artery. *Circulation* **97,** 1731–1737.

133. Yue, T. L., Ma, X. L., Wang, X., Romanic, A. M., Liu, G. L., Louden, C., et al. (1998) Possible involvement of stress-activated protein kinase signaling pathway and Fas receptor expression in prevention of ischemia/reperfusion-induced cardiomyocyte apoptosis by carvedilol. *Circ. Res.* **82,** 166–174.

134. Chesley, A., Lundberg, M. S., Asai, T., Xiao, R. P., Ohtani, S., Lakatta, E. G., et al. (2000) The beta(2)-adrenergic receptor delivers an antiapoptotic signal to cardiac myocytes through G(i)-dependent coupling to phosphatidylinositol 3'-kinase. *Circ. Res.* **87,** 1172–1179.

135. Hanford, D. S. and Glembotski, C. C. (1996) Stabilization of the B-type natriuretic peptide mRNA in cardiac myocytes by alpha-adrenergic receptor activation: Potential roles for protein kinase C and mitogen-activated protein kinase. *Mol. Endocrinol.* **10,** 1719–1727.

136. Cano, E., Doza, Y. N., Ben-Levy, R., Cohen, P., and Mahadevan, L. C. (1996) Identification of anisomycin-activated kinases p45 and p55 in murine cells as MAPKAP kinase-2. *Oncogene* **12,** 805–812.

137. Baines, C. P., Wang, L., Cohen, M. V., and Downey, J. M. (1998) Protein tyrosine kinase is downstream of protein kinase C for ischemic preconditioning's anti-infarct effect in the rabbit heart. *J. Mol. Cell Cardiol.* **30,** 383–392.

5

Development of Anti-Inflammatory Drugs for Cardiovascular Disease

Melanie B. Smith and David J. Lefer

CONTENTS

1. INFLAMMATION IN CARDIOVASCULAR DISEASE

Cardiovascular disease is the leading cause of death in the United States. One in three men and one in ten women develop severe cardiovascular disease before the age of 60, resulting in health expenditures of over $100 billion per year. Even though cardiovascular disease primarily affects people advanced in age, disease progression

From: *Cardiac Drug Development Guide*
Edited by: M. K. Pugsley © Humana Press Inc., Totowa, NJ

begins early. Initiation of atherogenesis via formation of fatty streaks can occur as early as infancy *(1)*.

With increased circulating low-density lipoproteins levels later in life, the inflammatory response induced by the first fatty streak progresses. Formation of atherosclerotic lesions is directed by inflammation. Once atheroscerotic plaques have been formed, the inflammatory response is heightened, and plaque stabilization is compromised. Plaque rupture promotes thrombosis, thereby increasing the likelihood of a coronary event, such as myocardial ischemia. Myocardial ischemia, and subsequently reperfusion, stimulates an even greater inflammatory response directing myocardial infarction. Often ischemic attacks are transient, with reperfusion following closely behind ischemia, but stimulation of full reperfusion may require percutaneous transluminal coronary angioplasty (PTCA). Angioplasty promotes reperfusion in exchange for endothelial damage and further heightening of the inflammatory response. Inflammation after these events frequently leads to restenosis.

Several events occur during the inflammatory process. Pro-inflammatory cytokines are released with the initial presence of fatty lesions. These molecules promote endothelial dysfunction, thereby decreasing endothelial nitric oxide (NO) production while increasing endothelial cell adhesion molecule and growth factor expression. Endothelial cell adhesion molecules mediate platelet and leukocyte aggregation at the site of inflammation, whereas growth factors stimulate vascular smooth muscle cell growth and proliferation. Thrombus formation and neointimal thickening direct pathology of these diseases. In addition, release of oxygen-derived free radicals by transmigrated neutrophils promotes further cellular damage enhancing endothelial dysfunction.

Several anti-inflammatory drug therapies to mitigate the pathology of cardiovascular diseases have been explored. Drug interventions may stimulate a reduction in release of detrimental cytokines and growth factors, inhibition of extracellular adhesion molecule expression, neutralization of reactive oxygen species, or inhibition of transcriptional activation of inflammatory mediators. The most useful drug therapies, however, may be those that target multiple cardiovascular disease factors.

2. ROLE OF INFLAMMATION IN ATHEROGENESIS

Inflammation occurs early in the progression of atherogenesis. Often, the first display of atherogenesis, the fatty streak, appears as early as childhood *(1)*. The fatty streak is characterized by the presence of inflammatory mediators, such as macrophages and T-lymphocytes *(2)*, which continue to direct inflammatory responses throughout atherosclerotic plaque development *(3,4)*.

Before plaque formation, endothelial dysfunction is evident *(5,6)*. Endothelial dysfunction results from a large host of factors, including dyslipidemia *(7,8)*, hypertension *(9,10)*, and elevated circulating homocysteine levels *(11–15)* in addition to other factors. The loss of endothelial function is characterized by a decrease in the release of endothelial-derived NO *(10,13,16)*, an increase in endothelial adhesiveness and permeability to leukocytes and platelets, and the release of cytokines and growth factors. It is this endothelial dysfunction that promotes plaque formation *(17,18)*.

3. CYTOKINES IN HYPERLIPIDEMIA AND ATHEROSCLEROSIS

Cytokines are released by a variety of cells in response to inflammatory stimuli. Cytokines important in the disease progression of atherosclerosis include interleukin-

1α (IL-1α) *(19,20)*, tumor necrosis factor-α (TNF-α; ref. *21*), and interferon γ (IFN-γ; ref. *22*). IL-1α is released from endothelial cells, smooth muscle cells, and monocytes and macrophages and plays a major role in cell proliferation *(19,20)*. It has been shown to promote smooth muscle cell proliferation in vitro *(23)* in addition to increasing the adhesiveness of leukocytes to endothelial cells by upregulating endothelial cell adhesion molecule expression *(23–26)*. In addition, IL-1 promotes the release of IL-6 *(27)*, IL-8 *(28)*, basic fibroblast growth factor *(29)*, platelet-derived growth factor *(20)*, and TNF-α *(30)*, thereby furthering the inflammatory response.

TNF-α is released by smooth muscle cells, monocytes and macrophages, and T-lymphocytes. TNF-α is responsible for cell proliferation *(21)* through the secre-tion of platelet-derived growth factor. TNF-α also plays an important role in the induction of cellular adhesion molecules. In addition, Galis et al. *(31)* have shown the importance of IL-1β and TNF-α in plaque stabilization. IL-1β and TNF-α both induce smooth muscle cells to synthesize and secrete collagenase into the interstitium. The resulting matrix degradation at inflammatory sites could promote plaque rupture.

IFN-γ contributes to smooth muscle cell proliferation at low levels *(32)*, but when present in excess as in inflammation, it inhibits hyperplasia *(33)*. IFN-γ also upregulates endothelial adhesion molecule expression, increasing the inflammatory response.

4. ROLE OF CELLULAR ADHESION MOLECULES IN ATHEROSCLEROSIS

During inflammation, cell adhesion molecule expression is enhanced on endothelial cells as well as on leukocytes and platelets. The expression of cell adhesion molecules and glycoprotein adhesion molecules in atherosclerosis will be considered.

Glycoprotein adhesion molecules (selectins) on the endothelium are significant in the process of leukocyte rolling along the inflamed endothelium *(34)*. E-selectin expression on activated endothelial cells is enhanced during inflammation via the presence of TNF-α *(32)*. P-selectin expression is induced in the presence of thrombin *(35)*, whereas, L-selectin expression is constitutive.

Cell adhesion molecules are necessary for leukocyte adhesion as well as extravasation. Endothelial cell adhesion molecules significant in atherosclerosis include intercellular adhesion molecule-1 (ICAM-1), vascular cellular adhesion molecule-1 (VCAM-1), athero-endothelial leukocyte adhesion molecule (athero-ELAM), and platelet endothelial cellular adhesion molecule (PECAM-1). ICAM-1 and PECAM-1 expression is constitutive on endothelial cells *(36)*, whereas VCAM-1 and arthero-ELAM are not constitutively expressed *(37–39)*. During inflammation, IL-1β and TNF-α induce production of arthero-ELAM and VCAM-1 *(38,39)*.

Adhesion molecules that bind endothelial adhesion molecules are present on leukocytes. These include three heterodimers of the CD11/CD18 integrin subfamily. Like ECAM expression, CD11b/CD18 and CD11c/CD18 expression on leukocytes are increased in the presence of TNF-α *(40,41)*. Leukocyte adhesion proteins are also induced by platelet-derived growth factor *(42)*.

5. ROLE OF MONOCYTES IN ATHEROSCLEROSIS

Monocytes adhere to inflamed endothelium in response to increased expression of cell adhesion molecules. Once a monocyte has migrated to the intima, it is converted to a macrophage. Macrophages release a number of cytokines, growth factors, and metalloproteinases *(43–45)*, which contribute to the pathogenesis of atherosclerosis.

Macrophages release IL-1β and TNF-α. These cytokines act on other macrophages and endothelial cells to promote the production and secretion of growth factors. In response to increased cytokine levels, endothelial cells release platelet-derived growth factor (PDGF) *(46)*. PDGF is directly responsible for the proliferation of smooth muscle cells characteristic of atherogenesis.

Growth factors released by macrophages include vascular endothelial growth factor, basic fibroblast growth factor, and transforming growth factors. These growth factors play a vital role in plaque growth and stability. Conversely, macrophage release of metalloproteinases results in extracellular matrix protein degradation, thereby contributing to plaque destabilization.

In addition to release of pro-inflammatory cytokines, growth factors, and metalloproteinases, macrophages also release reactive oxygen species that also contribute to cellular damage. Toxic oxygen radicals modify low-density lipoproteins that can then stimulate endothelial cells to release monocyte chemotactic protein *(47)*. Furthermore, these lipids can be ingested by monocyte-derived macrophages, resulting in foam cell formation.

Foam cells are lipid-laden macrophages. They are important in plaque core growth and plaque destabilization. Inflammatory mediators promote apoptosis of foam cells. As inflammatory mediators stimulate apoptosis, foam cells pour their lipid contents into the soft plaque core, enlarging it *(48,49)*. If apoptosis occurs in several foam cells simultaneously, the plaque core may grow enough to damage the fibrous cap, resulting in plaque rupture.

6. INFLAMMATION AND PLAQUE STABILITY

Dysfunctional endothelium characteristic of atherosclerotic plaques chronically promotes the recruitment of inflammatory mediators. Activated leukocytes and endothelial cells release pro-inflammatory cytokines (IL-1β, TNF-α and IFN-γ). These cytokines result in smooth muscle cell proliferation, and these smooth muscle cells increase the formation of plaque extracellular matrix proteins *(50)*.

Although the enhancement of cytokine release stimulates smooth muscle proliferation *(21,23)*, thereby resulting in plaque stability, cytokine release can also direct plaque instability. IFN-γ actually inhibits cellular proliferation at high concentrations, consequently promoting plaque destabilization *(34)*. IL-1β and TNF-α have also been shown to release matrix metalloproteinases that degrade extracellular matrix proteins produced by proliferating smooth muscle cells. Matrix metalloproteinases important in plaque destabilization include collagenase (MMP1), stromelysin (MMP3), and gelatinases (MMP2 and MMP9; refs. *51,52*).

In addition to inflammatory cytokine release affecting plaque stability, inflammatory mediators stimulate apoptosis of foam cells and smooth muscle cells *(48)*. When foam cells undergo apoptosis, they release lipids thereby enlarging the lipid core. In addition, apoptosis of smooth muscle cells decreases the production of extracellular matrix proteins. When challenged with increased degradation of matrix proteins by metalloproteinases and decreased protein production by smooth muscle cells, further loss of plaque stability occurs.

7. DRUGS IN DEVELOPMENT TO PREVENT THE INFLAMMATORY RESPONSES IN ATHEROGENESIS

Therapeutic intervention has attempted to target several steps of atherosclerotic inflammation. Therapies include cytokine inhibitors, blockade of PDGF, cholesterol acyltransferase (ACAT) inhibition, antioxidants, anti-inflammatory agents, and lipid-lowering drugs.

Cytokine inhibitors include anti-TNF-α antibodies that have been shown in some models to decrease leukocyte aggregation *(53)*. Other drugs that inhibit TNF-α activity include pentoxifylline *(54)*, theophylline, and 3-isobutyl-L-methylxanthine *(55)* by targeting TNF-α production. Furthermore, suppression of IL-1β production occurs in human monocytes with dexamethasone treatment *(56)*. In addition to cytokine blockade, the inhibition of molecules they stimulate is another possible route of therapy. Inhibition of cytokine-stimulated PDGF prevents accumulation of smooth muscle cells in atherosclerotic lesions and, therefore, plaque growth *(57)*.

Additional modes of therapy include inhibition of leukocyte adhesion to the endothelium and inhibition of ACAT. Antibodies against CD43 inhibit leukocyte adhesion to activated endothelial cells, whereas inhibition of ACAT decreases lipid absorption in the gastrointestinal tract. This decrease in lipid uptake results in reduction of fatty streak formation *(58)* or plaque stabilization via decreased foam cell formation.

Plaque stabilization has also been accomplished with antioxidants, antiplatelet and anti-inflammatory agents, as well as lipid-lowering drugs. Antioxidants, such as probucol and vitamin E, inhibit the oxidation of low-density lipoproteins *(59,60)*, thereby inhibiting disease progression. Anti-inflammatory drugs, such as aspirin, are beneficial in reducing atherosclerotic inflammation by reducing IL-1 levels and macrophage colony stimulating factor expression *(61)*. Aspirin also has antithrombotic effects.

Lipid-lowering drugs include bile acid-binding resins, nicotinic acid, fibric acid derivatives, probucol, and HMG CoA reductase inhibitors (statins). Statins are currently the drug of choice for elevated serum cholesterol because of their additional antioxidant, antiproliferative, anti-inflammatory, antiplatelet effects, and ability to prolong the half-life of endothelial NO synthase (NOS; refs. *62–66*).

8. INFLAMMATION IN ACUTE MYOCARDIAL ISCHEMIA

Inflammation after acute episodes of myocardial ischemia mediates myocardial necrosis. Inflammatory chemoattractants stimulate the aggregation of neutrophils to the ischemic area. Neutrophils then infiltrate the myocardium and release pro-inflammatory cytokines, proteinases, and reactive oxygen species, thereby furthering myocardial damage. In addition, the presence of free radicals activates nuclear factor κB (NFκB), which is responsible for transcription of several pro-inflammatory mediators. The resulting increase in the inflammatory response increases cellular damage, eventually resulting in necrosis.

9. CYTOKINES IN MYOCARDIAL ISCHEMIA–REPERFUSION

IL-1β, IL-6, and TNF-α are pro-inflammatory cytokines that contribute to the pathogenesis of myocardial ischemia and reperfusion. Released by adherent monocytes and neutrophils, cytokines exacerbate ischemia–reperfusion injury in the myocardium *(67,68)*. IL-1β, IL-6, and TNF-α also induce the myocardium to synthesize ICAM-1. Additional ICAM-1 is expressed on the surface of the endothelium and promotes leukocyte adherence *(69,70)*. IL-1β and TNF-α cause adhered leukocytes as well as endothelial cells to increase oxidant formation, further damaging the already impaired myocardium *(71)*. Furthermore, TNF-α decreases the release of NO from the endothelium *(72,73)*, which results in reduced vasodilatory ability and decreased myocardial contractility *(74)*.

10. EXTRACELLULAR ADHESION MOLECULES IN MYOCARDIAL ISCHEMIA–REPERFUSION (MI/R)

Like atherosclerosis, inflammation after MI/R results in increased expression of extracellular adhesion molecules on leukocytes and endothelial cells. To demonstrate the importance of PECAM-1 in MI/R, Gumina et al. *(75)* determined the effects of a PECAM-1 antibody. The reduction in MI/R injury they found suggests this constitutively expressed adhesion molecule acts significantly in MI/R injury. Jones et al. *(76)* demonstrated that endothelial expression of ICAM-1, E-selectin, and P-selectin levels increase subsequent to MI/R. The cellular expression of these adhesion molecules peaks at 24 h postischemia in the murine model, and deficiency of P-selectin, E-selectin, or ICAM-1 exerts cardioprotection.

In addition to the increase in endothelial cell adhesion molecules, leukocyte expression of CD-18 was prominent as well *(76)*. Mice deficient in CD-18 showed attenuation of myocardial necrosis after MI/R *(76)*. Also, GPIIb/IIIa, an integrin adhesion molecule on activated platelets, moves to the cell surface during inflammation, thereby increasing platelet aggregation.

11. LEUKOCYTES AND PLATELETS IN MI/R

Subsequent to MI/R, neutrophils are sequestered in the myocardium. Because of the induction of extracellular adhesion molecules on neutrophils and endothelial cells, neutrophil adherence to the endothelium is exacerbated. Cohered neutrophils stimulate endothelial activation through the production of cytokines, reactive oxygen species, and proteinases *(77–79)*. Reactive oxygen species can modify lipids, promoting lack of membrane integrity, whereas proteinases degrade cellular proteins.

Another role of neutrophils in the ischemic-reperfused myocardium is the stimulation of phospholipase A_2 thereby resulting in synthesis of leukotriene B_4 and platelet-activating factor (PAF; refs. *80,81*). These substances further increase neutrophil adhesion to the endothelium. In addition, PAF indirectly decreases coronary blood flow by promoting platelet aggregation *(82)*.

12. NFκB AND MI/R

In response to inflammatory stimuli, activation of the endothelium is dependent upon the transcription factor NFκB. NFκB plays a principle role in the gene expression of coagulation mediators, adhesion molecules, cytokines, and chemokines all of which are important in MI/R injury *(83)*.

After MI/R, there is increased free radical production and decreased myocardial antioxidant activity *(84,85)*. The resulting increase in the presence of free radicals in the myocardium stimulates the activation of NFκB *(86)*. Activation of NFκB promotes an increase in pro-inflammatory cytokines IL-1β, IL-6, and TNF-α *(86)*.

NFκB also regulates gene expression of the adhesion molecules E-selectin, VCAM-1, and ICAM-1. These, in addition to the chemokine IL-8, are responsible for neutrophil rolling, adhesion, and eventually transmigration into the already inflamed endothelium *(87)*. Once in the interstitium, neutrophils increase production of free radicals, further upregulating NFκB activation.

Finally, NFκB increases the expression of procoagulant factors, including plasminogen activator, tissue factor, PAF receptor, and P-selectin, making the vascular endothelium more prone to thrombus formation *(83)*.

13. OXIDANTS AND MI/R

The reduction of oxygen results in the formation of superoxide anions, hydroxide radicals, and hydrogen peroxides *(88,89)*. Antioxidants are normally present in the myocardium to prevent injury from constitutive free radical formation. Superoxide dismutase catalyzes the conversion of oxygen radicals to molecular oxygen and hydrogen peroxide *(84)*. Hydrogen peroxide is then reduced to water by either catalase or glutathione peroxidase *(84,85)*. After MI/R, antioxidant activity is decreased *(90,91)*, thereby rendering the remaining antioxidants unable to prevent myocardial damage resulting from increased free radical formation *(84,85)*. In the absence of the normal antioxidant levels, free radicals peroxidize lipids. These peroxidized lipids then are unable to maintain the integrity of the cellular membrane or the environment surrounding membrane proteins resulting in cellular damage *(92)*. Free radicals may also be responsible for the activation of transcription factor NFκB, which is thought to further propagate inflammatory responses subsequent to MI/R.

14. DRUGS TO ATTENUATE INFLAMMATION IN MI/R

Atherosclerotic drug therapies can decrease the risk of coronary heart disease, but MI/R drug therapies must focus on the reduction of injury after an ischemic attack. Neutrophil and platelet adhesion to the endothelium, oxidant production, and NFκB activation have all been targeted to attenuate MI/R injury.

Antibodies to extracellular adhesion molecules on endothelial cells, neutrophils, and platelets show promising results in reducing MI/R injury. Antibodies to PECAM-1 block neutrophil and monocyte migration in vitro and, more recently, PECAM-1 antibodies have been shown to decrease myocardial infarct size in rats *(75)*. Blockade of either ICAM-1 *(76,94,95)* or CD18 *(76,96,97)* also results in attenuated myocardial injury after MI/R.

Selectin inhibitors comprise a large group of therapies available to attenuate MI/R injury. Antibodies and other inhibitory molecules against E-selectin, P-selectin, and L-selectin have been shown to protect the ischemic-reperfused myocardium. E-selectin–specific inhibitors include CL-2 antibody and CY-1787 antibody, whereas inhibitors of E-selectin and P-selectin include sialyl-Lewis^x oligosaccharide (CY-1503) and a small molecule, TBC-1269. Inhibition of L-selectin has only been shown with the monoclonal antibody DREG-200. A complete review of cardioprotection by selectins is available *(98)*.

Agents have also been developed to protect the myocardium from the numerous roles neutrophils play in myocardial damage. Antineutrophil agents mitigate the deleterious effects of neutrophils, thereby attenuating injury after MI/R. This has been shown using cobra venom factor, prostaglandins, nonsteroidal anti-inflammatory drugs, lipoxygenase inhibitors, and PR-39, an antimicrobial peptide that also inhibits neutrophils *(99)*.

Activation of NFκB) results in transcription of a myriad of inflammatory mediators. Drug therapies that inhibit NFκB activation, and hence production of downstream inflammatory mediators, decrease inflammation after MI/R, preserving the myocardium. IRFI 042, an antioxidant, inhibits NFκB activation, thereby reducing MI/R-directed inflammation, whereas transfection of oligodeoxynucleotides specific for NFκB into endothelial and cardiomyocyte nuclei was also cardioprotective *(100,101)*.

Several antioxidants have been proposed to protect the myocardium from MI/R injury. CI-959, an inhibitor of free radical formation, reduces MI/R-directed damage *(102)*. Superoxide dismutase (SOD), glutathione peroxidase, and catalase administration have all been considered as therapeutic agents for the treatment of acute myocardial infarction; however, the findings are somewhat controversial. Gallagher et al. *(103)* showed no attenuation in myocardial infarct size in canines following administration of SOD or catalase. Jolly et al. *(104)* demonstrated that combined therapy of SOD and catalase reduced canine infarct size. Werns et al. *(105)* demonstrated that only SOD, and not catalase, administration resulted in cardioprotection against MI/R injury. Murine studies indicate a role for manganese SOD and glutathione peroxidase, but not copper–zinc SOD in reduction of MI/R injury *(105a)*.

Additional studies evaluating the effects of SOD and catalase have been reviewed *(106)*. Similarly, xanthine oxidase inhibitors, such as allopurinol, also show opposing results in attenuating MI/R injury *(107–109)*.

Nonspecific drug intervention to protect the myocardium is also available. Therapies, such as perfluorochemicals and adenosine, mediate cardiomyocyte protection at several levels. Perfluorochemical blood substitutes reduce neutrophil accumulation and adhesion to the endothelium as well as superoxide production *(110,111)*. Adenosine administration after MI/R targets several phases of the inflammatory response, thereby protecting the myocardium. It mediates coronary vasodilation *(112)*, reduces endothelial–neutrophil interactions *(113)*, and inhibits platelet aggregation and thromboxane release *(114)*.

15. INFLAMMATION AND RESTENOSIS

Restenosis is a common inflammatory response following one-third to one-half of all PTCA procedures *(115)*. Restenosis is characterized as an increased inflammatory response in a vessel that has already exhibited inflammation, such as those vessels containing atherosclerotic plaques *(116)*. Restenosis results in increased smooth muscle cell proliferation that is initiated approx 1 wk after angioplasty *(116,117)*. In addition to cellular proliferation and intimal thickening, vessels are prone to thrombosis because of the accumulation of platelets at the inflammatory site *(118)*.

16. CYTOKINES AND OTHER INFLAMMATORY MEDIATORS IN RESTENOSIS

Like in other inflammatory diseases, pro-inflammatory cytokines and growth factors are thought to mediate restenosis. Cytokines, such as IL-1α and IL-1β, and TNF-α are released from the endothelium during the inflammatory process. These cytokines act on the same endothelial cells to promote pro-inflammatory and prothrombotic responses *(119,120)*. Activated endothelial cells release PAF *(119,120)*, resulting in increased adherence of platelets to the vascular wall. The presence of IL-1β and TNF-α also increases the presence of von Willebrand factor in the presence of thrombin *(121)*.

Cytokines also play a role in leukocyte adhesion the vascular endothelium. The local concentration of IL-1β and TNF-α control leukocyte recruitment and adhesion *(122)*, and this aggregation contributes to vascular stenosis. In addition to cytokine levels increasing during restenosis, growth factors also promote neointimal formation. The accumulation of platelets at the inflamed endothelium results in increased release of PDGF *(123)*, which induces restenotic smooth muscle proliferation.

17. LEUKOCYTES IN RESTENOSIS

After PTCA, the endothelium is denuded promoting endothelial dysfunction. Endothelial dysfunction initiates an inflammatory response. Chemokines are released from the endothelium, resulting in chemotaxis of neutrophils, which further enhance inflammation through release of cytokines and reactive oxygen species and stimulation of leukotriene B_4 and PAF production *(80,81)*.

Cytokines, such as TNF-α and IL-1β, activate thrombus formation during restenosis via action on the endothelium *(119,120)*. Thrombus formation is also enhanced by neutrophilic activation of PAF. PAF recruits platelets to the inflammatory site, which promote progression of restenosis by releasing platelet-derived growth factor *(123)*. Together, leukotriene B_4 and PAF increase adhesion of neutrophils to the endothelium exacerbating inflammation.

In addition, release of free radicals from neutrophils stimulates oxidation of cellular lipids. The presence of these oxidized lipids in the endothelial cell membrane compromises cellular integrity, thereby enhancing endothelial dysfunction.

18. PLATELETS IN RESTENOSIS

Platelet endothelial cell interactions occur almost immediately after arterial injury and often result in thrombus formation *(118)*. In the presence of inflammatory stimuli, integrin adhesion molecule GPIIb/IIIa is activated, resulting in increased expression on the cellular membrane. Activation of this molecule increases platelet adhesion and consequently thrombus. Concurrent with tissue injury resulting from angioplasty is the exposure of cellular matrix proteins, including collagen and fibrin, and loss of the normal antithrombotic nature of the endothelium. Fibrin, platelets, and erythrocytes are the only substrates necessary in thrombus formation during this inflammatory state. In addition to thrombus formation, the adhesion of platelets to the vessel wall promotes the release of PDGF, epidermal growth factor, and transforming growth factor beta *(123)*. The release of PDGF from platelets as well as the surrounding endothelium propagates proliferation of smooth muscle cells. Once smooth muscle cells undergo proliferation, release of PDGF from platelets is no longer necessary to stimulate hyperplasia because smooth muscle cells are now capable of secreting an isoform of PDGF *(124)*. It is this smooth muscle proliferation that is thought to be directly responsible for intimal thickening characteristic of restenosis.

19. DRUGS TO REDUCE INFLAMMATION IN RESTENOSIS

Therapies currently used to protect individuals from restenosis mainly target thrombus formation by decreasing platelet adhesion to the endothelium as well as to other platelets. As in atherosclerosis, cytokine inhibitors may attenuate the inflammatory response that occurs in restenosis. Antibodies against TNF-α and IL-1β exhibit a reduction in thrombus formation by inhibiting the loss of endothelial antithrombotic properties. Inhibitors of platelet integrin adhesion molecule GPIIb/IIIa, such as abciximab (i.e., Reopro®), have demonstrated profound inhibition on platelet aggregation, resulting in decreased thrombus formation and eventually reduction in death. This reduction, however, shows no benefits greater than the use of aspirin *(125)*. Other antiplatelet drugs include the thrombin inhibitor hirudin, a PDGF receptor antagonist, and a direct platelet P2T receptor antagonist *(126–128)*. In addition to antiplatelet therapies, delivery of c-*myc* antisense oligomers during catheterization reduces neointimal growth thereby preventing restenosis *(129)*.

20. NO AND INFLAMMATION IN CARDIOVASCULAR DISEASE

NO, formally known as endothelial-derived relaxing factor *(130,131)*, is synthesized via NOS action on L-arginine *(131)*. NOS is present in three forms: endothelial NOS (eNOS or NOS 3), neuronal NOS, and inducible NOS. The first two of these are expressed constitutively, whereas the latter is induced during pathological states.

Hypercholesterolemia promotes endothelial dysfunction in the absence of atherosclerotic lesions *(132,133)*. Endothelial dysfunction results in a decrease in NO bioavailability either by decreasing eNOS activity or by reducing L-arginine availability. In addition to attenuated levels of NO release, endothelial dysfunction can also direct formation of atherosclerotic lesions.

Atherogenesis occurs when damaged endothelium stimulates inflammation. This is characterized by release of pro-inflammatory cytokines, growth factors, and reactive oxygen species. The presence of cytokines and growth factors promote inducible NOS expression whereas free radicals inactivate NO *(134)*. NO normally helps maintain hemostasis, but in the inflamed vessel, vasoconstriction occurs *(135)*. NO also protects from leukocyte adhesion and, indirectly, platelet aggregation during physiologic conditions *(136,137)*. In addition, NO inhibits smooth muscle cell proliferation via increased cyclic–guanosine monophosphate production *(138)* as well as decrease oxidation of low-density lipoproteins protecting the artery from lipid accumulation *(139)*. Attenuation of NO production increases likelihood of atherosclerotic plaque formation and rupture and, consequently, an acute attack of MI.

Subsequent to MI, there is increased free radical production by neutrophils and endothelial cells. Enhancement of circulating free radicals neutralizes eNOS production of NO *(140)*. Lefer et al. *(141)* demonstrated the importance of eNOS in leuko-cyte–endothelial interactions via the use of gene-targeted animals. Mice deficient in eNOS showed enhanced P-selectin expression and elevated leukocyte rolling and adhesion at baseline conditions. In addition, eNOS-deficient animals exhibited increased MI/R injury. Results of these studies clearly demonstrate the importance of eNOS-derived NO in vascular homeostasis. After acute MI, catheterization and PTCA is often necessary to achieve full reperfusion. Unfortunately, angioplasty often results in damage to vascular endothelium so severe that the inflammatory response is reinitiated directing restenosis. As in atherosclerosis, decline in NO availability pre-cipitates restenosis. In addition to NO stimulating vasoconstriction because of endot-helial damage, the lack of adequate amounts of NO result in vascular obstruction. Finally, NO has antiplatelet and antiproliferative effects *(138,142)* that are diminished following PTCA.

21. SUMMARY

Various levels of the inflammatory response have been targeted in attempt to rectify cardiovascular pathology. Drug interventions examined include inhibitors of inflam-matory mediator production through inhibition of NFκB, cytokine inhibitors, extracel-lular adhesion molecule inhibitors, antiplatelet and antineutrophil preparations, antioxidants, and lipid-lowering agents. The common goal, however, is preservation or reestablishment of functional endothelium. Under normal conditions, endothelial cells exert anti-inflammatory effects that are in part mediated through NO release. Physi-ologic levels of NO attenuate leukocyte-endothelial adhesion and platelet aggregation in addition to prevention of vascular smooth muscle proliferation.

REFERENCES

1. Napoli, C., D'Armiento, F. P., Mancini, F. P., Postiglione, A., Witztum, J. L., Palumbo, G., et al. (1997) Fatty streak formation occurs in human fetal aortas and is greatly enhanced by maternal hypercholesterolemia. Intimal accumulation of low density lipo-protein and its oxidation precede monocyte recruitment into early atherosclerotic lesions. *J. Clin Invest.* **100**, 2680–2690.
2. Stary, H. C., Chandler, A. B., Glagov, S., Guyton, J. R., Insull, W., Jr., Rosenfeld, M. E., et al. (1994) A definition of initial, fatty streak, and intermediate lesions of atherosclero-sis. A report from the Committee on Vascular Lesions of the Council on Arteriosclerosis, American Heart Association. *Circulation* **89**, 2462–2478.
3. Jonasson, L., Holm, J., Skalli, O., Bondjers, G., and Hansson, G. K. (1986) Regional accumulations of T cells, macrophages, and smooth muscle cells in the human athero-sclerotic plaque. *Arteriosclerosis* **6**, 131–138.
4. van der Wal, A. C., Das, P. K., Bentz, V. B., van der Loos, C. M., and Becker, A. E. (1989) Atherosclerotic lesions in humans. In situ immunophenotypic analysis suggesting an immune mediated response. *Lab. Invest.* **61**, 166–170.
5. McLenachan, J. M., Williams, J. K., Fish, R. D., Ganz, P., and Selwyn, A. P. (1991) Loss of flow-mediated endothelium-dependent dilation occurs early in the development of ath-erosclerosis. *Circulation* **84**, 1273–1278.
6. Kinlay, S. and Ganz, P. (1997) Role of endothelial dysfunction in coronary artery disease and implications for therapy. *Am. J. Cardiol.* **80**, 11I–16I.
7. Morel, D. W., Hessler, J. R., and Chisolm, G. M. (1983) Low density lipoprotein cytotox-icity induced by free radical peroxidation of lipid. *J. Lipid Res.* **24**, 1070–1076.

8. Griendling, K. K. and Alexander, R. W. (1997) Oxidative stress and cardiovascular disease. *Circulation* **96,** 3264–3265.

9. Swei, A., Lacy, F., DeLano, F. A., and Schmid-Schonbein, G. W. (1997) Oxidative stress in the Dahl hypertensive rat. *Hypertension* **30,** 1628–1633.

10. Vanhoutte, P. M. and Boulanger, C. M. (1995) Endothelium-dependent responses in hypertension. *Hypertens. Res.* **18,** 87–98.

11. Hajjar,K. A. (1993) Homocysteine-induced modulation of tissue plasminogen activator binding to its endothelial cell membrane receptor. *J. Clin Invest.* **91,** 2873–2879.

12. Harker, L. A., Ross, R., Slichter, S. J., and Scott, C. R. (1976) Homocystine-induced arteriosclerosis. The role of endothelial cell injury and platelet response in its genesis. *J. Clin Invest.* **58,** 731–741.

13. Upchurch, G. R., Jr., Welch, G. N., Fabian, A. J., Freedman, J. E., Johnson, J. L., Keaney, J. F., Jr., et al. (1997) Homocysteine decreases bioavailable nitric oxide by a mechanism involving glutathione peroxidase. *J. Biol. Chem.* **272,** 17012–17017.

14. Majors, A., Ehrhart, L. A., and Pezacka, E. H. (1997) Homocysteine as a risk factor for vascular disease. Enhanced collagen production and accumulation by smooth muscle cells. *Arterioscler. Thromb. Vasc. Biol.* **17,** 2074–2081.

15. Bellamy, M. F., McDowell, I. F., Ramsey, M. W., Brownlee, M., Bones, C., Newcombe, R. G., et al. (1998) Hyperhomocysteinemia after an oral methionine load acutely impairs endothelial function in healthy adults. *Circulation* **98,** 1848–1852.

16. Quyyumi, A. A., Dakak, N., Andrews, N. P., Husain, S., Arora, S., Gilligan, D. M., et al. (1995) Nitric oxide activity in the human coronary Circulation. Impact of risk factors for coronary atherosclerosis. *J. Clin Invest.* **95,** 1747–1755.

17. Gimbrone, M. A., Jr., Topper, J. N., Nagel, T., Anderson, K. R., and Garcia-Cardena, G. (2000) Endothelial dysfunction, hemodynamic forces, and atherogenesis. *Ann. N. Y. Acad. Sci.* **902,** 230–239.

18. Topper, J. N. and Gimbrone, M. A., Jr. (1999) Blood flow and vascular gene expression: Fluid shear stress as a modulator of endothelial phenotype. *Mol. Med. Today* **5,** 40–46.

19. Libby, P., Friedman, G. B., and Salomon, R. N. (1989) Cytokines as modulators of cell proliferation in fibrotic diseases. *Am. Rev. Respir. Dis.* **140,** 1114–1117.

20. Raines, E. W., Dower, S. K., and Ross, R. (1989) Interleukin-1 mitogenic activity for fibroblasts and smooth muscle cells is due to PDGF-AA. *Science* **243,** 393–396.

21. Old, L. J. (1985) Tumor necrosis factor (TNF). *Science* **230,** 630–632.

22. Amento, E. P., Ehsani, N., Palmer, H., and Libby, P. (1991) Cytokines and growth factors positively and negatively regulate interstitial collagen gene expression in human vascular smooth muscle cells. *Arterioscler. Thromb.* **11,** 1223–1230.

23. Libby,P, Warner, S. J., and Friedman, G. B. (1988) Interleukin 1: A mitogen for human vascular smooth muscle cells that induces the release of growth-inhibitory prostanoids. *J. Clin. Invest.* **81,** 487–498.

24. Cybulsky, M. I. and Gimbrone, M. A., Jr. (1991) Endothelial expression of a mononuclear leukocyte adhesion molecule during atherogenesis. *Science* **251,** 788–791.

25. Bevilacqua, M. P., Stengelin, S., Gimbrone, M. A., Jr., and Seed, B. (1989) Endothelial leukocyte adhesion molecule 1: An inducible receptor for neutrophils related to complement regulatory proteins and lectins. *Science* **243,** 1160–1165.

26. Pober, J. S. and Cotran, R. S. (1990) Cytokines and endothelial cell biology. *Physiol. Rev.* **70,** 427–451.

27. Loppnow, H. and Libby, P. (1990) Proliferating or interleukin 1-activated human vascular smooth muscle cells secrete copious interleukin 6. *J. Clin Invest.* **85,** 731–738.

28. Valente, A. J., Graves, D. T., Vialle-Valentin, C. E., Delgado, R., and Schwartz, C. J. (1988) Purification of a monocyte chemotactic factor secreted by nonhuman primate vascular cells in culture. *Biochemistry* **27,** 4162–4168.

29. Gay, C. G., and Winkles, J. A. (1991) Interleukin 1 regulates heparin-binding growth factor 2 gene expression in vascular smooth muscle cells. *Proc. Natl. Acad. Sci. USA* **88,** 296–300.

30. Warner, S. J., Friedman, G. B., and Libby, P. (1989) Regulation of major histocompatibility gene expression in human vascular smooth muscle cells. *Arteriosclerosis* **9,** 279–288.

31. Galis, Z. S., Muszynski, M., Sukhova, G. K., Simon-Morrissey, E., Unemori, E. N., Lark, M. W., et al. (1994) Cytokine-stimulated human vascular smooth muscle cells synthesize a complement of enzymes required for extracellular matrix digestion. *Circ. Res.* **75,** 181–189.

32. Battegay, E. J., Raines, E. W., Seifert, R. A., Bowen-Pope, D. F., and Ross, R. (1990) TGF-beta induces bimodal proliferation of connective tissue cells via complex control of an autocrine PDGF loop. *Cell* **63,** 515–524.

33. Moses, H. L., Yang, E. Y., and Pietenpol, J. A. (1990) TGF-beta stimulation and inhibition of cell proliferation: New mechanistic insights. *Cell* **63,** 245–247.

34. Butcher, E. C. (1991) Leukocyte-endothelial cell recognition: Three (or more) steps to specificity and diversity. *Cell* **67,** 1033–1036.

35. Lorant, D. E., Patel, K. D., McIntyre, T. M., McEver, R. P., Prescott, S. M., and Zimmerman, G. A. (1991) Coexpression of GMP-140 and PAF by endothelium stimulated by histamine or thrombin: A juxtacrine system for adhesion and activation of neutrophils. *J. Cell. Biol.* **115,** 223–234.

36. Dustin, M. L., Rothlein, R., Bhan, A. K., Dinarello, C. A., and Springer, T. A. (1986) Induction by IL 1 and interferon-gamma: Tissue distribution, biochemistry, and function of a natural adherence molecule (ICAM-1). *J. Immunol.* **137,** 245–254.

37. Bevilacqua, M. P., Pober, J. S., Mendrick, D. L., Cotran, R. S., and Gimbrone, M. A., Jr. (1987) Identification of an inducible endothelial-leukocyte adhesion molecule. *Proc. Natl. Acad. Sci. USA* **84,** 9238–9242.

38. Munro, J. M., Pober, J. S., and Cotran, R. S. (1989) Tumor necrosis factor and interferon-gamma induce distinct patterns of endothelial activation and associated leukocyte accumulation in skin of Papio anubis. *Am. J. Pathol.* **135,** 121–133.

39. Cotran, R. S., Gimbrone, M. A., Jr., Bevilacqua, M. P., Mendrick, D. L., and Pober, J. S. (1986) Induction and detection of a human endothelial activation antigen in vivo. *J. Exp. Med.* **164,** 661–666.

40. Lo, S. K., Detmers, P. A., Levin, S. M., and Wright, S. D. (1989) Transient adhesion of neutrophils to endothelium. *J. Exp. Med.* **169,** 1779–1793.

41. Gamble, J. R., Harlan, J. M., Klebanoff, S. J., and Vadas, M. A. (1985) Stimulation of the adherence of neutrophils to umbilical vein endothelium by human recombinant tumor necrosis factor. *Proc. Natl. Acad. Sci. USA* **82,** 8667–8671.

42. Miller, L. J., Bainton, D. F., Borregaard, N., and Springer, T. A. (1987) Stimulated mobilization of monocyte Mac-1 and p150,95 adhesion proteins from an intracellular vesicular compartment to the cell surface. *J. Clin. Invest.* **80,** 535–544.

43. Werb, Z. and Gordon, S. (1975) Secretion of a specific collagenase by stimulated macrophages. *J. Exp. Med.* **142,** 346–360.

44. Mainardi, C. L., Seyer, J. M., and Kang, A. H. (1980) Type-specific collagenolysis: a type V collagen-degrading enzyme from macrophages. *Biochem. Biophys. Res. Commun.* **97,** 1108–1115.

45. Werb, Z., Gordon, S. (1975) Elastase secretion by stimulated macrophages. Characterization and regulation. *J. Exp. Med.* **142,** 361–377.

46. Hajjar, K. A., Hajjar, D. P., Silverstein, R. L., and Nachman, R. L. (1987) Tumor necrosis factor-mediated release of platelet-derived growth factor from cultured endothelial cells. *J. Exp. Med.* **166,** 235–245.

47. Leonard, E. J. and Yoshimura, T. (1990) Human monocyte chemoattractant protein-1 (MCP-1). *Immunol. Today* **11,** 97–101.

48. Bjorkerud, S. and Bjorkerud, B. (1996) Apoptosis is abundant in human atherosclerotic lesions, especially in inflammatory cells (macrophages and T cells), and may contribute to the accumulation of gruel and plaque instability. *Am. J. Pathol.* **149**, 367–380.

49. Munro, J. M. and Cotran, R. S. (1998) The pathogenesis of atherosclerosis: Atherogenesis and inflammation. *Lab. Invest.* **58**, 249–261.

50. Campbell, G. R., Campbell, J. H., Manderson, J. A., Horrigan, S., and Rennick, R. E. (1988) Arterial smooth muscle. A multifunctional mesenchymal cell. *Arch. Pathol. Lab. Med.* **112**, 977–986.

51. Henney, A. M., Wakeley, P. R., Davies, M. J., Foster, K., Hembry, R., Murphy, G., et al. (1991) Localization of stromelysin gene expression in atherosclerotic plaques by in situ hybridization. *Proc. Natl. Acad. Sci. USA* **88**, 8154–8158.

52. Galis, Z.S, Sukhova, G. K., Lark, M. W., and Libby, P. (1994) Increased expression of matrix metalloproteinases and matrix degrading activity in vulnerable regions of human atherosclerotic plaques. *J. Clin Invest.* **94**, 2493–2503.

53. Windsor, A. C., Walsh,C. J., Mullen, P. G., Cook, D. J., Fisher, B. J., Blocher, C. R., et al. (1993) Tumor necrosis factor-alpha blockade prevents neutrophil CD18 receptor upregulation and attenuates acute lung injury in porcine sepsis without inhibition of neutrophil oxygen radical generation. *J. Clin Invest.* **91**, 1459–1468.

54. Han, J., Thompson, P., and Beutler, B. (1990) Dexamethasone and pentoxifylline inhibit endotoxin-induced cachectin/tumor necrosis factor synthesis at separate points in the signaling pathway. *J. Exp. Med.* **172**, 391–394.

55. Endres, S., Fulle, H. J., Sinha, B., Stoll, D., Dinarello, C. A., Gerzer, R., et al. (1991) Cyclic nucleotides differentially regulate the synthesis of tumour necrosis factor-alpha and interleukin-1 beta by human mononuclear cells. *Immunology* **72**, 56–60.

56. Kern, J. A., Lamb, R. J., Reed, J. C., Daniele, R. P., and Nowell, P. C. (1988) Dexamethasone inhibition of interleukin 1 beta production by human monocytes. Posttranscriptional mechanisms. *J. Clin Invest.* **81**, 237–244.

57. Sano, H., Sudo, T., Yokode, M., Murayama, T., Kataoka, H., Takakura, N., et al. (2001) Functional blockade of platelet-derived growth factor receptor-beta but not of receptor-alpha prevents vascular smooth muscle cell accumulation in fibrous cap lesions in apolipoprotein E-deficient mice. *Circulation* **103**, 2955–2960.

58. Nicolosi, R. J., Wilson, T. A., and Krause, B. R. (1998) The ACAT inhibitor, CI-1011 is effective in the prevention and regression of aortic fatty streak area in hamsters. *Atherosclerosis* **137**, 77–85.

59. Sasahara, M., Raines, E. W., Chait, A., Carew, T. E., Steinberg, D., Wahl, et al. (1994) Inhibition of hypercholesterolemia-induced atherosclerosis in the nonhuman primate by probucol. I. Is the extent of atherosclerosis related to resistance of LDL to oxidation? *J. Clin Invest.* **94**, 155–164.

60. Verlangieri, A. J. and Bush, M. J. (1992) Effects of d-alpha-tocopherol supplementation on experimentally induced primate atherosclerosis. *J. Am. Coll. Nutr.* **11**, 131–138.

61. Ikonomidis, I., Andreotti, F., Economou, E., Stefanadis, C., Toutouzas, P., and Nihoyannopoulos, P. (1999) Increased proinflammatory cytokines in patients with chronic stable angina and their reduction by aspirin. *Circulation* **100**, 793–798.

62. Ridker, P. M., Rifai, N., Pfeffer, M. A., Sacks, F., and Braunwald, E. (1999) Long-term effects of pravastatin on plasma concentration of C-reactive protein. The Cholesterol and Recurrent Events (CARE) Investigators. *Circulation* **100**, 230–235.

63. Bellosta, S., Bernini, F., Ferri, N, Quarato, P., Canavesi, M., Arnaboldi, L., et al. (1998) Direct vascular effects of HMG-CoA reductase inhibitors. *Atherosclerosis* **137(Suppl)**, S101–S109.

64. Lacoste, L., Lam, J. Y., Hung, J., Letchacovski, G., Solymoss, C. B., and Waters, D. (1995) Hyperlipidemia and coronary disease. Correction of the increased thrombogenic potential with cholesterol reduction. *Circulation* **92**, 3172–3177.

65. Ridker, P. M., Rifai, N., Pfeffer, M. A., Sacks, F. M., Moye, L. A., Goldman, S., et al. (1998) Inflammation, pravastatin, and the risk of coronary events after myocardial infarction in patients with average cholesterol levels. Cholesterol and Recurrent Events (CARE) Investigators. *Circulation* **98,** 839–844.

66. Kleinveld, H. A., Demacker, P. N., De Haan, A. F., and Stalenhoef, A. F. (1993) Decreased in vitro oxidizability of low-density lipoprotein in hypercholesterolaemic patients treated with 3-hydroxy-3-methylglutaryl- CoA reductase inhibitors. *Eur J. Clin Invest.* **23,** 289–295.

67. Gwechenberger, M., Mendoza, L. H., Youker, K. A., Frangogiannis, N. G., Smith, C. W., Michael, L. H., et al. (1999) Cardiac myocytes produce interleukin-6 in culture and in viable border zone of reperfused infarctions. *Circulation* **99,** 546–551.

68. Irwin, M. W., Mak, S., Mann, D. L., Qu, R., Penninger, J. M., Yan, A., et al. (1999) Tissue expression and immunolocalization of tumor necrosis factor-alpha in postinfarction dysfunctional myocardium. *Circulation* **99,** 1492–1498.

69. Entman, M. L., Youker, K., Shappell, S. B., Siegel, C., Rothlein, R., Dreyer, W. J., et al. (1990) Neutrophil adherence to isolated adult canine myocytes: Evidence for a CD18-dependent mechanism. *J. Clin Invest.* **85,** 1497–1506.

70. Smith, C. W., Entman, M. L., Lane, C. L., Beaudet, A. L., Ty, T. I., Youker, K., et al. (1991) Adherence of neutrophils to canine cardiac myocytes in vitro is dependent on intercellular adhesion molecule-1. *J. Clin Invest.* **88,** 1216–1223.

71. Das, U. N., Padma, M., Sagar, P. S., Ramesh, G., and Koratkar, R. (1990) Stimulation of free radical generation in human leukocytes by various agents including tumor necrosis factor is a calmodulin dependent process. *Biochem. Biophys. Res. Commun.* **167,** 1030–1036.

72. Aoki, N., Siegfried, M., and Lefer, A. M. (1989) Anti-EDRF effect of tumor necrosis factor in isolated, perfused cat carotid arteries. *Am. J. Physiol.* **256,** H1509–H1512.

73. Lefer, A. M. and Aoki, N. (1990) Leukocyte-dependent and leukocyte-independent mechanisms of impairment of endothelium-mediated vasodilation. *Blood Vessels* **27,** 162–168.

74. Cain, B. S., Harken, A. H., and Meldrum, D. R. (1999) Therapeutic strategies to reduce TNF-alpha mediated cardiac contractile depression following ischemia and reperfusion. *J. Mol. Cell Cardiol.* **31,** 931–947.

75. Gumina, R. J., Schultz, J., Yao, Z., Kenny, D., Warltier, D. C., Newman, P. J., et al. (1996) Antibody to platelet/endothelial cell adhesion molecule-1 reduces myocardial infarct size in a rat model of ischemia-reperfusion injury. *Circulation* **94,** 3327–3333.

76. Jones, S. P., Trocha, S. D., Strange, M. B., Granger, D. N., Kevil, C. G., Bullard, D. C., et al. (2000) Leukocyte and endothelial cell adhesion molecules in a chronic murine model of myocardial reperfusion injury. *Am. J. Physiol.* **279,** H2196–H2201.

77. Lucchesi, B. R. (1990) Modulation of leukocyte-mediated myocardial reperfusion injury. *Ann. Rev. Physiol.* **52,** 561–576.

78. Ferrer-Lopez, P., Renesto, P., Schattner, M., Bassot, S., Laurent, P., and Chignard, M. (1990) Activation of human platelets by C5a-stimulated neutrophils: A role for cathepsin G. *Am. J. Physiol.* **258,** C1100–C1107.

79. Suzuki , M., Asako, H., Kubes, P., Jennings, S., Grisham, M. B., and Granger, D. N. Neutrophil-derived oxidants promote leukocyte adherence in postcapillary venules. *Microvasc. Res.* **42,** 125–138.

80. Borgeat, P. and Samuelsson, B. Metabolism of arachidonic acid in polymorphonuclear leukocytes. Structural analysis of novel hydroxylated compounds. *J. Biol. Chem.* **254,** 7865–7869.

81. Lotner, G. Z., Lynch, J. M., Betz, S. J., and Henson, P. M. (1980) Human neutrophil-derived platelet activating factor. *J. Immunol.* **124,** 676–684.

82. Montrucchio, G., Alloatti, G., Tetta, C., De Luca, R., Saunders, R. N., Emanuelli ,G., Camussi, G. (1989) Release of platelet-activating factor from ischemic-reperfused rabbit heart. *Am. J. Physiol.* **256,** H1236–H1246.

83. Boyle, E. M., Jr., Canty, T. G., Jr., Morgan, E. N., Yun, W., Pohlman, T. H., and Verrier, E. D. (1999) Treating myocardial ischemia-reperfusion injury by targeting endothelial cell transcription. *Ann. Thorac. Surg.* **68**, 1949–1953.

84. Fridovich, I. (1983) Superoxide radical: An endogenous toxicant. *Annu. Rev. Pharmacol. Toxicol.* **23**, 239–257.

85. McCord, J. M., Fridovich, I. (1978) The biology and pathology of oxygen radicals. *Ann. Intern. Med.* **89**, 122–127.

86. Chandrasekar, B., Colston, J. T., Geimer, J., Cortez, D., and Freeman, G. L. (2000) Induction of nuclear factor kappaB but not kappaB-responsive cytokine expression during myocardial reperfusion injury after neutropenia. *Free Rad. Biol. Med.* **28**, 1579–1588.

87. Collins, T., Read, M. A., Neish, A. S., Whitley, M. Z., Thanos, D, and Maniatis, T. (1995) Transcriptional regulation of endothelial cell adhesion molecules: NF-kappa B and cytokine-inducible enhancers. *FASEB J.* **9**, 899–909.

88. Del Maestro, R. F. (1980) An approach to free radicals in medicine and biology. *Acta Physiol. Scand. Suppl.* **492**, 153–168.

89. McCord, J. M. (1985) Oxygen-derived free radicals in postischemic tissue injury. *N. Engl. J. Med.* **312**, 159–163.

90. Ferrari, R., Ceconi, C., Curello, S., Guarnieri, C., Caldarera, C. M., Albertini, A., Visioli, O. (1985) Oxygen-mediated myocardial damage during ischaemia and reperfusion: role of the cellular defences against oxygen toxicity. *J. Mol. Cell. Cardiol.* **17**, 937–945.

91. Guarnieri, C., Flamigni, F., and Caldarera, C. M. (1980) Role of oxygen in the cellular damage induced by re-oxygenation of hypoxic heart. *J. Mol. Cell. Cardiol.* **12**, 797–808.

92. Kako, K. J. (1987) Free radical effects on membrane protein in myocardial ischemia/reperfusion injury. *J. Mol. Cell. Cardiol.* **19**, 209–211.

93. Ohto, H., Maeda, H., Shibata, Y., Chen, R. F., Ozaki, Y., Higashihara, M., et al. (1985) A novel leukocyte differentiation antigen: Two monoclonal antibodies TM2 and TM3 define a 120-kd molecule present on neutrophils, monocytes, platelets, and activated lymphoblasts. *Blood* **66**, 873–881.

94. Ma, X. L., Lefer, D. J., Lefer, A. M., and Rothlein, R. (1992) Coronary endothelial and cardiac protective effects of a monoclonal antibody to intercellular adhesion molecule-1 in myocardial ischemia and reperfusion. *Circulation* **86**, 937–946.

95. Zhao, Z. Q., Lefer, D. J., Sato, H., Hart, K. K., Jefforda, P. R., and Vinten-Johansen, J. (1997) Monoclonal antibody to ICAM-1 preserves postischemic blood flow and reduces infarct size after ischemia-reperfusion in rabbit. *J. Leuk. Biol.* **62**, 292–300.

96. Arai, M., Lefer, D. J., So, T., DiPaula, A, Aversano, T., and Becker, L. C. (1996) An anti-CD18 antibody limits infarct size and preserves left ventricular function in dogs with ischemia and 48-hour reperfusion. *J. Am. Coll. Cardiol.* **27**, 1278–1285.

97. Aversano, T., Zhou, W., Nedelman, M., Nakada, M., and Weisman, H. (1995) A chimeric IgG4 monoclonal antibody directed against CD18 reduces infarct size in a primate model of myocardial ischemia and reperfusion. *J. Am. Coll. Cardiol.* **25**, 781–788.

98. Lefer, D. J. (2000) Pharmacology of selectin inhibitors in ischemia/reperfusion states. *Annu. Rev. Pharmacol. Toxicol.* **40**, 283–294.

99. Hoffmeyer, M. R., Scalia, R., Ross, C. R., Jones, S. P., and Lefer, D. J. (2000) PR-39, a potent neutrophil inhibitor, attenuates myocardial ischemia- reperfusion injury in mice. *Am. J. Physiol.* **279**, H2824–H2828.

100. Altavilla, D., Deodato, B., Campo, G. M., Arlotta, M., Miano, M., Squadrito, G., et al. (2000) IRFI 042, a novel dual vitamin E-like antioxidant, inhibits activation of nuclear factor-kappaB and reduces the inflammatory response in myocardial ischemia-reperfusion injury. *Cardiovasc. Res.* **47**, 515–528.

101. Sakaguchi, T., Sawa, Y., Fukushima, N., Nishimura, M., Ichikawa, H., Kaneda, Y., Matsuda, H. (2001) A novel strategy of decoy transfection against nuclear factor-kappaB in myocardial preservation. *Ann. Thorac. Surg.* **71**, 624–629.

102. Burke, S. E., Wright, C. D., Potoczak, R. E., Boucher, D. M., Dodd, G. D., Taylor, D. G., Jr., Kaplan, H. R. (1992) Reduction of canine myocardial infarct size by CI-959, an inhibitor of inflammatory cell activation. *J. Cardiovasc. Pharmacol.* **20**, 619–629.

103. Gallagher, K. P., Buda, A. J., Pace, D., Gerren, R. A., and Shlafer, M. (1986) Failure of superoxide dismutase and catalase to alter size of infarction in conscious dogs after 3 hours of occlusion followed by reperfusion. *Circulation* **73**, 1065–1076.

104. Jolly, S. R., Kane, W. J., Bailie, M. B., Abrams, G. D., and Lucchesi, B. R. (1984) Canine myocardial reperfusion injury. Its reduction by the combined administration of superoxide dismutase and catalase. *Circ. Res.* **54**, 277–285.

105. Werns, S. W., Shea, M. J., Driscoll, E. M., Cohen, C., Abrams, G. D., Pitt, B., Lucchesi, B. R. (1985) The independent effects of oxygen radical scavengers on canine infarct size. Reduction by superoxide dismutase but not catalase. *Circ. Res.* **56**, 895–898.

105a. Jones, S. P., Hoffmeyer, M. R., Sharp, B. R., Ho, Y. S., and Lefer, D. J. (2003) Role of intracellular antioxidant enzymes after in vivo myocardial ischemia and reperfusion. *Am. J. Physiol. Heart Circ. Physiol.* **284**, H277–H282.

106. Engler, R. and Gilpin, E. (1989) Can superoxide dismutase alter myocardial infarct size? *Circulation* **79**, 1137–1142.

107. Reimer, K. A. and Jennings, R. B. (1985) Failure of the xanthine oxidase inhibitor allopurinol to limit infarct size after ischemia and reperfusion in dogs. *Circulation* **71**, 1069–1075.

108. Werns, S. W., Shea, M. J., Mitsos, S. E., Dysko, R. C., Fantone, J. C., Schork, M. A., et al. (1986) Reduction of the size of infarction by allopurinol in the ischemic-reperfused canine heart. *Circulation* **73**, 518–524.

109. Puett, D. W., Forman, M. B., Cates, C. U., Wilson, B. H., Hande, K. R., Friesinger, G. C., Virmani, R. (1987) Oxypurinol limits myocardial stunning but does not reduce infarct size after reperfusion. *Circulation* **76**, 678–686.

110. Virmani, R, Fink, L. M., Gunter, K., and English, D. (1984) Effect of perfluorochemical blood substitutes on human neutrophil function. *Transfusion* **24**, 343–347.

111. Bajaj, A. K., Cobb, M. A., Virmani, R., Gay, J. C., Light, R. T., and Forman, M. B. (1989) Limitation of myocardial reperfusion injury by intravenous perfluorochemicals. Role of neutrophil activation. *Circulation* **79**, 645–656.

112. Berne, R. M. (1980) The role of adenosine in the regulation of coronary blood flow. *Circ. Res.* **47**, 807–813.

113. Cronstein, B. N., Levin, R. I., Belanoff, J., Weissmann, G., and Hirschhorn, R. (1986) Adenosine: an endogenous inhibitor of neutrophil-mediated injury to endothelial cells. *J. Clin Invest.* **78**, 760–770.

114. Tanabe, M., Terashita, Z., Nishikawa, K., and Hirata, M. (1984) Inhibition of coronary circulatory failure and thromboxane A2 release during coronary occlusion and reperfusion by 2-phenylaminoadenosine (CV-1808) in anesthetized dogs. *J. Cardiovasc. Pharmacol.* **6**, 442–448.

115. Ross, R., Raines, E. W., and Bowen-Pope, D. F. (1986) The biology of platelet-derived growth factor. *Cell* **46**, 155–169.

116. Ferrell, M., Fuster, V., Gold, H. K., and Chesebro, J. H. (1992) A dilemma for the 1990s. Choosing appropriate experimental animal model for the prevention of restenosis. *Circulation* **85**, 1630–1631.

117. Nobuyoshi, M., Kimura, T., Ohishi, H., Horiuchi, H., Nosaka, H., Hamasaki, N., et al. (1991) Restenosis after percutaneous transluminal coronary angioplasty: pathologic observations in 20 patients. *J. Am. Coll. Cardiol.* **17**, 433–439.

118. Harker, L. A. (1987) Role of platelets and thrombosis in mechanisms of acute occlusion and restenosis after angioplasty. *Am. J. Cardiol.* **60**, 20B–28B.

119. Pober, J. S. (1988) Warner-Lambert/Parke-Davis award lecture. Cytokine-mediated activation of vascular endothelium. Physiology and pathology. *Am. J. Pathol.* **133**, 426–433.

120. Mantovani, A. and Dejana, E. (1989) Cytokines as communication signals between leukocytes and endothelial cells. *Immunol. Today* **10,** 370–375.

121. Paleolog, E. M., Crossman, D. C., McVey, J. H., and Pearson, J. D. (1990) Differential regulation by cytokines of constitutive and stimulated secretion of von Willebrand factor from endothelial cells. *Blood* **75,** 688–695.

122. Springer, T. A. (1994) Traffic signals for lymphocyte re-Circulation and leukocyte emigration: The multi-step paradigm. *Cell* **76,** 301–314.

123. Baumgartner, H. R., and Muggli, R. Adhesion and aggregation: morphological demonstration and quantification in vivo and in vitro, in *Platelets in Biology and Pathology* (Gordon, J. L., ed.), Elsevier Press Inc, Amsterdam, 1976, pp. 23–39.

124. Walker, L. N., Bowen-Pope, D. F., Ross, R., and Reidy, M. A. (1986) Production of platelet-derived growth factor-like molecules by cultured arterial smooth muscle cells accompanies proliferation after arterial injury. *Proc. Natl. Acad. Sci. USA* **83,** 7311–7315.

125. Antiplatelet Trialists' Collaboration. (1994) Collaborative overview of randomised trials of antiplatelet therapy-I: Prevention of death, myocardial infarction, and stroke by prolonged antiplatelet therapy in various categories of patients. *Br. Med. J.* **308,** 81–106.

126. Maresta, A., Balducelli, M., Cantini, L., Casari, A., Chioin, R., Fabbri, M., et al. (1994) Trapidil (triazolopyrimidine), a platelet-derived growth factor antagonist, reduces restenosis after percutaneous transluminal coronary angioplasty. Results of the randomized, double-blind STARC study. Studio Trapidil versus Aspirin nella Restenosi Coronarica. *Circulation* **90,** 2710–2715.

127. Dosquet, C., Weill, D., and Wautier, J. L. (1995) Cytokines and thrombosis. *J. Cardiovasc. Pharmacol.* **25(Suppl 2),** S13–S19.

128. Huang, J., Driscoll, E. M., Gonzales, M. L., Park, A. M., and Lucchesi, B. R. (2000) Prevention of arterial thrombosis by intravenously administered platelet P2T receptor antagonist AR-C69931MX in a canine model. *J. Pharmacol. Exp. Ther.* **295,** 492–499.

129. Shi, Y., Fard, A., Galeo, A., Hutchinson, H. G., Vermani, P., Dodge, G. R., et al. (1994) Transcatheter delivery of c-myc antisense oligomers reduces neointimal formation in a porcine model of coronary artery balloon injury. *Circulation* **90,** 944–951.

130. Palmer, R. M., Ashton, D. S., and Moncada, S. (1988) Vascular endothelial cells synthesize nitric oxide from L-arginine. *Nature* **333,** 664–666.

131. Ignarro, L. J., Buga, G. M., Wood, K. S., Byrns, R. E., and Chaudhuri, G. (1987) Endothelium-derived relaxing factor produced and released from artery and vein is nitric oxide. *Proc. Natl. Acad. Sci. USA* **84,** 9265–9269.

132. Chowienczyk, P. J., Watts, G. F., Cockcroft, J. R., and Ritter, J. M. (1992) Impaired endothelium-dependent vasodilation of forearm resistance vessels in hypercholesterolaemia. *Lancet* **340,** 1430–1432.

133. Creager, M. A., Cooke, J. P., Mendelsohn, M. E., Gallagher, S. J., Coleman, S. M., Loscalzo, J., et al. (1990) Impaired vasodilation of forearm resistance vessels in hypercholesterolemic humans. *J. Clin Invest.* **86,** 228–234.

134. Rubanyi, G. M. (1988) Vascular effects of oxygen-derived free radicals. *Free Rad. Biol. Med.* **4,** 107–120.

135. Chu, A., Chambers, D. E., Lin, C. C., Kuehl, W. D., Palmer, R. M., Moncada, S., et al. (1991) Effects of inhibition of nitric oxide formation on basal vasomotion and endothelium-dependent responses of the coronary arteries in awake dogs. *J. Clin Invest.* **87,** 1964–1968.

136. Kubes, P., Suzuki, M., and Granger, D. N. (1991) Nitric oxide: An endogenous modulator of leukocyte adhesion. *Proc. Natl. Acad. Sci. USA* **88,** 4651–4655.

137. Bassenge, E. (1991) Antiplatelet effects of endothelium-derived relaxing factor and nitric oxide donors. *Eur. Heart J.* **12(Suppl E),** 12–15.

138. Assender, J. W., Southgate, K. M., Hallett, M. B., and Newby, A. C. (1992) Inhibition of proliferation, but not of Ca2+ mobilization, by cyclic AMP and GMP in rabbit aortic smooth-muscle cells. *Biochem. J.* **288,** 527–532.

139. Jessup, W., Mohr, D., Gieseg, S. P., Dean, R. T., and Stocker, R. (1992) The participation of nitric oxide in cell. *Biochim. Biophys. Acta.* **1180,** 73–82.

140. Ohlstein, E. H. and Nichols, A. J. (1989) Rabbit polymorphonuclear neutrophils elicit endothelium-dependent contraction in vascular smooth muscle. *Circ. Res.* **65,** 917–924.

141. Lefer, D. J., Jones, S. P., Girod, W. G., Baines, A., Grisham, M. B., Cockrell, A. S., et al. (1999) Leukocyte-endothelial cell interactions in nitric oxide synthase- deficient mice. *Am. J. Physiol.* **276,** H1943–H1950.

142. Barrett, M. L., Willis, A. L., and Vane, J. R. (1989) Inhibition of platelet-derived mitogen release by nitric oxide (EDRF). *Agents Actions* **27,** 488–491.

6

Development and Use of Platelet Glycoprotein Antagonists in Heart Disease

Joel S. Bennett

CONTENTS

1. INTRODUCTION

Platelets are not only responsible for primary hemostasis *(1)*, but also for the thrombi that produce the morbidity and mortality of arterial vascular disease *(2)*. Although considerable effort has been expended to associate augmented platelet function with arterial thrombosis, it is more likely that the formation of platelet thrombi simply represents normal platelet function in the wrong location. It follows then that a rational approach to treating atherosclerotic disease is to prevent the development of vascular lesions in the first place. Nonetheless, the administration of platelet-inhibitory drugs, such as aspirin *(3)*, has been of proven benefit to individuals with established vascular disease, providing the impetus to identify more effective clinically useful platelet function inhibitors. Moreover, there has been substantial progress in understanding the biochemical basis of platelet function, providing additional targets for drug development. However, clinical experience has shown that the therapeutic index for the existing potent platelet inhibitors is narrow, suggesting that new and novel approaches to impairing platelet function will be required.

2. PLATELET ADHESION

2.1. Role of von Willebrand Factor (vWf)

Circulating platelets are maintained in a nonreactive state until they are needed for hemostasis, at least in part by inhibitory molecules, such as nitric oxide and prostacyclin, which are secreted by endothelial cells. In addition, the endothelium lining blood cells is a barrier separating platelets from adhesive substrates in the subendothelial connective tissue matrix. Disruption of the endothelium by trauma or dis-

From: *Cardiac Drug Development Guide*
Edited by: M. K. Pugsley © Humana Press Inc., Totowa, NJ

ease allows platelets to interact with the subendothelial matrix. When this occurs in the venous circulation, where shear rates are low, platelets can interact with exposed collagen, fibronectin, and laminin via the integrins $\alpha2\beta1$, $\alpha5\beta1$, and $\alpha6\beta1$, respectively [4]. However, platelets are not thought to make major contributions to the initiation and propagation of venous thrombosis, which depends predominantly on intravascular production of a fibrin clot. However, platelets play a critical role in the initiation of thrombosis at the higher shear rates present in arteries and in the microcirculation. Under these conditions, platelet adhesion requires the presence of subendothelial vWf [5]. vWf, an elongated multimeric glycoprotein that is synthesized by endothelial cells and megakaryocytes [6,7], binds to the GPIb-IX-V complex on unactivated platelets [8] and to the GPIIb/IIIa (αIIbβ3) complex on activated platelets [9]. Although vWf is present in plasma, it is normally not present on the platelet surface. Exposing vWf in vitro to the antibiotic ristocetin and to the snake venom protein botrocetin induces vWf binding to GPIb-IX-V [10]. The factors that enable platelets to adhere to vWf in vivo are uncertain. Perfusion of whole blood or isolated platelets over surfaces coated with vWf results in shear rate-dependent platelet translocation (rolling) on the coated surface [11], suggesting that shear stress itself induces vWf binding by affecting the conformation of GPIb-IX-V, vWf, or both. It is also possible that changes in the conformation of vWf occur when it is incorporated into the subendothelium and enable it to bind to GPIb-IX-V [12].

Although platelet binding to vWf might appear to be a tempting target for antiplatelet therapy, congenital deficiency or abnormality of vWf results in von Willebrand disease, a common hemorrhagic diathesis [10]. von Willebrand disease is relatively mild in heterozygous individuals but can be a severe disorder in homozygous or doubly heterozygous patients (type III disease), suggesting that potent inhibitors of vWf binding to GPIb-IX-V could cause serious bleeding. Similarly, homozygosity for GPIb-IX deficiency, a rare condition known as the Bernard–Soulier syndrome, is a serious hereditary bleeding disorder [13]. Nonetheless, a number of agents that disrupt vWf binding to GPIb-IX-V have been studied in vitro and in animal models as either proof of principal or as potential antithrombotic drugs. These include aurin tricarboxylic acid [14], a negatively charged triphenylmethane derivative that is also a general endonuclease inhibitor with antiapoptotic properties [15,16] and perhaps an inhibitor of fibrinogen binding to GPIIb/IIIa [17]; AJW200, a humanized monoclonal antibody against vWf that has been reported to produce sustained inhibition of ex vivo ristocetin-induced platelet aggregation with only a moderate prolongation of the bleeding time and no change in plasma vWf concentrations in cynomolgus monkeys [18]; and several snake venom-derived proteins, echicetin [19], crotalin [20], and agkistin [21], that bind to GPIb. None of these agents have been used in humans, and their clinical utility is uncertain.

2.2. Collagen as an Adhesive Substrate and Platelet Agonist

Collagen is a unique matrix protein because it not only is a substrate for platelet adhesion but is also the binding site for vWf in the subendothelium [22] and functions as an agonist for platelet aggregation and secretion [23]. A number of platelet proteins have been reported to interact with collagen, including GPIIb (αIIb), GPIV, and two proteins, a 65,000 molecular weight protein that binds to type 1 collagen and an 85,000–90,000 molecular weight protein. However, there is a substantial and growing body of data indicating that only the integrin α2β1 (GPIa-IIa) and GPVI are physiological plate-let collagen receptors *(24–27)*. The relative importance of collagen as an adhesive sub-strate (as opposed to simply acting as a binding site for vWf) , as well as a platelet agonist, is uncertain, although it has generally been assumed to play a central role in platelet thrombus formation. The few reported patients lacking either α2β1 or GPVI were identified because they had mild bleeding disorders *(25,26,28,29)*, implying that these proteins are involved in normal hemostasis. Moreover, increased α2β1 expres-sion resulting from inherited polymorphisms in the *α2* gene have been associated with increased risks for stroke and nonfatal myocardial infarction in younger patients in some *(30,31)* although all *(32)* studies.

The relative contributions of α2β1 and GPVI to collagen-initiated platelet function is also unclear. α2β1 is a widely expressed integrin that binds with high affinity to type I collagen, as well as to collagen types II–V and to laminins 1 and 5, depending on the cellular context *(33)*. However, disruption of the *α2* gene in mice has had only a mini-mal effect on the interaction of platelets with fibrillar collagen and no effect on murine hemostasis *(33)*. By contrast, disruption of GPVI expression in mice abrogates platelet adhesion to, and activation by, collagen, indicating that GPVI is essential in this regard *(34)*. GPVI, a membrane protein of the immunoglobulin gene superfamily, appears to be expressed only in megakaryocytes and platelets *(24,35)*. Accordingly, GPVI would seem to be a desirable target for the development of platelet inhibitors, for use either alone or in concert with other antiplatelet agents.

3. PLATELET AGGREGATION

After adhesion, platelets aggregate to form a hemostatic plug or a platelet-rich throm-bus. In contrast with platelet adhesion, platelet aggregation is an active metabolic pro-cess in which platelet agonist binding to specific receptors initiates signaling pathways that enable the platelet membrane protein GPIIb/IIIa to bind soluble macromolecular ligands, such as fibrinogen or vWf *(36)*. The fibrinogen or vWf bound to GPIIb/IIIa crosslinks platelets into a hemostatic plug or thrombus.

3.1. GPIIb/IIIa, the Platelet Fibrinogen Receptor

GPIIb/IIIa (αIIbβ3), a member of the integrin superfamily of adhesion receptors, is expressed exclusively on platelets and megakaryocytes *(37)*. There are approx 80,000 copies of GPIIb/IIIa on the surface of unstimulated platelets and additional copies, which are present in the membranes of platelet granules, can be translocated to the platelet surface during platelet secretion *(38)*. Ultrastructural studies of GPIIb/IIIa purified from human platelets and soulublized in detergent micelles indicate that the heterodimer consists of an 8- × 12-nm nodular head containing a ligand binding site and two 18-nm flexible stalks extending from one side of the head containing trans-membrane and cytoplasmic domains *(39)*.

In contrast with most integrins, GPIIb/IIIa is unable to bind fibrinogen or vWf until platelets are stimulated by agonists, such as adenosine diphosphate (ADP) and throm-bin *(40,41)*. How agonist-induced signaling regulates ligand binding to GPIIb/IIIa is uncertain. The signals that shift GPIIb/IIIa to an active state do so by affecting its cytoplasmic domains *(42)*. There is no evidence that phosphorylation of either the GPIIb or the GPIIIa cytoplasmic domains at tyrosine, serine, or threonine residues is involved *(43)*. It has been proposed that the membrane proximal portions of the GPIIb and GPIIIa cytoplasmic domains interact via a salt-bridge to constrain GPIIb/IIIa activity *(44)*. Disruption of the salt-bridge by some type of integrin-activating agent would then shift GPIIb/IIIa to an active state. However, there is no compelling physical evidence that the cytoplasmic domains of GPIIb and GPIIIa actually interact when the proteins are present in a membrane-like environment *(45)*. Several molecules that interact with the cytoplasmic domains of either GPIIb and GPIIIa have been detected using yeast two-hybrid screens. These molecules include β3-endonexin *(46)* and ILK *(47)*, proteins that bind to the cytoplasmic domain of GPIIIa, and CIB *(48)*, a protein that binds to the cytoplasmic domain of GPIIb. Overexpressing β3-endonexin in Chinese hamster ovary (CHO) cells can shift GPIIb/IIIa to an active conformation *(49)*, and it has been reported that CIB can activate GPIIb/IIIa in vitro and in vivo *(50)*. In addition, several cytoskeletal proteins, including talin, α-actinin, filamin, and skelemin, have been reported to interact with the cytoplasmic domains of integrin β subunits, including GPIIIa *(51–53)*. These interactions have been implicated in cytoskeleton-mediated postreceptor binding events, such as cell spreading, cell migration, and clot retraction, and signaling events, including tyrosine phosphorylation of proteins, such as focal adhesion kinase *(54)*. In addition, binding of talin head domains to GPIIIa in CHO cells has been reported to induce GPIIb/IIIa activation *(55)*. This suggests that the interaction of GPIIb/IIIa with cytoskeletal proteins could be directly involved in GPIIb/IIIa activation as well.

The major GPIIb/IIIa ligand is fibrinogen. Fibrinogen is composed of pairs of α, β, and γ chains folded into three nodular domains. Although peptides corresponding to the carboxyl terminal 10–15 amino acids of the γ chain *(56)* or containing the arginine–glycine–aspartic acid (RGD) motif present at two sites in the α chain *(57)* inhibit fibrinogen binding to GPIIb/IIIa, fibrinogen binding to GPIIb/IIIa is actually mediated by the γ chain sequences *(58,59)*. However, clinical studies confirm that RGD-containing peptides inhibit GPIIb/IIIa function *(2)*. The structural basis for these observations is not clear, but competitive binding measurements indicate that the γ chain and RGD peptides cannot bind to GPIIb/IIIa at the same time *(60)*, implying that RGD peptides inhibit fibrinogen binding by preventing the interaction of GPIIb/IIIa with the γ chain sequence. Nonetheless, RGD peptides need not directly compete with fibrinogen for binding to GPIIb/IIIa. It is noteworthy in this regard that Hu et al. *(61)* used plasmon resonance spectroscopy to demonstrate that GPIIb/IIIa contains distinct but interacting sites for fibrinogen and RGD ligands.

Ligand binding to GPIIb/IIIa involves specific regions of the amino-terminal portions of both GPIIb and GPIIIa *(62)*. A region in GPIIIa encoded by the fourth and fifth exons of the GPIIIa gene that encompasses amino acids 95–223 *(63)*, including an RGD-crosslinking site located in the vicinity of amino acids 109–171 *(64)*, has been implicated in ligand binding. This region also contains an array of residues whose fold, as shown in the recently reported crystal structure of the extracellular portion of the integrin αvβ3, resembles that of the ligand-binding metal ion-dependent adhesion sites (MIDAS) in integrin I domains *(65)*.

The amino terminal portion of GPIIb, like the amino-terminal portion of other integrin a subunits is folded into a β propeller configuration *(65)*. Each blade of the propeller is composed of a β sheet formed from four antiparallel β strands. Loops connecting the strands are located on either the upper or low surface of the propeller. A number of naturally occurring and laboratory induced mutations involving GPIIb amino acids 145, 183, 184, 189, 190, 191, 193, and 224 impair GPIIb/IIIa function, suggesting that these residues interact with GPIIb/IIIa ligands *(66)*. Because the loops containing these amino acids are juxtaposed in one quadrant on the upper surface of the propeller, it is possible that this is the region of GPIIb that binds ligands *(66)*. In a comprehensive study of ligand binding to GPIIb/IIIa, Kamata et al. *(67)* replaced each of the 27 loops in the GPIIb propeller with the corresponding loops from the $\alpha 4$ or $\alpha 5$ integrin subunits. They found that eight replacements, all on located on the upper surface of the propeller, prevented fibrinogen binding to GPIIb/IIIa expressed in CHO cells, again suggesting that ligands bind to the upper surface of the propeller.

3.2. GPIIb/IIIa Antagonists as Antithrombotic Agents

Because ligand binding to GPIIb/IIIa on activated platelets is a prerequisite for platelet aggregation, and for the formation of arterial thrombi, GPIIb/IIIa has been a major target for antiplatelet drug development. Three intravenous GPIIb/IIIa antagonists (abciximab, eptifibatide, and tirofiban) have been shown in large multicenter clinical trials to be efficacious in reducing the incidence of a common endpoint of death, myocardial infarction, and urgent coronary artery revascularization in patients with acute coronary syndromes and have been approved for use in this setting.

3.2.1. Abciximab

Abciximab (c7E3, ReoPro), the Fab fragment of a human-murine chimeric monoclonal antibody, inhibits agonist-stimulated fibrinogen binding to GPIIb/IIIa and in vitro platelet aggregation *(68)*. Abciximab also binds to the vitronectin receptor $\alpha v \beta 3$ and to the leukocyte integrin $\alpha M \beta 2$ *(69)*. When administered to humans at a dose that results in >80% GPIIb/IIIa occupancy, ADP-stimulated platelet aggregation is reduced to <20% of baseline and there is marked prolongation of the skin bleeding time *(70)*. After abciximab administration is stopped, GPIIb/IIIa occupancy declines slowly and platelet aggregation is restored to normal by 24–36 h. Nonetheless, abciximab can detected on circulating platelets for up to 15 d, implying continuous redistribution of the drug throughout the platelet pool over time *(71)*.

The efficacy of abciximab in patients with acute coronary syndromes was tested in four large clinical trials. In Evaluation of Platelet IIb/IIIa Antibody for Preventing Ischemic Complications of High Risk Angioplasty (EPIC), patients undergoing angioplasty were given aspirin and heparin and randomized to either a placebo, an abciximab bolus, or an abciximab bolus followed by a 12-h abciximab infusion *(72)*. The subsequent Evaluation on PTCA to Improve Long-Term Outcome with Abciximab GPIIb/IIIa Blockade (EPILOG) trial tested the hypothesis that excessive heparin dosage was responsible for bleeding experienced by patients in EPIC by randomizing patients undergoing angioplasty to placebo plus standard dose weight-adjusted heparin, abciximab plus standard dose weight-adjusted heparin, or abciximab plus low dose weight-adjusted heparin *(73)*. In c7E3 Fab Antiplatelet Therapy in Unstable Refractory Angina (CAPTURE), patients undergoing angioplasty for refractory unstable angina were given aspirin and heparin and randomly assigned to either placebo or an abciximab bolus followed by an 18- to 24-h abciximab infusion beginning prior to angioplasty and continuing for 1 h afterward *(74)*. The Evaluation of Platelet IIb/IIIa Inhibitor for Stenting (EPISTENT) trial addressed whether abciximab also improved the safety and benefit of coronary artery stenting *(75)*. In each of these trials, abciximab significantly decreased the composite endpoint by 35%, 55%, 34%, and 51%, respectively. In addition, EPILOG demonstrated that abciximab could be administered safely along with low-dose weight-adjusted heparin.

3.2.2. Eptifibatide

Eptifibatide (Integrilin), a synthetic cyclic heptapeptide based on the Lys-Gly-Asp (KGD) motif of the snake venom disintegrin barbourin, binds exclusively to GPIIb/IIIa *(76)*. In humans, eptifibatide reversibly inhibits platelet aggregation with only a modest prolongation of the bleeding time *(77)*. Because eptifibatide binding to GPIIb/IIIa is enhanced at low calcium concentrations and because dosing in early trials was based on studies using blood samples anticoagulated with citrate, it is likely that the eptifibatide doses initially selected were suboptimal *(78)*. Thus, in the Integrilin to Minimize Platelet Aggregation and Coronary Thrombosis-II (IMPACT-II) trial of patients undergoing coronary intervention, eptifibatide doses were chosen to achieve 70–100% inhibition of ADP-stimulated platelet aggregation in citrate-anticoagulated plasma, but there was no statistical differences in outcome between patients receiving placebo and eptifibatide *(79)*. Higher eptifibatide doses were chosen for the Platelet Glycoprotein IIb-IIIa in Unstable Angina: Receptor Suppression Using Integrilin Therapy (PURSUIT) trial of patients with unstable angina or non-Q wave myocardial infarction (MI) *(80)*. The difference in the composite endpoint between patients receiving placebo and eptifibatide was small (15.7 vs 14.2%) but was now statistically significant ($p = 0.04$). An even higher dose of eptifibatide was given to patients undergoing coronary artery stent implantation in the recently reported Enhanced Suppression of the Platelet IIb/IIIa Receptor with Integrilin Therapy (ESPRIT) trial *(81)*. The efficacy of eptifibatide in this trial was comparable to that of abciximab in EPISTENT, implying that eptifibatide is an effective GPIIb/IIIa when appropriate doses are administered.

3.2.3. Tirofiban

Tirofiban (MK-0383, Aggrastat) is an RGD-based peptidomimetic analog of tyrosine that binds reversibly to GPIIb/IIIa on resting platelets with nanomolar affinity *(82)*. The efficacy and safety of iv tirofiban in patients with coronary artery disease was studied in three large clinical trials. In the Randomized Efficacy Study of Tirofiban for Outcomes and Restenosis (RESTORE) trial, patients undergoing balloon angioplasty or directional atherectomy for unstable angina or acute MI were given aspirin and heparin and randomized to receive placebo or tirofiban for 36 h *(83)*. The composite endpoint was reduced by 38% at 2 d ($p = 0.005$), 27% at 7 d ($p = 0.022$), 16% at 30 d ($p = 0.16$), and 11% ($p = 0.11$) at 6 mo in patients treated with tirofiban without significant differences in bleeding or thrombocytopenia *(84)*. The Platelet Receptor Inhibition in Ischemic Syndrome Management (PRISM) and Platelet Receptor Inhibition in Ischemic Syndrome Management in Patients Limited by Unstable Signs and Symptoms (PRISM-PLUS) trials examined the effect of tirofiban on patients with unstable angina and non-Q-wave MI. In PRISM, patients with unstable angina were given aspirin and randomized to receive either heparin or aspirin and tirofiban for 48 h *(85)*. At 48 h, there was a significant 32% decrease in the incidence of the composite endpoint, but the decrease was no longer significant at 7 and 30 d. In PRISM-PLUS, patients with unstable angina and non-Q-wave MI were given aspirin and randomly assigned to receive either tirofiban, heparin, or two-thirds the tirofiban dose given in PRISM and heparin for a minimum of 48 h *(86)*. The tirofiban only arm was stopped because of an increase in 7- d mortality. However, there was a significant 30% decrease in the composite endpoints at 7 d in the tirofiban with heparin arm, a difference that narrowed to 20% at 30 d and 16% at 6 mo but remained statistically significant.

The results of these trials have validated GPIIb/IIIa as a pharmacologic target, have demonstrated that GPIIb/IIIa antagonists are effective in decreasing the risk for acute events in patients with coronary artery syndromes, and have shown that GPIIb/IIIa antagonists can be safely administered for short periods of time without excessive bleeding. Nonetheless, there is little evidence that the beneficial effect of these agents persists beyond the acute period.

3.3. Oral GPIIb/IIIa Antagonists

A number of orally active GPIIb/IIIa antagonists have been developed to extend the benefit of the intravenous agents. These antagonists, including xemilofiban, sibrafiban, lamifiban, lefradafiban, orbofiban, and roxifiban, are based on the RGD sequence and are pro-drugs that must be converted metabolically into active forms. In general, they have limited bioavailability and steep dose–response curves *(87,88)*.

The efficacy and safety of three of these antagonists have been examined in three large randomized and blinded controlled trials with largely unexpected and disappointing results. In the Sibrafiban vs Aspirin to Yield Maximum Protection from Ischemic Heart Events Post-Acute Coronary Syndromes (SYMPHONY) trial, patients with stable angina pectoris were randomized to receive aspirin, low-dose sibrafiban, or high-dose sibrafiban for 90 d *(89)*. At the end of 90 d, there was no difference in the rate of death, nonfatal or recurrent myocardial infarction, or severe recurrent ischemia between the three groups, but there was substantially more bleeding in patients who received sibrafiban, although most of the bleeding was minor. In the Evaluation of Xemilofiban in Controlling Thrombotic Events (EXCITE) trial, patients undergoing percutaneous coronary revascularization were randomized to receive placebo or xemilofiban and then were maintained on either placebo or one of two doses of xemilofiban for up to 182 d *(90)*. No difference in the incidence of death, nonfatal MI, or urgent revascularization was observed between the groups, but again the majority of patients receiving xemilofiban experienced minor bleeding. In the Phase III International Randomized Double Blind Placebo-Controlled Trial Evaluating the Efficacy and Safety of Orbofiban in Patients with Unstable Coronary Syndromes (OPUS-TIMI 16) trial, patients with unstable angina were given aspirin and were randomized to receive one of two orbofiban regimens or placebo. A analysis of results at 30 and 300 d indicated that treatment with orbofiban did not reduce clinical events and may have been associated with a small excess in early mortality *(91)*. There was also increased bleeding in patients receiving orbofiban. Taken together, these studies confirm the expectation, based on the clinical course of patients with Glanzmann thrombasthenia *(92)*, that patients undergoing chronic GPIIb/IIIa blockade will experience bleeding. Surprisingly, they also suggest that the currently available oral GPIIb/IIIa antagonists are no more effective, and may even be worse, than other currently available antiplatelet agents, such as aspirin.

3.4. Potential Alternative Strategies
for Identifying GPIIb/IIIa Antagonists

Although available data suggest that there may little more to be gained from the development of additional GPIIb/IIIa antagonists, the currently available agents are essentially based on a single theme. Thus, except for the monoclonal antibody Fab fragment abciximab, they have been designed around the RGD motif (with the notable exception of RWJ-53308, which is based on the sequence of the carboxyl terminus of the fibrinogen γ chain; ref. *93*). However, the effect of RGD-containing agents on GPIIb/IIIa function is indirect and under the appropriate conditions, RGD-containing peptides can induce, rather than inhibit, GPIIb/IIIa function *(94)*. It has been reported that fibrinogen binding to rabbit and rat platelets is relatively insensitive to inhibition by RGD-containing peptides *(95,96)*. Accordingly, we have studied the effect of the tetrapeptide Arg-Gly-Asp-Ser (RGDS) on fibrinogen binding to chimeric GPIIb/IIIa molecules composed of portions of the rat and human proteins *(97)*. We found that fibrinogen binding to CHO cells expressing human GPIIb/IIIa or a human GPIIb/rat GPIIIa hybrid was equally sensitive to RGDS, whereas cells expressing rat GPIIb/IIIa and a rat GPIIb/human GPIIIa hybrid were equally resistant, indicating that the sequences regulating GPIIb/IIIa responsiveness to RGD peptides are located in GPIIb. The amino terminus of GPIIb consists of seven tandem repeats *(65,98)*. To localize the sites in GPIIb regulating RGD responsiveness, we replaced amino terminal repeats of rat GPIIb with the corresponding human sequences and coexpressed the resulting chimeras with human GPIIIa. We found that when the first four repeats of rat GPIIb were replaced by the human sequences, the resulting heterodimer was sensitive to RGDS. In contrast, when the first two repeats were of human origin, the chimera was resistant. A chimera in which the first three repeats were human was of intermediate sensitivity. Thus, these data indicate that the sequences regulating the response of GPIIb/IIIa to RGDS are located in the third and fourth amino terminal repeats of GPIIb.

There are two ways that RGDS could inhibit fibrinogen binding to GPIIb/IIIa. First, RGDS could bind at or near the third and fourth repeats and directly compete with fibrinogen for binding. Second, RGDS binding could exert an inhibitory allosteric effect on the third and fourth repeats. To differentiate between these possibilities, we measured the ability of RGDS to induce the binding of the human β3-specific monoclonal antibody 10-758 to RGDS-sensitive and RGDS-resistant forms of GPIIb/IIIa. Because we found that RGDS induced equivalent 10-758 binding to each form of GPIIb/IIIa, it is likely that the RGD effect on GPIIb/IIIa is indirect and is the result of the induction of an allosteric change in the third and fourth amino terminal repeats of GPIIb.

In the recently reported crystal structure of a cyclic RGD ligand bound to the extracellular domain of αvβ3 *(99)*, the Arg side chain of RGD was present in a groove on the upper surface of the β propeller formed by loops connecting the second and third and third and fourth propeller blades. This is precisely the region of GPIIb we perturbed in our human/rat GPIIb chimeras. Thus, this region of GPIIb appears to exert allosteric regulation on fibrinogen binding to GPIIb/IIIa. Alterations in integrin tertiary and/or quaternary structure regulate their affinity, and possibly their avidity, for ligands. Recent studies of the domain I of the leukocyte integrin subunit αL emphasize the importance of changes in the conformation of the α subunit amino-terminus in integrin function. Ligands for the integrins αLβ2 and αMβ2 ligands, such as intercellular adhesion molecule-1, -2, and -3, bind to a divalent cation-containing MIDAS motif on the upper I domain surface *(100)*. However, amino acids distal to the MIDAS motif, lining a cleft formed by the seventh α-helix and the central β sheet of the I domain, regulate ligand binding to αLβ2 in an allosteric fashion *(100,101)*. In addition, the cleft constitutes the binding site for lovastatin, which locks the αLβ2 in an inactive conformation *(100)*. Thus, by analogy, it may be possible to identify non-RGD–based compounds that bind to the amino terminus of GPIIb and affect GPIIb/IIIa function in a manner similar to the effect of lovastatin on αLβ2. Because such compounds would not necessarily be peptides or peptidomimetics, their bioavailability and dose–response curves might more favorable than currently available GPIIb/IIIa antagonists, thereby fulfilling the theoretical promise of GPIIb/IIIa antagonists.

3.5. Proteins Expressed on the Platelet Surface after Platelet Activation

Several glycoproteins not present on the surface of resting platelets are translocated to the platelet surface during platelet secretion. These proteins are not involved directly in the initiation of thrombosis but are involved in later, thrombosis-induced, inflammatory reactions. Thus, agents that inhibit these proteins may have salutary effects on the course of disease processes such as atherosclerosis.

3.5.1. P-Selectin

P-selectin, a type I membrane protein that is present in the membranes of platelet α granules and granules in unstimulated endothelial cells, is phosphorylated and translocated to the surface of activated cells *(102)*. P-selectin is composed of an amino terminal C-type lectin domain, an epidermal growth factor domain, a series of complement repeats, a transmembrane domain, and a carboxyl-terminal cytoplasmic tail *(102)*. The major P-selectin ligand on leukocytes is PSGL-1, a mucin-like transmembrane protein that is located on the tips of microvilli of neutrophils, eosinophils, basophils, monocytes, and lymphocytes and is highly enriched in the O-linked fucosylated, sialylated glucosamines that are essential for P-selectin binding *(103,104)*. PSGL-1 binding to the lectin domain of endothelial cell and platelet P-selectin under flow conditions is largely responsible for leukocyte tethering and rolling on stimulated endothelium *(105)* and activated platelets *(106)* and for the incorporation of leukocytes into platelet thrombi *(102)*. The latter interaction may play an important role in the fibrin formation characteristic of inflammatory lesions because P-selectin binding to monocyte PSGL-1 induces the expression of tissue factor *(102)*. Moreover, P-selectin binding to PSGL-1 on primed monocytes mobilizes the transcription factor nuclear factor κB and induces the synthesis of a variety of chemokines *(102)*. Thus, impairing P-selectin function and PSGL-1 could potentially inhibit the synthesis and/or release of substances that amplify both inflammation and thrombosis.

3.5.2. CD40 Ligand (CD40L, CD154)

CD40 ligand (CD40L, CD154) is a transmembrane protein related to TNK-α *(107)*. It is present on CD4-positive T cells, mast cells, basophils, eosinophils, and natural killer cells. CD40L is involved in isotype switching in the immune response and mutations in humans result in the X-linked hyper-IgM syndrome. CD40L is also present in platelet granules and is translocated to the surface of activated platelets *(107)*. CD40, the receptor for CD40L, is present on endothelial cells and CD40 engagement results in upregulation of E-selectin, vascular cellular adhesion molecule-1, and intercellular adhesion molecule-1, as well as secretion of interleukin-8 and monocyte chemoattractant protein-1 (MCP-1) *(107)*. Thus, expression of platelet CD40L can initiate a vascular inflammatory response. CD40L also contains a KGD motif and can bind to isolated GPIIb/IIIa and to GPIIb/IIIa on thrombin-stimulated platelets *(108)*. Studies of experimentally induced arterial thrombosis in CD40L-deficient mice suggest that CD40L may be involved in the formation of a stable thrombus, a function that appears to be independent of CD40 and may involve KGD-dependent CD40L binding to GPIIb/IIIa *(108)*. However, thromboembolism has been reported after the administration of a monoclonal antibody against CD40L to monkeys undergoing renal transplantation *(109)*. Thus, CD40L appears to be involved at some point in thrombus formation, but defining its role in thrombus and its potential as a therapeutic target in thrombotic disease will require additional study.

REFERENCES

1. Sixma, J. J. and Wester, J. (1977) The hemostatic plug. *Semin. Hematol.* **14,** 265–299.
2. Lefkovits, J., Plow, E. and Topol, E. (1995) Platelet glycoprotein IIb/IIIa receptors in cardiovascular medicine. *N. Engl. J. Med.* **332,** 1553–1559.
3. Patrono, C. (1994) Aspirin as an antiplatelet drug. *N. Engl. J. Med.* **330,** 1287–1294.
4. Hemler, M. E., Crouse, C., Takada, Y. and Sonnenberg, A. (1988) Multiple very late antigen (VLA) heterodimers on platelets. Evidence for distinct VLA-2, VLA-5 (fibronectin receptor), and VLA-6 structures. *J. Biol. Chem.* **263,** 7660–7665.
5. Turitto, V. T., Weiss, H. J., Zimmerman, T. S., and Sussman, II. (1985) Factor VIII/von Willebrand factor in subendothelium mediates platelet adhesion. *Blood* **65,** 823–831.
6. Wagner, D. D. and Marder, V. J. (1984) Biosynthesis of von Willebrand protein by human endothelial cells: Processing steps and their intracellular localization. *J. Cell Biol.* **99,** 2123–2130.
7. Sporn, L. A., Chavin, S. I., Marder, V. J., and Wagner, D. D. (1985) Biosynthesis of von Willebrand protein by human megakaryocytes. *J. Clin. Invest.* **76,** 1102–1106.
8. Coller, B. S., Peerschke, E. I., Scudder, L. E. and Sullivan, C. A. (1983) Studies with a murine monoclonal antibody that abolishes ristocetin-induced binding of von Willebrand factor to platelets: Additional evidence in support of GPIb as a platelet receptor for von Willebrand factor. *Blood* **61,** 99–110.
9. Ruggeri, Z. M., DeMarco, L., Gatti, L., Bader, R. and Montgomery, R. R. (1983) Platelets have more than one binding site for von Willebrand factor. *J. Clin. Invest.* **72,** 1–12.
10. Ruggeri, Z. M. and Zimmerman, T. S. (1987) von Willebrand factor and von Willebrand disease. *Blood* **70,** 895–904.
11. Savage, B., Saldivar, E., and Ruggeri, Z. M. (1996) Initiation of platelet adhesion by arrest onto fibrinogen or translocation on von Willebrand factor. *Cell* **84,** 289–297.
12. Roth, G. J. (1991) Developing relationships: Arterial platelet adhesion, glycoprotein Ib, and leucine-rich glycoproteins. *Blood* **77,** 5–19.
13. Weiss, H. J., Tschopp, T. B., Baumgartner, H. R., Sussman, I. I., Johnson, M. M., and Egan, J. J. (1974) Decreased adhesion of giant (Bernard-Soulier) platelets to subendothelium. Further implications on the role of von Willebrand factor in hemostasis. *Am. J. Med.* **57,** 920–925.
14. Matsuno, H., Kozawa, O., Niwa, M., and Uematsu, T. (1997) Inhibition of von Willebrand factor binding to platelet GP Ib by a fractionated aurintricarboxylic acid prevents restenosis after vascular injury in hamster carotid artery. *Circulation* **96,** 1299–1304.
15. Okada, N. and Koizumi, S. (1995) A neuroprotective compound, aurin tricarboxylic acid, stimulates the tyrosine phosphorylation cascade in PC12 cells. *J. Biol. Chem.* **270,** 16,464–16,469.

16. Rui, H., Xu, J., Mehta, S., Fang, H., Williams, J., Dong, F., and Grimley, P. M. (1998) Activation of the Jak2-Stat5 signaling pathway in Nb2 lymphoma cells by an anti-apoptotic agent, aurintricarboxylic acid. *J. Biol. Chem.* **273**, 28–32.

17. Azzam, K., Cisse-Thiam, M., and Drouet, L. (1996) The antithrombotic effect of aurin tricarboxylic acid in the guinea pig is not solely due to its interaction with the von Willebrand factor-GPIb axis. *Thromb. Haemost.* **75**, 203–210.

18. Kageyama, S., Yamamoto, H., Nakazawa, H., Matsushita, J., Kouyama, T., Gonsho, A., et al. (2002) Pharmacokinetics and pharmacodynamics of AJW200, a humanized monoclonal antibody to von Willebrand factor, in monkeys. *Arterioscler. Thromb. Vasc. Biol.* **22**, 187–192.

19. Peng, M., Lu, W., Beviglia, L., Niewiarowski, S., and Kirby, E. P. (1993) Echicetin: A snake venom protein that inhibits binding of vonWillebrand factor and alboaggregins to platelet glycoprotein Ib. *Blood* **81**, 2321–2328.

20. Chang, M. C., Lin, H. K., Peng, H. C., and Huang, T. F. (1998) Antithrombotic effect of crotalin, a platelet membrane glycoprotein Ib antagonist from venom of Crotalus atrox. *Blood* **91**, 1582–1589.

21. Yeh, C. H., Chang, M. C., Peng, H. C., and Huang, T. F. (2001) Pharmacological characterization and antithrombotic effect of agkistin, a platelet glycoprotein Ib antagonist. *Br. J. Pharmacol.* **132**, 843–850.

22. Savage, B., Almus-Jacobs, F., and Ruggeri, Z. M. (1998) Specific synergy of multiple substrate-receptor interactions in platelet thrombus formation under flow. *Cell* **94**, 657–666.

23. Charo, I. F., Feinman, R. D., and Detwiler, T. C. (1977) Interrelations of platelet aggregation and secretion. *J. Clin. Invest.* **60**, 866–873.

24. Clemetson, J. M., Polgar, J., Magnenat, E., Wells, T. N., and Clemetson, K. J. (1999) The platelet collagen receptor glycoprotein VI is a member of the immunoglobulin superfamily closely related to FcαR and the natural killer receptors. *J. Biol. Chem.* **274**, 29,019–29,024.

25. Moroi, M., Jung, S. M., Okuma, M., and Shinmyozu, K. (1989) A patient with platelets deficient in glycoprotein VI that lack both collagen-induced aggregation and adhesion. *J. Clin. Invest.* **84**, 1440–1445.

26. Nieuwenhuis, H. K., Akkerman, J. W. N., Houdijk, W. P. M., and Sixma, J. J. (1985) Human blood platelets showing no response to collagen fail to express surface glycoprotein Ia. *Nature* **318**, 470–472.

27. Arai, M., Yamamoto, N., Moroi, M., Akamatsu, N., Fukutake, K., and Tanoue, K. (1995) Platelets with 10% of the normal amount of glycoprotein VI have an impaired response to collagen that results in a mild bleeding tendency. *Br. J. Haematol.* **89**, 124–130.

28. Nieuwenhuis, H. K., Sakariassen, K. S., Houdijk, W. P. M., Nievelstein, P. F. E. M., and Sixma, J. J. (1986) Deficiency of platelet membrane glycoprotein Ia associated with a decreased platelet adhesion to subendothelium: A defect in platelet spreading. *Blood* **68**, 692–695.

29. Kehrel, B., Balleisen, L., Kokott, R., Mesters, R., Stenzinger, W., Clemetson, K. J., and van de Loo, J. (1988) Deficiency of intact thrombospondin and membrane glycoprotein Ia in platelets with defective collagen-induced aggregation and spontaneous loss of disorder. *Blood* **71**, 1074–1078.

30. Santoso, S., Kunicki, T. J., Kroll, H., Haberbosch, W., and Gardemann, A. (1999) Association of the platelet glycoprotein Ia C807T gene polymorphism with nonfatal myocardial infarction in younger patients. *Blood* **93**, 2449–2453.

31. Carlsson, L. E., Santoso, S., Spitzer, C., Kessler, C., and Greinacher, A. (1999) The alpha2 gene coding sequence T807/A873 of the platelet collagen receptor integrin alpha2beta1 might be a genetic risk factor for the development of stroke in younger patients. *Blood* **93**, 3583–3586.

32. Corral, J., Gonzalez-Conejero, R., Rivera, J., Ortuno, F., Aparicio, P., and Vicente, V. (1999) Role of the 807 C/T polymorphism of the alpha2 gene in platelet GP Ia collagen

receptor expression and function—effect in thromboembolic diseases. *Thromb. Haemost.* **81,** 951–956.

33. Holtkotter, O., Nieswandt, B., Smyth, N., Muller, W., Hafner, M., Schulte, V., et al. (2002) Integrin alpha 2-deficient mice develop normally, are fertile, but display partially defective platelet interaction with collagen. *J. Biol. Chem.* **277,** 10,789–10,794.

34. Nieswandt, B., Brakebusch, C., Bergmeier, W., Schulte, V., Bouvard, D., et al. (2001) Glycoprotein VI but not alpha2beta1 integrin is essential for platelet interaction with collagen. *EMBO J.* **20,** 2120–2130.

35. Jandrot-Perrus, M., Busfield, S., Lagrue, A. H., Xiong, X., Debili, N., Chickering, T., et al. (2000) Cloning, characterization, and functional studies of human and mouse glycoprotein VI: A platelet-specific collagen receptor from the immunoglobulin superfamily. *Blood* **96,** 1798–1807.

36. Bennett, J. S. (1996) Structural biology of glycoprotein IIb-IIIa. *Trends Cardiovasc. Med.* **6,** 31–37.

37. Poncz, M., Eisman, R., Heidenreich, R., Silver, S. M., Vilaire, G., Surrey, S., et al. (1987) Structure of the platelet membrane glycoprotein IIb. *J. Biol. Chem.* **262,** 8476–8482.

38. Wagner, C. L., Mascelli, M. A., Neblock, D. S., Weisman, H. F., Coller, B. S., and Jordan, R. E. (1996) Analysis of GPIIb/IIIa receptor number by quantitation of 7E3 binding to human platelets. *Blood* **88,** 907–914.

39. Weisel, J. W., Nagaswami, C., Vilaire, G., and Bennett, J. S. (1992) Examination of the platelet membrane glycoprotein IIb/IIIa complex and its interaction with fibrinogen and other ligands by electron microscopy. *J. Biol. Chem.* **267,** 16,637–16,643.

40. Bennett, J. S. and Vilaire, G. (1979) Exposure of platelet fibrinogen receptors by ADP and epinephrine. *J. Clin. Invest.* **64,** 1393–1401.

41. Litvinov, R. I., Shuman, H., Bennett, J. S., and Weisel, J. W. (2002) Binding strength and activation state of single fibrinogen-integrin pairs on living cells. *Proc. Natl. Acad. Sci. USA* **99,** 7423–7431.

42. O'Toole, T. E., Katagiri, Y., Faull, R. J., Peter, K., Tamura, R., Quaranta, V., et al. (1994) Integrin cytoplasmic domains mediate inside-out signal transduction. *J. Cell. Biol.* **124,** 1047–1059.

43. Hillery, C. A., Smyth, S. S., and Parise, L. V. (1991) Phosphorylation of human platelet glycoprotein IIIa (GPIIIa) Dissociation from fibrinogen receptor activation and phosphorylation of GPIIIa in vitro. *J. Biol. Chem.* **266,** 14,663–14,669.

44. Hughes, P. E., Diaz-Gonzales, F., Leong, L., Wu, C., McDonald, J. A., Shattil, S. J., et al. (1996) Breaking the integrin hinge. A defined structural constraint regulates integrin signaling. *J. Biol. Chem.* **271,** 6571–6574.

45. Li, R., Babu, C. R., Lear, J. D., Wand, A. J., Bennett, J. S., and DeGrado, W. F. (2001) Oligomerization of the integrin alphaIIbbeta3: Roles of the transmembrane and cytoplasmic domains. *Proc. Natl. Acad. Sci. USA* **98,** 12,462–12,467.

46. Shattil, S. J., O'Toole, T., Eigenthaler, M., Thon, V., Williams, M., Babior, B. M., Ginsberg, M. H. (1995) β3-endonexin, a novel polypeptide that interacts specifically with the cytoplasmic tail of the integrin β3 subunit. *J. Cell. Biol.* **131,** 807–816.

47. Hannigan, G. E., Leung-Hagesteijn, C., Fitz-Gibbon, L., Coppolino, M. G., Redeva, G., Filmus, J., et al. (1996) Regulation of cell adhesion and anchorage-dependent growth by a new β1-integrin-linked protein kinase. *Nature* **379,** 91–95.

48. Naik, U. P., Patel, P. M., and Parise, L. V. (1997) Identification of a novel calcium-binding protein that interacts with the integrin αIIβ cytoplasmic domain. *J. Biol. Chem.* **272,** 4651–4654.

49. Kashiwagi, H., Schwartz, M. A., Eigenthaler, M., Davis, K. A., Ginsberg, M. H., and Shattil, S. J. (1997) Affinity modulation of platelet integrin αIIbβ3 by β3-endonexin, a selective binding partner of the β3 integrin cytoplasmic tail. *J. Cell Biol.* **137,** 1433–1443.

50. Tsuboi, S. (2002) Calcium integrin-binding protein activates platelet integrin alpha IIbbeta 3. *J. Biol. Chem.* **277,** 1919–1923.

51. Pfaff, M., Liu, S., Erle, D. J., and Ginsberg, M. H. (1998) Integrin beta cytoplasmic domains differentially bind to cytoskeletal proteins. *J. Biol. Chem.* **273,** 6104–6109.

52. Calderwood, D. A., Shattil, S. J., and Ginsberg, M. H. (2000) Integrins and actin filaments: Reciprocal regulation of cell adhesion and signaling. *J. Biol. Chem.* **275,** 22,607–22,610.

53. Reddy, K. B., Bialkowska, K., and Fox, J. E. (2001) Dynamic modulation of cytoskeletal proteins linking integrins to signaling complexes in spreading cells. Role of skelemin in initial integrin-induced spreading. *J. Biol. Chem.* **276,** 28,300–28,308.

54. Shattil, S. J., Kashiwagi, H., and Pampori, N. (1998) Integrin signaling: the platelet paradigm. *Blood* **91,** 2645–2657.

55. Calderwood, D. A., Zent, R., Grant, R., Rees, D. J., Hynes, R. O., and Ginsberg, M. H. (1999) The Talin head domain binds to integrin beta subunit cytoplasmic tails and regulates integrin activation. *J. Biol. Chem.* **274,** 28,071–28,074.

56. Hawiger, J., Kloczewiak, M., Bednarek, M. A., and Timmons, S. (1989) Platelet receptor recognition domains on the a chain of human fibrinogen: Structure-function analysis. *Biochemistry* **28,** 2929–2914.

57. Gartner, T. K. and Bennett, J. S. (1985) The tetrapeptide analogue of the cell attachment site of fibronectin inhibits platelet aggregation and fibrinogen binding to activated platelets. *J. Biol. Chem.* **260,** 11,891–11,894.

58. Farrell, D. H., Thiagarajan, P., Chung, D. W., and Davie, E. W. (1992) Role of fibrinogen α and γ chain sites in platelet aggregation. *Proc. Natl. Acad. Sci. USA* **89,** 10729–10732.

59. Farrell, D. H. and Thiagarajan, P. (1994) Binding of recombinant fibrinogen mutants to platelets. *J. Biol. Chem.* **269,** 226–231.

60. Bennett, J. S., Shattil, S. J., Power, J. W., and Gartner, T. K. (1988) Interaction of fibrinogen with its platelet receptor. Differential effects of a and g chain fibrinogen peptides on the glycoprotein IIb-IIIa complex. *J. Biol. Chem.* **263,** 12,948–12,953.

61. Hu, D. D., White, C. A., Panzer-Knodle, S., Page, J. D., Nicholson, N., and Smith, J. W. (1999) A new model of dual interacting ligand binding sites on integrin αIIbβ3. *J. Biol. Chem.* **274,** 4633–4639.

62. Puzon-McLaughlin, W., Kamata, T., and Takada, Y. (2000) Multiple discontinuous ligand-mimetic antibody binding sites define a ligand binding pocket in integrin αaIIbβ3. *J. Biol. Chem.* **275,** 7795–7802.

63. Lin, E. C. K., Ratnikov, B. I., Tsai, P. M., Carron, C. P., Myers, D. M., Barbas, C. F., III, and Smith, J. W. (1997) Identification of a region in the integrin β3 subunit that confers ligand binding specificity. *J. Biol. Chem.* **272,** 23,912–23,920.

64. D'Souza, S. E., Ginsberg, M. H., Lam, S. C., and Plow, E. F. (1988) Chemical cross-linking of arginyl-glycyl-aspartic acid peptides to an adhesion receptor on platelets. *J. Biol. Chem.* **263,** 3943–3951.

65. Xiong, J. P., Stehle, T., Diefenbach, B., Zhang, R., Dunker, R., Scott, D. L., et al. (2001) Crystal structure of the extracellular segment of integrin alpha Vbeta3. *Science* **294,** 339–345.

66. Basani, R. B., French, D. L., Vilaire, G., Brown, D. L., Chen, F., Coller, B. S., et al. (2000) A naturally occurring mutation near the amino terminus of aIIb defines a new region involved in ligand binding to aαibβ3. *Blood* **95,** 180–188.

67. Kamata, T., Tieu, K. K., Irie, A., Springer, T. A., and Takada, Y. (2001) Amino acid residues in the alpha IIb subunit that are critical for ligand binding to integrin alpha IIbbeta 3 are clustered in the beta-propeller model. *J. Biol. Chem.* **276,** 44,275–44,283.

68. Coller, B. S. (1985) A new murine monoclonal antibody reports an activation-dependent change in the conformation and/or microenvironment of the platelet glycoprotein IIb-IIIa complex. *J. Clin. Invest.* **76,** 101–108.

69. Coller, B. S. (1999) Binding of abciximab to αVβ3 and activated αMβ2 receptors: With a review of platelet-leukocyte interactions. *Thromb. Haemost.* **82,** 326–336.

70. Tcheng, J., Ellis, S., George, B., Kereiakes, D., Kleiman, N., Talley, J., et al. (1994) Pharmacodynamics of chimeric glycoprotein IIb/IIIa integrin antiplatelet antibody Fab 7E3 in high-risk coronary angioplasty. *Circulation* **90,** 1757–1764.

71. Mascelli, M. A., Lance, E. T., Damaraju, L., Wagner, C. L., Weisman, H. F., and Jordan, R. E. (1998) Pharmacodynamic profile of short-term abciximab treatment demonstrates prolonged platelet inhibition with gradual recovery from GP IIb/IIIa receptor blockade. *Circulation* **97,** 1680–1688.

72. EPIC Investigators. (1994) Use of a monoclonal antibody directed against the platelet glycoprotein IIb/IIIa receptor in high-risk coronary angioplasty. *N. Engl. J. Med.* **330,** 956–961.

73. EPILOG Investigators. (1997) Platelet glycoprotein IIb/IIIa receptor blockade and low-dose heparin during percutaneous coronary revascularization. The EPILOG Investigators. *N. Engl. J. Med.* **336,** 1689–1696.

74. CAPTURE Investigators. (1997) Randomised placebo-controlled trial of abciximab before and during coronary intervention in refractory unstable angina: the CAPTURE Study. *Lancet* **349,** 1429–1435.

75. EPISTENT Investigators. (1998) Randomised placebo-controlled and balloon-angioplasty-controlled trial to assess safety of coronary stenting with use of platelet glycoprotein-IIb/IIIa blockade. *Lancet* **352,** 87–92.

76. Phillips, D. R. and Scarborough, R. M. (1997) Clinical pharmacology of eptifibatide. *Am. J. Cardiol.* **80,** 11B–20B.

77. Harrington, R. A., Kleiman, N. S., Kottke-Marchant, K., Lincoff, A. M., Tcheng, J. E., Sigmon, K. N., et al. (1995) Immediate and reversible platelet inhibition after intravenous administration of a peptide glycoprotein IIb/IIIa inhibitor during percutaneous coronary intervention. *Am. J. Cardiol.* **76,** 1222–1227.

78. Phillips, D. R., Teng, W., Arfsten, A., Nannizzi-Alaimo, L., White, M. M., Longhurst, C., et al. (1997) Effect of Ca^{2+} on GP IIb-IIIa interactions with integrilin: enhanced GP IIb-IIIa binding and inhibition of platelet aggregation by reductions in the concentration of ionized calcium in plasma anticoagulated with citrate. *Circulation* **96,** 1488–1494.

79. IMPACT-II Investigators. (1997) Randomised placebo-controlled trial of effect of eptifibatide on complications of percutaneous coronary intervention: IMPACT-II. *Lancet* **349,** 1422–1428.

80. Harrington, R. A. (1997) Design and methodology of the PURSUIT trial: Evaluating eptifibatide for acute ischemic coronary syndromes. Platelet Glycoprotein IIb-IIIa in Unstable Angina: Receptor Suppression Using Integrilin Therapy. *Am. J. Cardiol.* **80,** 34B–38B.

81. ESPRIT Investigators. (2000) Novel dosing regimen of eptifibatide in planned coronary stent implantation (ESPRIT): A randomised, placebo-controlled trial. *Lancet* **356,** 2037–2044.

82. Cook, J. J., Bednar, B., Lynch, J. L., Jr., Gould, R. J., Egbertson, M. S., Halczenko, W., et al. (1999) Tirofiban (Aggrastat®). *Cardiovasc. Drug Rev.* **17,** 199–224.

83. RESTORE Investigators. (1997) Effects of platelet glycoprotein IIb/IIIa blockade with tirofiban on adverse cardiac events in patients with unstable angina or acute myocardial infarction undergoing coronary angioplasty. The RESTORE Investigators. Randomized Efficacy Study of Tirofiban for Outcomes and REstenosis. *Circulation* **96,** 1445–1453.

84. Gibson, C. M., Goel, M., Cohen, D. J., Piana, R. N., Deckelbaum, L. I., Harris, K. E., and King, S. B., 3rd. (1998) Six-month angiographic and clinical follow-up of patients prospectively randomized to receive either tirofiban or placebo during angioplasty in the RESTORE trial. Randomized Efficacy Study of Tirofiban for Outcomes and Restenosis. *J. Am. Coll. Cardiol.* **32,** 28–34.

85. PRISM Investigators. (1998) A comparison of aspirin plus tirofiban with aspirin plus heparin for unstable angina. *N. Engl. J. Med.* **338,** 1498–1505.

86. PRISM-PLUS Investigators. (1998) Inhibition of the platelet glycoprotein IIb/IIIa receptor with tirofiban in unstable angina and non-Q-wave myocardial infarction. *N. Engl. J. Med.* **338,** 1488–1497.

87. Theroux, P. (1998) Oral inhibitors of platelet membrane receptor glycoprotein IIb/IIIa in clinical cardiology: Issues and opportunities. *Am. Heart J.* **135**, S107–S112.
88. Kereiakes, D. J. (1999) Oral blockade of the platelet glycoprotein IIb/IIIa receptor: Fact or fancy? *Am. Heart J.* **138**, S39–46.
89. SYMPHONY Investigators. (2000) Comparison of sibrafiban with aspirin for prevention of cardiovascular events after acute coronary syndromes: A randomized trial. *Lancet* **355**, 337–345.
90. O'Neill, W. W., Serruys, P., Knudtson, M., Van Es, G.-A., Timmis, G. C., van der Zwaan, C., et al. (2000) Long-term treatment with a platelet glycoprotein-receptor antagonist after percutaneous coronary revascularization. *N. Engl. J. Med.* **342**, 1316–1324.
91. Cannon, C. P., McCabe, C. H., Wilcox, R. G., Langer, A., Caspi, A., Berink, P., et al. (2000) Oral glycoprotein IIb/IIIa inhibition with orbofiban in patients with unstable coronary syndromes (OPUS-TIMI 16) trial. *Circulation* **102**, 149–56.
92. George, J. N., Caen, J. P., and Nurden, A. T. (1990) Glanzmann's thrombasthenia: The spectrum of clinical disease. *Blood* **75**, 1383–1395.
93. Damiano, B. P., Mitchell, J. A., Giardino, E., Corcoran, T., Haertlein, B. J., de Garavilla, L., et al. (2001) Antiplatelet and antithrombotic activity of RWJ-53308, a novel orally active glycoprotein IIb/IIIa antagonist. *Thromb. Res.* **104**, 113–126.
94. Du, X. P., Plow, E. F., Frelinger, A. L., III, OToole, T. E., Loftus, J. C., and Ginsberg, M. H. (1991) Ligands "activate" integrin alpha IIb beta 3 (platelet GPIIb/IIIa) *Cell* **65**, 409–416.
95. Harfenist, E. J., Packham, M. A., and Mustard, J. F. (1988) Effects of cell adhesion peptide, Arg-Gly-Asp-Ser, on responses of washed platelets from humans, rabbits, and rats. *Blood* **71**, 132–136.
96. Jennings, L. K., White, M. M., and Mandrell, T. D. (1995) Interspecies comparison of platelet aggregation, LIBS expression and clot retraction: Observed differences in GPIIb/IIIa functional activity. *Thromb. Haemostas.* **74**, 1551–1556.
97. Basani, R. B., D'Andrea, G., Mitra, N., Vilaire, G., Richberg, M., Kowalska, M. A., et al. (2001) RGD-containing peptides inhibit fibrinogen binding to platelet alpha(IIb)beta3 by inducing an allosteric change in the amino-terminal portion of alpha(IIb) *J. Biol. Chem.* **276**, 13,975–13,981.
98. Springer, T. A. (1997) Folding of the N-terminal, ligand-binding region of integrin a-subunits into a β-propeller domain. *Proc. Natl. Acad. Sci., USA* **94**, 65–72.
99. Xiong, J. P., Stehle, T., Zhang, R., Joachimiak, A., Frech, M., Goodman, S. L., and Arnaout, M. A. (2002) Crystal structure of the extracellular segment of integrin alpha Vbeta3 in complex with an Arg-Gly-Asp ligand. *Science* **296**, 151–155.
100. Kallen, J., Welzenbach, K., Ramage, P., Geyl, D., Kriwacki, R., Legge, G., et al. (1999) Structural basis for LFA-1 inhibition upon lovastatin binding to the CD11a I-domain. *J. Mol. Biol.* **292**, 1–9.
101. Huth, J. R., Olejniczak, E. T., Mendoza, R., Liang, H., Harris, E. A., Lupher, M. L., Jr., et al. (2000) NMR and mutagenesis evidence for an I domain allosteric site that regulates lymphocyte function-associated antigen 1 ligand binding. *Proc. Natl. Acad. Sci. USA* **97**, 5231–5236.
102. Furie, B., Furie, B. C., and Flaumenhaft, R. (2001) A journey with platelet P-selectin: The molecular basis of granule secretion, signalling and cell adhesion. *Thromb. Haemost.* **86**, 214–221.
103. Yang, J., Furie, B. C., and Furie, B. (1999) The biology of P-selectin glycoprotein ligand-1: Its role as a selectin counterreceptor in leukocyte-endothelial and leukocyte-platelet interaction. *Thromb. Haemost.* **81**, 1–7.
104. McEver, R. P. (2002) P-selectin and PSGL-1: Exploiting connections between inflammation and venous thrombosis. *Thromb. Haemost.* **87**, 364–365.
105. Mayadas, T. N., Johnson, R. C., Rayburn, H., Hynes, R. O., and Wagner, D. D. (1993) Leukocyte rolling and extravasation are severely compromised in P selectin-deficient mice. *Cell* **74**, 541–554.

106. Subramaniam, M., Frenette, P. S., Saffaripour, S., Johnson, R. C., Hynes, R. O., and Wagner, D. D. (1996) Defects in hemostasis in P-selectin-deficient mice. *Blood* **87,** 1238–1242.

107. Henn, V., Slupsky, J. R., Grafe, M., Anagnostopoulos, I., Forster, R., Muller-Berghaus, G., and Kroczek, R. A. (1998) CD40 ligand on activated platelets triggers an inflammatory reaction of endothelial cells. *Nature* **391,** 591–594.

108. Andre, P., Prasad, K. S., Denis, C. V., He, M., Papalia, J. M., Hynes, R. O., et al. (2002) CD40L stabilizes arterial thrombi by a beta3 integrin-dependent mechanism. *Nat. Med.* **8,** 247–252.

109. Kawai, T., Andrews, D., Colvin, R. B., Sachs, D. H., and Cosimi, A. B. (2000) Thromboembolic complications after treatment with monoclonal antibody against CD40 ligand. *Nat. Med.* **6,** 114.

7

The Sodium–Hydrogen Exchange System in the Heart

A Target for the Protection of the Ischemic and Reperfused Heart and Inhibition of Heart Failure

Morris Karmazyn

CONTENTS

1. INTRODUCTION

Sodium–hydrogen exchange (NHE) is among the most important processes involved in pH regulation in the cardiac cell, especially under ischemic conditions. There is now excellent evidence that stimulation of NHE contributes to paradoxical induction of cell injury. The mechanism for this is related to the fact that activation of the exchanger is closely coupled to sodium influx and, therefore, to elevation in intracellular calcium concentrations through the Na–Ca exchange. The NHE is exquisitely sensitive to intracellular acidosis, however, other factors can also stimulate the exchanger through phosphorylation-dependent as well as independent processes. Seven NHE isoforms have been identified and designated as NHE-1 through NHE-7. NHE-1 to NHE-5 are found in the cell membrane, whereas NHE-6 and NHE-7 are located intracellularly. NHE-1 is the major subtype in the mammalian myocardium. The predominance of NHE-1 in the myocardium is of some importance because pharmacological development of NHE

From: *Cardiac Drug Development Guide*
Edited by: M. K. Pugsley © Humana Press Inc., Totowa, NJ

inhibitors for cardiac therapeutics has concentrated specifically on those agents that are selective for NHE-1. These agents, as well as the earlier nonspecific amiloride derivatives have now been extensively demonstrated to possess excellent cardioprotective properties. The salutary effects of NHE inhibitors have been demonstrated using a variety of experimental models as well as animal species, suggesting that the role of the NHE in mediating injury is not species-specific. The success of NHE inhibitors in experimental studies has led to clinical trials for the evaluation of these agents in high-risk patients with coronary artery disease as well as in patients with acute myocardial infarction. Recent evidence also suggests that NHE inhibition inhibits the remodeling process after myocardial infarction, independently of infarct size reduction, and also heart failure caused by other factors. As such, inhibitors of NHE offer substantial promise for clinical development for attenuation of both acute responses to myocardial as well as chronic postinfarction responses resulting in the evolution to heart failure.

Changes in intracellular pH can have profound effects on cardiac contractility through complex mechanisms. It is therefore critical that the cell possesses mechanisms by which intracellular (pH_i) is regulated especially after intracellular acidosis as a consequence of myocardial ischemia. Although the regulation of pH_i is very complex and reflects a net balance of alkalinizing and acidification processes, the two major alkalinizing exchangers that are important for controlling intracellular acidosis are the Na–H exchanger (NHE) and a Na–HCO_3^- symport *(1)*. The NHE represents one of the key mechanisms for restoring pH_i following ischemia-induced acidosis by extruding protons concomitantly with Na influx in an electroneutral process. At present, seven NHE isoforms have been identified (termed NHE-1 to NHE-7) with the NHE-1 subtype representing the ubiquitous isoform, although it appears that it is the primary one found in the mammalian heart. When NHE is activated, the simultaneous entry of Na during NHE activation likely represents an important route for increasing intracellular Na concentrations during various conditions. In the ischemic cell particularly, the activation of NHE by intracellular proton generation and the resultant entry of Na results in a potential disastrous consequence because of the fact that the excess Na cannot be extruded because of depressed Na-K ATPase activity. As a result, the reduction in the transmembrane Na gradient will result in increased intracellular Ca levels via the Na–Ca exchanger, producing intracellular Ca overload and cell death. Pharmacological studies with NHE inhibitors have extensively and repeatedly demonstrated protective effects in a large number of experimental models. Inhibition of NHE as a therapeutic tool has now entered the clinical arena as reflected by substantial effort by the pharmaceutical industry to develop potent NHE-1–specific inhibitors with potential as effective therapeutic agents in patients with coronary artery disease. Indeed, some of these agents have either undergone or are currently in the process of clinical evaluation. Importantly, it is now emerging that in addition to its potential role in mediating ischemic and reperfusion injury, NHE also contributes to the postinfarction hypertrophic and remodeling process, which can lead to the eventual development of heart failure. As such, a potential added benefit of NHE-1 inhibitors may include attenuation of the evolution of infarcted myocardium to failure. The aim of this review is to summarize our current knowledge of NHE-1 in the heart in terms of its structure and regulation, and of particular relevance, the importance of NHE-1 in cardiac pathology. The role of NHE-1 in the ischemic and reperfused heart has now been firmly established and reviewed in a number of recent publications *(2,3)*.

Accordingly, heavier emphasis will be placed on the emerging role of NHE-1 in the heart failure process that could represent a completely novel approach toward treating heart failure.

2. NHE ISOFORMS

As alluded to in the previous section, to date seven isoforms of NHE have been identified in mammalian cells. They represent distinct gene products and exhibit distinct differences in their primary structures, patterns of tissue expression, membrane localization, the number of transmembrane spanning regions, functional properties, physiological roles, and sensitivities to pharmacological inhibition *(4,5)*. NHE-1 is expressed in virtually all mammalian cells, whereas NHE-2 to NHE-5 show a more restricted pattern of expression. NHE-6 is intracellularly localized *(6,7)* and could be an important modulator of intramitochondrial Na and H levels as well mitochondrial Ca levels, particularly in pathological conditions *(6)*; however, substantial research in necessary to delineate the potential role of NHE6 in the heart either under normal or pathological conditions. NHE7 is located within the Golgi network *(8)*.

3. STRUCTURE AND CELLULAR LOCALIZATION OF NHE-1

As depicted in Fig. 1, NHE-1 contains 815 amino acids and can be separated into two distinct functional domains: a 500-amino acid transmembrane domain, made up of 12 transmembrane spanning segments, and a 315-amino acid hydrophilic cytoplasmic carboxy-terminal domain. The 500-amino acid transmembrane domain is primarily responsible for proton extrusion, and the 315-amino acid C-terminal domain is responsible for modulation of NHE-1 activity, primarily via phosphorylation-dependent reactions *(4,9)*. Although the predicted molecular weight of the exchanger is 91 kDa, the actual weight is 110 kDa because it is glycosylated, although this does not appear to be essential for transport function *(10)*.

Immunohistochemical studies have revealed that NHE-1 is predominantly localized at the intercalated disk region of atrial and ventricular myocytes in close proximity to the gap junction protein, connexin 43 and, to a lesser extent, along the transverse tubular system *(11)*. Connexin 43 and the sarcoplasmic reticulum Ca release channel (i.e., ryanodine receptor) are highly pH_i sensitive. Thus, it has been speculated that because of its apparent localization, NHE-1 regulates the pH microenvironment of these pH_i-sensitive proteins and thereby influences cell-to-cell ion dependent communication and intracellular Ca levels *(11)*.

4. REGULATION OF NHE-1 ACTIVITY

4.1. Role of pH_i

The major stimulus that regulates NHE-1 activity under normal physiological conditions is pH_i *(12)*. Within the normal physiological pH range (pH 7.1–7.3), NHE-1 activity is negligible, but as pH_i decreases, the exchanger becomes rapidly activated. The reason for this rapid activation is caused by the so-called H sensor, which is found on the cytoplasmic surface of the exchanger and accounts for the sensitivity of the exchanger to pH_i. Although the exact nature of the molecular mechanisms involved in

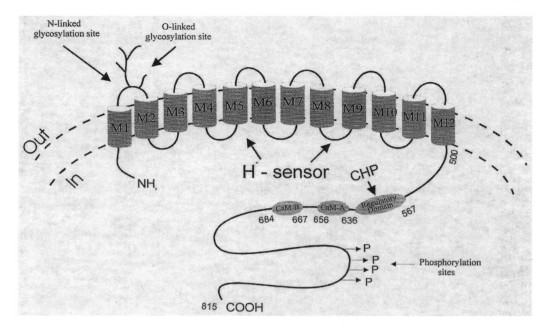

Fig. 1. Putative topological model of 815 amino acid NHE-1 showing 12 transmembrane spanning segments and hydrophilic carboxyl terminus with indications of proposed regulatory sites. *See* text for details.

activation by the H sensor is poorly understood, it is believed that binding of H to this site induces a conformational change of the NHE oligomer, resulting in an increase in NHE activity *(13)*. Extrinsic factors, such as hormones, growth factors, cytokines, and autocrine/paracrine regulators, modulate NHE-1 activity by increasing the sensitivity of the H sensor to pH_i, thus causing a shift of NHE-1 activity toward an alkaline range; that is, NHE-1 activity increases at a less acidic pH_i. This shift in pH_i dependence is accomplished mainly via phosphorylation reactions of the C-terminal domain of the exchanger, which is responsible for determining the pH_i set point value of the H sensor *(9,14)*.

4.2. Activation by Paracrine and Autocrine Factors

Various signaling pathways can modulate cardiac NHE-1 activity, including endothelin-1 *(15,16)*, angiotensin II *(17,18)*, α_1-adrenergic agonists *(19,20)*, thrombin *(21)*, and growth factors *(14,22,23)*. Accordingly, it is important to stress that these stimulatory factors are modulators of normal cardiac activity and are also potential contributors to cardiac pathology. The effects of these agonists generally involve phosphoinositide hydrolysis and activation of kinases, such as protein kinase C (PKC), resulting in NHE-1 activation *(4,9,23,24)*. In addition, cardiotoxic ischemic metabolites, such as hydrogen peroxide *(25)* and lysophosphatidylcholine *(26)*, have also been demonstrated to stimulate NHE-1 activity, a phenomenon that likely contributes to the cardiotoxic effects of these factors.

4.3. Phosphorylation-Dependent Regulation

Structure–function studies have indicated that NHE-1 contains consensus sequences for mitogen-activated protein (MAP) kinases, which have been implicated in NHE-1 phosphorylation and activation *(25,27)*, and it has been established, using rabbit skeletal muscle, that MAP kinases can directly phosphorylate the C-terminal domain of NHE-1 *(27)*. Recently, a role for p90[rsk] in MAP kinase-dependent phosphorylation of NHE-1 has been demonstrated in rat myocardium *(28)*. In addition, hypoxia, hypoxia with reoxygenation *(29)*, hydrogen peroxide *(25)*, and other reactive oxygen species *(30)* have been known to stimulate the MAP kinase signaling pathway, which can contribute to NHE-1 activation.

4.4. Phosphorylation-Independent Regulation

NHE-1 activity can also be regulated via phosphorylation-independent mechanisms *(31,32)*. For example, deletion of the cytoplasmic C-terminal domain at residue 635 removes all phosphorylation sites, although this reduces growth factor activation of NHE-1 by only 50% *(27)*. In addition, NHE-1 activity can be completely eliminated after deletion of residues 567–635, while at the same time preserving mitogen-stimulated phosphorylation *(32)*. These studies therefore strongly implicate factors other than phosphorylation, which may be involved in NHE-1 activation. Bertrand et al. *(31)* reported that the cytoplasmic C-terminal tail of NHE-1 contained two domains capable of binding calmodulin with either high (CaM-A residues 636–656) or low (CaM-B residues 567–635) affinity. The high affinity CaM-A site is believed to be important in transport regulation. Deletions of residues 636–656 render NHE-1 constitutively active, as if cytosolic Ca levels were continuously elevated. Based on these observations, it was suggested that at basal intracellular Ca levels, the unoccupied CaM-A binding domain exerts an autoinhibitory effect that is relieved upon Ca/calmodulin binding *(32)*. Although this has yet to be demonstrated in the myocardium, it nevertheless suggests an alternative method for NHE-1 activation in pathological conditions in which intracellular Ca levels are elevated.

4.5. Role of ATP in Regulating NHE-1 Activity

ATP has also been demonstrated to regulate NHE-1 activity. Depletion of cytoplasmic ATP results in reduced transport activity of the exchanger *(33,34)*, although it appears that this is unlikely related to changes in the phosphorylation state of the exchanger *(34)*. It has been hypothesized that a yet-to-be-identified ancillary protein may mediate the effect of ATP depletion on NHE-1 activity. It is believed that an ATP-dependent reversible association of a cofactor may regulate the exchanger and that upon binding of ATP, this cofactor will dissociate from the exchanger and remove its inhibitory effect *(34)*. Whether this has relevance to the regulation of NHE-1 in the ischemic myocardium is not known, particularly because ATP depletion during ischemia is a relatively slow process. However, the possibility exists that very low levels of the nucleotide in ischemic myocytes could potentially counter the stimulatory effect of intracellular acidosis on NHE-1 activity *(2)*.

4.6. NHE-1 Activation by G Proteins

It is also worth mentioning that a number of G proteins can modulate NHE-1 activity, although they have only been demonstrated to do so in noncardiac tissue. The mechanisms by which G proteins stimulate NHE-1 activity are very complex and vary depending on the G protein type. For example, $G_{\alpha q}$ and $G_{\alpha 12}$ have been shown to regulate NHE-1 activity primarily via a PKC-dependent pathway, whereas $G_{\alpha 13}$ mediates

NHE-1 activity via a PKC-independent pathway *(35–37)*. $G_{\alpha 13}$ uses a distinct kinase cascade, using the Rho family of GTPases (Cdc42 and RhoA) to activate NHE-1 through MAP/extracellular signal-regulated kinase kinase 1–dependent (Cdc42) and – independent (RhoA) pathways *(38)*.

5. REGULATION OF NHE-1 EXPRESSION

Another important level of regulation of NHE-1 deals with the number of available exchanger units available on the plasma membrane. Although the majority of the studies published on the regulation of NHE-1 have focused on regulation of activity, only a few studies have focused on the regulation of expression of the exchanger. This primarily reflects the fact that the promoter region of NHE-1 has only been recently cloned. Kolyada et al *(39)* used footprinting analysis to identify the existence of four protected sites that were able to bind to hepatic proteins and that two of these binding regions (B and C) contained a binding site for the activator protein-2 (AP-2) or the AP-2-like transcription factor *(39)*. Although the AP-2 site contributes to the transcriptional regulation of NHE-1 in cardiomyocytes, a majority of NHE-1 promoter activity has been demonstrated to be caused by elements distal to the AP-2 site, primarily a poly(d·>dT)-rich region *(40,41)*. Irrespective of exact mechanism for transcriptional regulation of NHE-1, it is nonetheless relevant that many factors that produce cell injury, including myocardial ischemia or the direct administration of cardiotoxic compounds, including lysophosphatidylcholine or hydrogen peroxide, can all increase tissue levels of NHE-1 mRNA, suggesting that the exchanger may be stimulated by both increased activity as well as turnover *(42)*.

6. MECHANISMS UNDERLYING NHE INVOLVEMENT IN MYOCARDIAL ISCHEMIC AND REPERFUSION INJURY

The primary basis for NHE-1 involvement in acute injury reflects the inability to extrude sodium by the ischemic cardiac cell because of Na-K ATPase inhibition, which occurs in concert with NHE-1 activation, the latter occurring as a consequence of increased proton generation during ischemia. Indeed, it could be stated that inhibition of Na-K ATPase is a prerequisite for NHE-1 involvement in ischemic and reperfusion injury and that in the absence of such inhibition NHE-1 activation would be unlikely to represent a deleterious influence on the myocardium. In addition, as noted above, NHE-1 is further activated by various hormonal, autocrine, or paracrine factors as well as metabolites produced either extracellularly or intracellularly during myocardial ischemia, including hydrogen peroxide and lysophosphatidylcholine. Thus, the net result is a multifactorial stimulation of NHE under pathological conditions, not only because of increased intracellular acidosis but also because of activation by external factors. Such marked NHE-1 stimulation increases an elevation in intracellular sodium levels, which in turn increases intracellular calcium levels via Na–Ca exchange resulting in cell injury.

It should be noted that an alternate concept regarding a reperfusion-induced NHE-dependent injury through Ca-independent mechanisms has also been proposed that has been termed the pH paradox. This hypothesis proposes that the reduction in intracellular ATP levels during myocardial ischemia results in phospholipase and protease activation, which would normally produce cell membrane injury; however, because these enzymes possess pH optima in the alkaline range their detrimental effects are attenuated by ischemia-induced acidosis. Upon reperfusion the rapid restoration of pH_i reverses the suppression of proteases and other enzymes seen during the ischemic period and results in cell death *(43)*. In addition, the restoration of pH_i stimulates the formation of the mitochondrial membrane permeability transition, which results in depression of ATP resynthesis via oxidative phosphorylation pathways *(43)*. The relative contribution of this process to NHE-1–dependent cardiac injury is, however, not certain but is supported by studies using individual myocytes illustrating a protective effect of NHE inhibition against reoxygenation, which can be dissociated from intracellular Ca levels *(44)*. It is possible that this mechanism may contribute specifically to reperfusion injury per se but obviously would not account for the potential role of NHE-1 inhibition during ischemia in the absence of reperfusion where the exchanger plays a critical role.

7. PHARMACOLOGICAL MODULATION OF NHE ACTIVITY

The first series of drugs that have been demonstrated to inhibit NHE are the potassium-sparing diuretic amiloride and, more specifically, the N-5–disubstituted derivatives of amiloride, which exhibit greater potency and specificity than the parent compound *(45)*. Despite the ability of these agents to inhibit NHE, their eventual therapeutic development has been restricted by various nonspecific actions, lack of selectivity against NHE-1, and relatively low potency. This has led to the development of novel benzoylguanidine compounds targeted specifically against NHE-1, thereby increasing potential for treatment in patients with coronary artery disease *(46–48)*. The first such compound was 3-methylsulphonyl-4-piperidinobenzoyl-guanidine methanesulphonate (HOE 694), developed by Hoechst Marion Roussel (now Aventis), which was followed by 4-isopropyl-3-methylsulphonylbenzoyl-guanidine methanesulphonate (HOE 642, cariporide), the latter, as discussed below currently undergoing clinical trials. Cariporide is a selective inhibitor of the cardiac-specific NHE-1 isoform, rendering it particularly attractive for therapeutic interventions for cardiac disorders while minimizing the potential for side effects. The mechanism of action of NHE-1 inhibitors is not known precisely, although their effects on the antiporter involve binding to sites on the lipophilic transmembrane region. After the construction of a variety of chimeric NHE constructs, Orlowski and Kandasamy *(49)* demonstrated potential sites on a number of transmembrane units to which these drugs can bind with the M4 and M9 regions of particular importance.

8. MYOCARDIAL PROTECTION BY NHE-1 INHIBITORS

The extensive documentation demonstrating cardioprotective effects of NHE inhibitors has strongly supported the concept of the antiporter's involvement in cardiac injury, especially under conditions of ischemia and reperfusion. The earlier studies used amiloride or amiloride analogs to demonstrate cardioprotective properties; however, more recent data using drugs targeted for clinical development reported excellent and consistent protection in a wide variety of experimental models and animal species that is likely unmatched in the cardioprotection literature. A number of such agents are either in clinical or preclinical development and all have been show to protect the myocardium against either ischemia or reperfusion or against the direct deleterious effects of cardiotoxic compounds produced by the ischemic myocardium. Moreover, there appear to be no discrepant results that fail to show protective effects of NHE-1 inhibitors. In addition, the protective effects of NHE-1 inhibitors appear to be species independent. A particularly striking feature of NHE-1 inhibitors is their ability to protect against various forms of dysfunctions, including reduced mortality, limitation of infarct size, improvement of functional recovery after reperfusion, reduction of arrhythmias, attenuation of calcium and sodium dyshomeostasis, reduction of apoptosis, as well as the preservation of metabolic status such as attenuation of high energy phosphate depletion. Many of the newer drugs have been tested for their ability to protect the myocardium when administered only at reperfusion, a property that would be important in terms of treatment of patients who present with acute myocardial infarction. Most agents do indeed demonstrate protective effects when administered at this period, although it should be stated that, in general, such protection is less than that seen with pre-ischemia drug administration. From a mechanistic perspective, these findings are not surprising because NHE-1 activation during ischemia contributes substantially to the sodium and calcium overloading conditions and resultant cell injury with further NHE-1 activation occurring immediately upon reflow. As such, optimum protective effects of NHE-1 inhibitors are likely realized when treatment can be maintained during both ischemia and reperfusion.

It is also interesting to note that the potential for toxicity or untoward side effects of NHE-1 inhibitors is relatively low in view of the specificity of newer agents. Moreover, it is important to point out that drugs targeted at NHE-1 inhibition have limited potential for disruption of normal cell homeostasis because NHE-1 activity is generally restricted under normal conditions, thus, these drugs have the potential for selectivity inhibiting a process associated primarily with pathology. Indeed, clinical evaluation of both cariporide and eniporide revealed excellent tolerance. For a fuller discussion of the role of NHE-1 in the ischemic reperfused heart, readers are referred to a number of recent reviews *(2,3)*.

9. CLINICAL EVALUATION OF NHE-1 INHIBITORS IN PATIENTS WITH CORONARY HEART DISEASE

A number of clinical studies have been performed with varying degrees of success. For example, the Guard During Ischemia Against Necrosis (GUARDIAN) study revealed no overall beneficial effects of the NHE-1 inhibitor cariporide in patients with acute coronary syndromes, although significant protection was observed with the highest cariporide dose, particularly in high-risk patients undergoing coronary artery bypass surgery *(50,51)*. Administering an NHE-1 inhibitor to patients at reperfusion after acute myocardial infarction has produced mixed results. In one study, the NHE-1 inhibitor eniporide failed to reduce injury as determined by enzyme values *(52)*. However, in a much smaller study, cariporide was found to improve ventricular function and decrease enzyme release when administered to patients prior to angioplasty *(53)*. The discrepant findings may be related to dosing levels, particularly because animal data revealed that NHE-1 inhibitors are less effective when administered at reperfusion and then only at concentrations substantially higher than those used when administered before ischemia.

Further assessment of clinical results with NHE-1 inhibitors can be obtained in a recent review *(54)*.

10. ROLE OF NHE-1 IN CARDIAC HYPERTROPHY AND HEART FAILURE

10.1. The Need for New Therapeutic Strategies for the Treatment of Heart Failure

The past number of years have seen substantial improvement in the therapeutic approaches for the treatment of heart failure (reviewed in ref. *55*) The introduction of angiotensin-converting enzyme (ACE) inhibitors and increased use of β adrenoceptor blockers have added to the armamentarium treating this complex syndrome. The incidence of heart failure is expanding rapidly primarily because of an aging population and also to increased survival rates after myocardial infarction. Indeed, in up to 70% of patients with heart failure its causative factors can be related to myocardial infarction. In the United States alone, more than 500,000 new cases of heart failure are diagnosed yearly. Yet, despite improved therapeutic strategies, mortality rates in patients with heart failure continue to be high. Understanding the fundamental underlying mechanisms for the development of heart failure, particularly in terms in the chronic maladaptive responses or remodeling likely holds the key for potentially effective heart failure management. As discussed below, NHE-1 may represent one such key target.

10.2. Theoretical Considerations for NHE-1 Involvement in Hypertrophy and Heart Failure

Myocardial hypertrophy, remodeling, and heart failure represent many complex events but in general involve initiating factors, such as increase in mechanical load and upregulation of a large number of hormonal, paracrine, and autocrine factors that contribute to the process through receptor-mediated changes in intracellular signaling *(55)*. As illustrated in Fig. 2, one of the major reasons for considering NHE-1 as a potentially important contributor to the heart failure process is based on the fact that, already alluded to in Section 4.2., the antiporter represents a key downstream factor activated by many such factors including α_1 adrenoceptor agonists, angiotensin II, and endothelin-1. Indeed, in cardiac cells, NHE inhibitors block hypertrophic responses to various stimuli. Stretch-induced stimulation in protein synthesis in neonatal cardiac myocytes as well as stretch-induced alkalinization in feline papillary muscles can be blocked by NHE inhibitors *(56,57)* as can norepinephrine-induced protein synthesis in cultured rat cardiomyocytes *(58)*. These studies reveal a commonality in terms of responses to a wide array of hypertrophic factors. Indeed, it has been suggested that NHE-1 activation represents a common response to mechanical stretch and a key player in the hypertrophic process *(59)*. Thus, cellular deformation under pathological conditions could lead to a cascade of events, resulting in cell hypertrophy and eventual myocardial remodeling. It has been proposed that this occurs as a consequence of the activation of both angiotensin II AT_1 receptors as well as the endothelin-1 ET_A receptor, which then activate intracellular signal transduction pathways, leading to increased NHE-1 activity and cell growth *(59,60)*. This may occur in an autocrine or paracrine fashion in which stretch stimulates the local release of these peptides, which then act on their respective receptor.

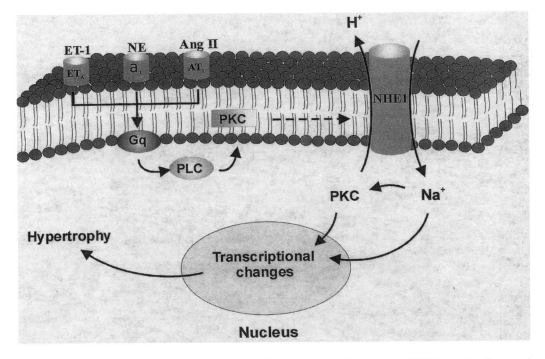

Fig. 2. A simplified illustration of possible pathways leading to NHE-1 activation and potential relevance to cell growth. Briefly, activation of NHE-1 can occur via a phospholipase C (PLC) resulting in increased phosphoinositide hydrolysis (not shown) via a G_q protein-dependent pathway. This would eventually lead to PKC activation, which would produce a stimulation of NHE-1 (dashed arrow), directly through PKC-dependent phosphorylation or phosphorylation through other kinases, such as MAP kinase. Irrespective of the exact mechanism, the resultant increased entry of Na ions through NHE-1 would cause transcriptional changes within the nucleus either through direct effect of the ions or secondary to PKC activation resulting in increased protein synthesis and hypertrophy. Various factors can activate this series of events including endothelin-1 (ET-1) acting on the ET_A receptors, norepinephrine (NE) acting on the $\alpha 1$ adrenergic receptor or angiotensin II (Ang II) through the AT_1 receptor. Thus, blocking NHE-1 would attenuate the hypertrophic effects of at least three factors, rendering it an attractive therapeutic strategy.

10.3. Experimental Evidence for NHE Involvement in Cell Hypertrophy and Heart Failure

Although experimental studies are still in their relative infancy, initial findings using NHE-1 inhibitors have been encouraging and support the concept that inhibition of NHE-1 is conducive to attenuation of the remodeling process and heart failure. Such findings have been observed in both in vitro and in vivo models of hypertrophy and heart failure. As already noted in Section 10.2., NHE inhibitors block norepinephrine induced protein synthesis in cultured neonatal rat ventricular myocytes, although in that particular study, the nonspecific inhibitor amiloride was used to inhibit the antiporter *(58)*. However, similar effects have been reported with HOE 694, a much more selective NHE-1 inhibitor *(61)*.

In vivo studies using clinically relevant animal models have further advanced the concept of NHE-1–mediated hypertrophy and heart failure and have provided very strong evidence for the antiporter's involvement in these processes. For example, early studies have shown that orally administered amiloride, a nonspecific NHE inhibitor, reduces fiber diameter in rat coronary ligation *(62)* and murine dilated cardiomyopathy models *(63)*. Dietary administration of the NHE-1–specific inhibitor cariporide completely abrogates the increased length of surviving myocytes after 1 wk after coronary artery occlusion and ameliorates contractile dysfunction in the absence of afterload reduction, thereby implicating a direct effect of the drug on myocardial remodeling *(64)*. Furthermore, more severe hypertrophy and heart failure observed at 3-mo postinfarction follow-up are reduced by approx 50% in animals treated with the NHE-1 inhibitor cariporide *(65)*. As noted, these effects of cariporide were observed in the absence of afterload reduction or reduction in infarct size, although others have reported a moderate infarct size reduction in cariporide-treated rats subjected to coronary ligation *(66)*. The evidence for a direct antiremodeling influence of NHE-1 inhibition is further reinforced by the findings that heart failure not associated with myocardial ischemia is also attenuated by NHE-1 inhibition. One such model involves the acute administration of monocrotaline to rats, which produces pulmonary neointimal thickening and compensatory right ventricular hypertrophy. We have recently reported that cariporide can effectively attenuate the right ventricular hypertrophic response as well as the accompanying hemodynamic defects whereas the pulmonary artery responses were unaffected *(67)*. Further such evidence stems from the spontaneously hypertensive rat, which develops left ventricular hypertrophy. It has recently been reported that cariporide causes a regression of left ventricular hypertrophy similarly to that seen with the vasodilators enalapril and nifedipine, but with no decrease in blood pressure *(68)*. Lastly, in a very recent study, it was reported that cariporide inhibits interstitial fibrosis, hypertrophy, and heart failure in transgenic mice that overexpress the cardiac β_1 adrenergic receptor *(69)*. Thus, it appears that NHE-1 inhibition may have the potential to favorably influence heart failure related to multiple initiating factors. A summary of the evidence for NHE-1 involvement on heart failure is provided in Table 1.

NHE-1 inhibitors appear also to have the ability to reverse the heart failure process when administered weeks after coronary artery ligation. In unpublished results, we have been able to observe a marked reduction in both myocardial hypertrophy as well as hemodynamic abnormalities when treatment was delayed by up to 6 wk after ligation. These effects were seen with cariporide as well as with newly developed potent NHE-1–selective inhibitor EMD 87580 (developed by Merck KgaA, Germany). As with other studies, these salutary effects were seen in the absence of afterload reduction. The ability to reverse remodeling and heart failure by NHE-1 inhibitors is a particularly exciting finding because it offers the prospect of potential reversal of the disease process in patients with established heart failure. At present, we have observed such reversal with up to 6-wk treatment delay, although it remains to be determined as to how long treatment can be withheld before the protective effects of NHE-1 inhibitors are lost.

10.4. Potential Mechanisms

Despite the emerging strong evidence for NHE-1 involvement in the heart failure process and the prospect for novel therapeutic interventions, the mechanisms underlying

Table 1
Summary of Experimental Evidence Linking NHE-1 to Heart Failure

---

NHE-1 is a common downstream mediator for various hypertrophic and promyocardial
    remodeling factors
NHE-1 activity or expression are increased in a number of models of hypertrophy
    and heart failure
NHE-1 activity is increased in clinical end-stage heart failure
NHE-1 inhibitors attenuate myocyte hypertrophy in vitro in response to hypertrophic factors
NHE-1 inhibitors prevent hypertrophy and heart failure

---

the role of NHE-1 is presently unknown. Although NHE-1–dependent intracellular pH changes may be proposed in view of the role of pH in protein synthesis, this is unlikely because it would be expected that under long-term NHE-1 blockade other intracellular pH regulatory processes would likely compensate to ensure maintenance of physiological pH levels. Recently, it has been suggested that NHE-1 activation results in the influx of sodium ions, which then in turn activate various PKC isozymes which then alter gene expression and protein synthesis *(70)*. However, the precise mechanism for NHE-1 involvement in myocardial remodeling and hypertrophy requires elucidation.

11. SUMMARY

The past number of years have seen substantial progress and advances with respect to the understanding of NHE-1 in the heart, particularly its role in mediating myocardial ischemic and reperfusion injury, and more recently, its potential role in long-term myocardial adaptation and development of heart failure. In terms of ischemic injury and cardiac protection these advances have lead, relatively rapidly, to the establishment of clinical trials aimed at determining whether selective NHE-1 inhibition protects high-risk patients with coronary artery disease or those with acute myocardial infarction. It is very likely and hopeful that new therapeutic strategies will emerge, based on both the clinical trials that have been or are currently being undertaken, as well as the obvious rapid development of a large number of new NHE-1 inhibitors. Major attention should be paid for developing novel strategies for treating heat failure since this is emerging as a major epidemic of the 21st century and the development of new effective therapeutic strategies is an urgent priority. The past 20 yr or so have seen important developments in the treatment of heart failure, but nonetheless mortality remains high. American Heart Association statistics reveal a 80% and 70% mortality rate, respectively, for men and women under the age of 65 within 8 yr after diagnosis. Among emerging therapies, the growth of molecular biology may have an important impact on the design of new strategies for the treatment of heart failure potentially involving gene therapy as a treatment modality. Yet classic pharmacological therapeutic approaches will likely remain the mainstay for heart failure therapy for some years to come. NHE-1 appears to be a highly attractive therapeutic target for heart failure, made more so by the availability of highly potent and NHE-1 selective inhibitors developed by various pharmaceutical houses. The initial impetus for this development was the potential of NHE-1 inhibitors as cardioprotective agents against ischemic or reperfusion injury and indeed, as previously alluded to, a number of these drugs have entered into clinical trials and are still currently under evaluation. The potential of NHE-1 inhibitors as agents for the treatment of heart failure is attractive for a number of reasons. First, from the clinical studies, NHE-1 inhibitors appear to have a good safety profile *(50–52)*, although this needs to be confirmed in chronic studies. The apparent good safety profile of NHE-1 inhibitors likely reflects the fact that these drugs target a system, which is upregulated under pathological conditions and is essentially inactive, or at least weakly active, in the normal cell. Moreover, there is now strong evidence that NHE-1 mediates the effects of many factors implicated in myocardial remodeling. As such, NHE-1 inhibitors have potentially greater efficacy than agents targeting a specific factor alone. Furthermore, NHE-1 inhibitors have very little if any hemodynamic effects, thus precluding excessive vasodilation, which would be undesirable in heart failure patients. Lastly, initial animal studies with NHE-1 inhibitors are highly encouraging and demonstrate a beneficial effect in terms of improving hemodynamics and reducing hypertrophy. Moreover, the effects are seen with substantial treatment delay, indicating that these agents have the ability to reverse the hypertrophy and heart failure processes. Despite the overall promising approach in terms of the beneficial effects of NHE-1 inhibitors, a number of key questions require resolution. Of importance is the question whether NHE-1 inhibition is superior to other approaches such as ACE inhibition or β receptor blockade or whether it offers additional beneficial effects to these treatment modalities. NHE-1 inhibition offers the potential to treat the heart failure process in the absence of undesirable effects, such as afterload reduction seen with ACE inhibitors. It has recently been reported that cariporide exerted less marked beneficial effects on postinfarction remodeling and hypertrophy in female rats compared to the angiotensin AT_1 receptor blocker losartan *(71)*. This needs to be addressed further, particularly in terms of the potential gender differences to NHE-1 inhibitor administration in heart failure.

ACKNOWLEDGMENTS

Studies cited from the author's laboratory are supported by the Canadian Institutes of Health Research. The author is a Career Investigator of the Heart and Stroke Foundation of Ontario.

REFERENCES

1. Leem, C. H., Lagadic-Gossmann, D., and Vaughan-Jones, R. D. (1999) Characterization of intracellular pH in the guinea-pig ventricular myocyte. *J. Physiol. (Lond)* **517,** 159–180.
2. Karmazyn, M., Gan, X. T., Humphreys, R. A., Yoshida, H., and Kusumoto, K. (1999) The myocardial Na+-H+ exchange: Structure, regulation and its role in heart disease. *Circ. Res.* **85,** 777–786.
3. Karmazyn, M. and Moffat, M. P. (1993) Role of Na+/H+ exchange in cardiac physiology and pathophysiology: Mediation of myocardial reperfusion injury by the pH paradox. *Cardiovasc. Res.* **27,** 915–924.
4. Wakabayashi, S., Shigekawa, M., and Pouysségur J. (1997) Molecular physiology of vertebrate Na+/H+ exchangers. *Physiol. Rev.* **77,** 51–74.
5. Orlowski, J. and Grinstein, S. (1997) Na+/H+ exchangers of mammalian cells. *J. Biol. Chem.* **272,** 22,373–22,376.

6. Numuta, M., Petrecca, K., Lake, N., and Orlowski J. (1998) Identification of a mitochondrial Na+/H+ exchanger. *J. Biol. Chem.* **273,** 6951–6959.

7. Nass, R. and Rao R. (1998) Novel localization of a Na+/H+ exchanger in a late endosomal compartment of yeast. Implications for vacuole biogenesis. *J. Biol. Chem.* **273,** 21,054–21,060.

8. Numata, M. and Orlowski, J. (2001) Molecular cloning and characterization of a novel (Na+,K+)/H+ exchanger localized to the trans-Golgi network. *J. Biol. Chem.* **276,** 17,387–17,394.

9. Bianchini, L. and Pouysségur J. (1996) Regulation of the Na+/H+ exchanger isoform NHE1: Role of phosphorylation. *Kidney Int.* **49,** 1038–1041.

10. Fliegel, L. and Fröhlich O. (1993) The Na+/H+ exchanger: An update on structure, regulation and cardiac physiology. *Biochem. J.* **296,** 273–285.

11. Petrecca, K., Atanasiu, R., Grinstein, S., Orlowski. J., and Shrier A. (1999) Subcellular localization of the Na+/H+ exchanger NHE1 in rat myocardium. *Am. J. Physiol.* **276,** H709–H717.

12. Wu, M. L. and Vaughan-Jones, R. D. (1997) Interaction between Na+ and H+ ions on Na-H exchange in sheep cardiac Purkinje fibers. *J. Mol. Cell. Cardiol.* **29,** 1131–1140.

13. Kinsella, J. L., Heller, P., and Fröhlich, J. P. (1998) Na+/H+ exchanger: Proton modifier site regulation of activity. *Biochem. Cell. Biol.* **76,** 743–749.

14. Wakabayashi, S., Fafournoux, P., Sardet, C., and Pouyéssgur J. (1992) The Na+/H+ antiporter cytoplasmic domain mediates growth factor signals and controls 'H' sensing. *Proc. Natl. Acad. Sci. USA* **89,** 2424–2428.

15. Khandoudi, N., Ho, J., and Karmazyn, M. (1994) Role of sodium/hydrogen exchange in mediating the effects of endothelin-1 on the normal and ischemic and reperfused heart. *Circ. Res.* **75,** 369–378.

16. Woo, S. H. and Lee, C. O. (1999) Effects of endothelin-1 on Ca2+ signaling in guinea pig ventricular myocytes: role of protein kinase C. *J. Mol. Cell. Cardiol.* **31,** 631–643.

17. Matsui, H., Barry, W. H., Livsey, C., and Spitzer, K. W. (1995) Angiotensin II stimulates sodium-hydrogen exchange in adult rabbit ventricular myocytes. *Cardiovasc. Res.* **29,** 215–221.

18. Gunasegaram, S., Haworth, R. S., Hearse, D. J., and Avkiran, M. (1999) Regulation of sarcolemmal Na+/H+ exchanger activity by angiotensin II in adult rat ventricular myocytes: opposing actions via AT1 versus AT2 receptors. *Circ. Res.* **85,** 919–930.

19. Wallert, M. A. and Fröhlich, O. (1992) α1-adrenergic stimulation of Na-H exchange in cardiac myocytes. *Am. J. Physiol.* **263,** C1096–C1102.

20. Yokoyame, H., Yasutake, M., and Avikran, M. (1998) α1-adrenergic stimulation of sarcolemmal Na+/H+ exchanger activity in rat ventricular myocytes: Evidence for selective mediation by the α1A-adrenoceptor subtype. *Circ. Res.* **82,** 1078–1085.

21. Yasutake, M., Haworth, R. S., King, A., and Avkiran, M. (1996) Thrombin activates the sarcolemmal Na+/H+ exchanger: Evidence for a receptor-mediated mechanism involving protein kinase C. *Circ. Res.* **79,** 705–715.

22. Bianchini, L., L'Allemain, G., and Pouysségur, J. (1996) The p42/p44 mitogen-activated protein kinase cascade is determinant in mediating activation of the Na+/H+ exchanger (NHE1 isoform) in response to growth factors. *J. Biol. Chem.* **272,** 271–279.

23. Counillon, L. and Pouysségur, J. (1995) Structure-function studies and molecular regulation of the growth factor activatable sodium-hydrogen exchanger (NHE-1). *Cardiovasc. Res.* **29,** 147–154.

24. Siczkowski, M. and Ng, L. L. (1996) Phorbol ester activation of the rat vascular myocyte Na+/H+ exchanger isoform 1. *Hypertension* **27,** 859–866.

25. Sabri, A., Byron, K. L., Samarel, A. M., Bell, J., and Lucchesi, P. A. (1998) Hydrogen peroxide activates mitogen-activated protein kinases and Na^+/H^+ exchange in neonatal rat cardiac myocytes. *Circ. Res.* **82,** 1053–1062.

26. Hoque, A. N.E, Haist. J. V., and Karmazyn, M. (1997) Na⁺/H⁺ exchange inhibition protects against mechanical, ultrastructural, and biochemical impairment induced by low concentrations of lysophosphatidylcholine in isolated rat hearts. *Circ. Res.* **80,** 95–102.

27. Wang, H., Silva, N. L., Lucchesi, P. A., Haworth, R., Wang, K., Michalak, M., et al. (1997) Phosphorylation and regulation of the Na⁺/H⁺ exchanger through mitogen-activated protein kinase. *Biochemistry* **29,** 9151–9158.

28. Moor, A. N. and Fliegel, L. (1999) Protein kinase-mediated regulation of the Na⁺/H⁺ exchanger in the rat myocardium by mitogen-activated protein kinase-dependent pathways. *J. Biol. Chem.* **274,** 22,985–22,992.

29. Seko, Y., Tobe, K, Ueki, K., Kadowaki, T., and Yazaki, Y. (1996) Hypoxia and hypoxia/ reoxygenation activate Raf-1, mitogen-activated protein kinase kinase, mitogen-activated protein kinases, and S6 kinase in cultured rat cardiac myocytes. *Circ. Res.* **78,** 82–90.

30. Takeishi, Y., Abe, J., Lee, J., Kawakatsu, H., Walsh, R. A., and Berk, B. C. (1999) Differential regulation of p90 ribosomal S6 kinase and big mitogen-activated protein kinase 1 by ischemia/reperfusion and oxidative stress in perfused guinea pig hearts. *Circ. Res.* **85,** 1164–1172.

31. Bertrand, B., Wakabayashi, S., Ikeda, T., Pouysségur, J., and Shigekawa, M. (1994) The Na+/H+ exchanger isoform 1 (NHE1) is a novel member of the calmodulin-binding proteins: identification and characterization of calmodulin-binding sites. *J. Biol. Chem.* **269,** 13,703–13,709.

32. Wakabayashi, S., Bertrand, B., Ikeda, T., Pouysségur, J., and Shigekawa, M. (1994) Mutation of calmodulin-binding site renders the Na⁺/H⁺ exchanger (NHE1) highly H⁺-sensitive and Ca²⁺ regulation-defective. *J. Biol. Chem.* **269,** 13,710–13,715.

33. Goss, G. G., Woodside, M., Wakabayashi, S., Pouysségur, J., Waddell, T., Downey, G. P., et al. (1995) ATP dependence of NHE-1, the ubiquitous isoform of the Na⁺/H⁺ antiporter: Analysis of phosphorylation and subcellular localization. *J. Biol. Chem.* **269,** 8741–8748.

34. Aharonovitz, O., Demaurex, N., Woodside, M. ,and Grinstein S. (1999) ATP dependence is not an intrinsic property of Na⁺/H⁺ exchanger NHE1: Requirement for an ancillary factor. *Am. J. Physiol.* **276,** C1303–C1311.

35. Dhanasekaran, N., Prasad, M, V., Wadsworth, S. J., Dermott, J. M., and van Rossum, G. (1994) Protein kinase C-dependent and -independent activation of Na⁺/H⁺ exchanger by G$_{α12}$ class of G proteins. *J. Biol. Chem.* **269,** 11,802–11,806.

36. Kitamura, K., Singer, W. D., Cano, A., and Miller, R. T. (1995) G$_{αq}$ and G$_{α13}$ regulate NHE-1 and intracellular calcium in epithelial cells. *Am. J. Physiol.* **268,** C101–C110.

37. Voyno-Yasenetskya, T., Conklin, B. R., Gilbert, R. L., Hooley, R., Bourne, H. R., and Barber, D. L. (1994) G$_{α13}$ stimulates Na-H exchange. *J. Biol. Chem.* **269,** 4721–4724.

38. Hooley, R., Yu, C., Symons, M., and Barber, D. L. (1996) G$_{α13}$ stimulates Na⁺/H⁺ exchange through distinct cdc41-dependent and RhoA-dependent pathways. *J. Biol. Chem.* **271,** 6152–6158.

39. Kolyada, A. Y., Lebedeva, T. V., Johns, C. A., and Madias, N. E. (1994) Proximal regulatory elements and nuclear activities required for transcription of the human Na⁺/H⁺ exchanger (NHE-1) gene. *Biochem. Biophys. Acta* **1217,** 54–64.

40. Yang, W., Dyck, J. R. B., Wang, H., and Fliegel, L. (1996) Regulation of the NHE-1 promoter in mammalian myocardium. *Am. J. Physiol.* **270,** H259–H266.

41. Wang, H., Yang, W., and Fliegel, L. (1997) Identification of an HMG-like protein involved in regulation of Na⁺/H⁺ exchanger expression. *Mol. Cell. Biochem.* **176,** 99–106.

42. Gan, X. T., Chakrabarti, S., and Karmazyn, M. (1999) Modulation of Na⁺/H⁺ exchange isoform 1 mRNA expression in isolated rat hearts. *Am. J. Physiol.* **277,** H993–H998.

43. Lemasters, J. J., Bond, J. M., Chacon, E., Harper, I. S., Kaplan, S. H., Ohata, H., et al. (1996) The pH paradox in ischemia-reperfusion injury to cardiac myocytes, in *Myocardial Ischemia: Mechanisms, Reperfusion, Protection* (Karmazyn, M., ed.), Birkhäuser, Basel, pp. 99–114.

44. Harper, I. S., Bond, J. M., Chacon, E., Reece, J. M., Herman, B., and Lemasters, J. J. (1993) Inhibition of Na+/H+ exchange preserves viability, restores mechanical function, and prevents the pH paradox in reperfusion injury to rat neonatal myocytes. *Basic Res. Cardiol.* **88,** 430–442.

45. Kleyman, T. R. and Cragoe, E. J. (1988) Amiloride and its analogs as tools in the study of ion transport. *J. Membr. Biol.* **105,** 1–21.

46. Baumgarth, M., Beier, N., and Gericke, R. (1997) (2-Methyl-5-(methylsulfonyl)benzoyl) guanidine Na/H antiporter inhibitors. *J. Med. Chem.* **40,** 2017–2034.

47. Baumgarth, M., Beier, N., and Gericke, R. (1998) Bicyclic acylguanidine Na+/H+ antiporter inhibitors. *J. Med. Chem.* **41,** 3736–3747.

48. Kleeman, H. W. and Weichert, A. G. (1999) Recent developments in the field of inhibitors of the Na+/H+ exchanger. *Drugs* **2,** 1009–1025.

49. Orlowski, J. and Kandasamy, R. A. (1996) Delineation of transmembrane domains of the Na+/H+ exchanger that confer sensitivity to pharmacological antagonists. *J. Biol. Chem.* **271,** 19,922–19,927

50. Karmazyn, M. (2000) Pharmacology and clinical assessment of cariporide for the treatment coronary artery diseases. *Expert. Opin. Investig. Drugs.* **9,** 1099–1108.

51. Théroux, P., Chaitman, B. R., Danchin, N., Erhardt, L., Meinertz, T., Schroeder, J. S., et al. (2000) Inhibition of the sodium-hydrogen exchanger with cariporide to prevent myocardial infarction in high-risk ischemic situations. Main results of the GUARDIAN trial. Guard during ischemia against necrosis (GUARDIAN) Investigators. *Circulation* **102,** 3032–3038.

52. Zeymer, U., Suryapranata, H., Monassier, J. P., Opolski, G., Davies, J., Rasmanis, G., et al. (2001) The Na+/H+ exchange inhibitor eniporide as an adjunct to early reperfusion therapy for acute myocardial infarction. Results of the evaluation of the safety and cardioprotective effects of eniporide in acute myocardial infarction (ESCAMI) trial. *J. Am. Coll. Cardiol.* **38,** 1644–1650.

53. Rupprecht, H. J., vom Dahl, J., Terres, W., Seyfarth, K. M., Richardt, G., Schultheibeta, H. P., et al. (2002) Cardioprotective effects of the Na+/H+ exchange inhibitor cariporide in patients with acute anterior myocardial infarctionundergoing direct PTCA. *Circulation* **101,** 2902–2908.

54. Avkiran, M. and Marber, M. S. (2002) Na+/H+ exchange inhibitors for cardioprotective therapy: Progress, problems and prospects. *J. Am. Coll. Cardiol.* **39,** 747–753.

55. Katz, A. M. (2000) *Heart Failure. Pathophysiology, Molecular Biology, and Clinical Management.* Lippincott Williams & Wilkins, Philadelphia, PA.

56. Yamazaki, T., Komuro, I., Kudoh, S., Zou, Y., Nagair, R., Aikawa, R., et al. (1998) Role of ion channels and exchanger in mechanical stretch-induced cardiomyocyte hypertrophy. *Circ. Res.* **82,** 430–437.

57. Cingolani, H. E., Alvarez, B. V., Ennis, I. L., and Camilión de Hurtado, M. C. (1998) Stretch-induced alkalinization of feline papillary muscle. An autocrine-paracrine system. *Circ. Res.* **83,** 775–780.

58. Hori, M., Nakatsubo, N., Kagiya, T., Iwai, K., Sato, H., Iwakura, K., et al. (1990) The role of Na+/H+ exchange in norepinephrine-induced protein synthesis in neonatal cultured cardiomyocytes. *Jpn. Circ. J.* **54,** 535–539.

59. Dostal, D. E. and Baker, K. M. (1998) Angiotensin and endothelin: messengers that couple ventricular stretch to the Na+/H+ exchanger and cardiac hypertrophy. *Circ. Res.* **83,** 870–873.

60. Cingolani, H. E. (1999) Na+/H+ exchange hyperactivity and myocardial hypertrophy: Are they linked phenomena? *Cardiovasc. Res.* **44,** 462–467.

61. Schluter, K. D., Schafer, M., Balser, C., Taimor, G., and Piper, H. M. (1998) Influence of pHi and.creatine phosphate on α-adrenoceptor-mediated cardiac hypertrophy. *J. Mol. Cell. Cardiol.* **30,** 763–771.

62. Hasegawa, S., Nakano, M., Taniguchi, Y., Imai, S., Murata, K., and Suzuki, T. (1995) Effects of Na(+)-H+ exchange blocker amiloride on left ventricular remodelling after anterior myocardial infarction in rats. *Cardiovasc. Drugs. Ther.* **9**, 823–826.
63. Taniguchi, Y., Nakano, M., Hasegawa, S., Kanda, T., Imai, S., Suzuki, T., Kobayashi, I. and Nagai, R. (1996) Beneficial effect of amiloride, a Na(+)-H+ exchange blocker, in a murine model of dilated cardiomyopathy. *Res. Commun. Chem. Pathol. Pharmacol.* **92**, 201–210.
64. Yoshida, M. and Karmazyn, M. (2000) Na+/H+ exchange inhibition attenuates hypertrophy and heart failure in 1-wk postinfarction rat myocardium. *Am. J. Physiol.* **278**, H300–H304.
65. Kusumoto, K., Haist, J. V., and Karmazyn, M. (2001) Na+/H+ exchange inhibition reduces hypertrophy and heart failure after myocardial infarction in rats. *Am. J. Physiol.* **280**, H738–H745.
66. Spitznagel, H., Chung, O., Xia, Q., Rossius, B., Illner, S., Jahnichen, G., et al. (2000) Cardioprotective effects of the Na+/H+-exchange inhibitor cariporide in infarct-induced heart failure. *Cardiovasc. Res.* **46**, 102–110.
67. Chen, L., Gan, X. T., Haist, J. V., Feng, Q., Lu, X., Chakrabarti, S., and Karmazyn, M. (2001) Attenuation of compensatory right ventricular hypertrophy and heart failure following monocrotaline-induced pulmonary vascular injury by the Na(+)-H+ exchange inhibitor cariporide. *J. Pharmacol. Exp. Ther.* **298**, 469–476.
68. Ennis, I. L., Alvarez, B. V., Camilión de Hurtado, M. C., and Cingolani, H. E. (1998) Enalapril induces regression of cardiac hypertrophy and normalization of pHi regulatory mechanisms. *Hypertension* **31**, 961–967.
69. Engelhardt, S., Hein, L., Keller, U., Klambt, K., and Lohse, M. J. (2002) Inhibition of Na(+)-H+ exchange prevents hypertrophy, fibrosis, and heart failure in β_1-adrenergic receptor transgenic mice. *Circ. Res.* **90**, 814–819.
70. Hayasaki-Kajiwara, Y., Kitano, Y., Iwasaki, T., Shimamura, T., Naya, N., Iwaki, K., and Nakajima M. (1999) Na+ influx via Na+/H+ exchange activates protein kinase C isozymes δ and ϵ in cultured neonatal rat cardiac myocytes. *J. Mol. Cell. Cardiol.* **31**, 1559–1572.
71. Loennechen, J. P., Wisloff, U., Falck, G., and Ellingesen, Ø. (2002) Effects of cariporide and losartan on hypertrophy, calcium transients, contractility, and gene expression in congestive heart failure. *Circulation* **105**, 1380–1386.

8

Nitric Oxide and Cardiac Ischemia

Mariarosaria Bucci, Inmaculada Posadas Mayo, and Giuseppe Cirino

CONTENTS

INTRODUCTION
NO
MYOCARDIAL ISCHEMIA–REPERFUSION (I–R) INJURY
MYOCARDIAL ISCHEMIA CONDITIONING
CONCLUSIONS
REFERENCES

1. INTRODUCTION

In a healthy heart, an increase in myocardial oxygen demand induces an increase in coronary artery blood flow and oxygen delivery. When obstructive coronary artery disease occurs, there is an abnormal diminished coronary blood supply relative to the myocardial oxygen demand known as hypoxia. The reduction in cardiac output is accompanied by increased systemic and pulmonary vascular resistance. These events are responsible for acute myocardial ischemia, which is manifested clinically by angina pectoris. Besides hypoxia, other disorders, such as a reduced delivery of substrates, accumulation of tissue metabolites, and reduction in vascular reactivity, can contribute to induce myocardial ischemia (Fig. 1). It is widely accepted that hypercholesterolemia, hypertension, diabetes mellitus, and cigarette smoking are important risk factors for the development of obstructive coronary atherosclerosis. These pathologies show, as a common pattern, an impaired endothelium-dependent vasorelaxation of the large coronary arteries that often is evident even before the formation of the atherosclerotic lesions *(1–5)*. These findings constitute an important issue because acute myocardial ischemia, resulting mainly from atherosclerotic coronary artery disease, occurs in as many as six millions persons, and approx 28 million people suffer obstructive coronary artery disease in the United States alone *(6,7)*. Over the last decade, it has been recognized the physiological and pathophysiological roles of endothelium in the cardiovascular system. Several substances released or metabolized by cardiac endothelial cells have direct effects on cardiac myocytes function, including nitric oxide (NO), prostanoids, endothelins, kinins, angiotensin II, reactive oxygen species (ROS), adenylpurines (for review, *see* ref. *8*). In particular in the heart, NO is the main vasodi-

From: *Cardiac Drug Development Guide*
Edited by: M. K. Pugsley © Humana Press Inc., Totowa, NJ

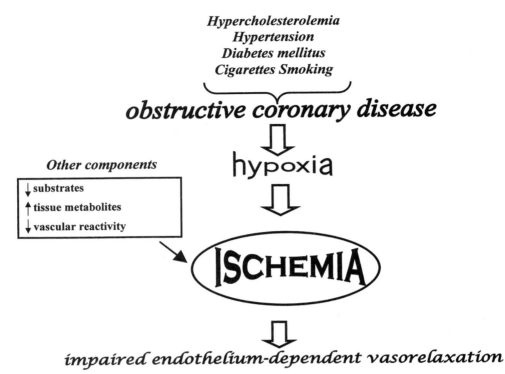

Fig. 1. Disparate risk factors (from pathologies to lifestyle habitudes) converge on obstructive coronary atherosclerosis. The main event raising from these coronary conditions is the blood supply reduction that in turn provokes hypoxia. This latter event is responsible for myocardial ischemia. However, other components, such as reduction in vascular reactivity, substrates availability and accumulation of tissue metabolites, can concur to myocardial ischemia genesis. The final outcome is an impaired endothelium-dependent vasorelaxation.

lator molecule produced and released by the coronary endothelium. The purpose of this chapter is to analyze the involvement of NO in cardiac function with particular regards to ischemia–reperfusion and preconditioning.

2. NO

NO is a small membrane-permeable molecule that serves as a mediator of many biological activities. It is produced in physiological and pathophysiological conditions by three different isoforms of NO synthase (NOS): endothelial NOS (eNOS), neuronal NOS (nNOS), and inducible NOS (iNOS; refs. *9,10*). eNOS and nNOS isoenzymes are constitutive and calcium–calmodulin-dependent enzymes *(11)*, in particular eNOS, are involved in the regulation of blood pressure and organ blood flow distribution. Endothelium-derived NO inhibits platelet aggregation, leukocyte adherence, and vascular smooth muscle cell proliferation *(12)*. Conversely, neuronal-derived NO has an important physiological role as neurotransmitter and as a potential mediator of the metabolism/blood flow coupling into the brain *(13)*. iNOS isoform can be induced by pro-inflammatory agents, such as endotoxin, cytokines, and bacterial products in several cells, including macrophages and smooth muscle cells *(14)*. NO production after the induction of iNOS has been implicated in the pathogenesis of various forms of septic shock *(15–18)* and inflammation (for recent review, *see* refs. *19–21*).

NO is synthesized from amino acid L-arginine to L-citrulline through a five-electron oxidation step via the formation of the intermediate N^G-hydroxy-L-arginine *(22–24)*. NOS-mediated NO production also requires oxygen and nicotinamide adenine dinucleotide phosphate, reduced form, and several cofactors, such as tetrahydro-biopteridin, flavin adenine dinucleotide, and flavine mononucleotide *(25)*. NO induces vasodilatation, and in particular coronary dilatation, by increasing cyclic guanosine monophosphate (cGMP) in vascular smooth muscle cells *(26)*. This cyclic molecule blunts the affinity of the troponin–tropomyosin complex on actin for calcium and promotes the calcium re-uptake by the sarcoplasmatic reticulum in vascular muscle cells inducing vasorelaxation *(26)*.

2.1. Physiology of NO in the Heart

Under resting condition, NO released from endothelium is constant and contributes to maintain coronary arteries in homeostatic state *(27)*; the force imposed on the coronary endothelium by flowing blood, defined "radial strain," is the main stimulus for NO release *(28–31)*. The rhythmic change in vessels caliber, as a result of the alternation of systole and diastole, results in the transient increase in intracellular calcium influx in the endothelial cells through the activation of phospholipase C pathway *(32,3)*. Increased calcium concentration in endothelium activates eNOS that in turn causes NO production *(34)*. Different endogenous molecules induce NO release from coronary endothelium, as acetylcholine, bradykinin, serotonin, adenosine triphosphate (ATP), and diphosphate (ADP), histamine, and substance P *(26,30,35)*. The most common dysfunction found in patients with atherosclerotic coronary artery disease is an impaired endothelium functionality *(2,3,5,36)*. Alterations in coronary vascular endothelial function were first described by Ludmer and coworkers in 1986 *(37)*. They observed a vasoconstriction of atherosclerotic segments after infusing acetylcholine into the left coronary artery of patients with atypical chest pain. Because coronary functionality is regulated by mechanical and agonist-mediated stimuli and both converge on NO production and release, endothelium dysfunction results as a decrease of NO concentration in vascular smooth muscle cells *(38)*. NO release is modulated at different levels by (1) availability of the precursor L-arginine; (2) alterations of eNOS function; and (3) interaction of NO with ROS, resulting in $ONOO^-$, $ONOO^-$, $NO_2\cdot$, and $OH\cdot$ formation *(39,40)*.

3. MYOCARDIAL ISCHEMIA–REPERFUSION (I–R) INJURY

Organ injury caused by transient ischemia followed by reperfusion is widely recognized as a significant source of morbidity and mortality in many clinical disorders, including myocardial infarction and cerebrovascular diseases *(41,42)*. Recently, with the introduction of organs transplantation, the impairment of graft organ function as a consequence of I–R has also become the goal of extensive scientific and clinical efforts *(43)*. In the heart, the major determinant of ischemic injury is the duration and the degree of reduction in myocardial perfusion relative to cardiac work. Brief ischemia (<20 min) results in contractile dysfunction during the ischemic episode, but it is usually followed by a complete recovery of function. Conversely, a more prolonged ischemia, results in permanent damage as a result of the myocardial cell death *(44,45)*. This irreversible damage is termed "wavefront phenomenon" of myocardial cell death *(46)*. Reperfusion, especially early after ischemia, seems to be the only way to salvage the myocardium from necrosis because restores blood supply, even though it is well established that reperfusion itself can bring nocuous effects, inducing several abnormalities in heart function. Coronary endothelium dysfunction *(47)*, upregulation of adhesion molecules on the endothelial cell surface (i.e., P-selectin) leading to polymorphonuclear leukocyte (PMN) rolling, and adherence to the endothelium *(48,49)* represent the early events that occur after 2.5–5 min from reperfusion. After 20 min of re-oxygenation, PMNs start to transmigrate from the coronary vasculature and to infiltrate into cardiac tissue *(47,49,50)*. Once in the cardiac tissue, PMNs release cytotoxic substances, such as oxygen free radicals, inflammatory cytokines, and proteolytic enzymes, inducing endothelial and myocardial injury *(51–53)*. In addition, several studies have showed that reperfusion induces cellular Ca^{2+} overload *(54)*, acute diastolic dysfunction, transient impairment of left ventricular systolic contractile function or "myocardial stunning" *(55)*, and arrhythmia. For this reason the cardiac dysfunction after an ischemic episode can be defined as ischemia-reperfusion injury (Fig. 2).

3.1. Involvement of ROS in I–R Injury

One of the main events involved in I–R injury resides in the generation of a ROS burst, in particular superoxide anion (O_2^-), that takes place just upon reperfusion *(54,56,57)*. NO can react with equimolar amount of O_2^- in irreversible manner to form peroxynitrite ($ONOOO^-$; ref. *58*), a toxic molecule that may play a role in the pathophysiology of myocardial I–R injury. Potential sources of ROS include myocytes, mitochondria, activated neutrophils and several endothelial enzymes (such as xanthine oxidase, nicotinamide adenine dinucleotide phosphate, reduced form, cyclooxygenase and NOSs *(45,59)*. Some studies have reported that during early reperfusion period, peroxynitrite formation occurs parallel to superoxide production *(57)*. In particular, Yasmin and coworkers have demonstrated that in isolated rat hearts there is an increase in peroxynitrite formation that is maximal 30 s after reperfusion *(60)*. This increase was accompanied by left ventricular alterations that were improved by treatment with the NOS inhibitor L-NMMA. In the same experimental setting, Wang and coworkers *(61)* found an increment of peroxynitrite during the early period of reflow, which results in amino acid nitration and cellular damage. Conversely, it has been shown that removal of O_2^- by reaction with NO may be considered beneficial *(62)*; indeed, in isolated perfused hearts, the administration of exogenous peroxynitrite at low concentration (0.4 µ*M*) reduced significantly the incidence of ventricular fibrillation after 10 min of I–R, whereas a higher concentration of $ONOOO^-$ (4–40 µ*M*) induced arrhythmias *(63)*. In contrast, it has been shown that from nano to micromolar concentration, $ONOO^-$ exerts beneficial effects similar to those of NO, inducing vasorelaxation in human coronary arteries *(64)* and in isolated rat aortic rings *(65)*. In addition, this reactive molecule attenuated the accumulation of PMNs in isolated rat heart *(65)* and in isolated perfused cat heart *(66)*. However, a potential molecular mechanism that could contribute to the beneficial effects of peroxynitrite is the *S*-nitrosation of cellular thiols, as shown in

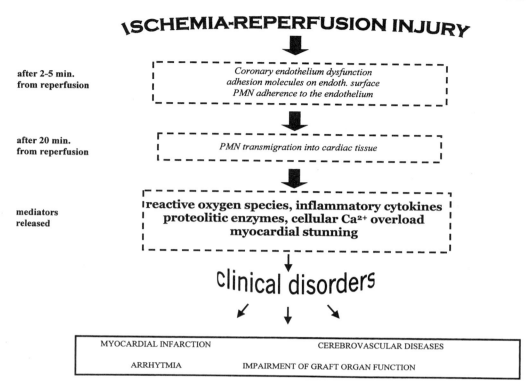

Fig. 2. Temporal events leading to I–R damage. Once PMNs infiltrate the cardiac tissue, ROS, cytokines, and enzymes release occurs, at the same time there is an increase in intracellular Ca^{2+}. All these events are involved in clinical disorders appearance.

isolated bovine pulmonary arterial rings *(67)*. *S*-nitrosothiols groups have been shown to stimulate purified soluble guanylyl cyclase in vascular smooth muscle cells *(68)* and in porcine aortic endothelial cells *(69)*, leading to NO-mediated cGMP accumulation. Elevation of cGMP content can decrease the cAMP levels, and this could account for the cardioprotective effects *(70)*. In addition, $ONOO^-$ reacts with compounds containing alcohol groups to form intermediate molecules that can act as NO donors producing vasodilatation and inhibition of platelet aggregation *(71)*. Thus, the exact role of $ONOO^-$ is not yet clearly identified.

4. MYOCARDIAL ISCHEMIC CONDITIONING

The term ischemic preconditioning (PC) was firstly applied to canine myocardium subjected to brief episodes of I–R that tolerated a more prolonged episode of ischemia better than myocardium not previously exposed *(72)*. A protective effect of myocardial ischemic PC has been demonstrated in several animal species, resulting in the strongest endogenous form of protection against myocardial injury, jeopardized myocardium, infarct size, and arrhythmias other than early reperfusion. New-onset angina before acute myocardial infarction, episodes of myocardial ischemia during coronary angioplasty or bypass surgery, and the "warm-up" phenomenon may represent the clinical counterparts of the PC phenomenon in humans. The results of the outstanding study of Murry and colleagues *(72)* undeniably represent a significant advance in our broad understanding of tissue ischemia pathophysiology. More recently, ischemic PC has also been shown to occur in a variety of organ systems, including brain, spinal cord, retina, liver, lung, and skeletal muscle, suggesting that this is an endogenous protective mechanism whereby tissues protect themselves from an impending threat. In particular, myocardial ischemic PC is the phenomenon by which a brief episode(s) of myocardial ischemia increases the ability of the heart to tolerate a subsequent prolonged ischemic injury. PC has an immediate beneficial effect known as early phase or first window of protection and a delayed effect known as the late phase or second window of protection, whose importance varies between species and organ systems *(73–81)*. Although the exact mechanisms of both protective components are still unclear, ischemic PC could be defined as a multifactorial pathophysiological process, requiring the interaction of numerous cellular signals, second messengers, and end-effector mechanisms, in which NO plays a central role.

4.1. Early-Phase PC

The early phase of PC or first window of protection develops within minutes from the initial ischemic insult, dissipates 2–3 h later and it is associated with post-translational modifications of pre-existing proteins. In several experimental settings, the role of NO in the early phase of PC has been investigated. The administration of the NOS inhibitor L-NNA to rabbits subjected to I–R injury has been shown to increase the infarct size *(82)*. Similarly, the changes observed in coronary vascular reactivity induced by ischemic PC in goat were prevented by L-NNA pretreatment *(83)*. Recent studies, have demonstrated an enhanced production of NO in myocardium subjected to brief episodes of I–R *(84)* in first window, confirming an important role for NO in this phase. The source of NO during early PC seems to be eNOS because the nonselective inhibitor L-NNA blocked early PC in rabbits, but a more selective iNOS inhibitor *s*-methylisothiourea was ineffective in this phase *(85)*. In addition, it has been proposed that in brief ischemia eNOS-derived NO leads to the activation of protein kinase C (PKC; refs. *86,87*). Indeed, after PC ischemia, NO can react with superoxide anion, leading to $ONOO^-$ formation, which in turn has been shown to activate the ε isoform of PKC *(40)*. Activation of PKC is reported to activate ATP-sensitive potassium (K_{ATP}) channels that could be both sarcolemmal and/or mitochondrial *(88,89)*. In this respect, it has been demonstrated that activation of sarcolemmal channels results in a reduction of the action potential duration with attenuation of Ca^{2+} influx and Ca^{2+} overload *(90)*, which occurs after a prolonged ischemia, whereas activation of mitochondrial channels attenuates Ca^{2+} overload at this level *(91,92)*. However, recent studies attribute to mitochondrial K_{ATP} channel activation, the main cardioprotective effects *(89,91,92)*.

4.2. Late-Phase PC

The late phase of PC or second window of protection becomes apparent 12–24 h after the ischemic insult and it is sustained up to 3 to 4 d *(93,94)*. Unlike the early phase, late PC requires increase synthesis of new proteins *(95)*. NO plays a prominent role also in this phase by mediating the cardioprotective effect of PC. The importance of NO as the key trigger or mediator of delayed protection of PC induced by pacing *(96)*, acetylcholine *(97)*, or brief episodes of ischemia *(85)* has been well documented in the last years. In this

respect, it has been demonstrated that exposure to exogenous NO is sufficient to repro-
duce late PC, e.g., administration of nitroglycerine can elicit second window of protection *(98)*. Similarly, treatment of rabbits with the NOS inhibitor L-NA 24 h after ischemic
PC completely abrogates the delayed protection against myocardial infarction *(99)*. Similar effects were observed when the selective inhibitors of iNOS, aminoguanidine, and
s-methylisothiourea, were administered to rabbits *(85,99)*. These results suggest that
iNOS is the specific isoform implicated in the second window of protection. This hypothesis has been challenged using iNOS knockout mice. PC of iNOS knockout mice 24 h
before coronary occlusion resulted in a nonreduction of infarct size whereas wild-type
mice experienced a profound protection against I–R injury *(100)*. In addition, Guo and
coworkers *(100)* demonstrated that late PC is associated with upregulation of myocardial
iNOS in mouse whereas eNOS remains unchanged. Further studies have demonstrated
that cardiac myocytes are the specific cells that express this protein during this phase
(61). Indeed, disruption of the iNOS gene, although completely abrogates the late PC
effect in mice, has no effect on early PC and on infarct size in the absence of PC *(101)*,
further confirming a key role of iNOS in late PC. Thus, PC is characterized by a biphasic
regulation of NOS activity (Fig. 3) with an increase of eNOS activity in the first window
followed by an increase of iNOS expression and activity in the second window. Also, in
this case, the mechanism participating in the second window of protection mediated by
NO seems to involve the activation of PKC *(102)*. A role for PKC and downstream signal
has been shown by Banerjee and colleagues *(102)*, they demonstrated that administration
of nitroglycerine to conscious rabbits mitigates myocardial stunning 24 h after ischemia,
and this effect was removed by chelerytrine, an inhibitor of PKC.

Thus, NO generated during initial ischemic stress can react with superoxide anion,
producing $ONOO^-$ which in turn activates the ε isoform of PKC. This activation may
trigger a signaling cascade including tyrosine–kinase and other kinases, such as MAP
kinases, ending with the activation of iNOS in the second window implying that the
two phases are intimately related *(40)*.

4.3. Pharmacological Modulation of PC

There are several mediators or endogenous substances that have been implicated in
PC. A complete overview of these substances goes beyond the scope of this chapter.
(For recent reviews, *see* refs. *8,73,101,103*.)

4.3.1. Cardioprotection by Heat Shock Proteins (HSPs)

Thermal stress is known to protect the myocardium against I–R injury and necrosis
by preserving mechanical function both in vivo and in vitro (for review, *see* ref. *104*).
In 1988, Currie and coworkers *(105)* demonstrated that rats exposed to 15 min of
hypertermia significantly improved recovery of contractile force, rate of contraction,
and rate of relaxation heart. Similar evidences were found in rabbit hearts exposed for
15 min to hyperthermia and then subjected to I–R *(106)*.

When cells are subjected to an increase in temperature, the expression of several
proteins, known as HSPs, is induced (for review, *see* refs. *107,108*). Among the various members of the HSPs family, the protein mainly induced in myocardium under
heat stress *(106)* or after brief hypoxia *(109)* seems to be heat shock protein 72
(HSP72). Recently, it has been described that rat hearts transfected with human
HSP70 (the constitutive isoform of HSP72) gene presented elevated levels of HSP70
in the myocardium *(110)*.

eNOS/iNOS switch in PC

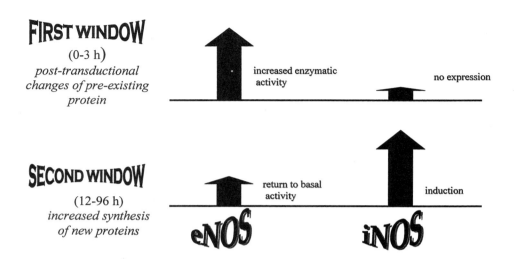

FIRST WINDOW

(0-3 h)
post-transductional changes of pre-existing protein

increased enzymatic activity

no expression

SECOND WINDOW

(12-96 h)
increased synthesis of new proteins

return to basal activity

induction

eNOS   iNOS

Fig. 3. Involvement of endothelial and inducible isoforms of nitric oxide synthase in myocardial preconditioning (PC). In the early phase of PC (first window of protection) eNOS activity is increased whereas iNOS is virtually absent. Conversely, in the late phase of PC (second window of protection) eNOS activity return at basal level while iNOS expression is enhanced.

This elevated expression was coupled to an enhanced recovery of both systolic and diastolic functions and less myocardial injury after I–R *(110)*. In addition it has been also shown that in transfected isolated rat hearts with *HSP70* gene, there is protection of mitochondrial respiration and improved ventricular function after I–R injury *(111)*. These data suggest that overexpression of *HSP70* plays a role in the enhancement of myocardial tolerance and may contribute to myocardial protection during treatment of acute myocardial infarction, cardiac surgery, or heart transplantation. Besides, it is known that heat stress or ischemia induce the increase of other members of the *HSPs* family; hearts from rabbits exposed to either ischemic or thermal stress showed an increase in the HSPs content in cardiac tissue *(94)*. In particular, myocardial *HSP72* is elevated by both ischemic and thermal pretreatments whereas *HSP60* is found preferentially elevated by ischemic pretreatment *(94)*. In both cases, overexpression of *HSPs* were accompanied by a reduction in infarct size *(94)*. Recently, Valen and coworkers *(112)* found an enhancement in the expression of *HSP72* and eNOS in biopsies from the right atrium of patients with unstable angina. In addition, it has been observed that heat shock sharply increases NO production in different rat organs and this precedes the increase in *HSP* synthesis *(113)*. These authors also reported that inhibition of NO synthesis with L-NNA is accompanied by a reduction of *HSPs* levels 24 h after heat shock, suggesting that NO is involved in the heat shock-induced activation of *HSP* synthesis. Conversely, studies on isolated hearts from rats subjected to heat stress for 15 min and 24 h after I–R show an increase of the *HSP72* and *HSP27* by immunohistochemical analysis that was not modified by pretreatment with the NOS inhibitor

L-NAME *(114)*. Because treatment with this inhibitor abolished myocardial ischemic tolerance without affecting HSP levels, seems that NO-mediated myocardial protection by heat stress is independent from *HSP72* and *HSP27* expression *(114)*. Thus, the crosstalk between heat stress and NO pathway is still unclear and needs further studies to better clarify at molecular level the possible interaction.

4.3.2. NO, Cardiomyocytes, and Apoptosis

Cell death may be classified into two different kinds: apoptosis and necrosis. Apoptosis, which is programmed cell death, differs from necrosis in terms of structural and biochemical features, including cytoplasmatic and nuclear condensation, subsequent formation of membrane-bound apoptotic bodies, and oligonucleosomal DNA degradation *(115)*. Apoptotic cell death of cardiomyocytes has been described in human heart failure *(116)* and in mouse I–R injury *(117)*. Apoptosis is mainly regulated by a proteolytic system involving a family of proteases called caspases, in which at least three families of genes are involved: ced-3, ced-4, and ced-9 *(118)*. The mammalian homologues of ced-3 encode for the family of cysteine proteases that constitute an enzymes cascade culminating in activation of caspase-3 *(119)*.

NO has been reported to induce apoptotic cell death in various cell types, including myocytes *(120,121)*. In particular, the injection of the human eNOS gene into the left ventricular wall of the rat heart in vivo caused an overexpression of eNOS accompanied by cell degeneration, including a reduction in myoplasm volume, mitochondrial accumulation, collagen deposition, and macrophage infiltration *(120)*. Terminal deoxynucleotidyl transferase-mediated deoxyuridine triphosphate-digoxigenin nick end labeling analysis for apoptosis and AZAN staining for necrosis revealed in myocardial cell necrosis and apoptosis; both phenomena were ameliorated by L-NAME pretreatment suggesting a role of NO in triggering this effect *(120)*. However, antiapoptotic effect of NO has also been reported in vitro. It has been shown that overstretching of papillary muscles produce an increase in apoptotic myocytes that is prevented by the NO donor C87-3754 *(122)*. Similarly, in human umbilical vein endothelial cells , tumor necrosis factor-α–induced apoptosis has been shown to be completely blocked by shear stress and this effect abrogated by inhibition of NOS; co-administration of the NO donors sodium nitroprusside (SNP) or S-nitroso-N-acetylpenicillamine (SNAP) with tumor necrosis factor-α mimicked the shear stress action *(123)*. In addition, more recently, Weiland and co-workers *(124)* showed that in isolated and perfused rat hearts subjected to I–R, inhibition of endogenous NO synthesis increased apoptosis during ischemia. This increased apoptosis is coupled to an enhanced expression of the active p17 subunit of caspase-3, strongly implying that NO suppresses apoptosis of cardiomyocytes by interfering with the caspase cascade *(124)*. These data also well fit with the finding that NO inhibits caspase-3 activity as a result of *S*-nitrosation of the essential cysteine residue in vitro *(123)*.

Concerning NO, apoptosis and I–R/PC, there are still too many diverging data, thus, at the present stage, the "state of the art" does not warrant any firm conclusion and does not even allow us to put forward any possible hypothesis.

4.3.3. Cardioprotection of Exercise Training

Physical exercise has been associated with a reduction in cardiovascular morbidity and mortality *(125–127)*. It has been thought to play an important role in cardiac rehabilitation and prevention of coronary artery disease through an improvement of coronary stenosis and microvascular dysfunction *(38,128,129)*. This beneficial effect involves an upregulation of eNOS with a consequent increase of NO release *(130)*.

The Lifestyle Heart Trial analyzed the effect of lifestyle changes, including vegetarian diet, stress-management techniques, smoking cessation, and 3 h of exercise training per week on the degree of coronary stenosis. After a 5-yr follow-up, they founded a significant regression of stenosis associated with a reduction in cardiac events *(131)*. Similar findings were described previously in the Stanford Coronary Risk Intervention Project. Patients receiving multiple risk reduction therapy (low-fat diet, lipid-lowering medication, and exercise training) showed an attenuation of the disease progression over the 4-yr study period *(132)*. Besides these effects described on coronary stenosis, exercise training may also improve myocardial perfusion via collateral vessels formation. Indeed, several studies on animals suggest that long-term intensive physical exercise increases coronary collateral vessels growth *(133,134)*.

To better understand the effect of exercise training on coronary endothelial dysfunction, it is essential to consider that coronary vasomotion is influenced by mechanical and agonist-mediated stimuli, both of which converge on endothelial NO production. Shear stress represents an important component of the beneficial effect of physical exercise that increases vascular NO concentration. When there is an endothelial dysfunction, a decreased NO concentration occurs at vascular smooth muscle cells level. Indeed, it is known that shear stress selectively activates uptake of L-arginine in porcine aortic endothelial cells *(135)*. Similarly, in bovine aortic endothelial cells subjected to shear stress, it has been observed a short-term enhancement of eNOS activity and expression *(136)*. Likewise, human umbilical vein endothelial cells exposed to fluid shear stress showed an overexpression of eNOS *(137)*. In addition, it has been also demonstrated that endothelium-derived NO increases the expression of extracellular superoxide dismutase (ecSOD) in human aortic smooth muscle cells *(138)*. ecSOD is one of the major antioxidant enzymatic system of the arterial wall, located between endothelium and vascular smooth muscle cells *(139)*. Inhibition of vascular SOD results in an impairment of endothelium-dependent dilation in bovine coronary arteries in vitro, implying that SOD levels are critical for the availability of NO *(140)*. This increase of ecSOD expression could in turn induce a reduction in ROS levels, resulting in an increase of vascular NO-mediated vasodilatation, since it is well known that ROS accelerate the extracellular degradation of NO. At the same time, it has been described that long-term exercise training also increases the resistance vessel sensitivity in dogs *(141)* and attenuates platelet function and increases platelet cGMP content in human *(142)*.

In summary, exercise training improves myocardial perfusion and NO seems to play a central role. It may be considered as a preventive strategy with long term benefits.

4.3.4. Role of Monophosphoryl Lipid A and RC-552 in PC

It is documented that lipopolysaccharide (LPS) can trigger endogenous protective mechanisms against I–R injury. This protective effect is evident 24 h after the ischemic insult and lasts for several days *(143)*. Moreover, LPS-induced delayed cardioprotection is reported to involve induction of NOS and this effect is comparable, in magnitude, to the second window of protection observed in ischemic PC *(144,145)*. These evidences have lead to the identification of monophosphoryl lipid A (MLA). MLA is a detoxified derivative from LPS of several Gram-negative strains *(146)* and it represents a novel agent capable of enhancing myocardial tolerance to I–R injury. MLA has cardioprotective activity, reduces infarct size, myocardial stunning, and dysrhythmia in several animal species (for review, *see* refs. *147,148*). MLA has been shown to be effective at doses ranging from 10–5000 μg/kg depending on animal species and experimental models *(149–151)*. Although MLA may induce ischemic tolerance through multifactorial mechanisms, current evidence suggests that MLA cardioprotective effect involves myocardial iNOS activation with NO coupled activation of myocardial K_{ATP} channels *(147,148,152)*. The role of the opening of K_{ATP} channel in MLA-induced myocardial protection after I–R has been evaluated using an inhibitor of K_{ATP} channel, 5-hydroxydecanoate *(153)*. Pretreatment with 5-hydroxydecanoate reverted MLA cardioprotective action confirming that MLA exerts its protective effect also through activation of K_{ATP} channel.

Recent studies have also hypothesized that delayed PC induced by MLA is related to stimulation of calcitonin gene-related peptide (CGRP; refs. *150,154*). CGRP is the main transmitter in capsaicin-sensitive sensory nerves and it has been demonstrated to participate in delayed PC *(155–157)*. Because it has been recently proposed that NO cardioprotection is also related to CGRP release *(158)* and MLA-induced PC is mediated by NO *(159)*, the involvement of CGRP in MLA-induced PC it has been investigated. In particular, He and co-workers *(150)* have demonstrated that in isolated rat hearts, cardioprotection exerted by pre-treatment with MLA, 24 h before the I–R injury, is linked to both an increase in NO synthesis and CGRP release. Pretreatment with L-NAME or with capsaicin, which selectively depletes the neurotransmitters in sensory nerves, abolished these protective effects *(150)*, supporting the hypothesis that MLA-cardioprotection is mediated by both CGRP and NO. More recently, it has been demonstrated that RC-552, a novel synthetic glycolipid related in chemical structure to MLA *(160)*, induces delayed cardioprotection via an inducible NOS-dependent pathway *(148,161)*.

In summary, although further clinical testing are necessary to establish the utility of MLA or structural analogues as a cardioprotective agents against I–R injury, presently this agent is proving very useful in expanding our understanding of mechanisms responsible for delayed cardiac PC against I–R injury.

5. CONCLUSIONS

The data reviewed in this chapter ascribe NO a central role in modulating physiological and pathophysiological myocardial function. The radial strain imposed by flowing blood on coronary endothelium, together with several endogenous molecule, constitute the stimulus for NO release. In the heart, NO is the main vasodilator molecule produced and released by the coronary endothelium. In presence of an atherosclerotic coronary artery disease there is an impaired endothelium dependent vasorelaxation of the large coronary arteries leading to a condition of hypoxia that culminate in acute myocardial ischemia. A large amount of studies, in vivo and in vitro, confirm the regulatory role of coronary endothelium-derived NO on myocardial function in different species and experimental settings. Even if from 1986 it is known the concept that brief episode of ischemia and reperfusion increases the ability of the heart to tolerate a subsequent prolonged ischemic event (ischemic preconditioning), only in the last years a specific role for NO has been investigated extensively. The data indicate that NO plays a central role in PC. In particular it seems that eNOS activity is enhanced in the early phase of PC whereas iNOS expression and activity is upregulated in the late phase of PC. This result should not be surprising because the events of the early phase of PC (0–3 h) prepare a pathological condition that allow the induction of iNOS in the late phase (12–96 h). In conclusion, even if the beneficial or detrimental role of NO is in some cases still to be clearly defined, as outlined is this chapter, undoubtedly NO has a key role in the heart function. Nevertheless, this molecule may does not warrant the development of new drugs being at the same time a too simple but complex therapeutic target. At any rate, NO and pathway leading to NO formation represent an important framework to define therapeutic target necessary to the development of new and more efficient drugs. More time is needed to further unravel the complex network of signal involved but some promising preclinical and early clinical data have been already shown.

REFERENCES

1. Metais, C., Li, J., Simons, M., and Sellke, F. W. (1998) Effect of coronary artery disease on expression and microvascular response to VEGF. *Am. J. Physiol.* **275**, H1411–H1418.
2. Zeiher, A. M., Drexler, H., Wollschalger, H., and Just, H. (1991) Endothelial dysfunction of the coronary microvasculature is associated with impaired coronary blood flow regulation in patients with early atherosclerosis. *Circulation* **84**, 1984–1992.
3. Drexler, H., Zeiher, A. M., Meinzer, K., and Just, H. (1991) Correction of endothelial dysfunction in coronary microcirculation of hypercholesterolaemic patients by L-arginine. *Lancet* **338**, 1546–1550.
4. Treasure, C. B., Klein, J. L., Vita, J. A., Manoukian, S. U., Remwick, G., Selwyn, A., et al. (1993) Hypertension and left ventricular hypertrophy are associated with impaired endothelium-mediated relaxation in human coronary resistance vessels. *Circulation* **87**, 86–93.
5. Liao, J. K. (1998) Nitric oxide and vascular disease. *Cardiol. Raunds* **2**, 1–7.
6. Feliciano, L. and Henning, R. J. (1999) Coronary artery blood flow: physiologic regulation. *Clin. Cardiol.* **22**, 775–786.
7. National Heart, Lung and Blood Institute (1990) Morbidity from coronary heart disease in the United States. NHLBI Data Fact Sheet, NIH Publication No. 93-2265, P.O. Box 30105, Bethesda, MD.
8. Shah, A. M. and MacCarthy, P. A. (2000) Paracrine and autocrine effects of nitric oxide on myocardial function. *Pharmacol. Ther.* **86**, 49–86.
9. Nathan, C. (1992) Nitric oxide as a secretory product of mammalian cells. *FASEB J.* **6**, 3051–3064.
10. Marletta, M. A. (1993) Nitric oxide synthase structure and mechanism. *J. Biol. Chem.* **268**, 12,231–12,234.
11. Snyder, S. H. (1992) Nitric oxide: first in a new class of neurotransmitters. *Science* **25**, 494–496.
12. Moncada, S., Palmer, R. M. and Higgs, E. A. (1991) Nitric oxide: Physiology, pathophysiology and pharmacology. *Pharmacol. Rev.* **43**, 109–141.
13. Southan, G. J. and Szabo C. (1996) Selective pharmacological inhibition of distinct nitric oxide synthase isoforms. *Biochem. Pharmacol.* **51**, 383–394.
14. Xie, Q. and Nathan, C. (1994) The high-output nitric oxide pathway: Role and regulation. *J. Leukoc. Biol* **56**, 576–582.
15. Kilbourn, R. G. and Griffith, O. W. (1992) Overproduction of nitric oxide in cytokines-mediated and septic shock. *J. Natl. Cancer Inst.* **84**, 827–831.
16. Palmer, R. M. J. (1993) The discovery of nitric oxide in the vessels wall. A unifying concept in the pathogenesis of sepsis. *Arch. Surg.* **128**, 396–401.

17. Szabo, C. (1995) Alterations in nitric oxide production in various forms of circulatory shock. *New Horizons* **3**, 2–32.
18. Szabo, C. and Thiemermann, C. (1994) Invited opinion: role of nitric oxide in hemorrhagic, traumatic and anaphylactic shock and in thermal injury. *Shock* **2**, 145–155.
19. Bredt, D. S. (1999) Endogenous nitric oxide synthesis: Biological function and pathophysiology. *Free Rad. Res.* **31**, 577–596.
20. Kubes, P. (2000) Inducible nitric oxide synthase: a little bit of good in all of us. *Gut* **47**, 6–9.
21. Alderton, W. K., Cooper, C. E., and Knowles, R. G. (2001) Nitric oxide synthases: A structure, function and inhibition. *Biochem. J.* **357**, 593–615.
22. Palmer, R. M., Ashston, D. S., and Moncada, S. (1988) Vascular endothelial cells synthesised nitric oxide from L-arginine. *Nature* **333**, 664–666.
23. Zembowicz, A., Hecker, M., Macarthur, H., Sessa, W. C., and Vane, J. R. (1991) Nitric oxide and another potent vasodilator are formed from N^G-hydroxy-L-arginine by cultured endothelial cells. *Proc. Natl. Acad. Sci. USA* **88**, 11,172–11,176.
24. Papapetropoulos, A., Rudic, R. D., and Sessa, W. C. (1999) Molecular control of nitric oxide synthases in the cardiovascular system. *Cardiovasc. Res.* **43**, 509–520.
25. Govers, R. and Rabelink T. J. (2001) Cellular regulation of endothelial nitric oxide synthase. *Am. J. Physiol. Renal. Physiol.* **280**, F193–F206.
26. Losano, G., Pagliaro, P., Gattullo, D., and Marsh, N. A. (1994) Contorl of coronary blood flow by endothelial release of nitric oxide. *Clin. Experim. Pharmacol. Physiol.* **21**, 783–789.
27. Kelm, M. and Schrader, J. (1990) Control of coronary vascular tone by nitric oxide. *Circ. Res.* **66**, 1561–1575.
28. Quyyumi, A. A., Dakak, N., Andrews, N. P., Gilligan, D. M., Panza, G. A., and Cannon, R. O. (1995) Contribution of nitric oxide to metabolic coronary vasodilatation in human heart. *Circulation* **92**, 320–326.
29. Kuo, L., Chilian, W. M., and Davis, M. J. (1991) Interaction of pressure- and flow-induced responses in porcine coronary resistance vessels. *Am. J. Physiol.* **261**, H1706–1715.
30. Furchgott, R. F. and Zawadzki, J. V. (1980) The obligatory role of endothelial cells in the relaxation of arterial smooth muscle by acetylcholine. *Nature* **288**, 373–376.
31. Kuo, L., Davis, M. G., Cannon, M. S., and Chilian, W. M. (1992) Pathophysiological consequences of atherosclerosis extend to the microcirculation. *Circ. Res.* **70**, 465–476.
32. Pohl, U., Busse, R., Kuon, E., and Bassenge, E. (1986) Pulsatile perfusion stimulates the release of endothelial autacoids. *J. Appl. Cardiol.* **1**, 215–235.
33. Shen, J., Luscinkas, F. W., Connolly, A., Dewey, C. F., and Gimbrone, M. A. (1992) Fluid shear stress modulates cytosolic free calcium in vascular endothelial cells. *Am. J. Physiol.* **262**, C384–C390.
34. Chilian, W. M., Kuo, L., De Fily, D. V., Jones, C. J. H., and Davis M. J. (1993) Endothelial regulation of coronary microvascular tone under physiological and pathophysiological conditions. *Eur. Heart J.* **14**, 55–59.
35. Bassenge, E. (1995) Control of coronary blood flow by autacoids. *Basic Res. Cardiol.* **90**, 125–141.
36. Treasure, C. B., Vita, J. A., Cox, D. A., Fish, R. D., Gordon, G. B., Mudge, G. H., et al. (1990) Endothelium-dependent dilation of the coronary microvasculature is impaired in dilated cardiomyopathy. *Circulation* **81**, 772–779.
37. Ludmer, P. L., Selwyn, A. P., Shook, T. L., Wayne, R. R., Mudge, G. H., Alexander, R. W. and Ganz, P. (1986) Paradoxical vasoconstriction induced by acetylcholine in atherosclerotic coronary arteries. *N. Engl. J. Med.* **315**, 1046–1051.
38. Gielen, S., Schuler, G., and Hambrecht, R. (2001) Exercise training in coronary artery disease and coronary vasomotion. *Circulation* **103**, 1–6.
39. Becker, B. F., Kupatt, C., Massoudy, P., and Zahler, S. (2000) Reactive oxygen species and nitric oxide in myocardial ischemia and reperfusion. *Z. Cardiol.* **89**, IX/88–IX/91.

40. Bolli, R., Dawn, B., Tang, X. L., Qiu, Y., Ping, P., Xuan, Y. T., et al. (1998) The nitric oxide hypothesis of late preconditioning. *Basic Res. Cardiol.* **93,** 325–338.

41. Szabo, A. and Heemann, U. (1998) Ischemia reperfusion injury and chronic allograft rejection. *Transplant. Proc.* **30,** 4281–4284.

42. Fan, C., Zwacka, R. M., and Engelhardt, J. F. (1999) Therapeutic approaches for ischemia/reperfusion injury in the liver. *J. Mol. Med.* **77,** 577–596.

43. Hammerman, C. and Kaplan, M. (1998) Ischemia and reperfusion injury. The ultimate pathophysiologic paradox. *Clin. Perinatol.* **25,** 757–777.

44. Reimer, K. A. and Jennings, R. B. (1979) The "wavefront phenomenon" of myocardial ischaemic cell death. II. Transmural progression of necrosis within the framework of ischaemic bed size (myocardium at risk) and collateral flow. *Lab. Invest.* **40,** 633–644.

45. MacCarthy, P. A. and Shah, A. M. (2000) The role of nitric oxide in cardiac ischaemia-reperfusion, in *Nitric Oxide* (Mayer B., ed.), Springer, London, pp. 545–570.

46. Reimer, K. A., Lowe, J. E., Rasmussen, M. M., and Jennings, R. B. (1977) The wavefront phenomenon of ischemic cell death. 1. Myocardial infarct size vs duration of coronary occlusion in dogs. *Circulation* **56,** 786–794.

47. Tsao, P. S. and Lefer, A. M. (1990) Time course and mechanism of endothelial dysfunction in isolated ischemic- and hypoxic-perfused rat hearts. *Am. J. Physiol. Heart Circ. Physiol.* **259,** H1660–H1666.

48. Inauen, W., Granger, D. N., Meininger, C. J., Schelling, M. E., Granger, H. J., and Kvietys, P. R. (1990) Anoxia-reoxygenation-induced, neutrophil-mediated endothelial cell injury: Role of elastase. *Am. J. Physiol.* **259,** H925–H931.

49. Lefer, A. M. and Lefer, D. J. (1996) The role of nitric oxide and cell adhesion molecules on the microcirculation in ischemia-reperfusion. *Cardiovasc. Res.* **32,** 743–751.

50. Weyrich, A. S., Buerke, M., Albertine, K. J., and Lefer, A. M. (1995) Time course of coronary vascular endothelial adhesion molecule expression during reperfusion of the ischemic feline myocardium. *J. Leukoc. Biol* **57,** 45–55.

51. Buerke, M., Weyrich, A. S., and Lefer A. M. (1994) Isolated cardiac myocytes are sensitised by hypoxia-reoxygenation to neutrophils released mediators. *Am. J. Physiol. Heart Circ. Physiol.* **266,** H128–H136.

52. Tsao, P. S. and Lefer, A. M. (1991) Recovery of endothelial function following myocardial ischemia and reperfusion in rat. *J. Vasc. Med. Biol.* **3,** 5–10.

53. Weiss, S. J. (1989) Tissue destruction by neutrophils. *N. Engl. J. Med.* **320,** 365–376.

54. Bolli, R., Jeroudi, M. O., Patel, B. S., Aruoma O. I., Halliwell, B., Lai, E. K. and McCay, P. B. (1989) Marked reduction of free radical generation and contractile dysfunction by antioxidant therapy begun at the time of reperfussion. *Circ. Res.* **65,** 607–622.

55. Braunwald, E. and Kloner, R. A. (1982) The stunned myocardium: Prolonged, post-ischaemic ventricular dysfunction. *Circulation* **66,** 1146–1149.

56. Zweier, J. L. (1988) Measurement of superoxide-derived free radicals in the reperfused heart. Evidence for a free radical mechanism of reperfusion injury. *J. Biol. Chem.* **263,** 1353–1357.

57. Wang, P. and Zweier, J. L. (1996) Measurement of nitric oxide and peroxynitrite generation in the postischemic heart. *J. Biol. Chem.* **271,** 29,223–29,230.

58. Beckman, J. S. and Koppenol, W. H. (1996) Nitric oxide, superoxide and peroxynitrite: The good, the bad and the ugly. *Am. J. Physiol.* **271,** C1424–C1437.

59. Darley-Usmar, V. and Halliwell, B. (1996) Reactive nitrogen species, reactive oxygen species, transition metal ions, and the vascular system. *Pharmaceut. Res.* **13,** 649–662.

60. Yasmin, W., Strynadka, K. D., and Schulz, R. (1997) Generation of peroxynitrite contributes to ischaemia-reperfusion injury in isolated rat hearts. *Cardiovasc. Res.* **33,** 422–432.

61. Wang, D., Yangm X. P., Lium Y. H., Carretero, O. A., and LaPointe, M. C. (1999) Reduction of myocardial infarct size by inhibition of inducible nitric oxide synthase. *Am. J. Hypertens.* **12,** 174–182.

62. Wink, D. A., Hanbauer, I., Krishna, M. C., DeGraff, W., Gamson, J., and Mitchell, J. B. (1993) Nitric oxide protects against cellular damage and cytotoxicity from reactive oxygen species. *Proc. Natl. Acad. Sci. USA* **90,** 9813–9817.

63. Sedat, A., Demiryürek, A. T., Çakici, I., and Kanzik, I. (1999) The beneficial effects of peroxynitrite on ischemia-reperfusion arrhythmias in rat isolated hearts. *Eur. J. Pharmacol.* **384,** 157–162.

64. Ku, D. D., Liu, S., and Dai, J. (1995) Coronary vascular and antiplatelet effects of peroxynitrite in human tissues. *Endothelium* **3,** 309–319.

65. Lefer, D. J., Scalia, R., Campbell, B., Nossuli, T. O., Hayward, R., Salamon, M., et al. (1997) Peroxynitrite inhibits leukocyte endothelial cell interactions and protects against ischemia-reperfusion injury in rats. *J. Clin. Invest.* **99,** 684–691.

66. Nossuli, T. O., Hayward, R., Scali, R., and Lefer, A. M. (1997) Peroxynitrite reduces myocardial infarct size and preserves coronary endothelium after ischemia and reperfusion in cats. *Circulation* **96,** 2317–2324.

67. Wu, M., Pritchard, K. A., Kaminski, P. M., Fayngersh, R. P., Hintze, T. H., and Woli, M. S. (1994) Involvement of nitric oxide and nitrosothiols in relaxation of pulmonary arteries to peroxynitrite. *Am. J. Physiol.* **266,** H2108–H2113.

68. Szabo, C., Zingarelli, B., and Salzman A. L. (1996) Role of poly-ADP ribosiltransferase activation in the vascular contractile and energetic failure elicited by exogenous nitric oxide and peroxynitrite. *Circ. Res.* **78,** 1051–1063.

69. Mayer, B., Scharammel, A., Klatt, P., Koesling, D., and Schmidt, K. (1995) Peroxynitrite-induced accumulation of cyclic GMP in endothelial cells and stimulation of purified soluble guanylyl cyclase: dependence on glutathione and possible role of S-nitrosation. *J. Biol. Chem.* **270,** 17,355–17,360.

70. Have-Madsen, L., Merry, P. F., Jurevicius, J., Skeberdis, A. V., and Fischmeister, R. (1996) Regulation of myocardial calcium channels by cyclic AMP metabolism. *Basic Res. Cardiol.* **91,** 1–8.

71. Moro, M. A., Darley-Usmar, V. M., Lizasoin, I., Su, Y., Knowles, R. G., Radomski, M. W., and Moncada, S. (1995) The formation of nitric oxide donors from peroxynitrite. *Br. J. Pharmacol.* **116,** 1999–2004.

72. Murry, C. E., Jennings, R. B., and Reimer K. A. (1986) Preconditioning with ischemia: A delay of lethal cell injury in ischemic myocardium. *Circulation* **74,** 1124–1136.

73. Napoli, C., Pinto, A., and Cirino, G. (2000) Pharmacological modulation, preclinical studies, and new clinical features of myocardial ischemic preconditioning. *Pharmacol. Ther.* **88,** 311–331.

74. Li, G., Vasquez, J. A., Gallagher, K. P., and Lucchesi, B. R. (1990) Myocardial protection with preconditioning. *Circulation* **82,** 609–619.

75. Downey, J. M. (1992) Ischemic preconditioning: Nature's own cardioprotective intervention. *Trends Cardiovasc. Med.* **2,** 170–176.

76. Walker, D. M. and Yellon, D. M. (1992) Ischemic preconditioning: From mechanism to exploitation. *Cardiovasc. Res.* **26,** 734–739.

77. Kloner, R. A. and Yellon, D. (1994) Does ischemic preconditioning occur in patients? *J. Am. Coll. Cardiol.* **24,** 1133–1142.

78. Yellon, D. M. and Baxter, G. F. (1995) "A second window protection" or delayed preconditioning phenomenon: Future horizons for myocardial protection? *J. Mol. Cell. Cardiol.* **27,** 1023–1024.

79. Bolli, R. (1996) The early and late phase of preconditioning against myocardial stunning and essential role of oxyradicals in the late phase: An overview. *Basic Res. Cardiol.* **91,** 57–63.

80. Connaughton, M. and Hearse, D. J. (1996) Three questions about preconditioning. *Basic Res. Cardiol.* **91,** 12–15.

81. Kloner, R. A., Bolli, R., Marban, E., Reinlib, L., and Braunwald E. (1998) Medical and cellular implications of stunning, hibernation and preconditioning. An NHLBI workshop. *Circulation* **97,** 1848–1867.

82. Williams, M. W., Taft, C. S., Ramnauth, S., Zhao, Z. Q., and Vinten-Johansen, J. (1995) Endogenous nitric oxide protects against ischemia-reperfusion injury in the rabbit. *Cardiovasc. Res.* **30,** 79–86.

83. Gattullo, D., Linden, R. J., Losano, G., Pagliaro, P., and Westerhof, N. (1999) Ischemic preconditioning changes the pattern of coronary reactive hyperemia in the goat: Role of adenosine and nitric oxide. *Cardiovasc. Res.* **42,** 57–64.

84. Xuan, Y. T., Tang, X. L., Qiu, Y., Banerjee, S., Takano, H., Han, H., et al. (2000) Biphasic response of cardiac nitric oxide synthase to ischemic preconditioning in conscious rabbits. *Am. J. Physiol.* **279,** H2360–H2371.

85. Bolli, R., Manchikalapudi, S., Tang, X. L., Takano, H., Qiu, Y., Guo, Y., et al. (1997) The protective effect of late preconditioning against myocardial stunning in conscious rabbits is mediated by nitric oxide synthase: Evidence that nitric oxide acts both as trigger and as a mediator of the late phase of ischemic preconditioning. *Circ. Res.* **81,** 1094–1107.

86. Lowenstein, C. J. (1999) Nitric oxide news is good news. *Proc. Natl. Acad. Sci. USA* **96,** 10,953–10,954.

87. Rakhit, R. D., Edwards, R. J., and Marber, M. S. (1999) Nitric oxide, nitrate and ischemic preconditioning. *Cardiovasc. Res.* **43,** 621–627.

88. Downey, J. M. and Cohen, M. V. (1997) Signal transduction in ischemic preconditioning. *Adv. Exp. Med. Biol.* **430,** 39–55.

89. Sasaki, N., Sato, T., Ohler, A., O'Rurke, B., and Marban, E. (2000) Activation of mitochondrial ATP-dependent potassium channels by nitric oxide. *Circulation* **101,** 439–445.

90. Gross, G. J. and Fryer, R. M. (1999) Sarcolemmal versus mitochondrial ATP-sensitive K^+ channels and myocardial preconditioning. *Circ. Res.* **84,** 973–979.

91. Baines, C. P., Liu, G. S., Birincioglu, M., Critz, S. D., Cohen, M. V., and Downey, J. M. (1999) Ischemic preconditioning depends on interaction between mitochondrial K_{ATP} channels and actin cytoskeleton. *Am. J. Physiol.* **276,** H1361–H1368.

92. Takashi, E., Wang, Y., and Ashraf M. (1999) Activation of mitochondrial K(ATP) channel elicits late preconditioning against myocardial infarction via protein kinase C signalling pathway. *Circ. Res.* **85,** 1146–1153.

93. Kuzuya, T., Hoshida, S., Yamashita, N., Fuji, H., Oe, H., Hori, M., et al. (1993) Delayed effects of sublethal ischemia on the acquisition of tolerance to ischemia. *Circ. Res.* **72,** 1293–1299.

94. Marber, M. S., Latchman, J. M., Walker, J. M., and Yellon, D. M. (1993) Cardiac stress protein elevation 24 hours after brief ischemia or heat stress is associated with resistance to myocardial infarction. *Circulation* **88,** 1264–1272.

95. Rizvi, A., Tang, X. L., Qiu, Y., Xuan, Y. T., Takano, H., Jadoon, A. K., et al. (1999) Increased protein synthesis is necessary for the development of late preconditioning against myocardial stunning in conscious rabbits. *Am. J. Physiol.* **277,** H874–H884.

96. Vegh, A., Papp, J. G., and Parratt, J. R. (1994) Prevention by dexamethasone of the marked antiarrhythmic effects of preconditioning induced 20 h after rapid cardiac pacing. *Br. J. Pharmacol.* **113,** 1081–1082.

97. Richard, V., Blanc, T., Kaeffer, N., Tron, C., and Thuillez, C. (1995) Myocardial and coronary endothelial protective effects of acetylcholine after myocardial ischaemia and reperfusion in rats: Role of nitric oxide. *Br. J. Pharmacol.* **115,** 1532–1538.

98. Hill, M., Takano, H., Tang, X. L., Kodani, E., Shirk, G., and Bolli, R. (2001) Nitroglycerin induces late preconditioning against myocardial infarction in conscious rabbits despite development of nitrate tolerance. *Circulation* **104,** 694–699.

99. Takano, H., Manchikalapudi, S., Tang, X. L., Qiu, Y., Rizvi, A., Jadoon, A. K., et al. (1998) Nitric oxide synthase is the mediator of late preconditioning against myocardial infarction in conscious rabbits. *Circulation* **98,** 441–449.

100. Guo, Y., Jones, W. K., Xuan, Y. T., Tang, X. L., Bao, W., Wu, W. J., et al. (1999) The late phase of ischemic preconditioning is abrogated by targeted disruption of the inducible NO synthase gene. *Proc. Natl. Acad. Sci. USA* **96,** 11,507–11,512.

101. Bolli, R. (2000) The late phase of preconditioning. *Circ. Res.* **87,** 972–983.

102. Banerjee, S., Tang X. L., Qiu, Y., Takano, H., Manchikalapudi, S., Dawn, B., et al. (1999) Nitroglycerine induces late preconditioning against myocardial stunning via a PKC-dependent pathway. *Am. J. Physiol.* **277,** H2488–H2494.

103. Pagliaro, P., Gattullo, D., Rastaldo, R., and Losano, G. (2001) Ischemic preconditioning from the first to second window of protection. *Life Sci.* **69,** 1–15.

104. Joyeux, M., Godin-Ribuot, D., Yellon, D. M., Demenge, P., and Ribuot, C. (1999) Heat stress response and myocardial protection. *Fundam. Clin. Pharmacol.* **13,** 1–10.

105. Currie, R. W., Karmazyn, M., Kloc, M., and Mailer, K. (1988) Heat-shock response is associated with enhanced postischemic ventricular recovery. *Circ. Res.* **63,** 543–549.

106. Yellon, D. M., Pasini, E., Caranoni, A., Marber, M. S., Latchman, D. S., and Ferrari, R. (1992) The protective role of heat stress in the ischemic and reperfused rabbit myocardium. *J. Mol. Cell. Cardiol.* **24,** 895–907.

107. Benjamin, I. J. and McMillan, D. R. (1998) Stress (heat shock) proteins molecular chaperones in cardiovascular biology and disease. *Circ. Res.* **83,** 117–132.

108. Kuhl, N. M. and Rensing, L. (2000) Heat shock effects on cell cycle progression. *Cell. Mol. Life Sci.* **57,** 450–463.

109. Knowlton, A. A., Brecher, P., and Apstein, C. S. (1991) Rapid expression of heat shock protein in the rabbit after brief ischemia. *J. Clin. Invest.* **87,** 139–147.

110. Suzuki, K., Sawa, Y., Kaneda, Y., Ichikawa, H., Shirakura, R., and Matsuda, H. (1997) In vivo gene transfection with heat shock protein 70 enhances myocardial tolerance to ischemia-reperfusion injury in rat. *J. Clin. Invest.* **99,** 1645–1650.

111. Jayakumar, J., Suzuki, K., Sammut, I. A., Smolenski, R. T., Khan, M., Latif, N., et al. (2001) Heat shock protein 70 gene transfection protects mitochondrial and ventricular function against ischemia-reperfusion injury. *Circulation* **104,** I303–I307.

112. Valen, G., Hansson, G. K., Dumitrescu, A., and Vaage, J. (2000) Unstable angina activates myocardial heat shock protein 72, endothelial nitric oxide synthase, and transcription factors NFKappaB and AP-1. *Cardiovas. Res.* **47,** 49–56.

113. Malyshev, I. Y., Manukhina, E. B., Mikoyan, V. D., Kubrina, L. N., and Vanin, A. F. (1995) Nitric oxide is involved in heat-induced HSP70 accumulation. *FEBS Lett.* **370,** 159–162.

114. Arnaud, C., Laubriet, A., Joyeux, M., Godin-Ribuot, D., Rochette, L., Demenge, P., and Ribuot, C. (2001) Role of nitric oxide synthases in the infarct size-reducing effect conferred by heat stress in isolated rat hearts. *Br. J. Pharmacol.* **132,** 1845–1851.

115. Searle, J., Kerr, J. F. R., and Bishop, C. J. (1982) Necrosis and apoptosis: Distinct modes of cell death with fundamentally different significance. *Pathol. Annu.* **17,** 229–259.

116. Narula, J., Haider, N., Virmani, R., DiSalvo, T. G., Kolodgie, F. D., Hajjar, R. J., et al. (1996) Apoptosis in myocytes in end-stage heart failure. *N. Engl. J. Med.* **335,** 1182–1189.

117. Bialik, S., Geenen, D. L., Sasson, I. E., Cheng, R., Horner, J. W., Evans, S. M., et al. (1997) Myocyte apoptosis during myocardial infarction in the mouse localizes to hypoxic regions but occurs independently of p53. *J. Clin. Invest.* **100,** 1363–1372.

118. White, E. (1996) Life, death, and the pursuit of apoptosis. *Gen. Dev.* **10,** 1–15.

119. Nagata, S. (1997) Apoptosis by Death Factor. *Cell* **88,** 355–365.

120. Kawaguchi, H., Shin, W. S., Wang, Y., Inukai, M., Kato, M., Matsuo-Okai, Y., et al. (1997) In vivo gene transfection of human endothelial cell nitric oxide synthase in cardiomyocytes causes apoptosis-like cell death. Identification using Sendai virus-coated liposomes. *Circulation* **95,** 2441–2447.

121. Albina, J., Cui, S., Mateo, R., and Reichner, J. (1993) Nitric oxide-mediated apoptosis in murine peritoneal macrophages. *J. Immunol.* **150,** 5080–5085.

122. Cheng, W., Li, B., Kajustra, J., Li, P., Wolin, M. S., Sonnebick, E. H., et al. (1995) Strech-induced programmed myocyte cell death. *J. Clin. Invest.* **96,** 2247–2259.

123. Dimmeler, S., Haendeler, J., Nehls, M., and Zehier, A. M. (1997) Suppression of apoptosis by nitric oxide via inhibition of ICE-like and CPP32-like proteases. *J. Exp. Med.* **185,** 601–608.

124. Weiland, U., Haendeler, J., Ihling, C., Albus, U., Scholz, W., Ruetten, H., et al. (2000) Inhibition of endogenous nitric oxide synthase potentiates ischemia-reperfusion-induced myocardial apoptosis via a caspase-3 dependent pathway. *Cardiovasc. Res.* **45,** 671–678.

125. Ekelund, L. G., Haskell, W. L., Johnson, J. L., Whaley, F. S., Criqui, M. H., and Sheps, D. S. (1988) Physical fitness as a predictor of cardiovascular mortality in asymptomatic North American men. The Lipid Research Clinics Mortality Follow-up Study. *N. Engl. Med.* **319,** 1379–1384.

126. Paffenbarger, R. S. Jr., Hyde, R. T., Wing, A. L., Lee, I. M., Jung, D. L., and Kampert, J. B. (1993) The association of changes in physical-activity level and other lifestyle characteristics with mortality among men. *N. Engl. Med.* **328,** 538–545.

127. Blair, S. N., Khol, H. W. III, Barlow, C. E., Paffenbarger, R. S. Jr., Gibbons, L. W., and Macera, C. A. (1995) Changes in physical fitness and all-cause mortality. A prospective study of healthy and unhealthy men. *JAMA* **273,** 1093–1098.

128. Schuler, G., Hambrecht, R., Schlierf, G., Grunze, M., Methfessel, S., Hauer, K., et al. (1992) Myocardial perfusion and regression of coronary artery disease in patients on a regimen of intensive physical exercise and low fat diet. *J. Am. Coll. Cardiol.* **19,** 34–42.

129. Ehsani, A. A., Heath, G. W., Hagberg, J. M., Sobel, B. E., and Holloszy, J. O. (1981) Effects of 12 months of intense exercise training on ischemic ST-segment depression in patients with coronary artery disease. *Circulation* **64,** 1116–1124.

130. Sessa, W. C., Pritchard, K., Seyedi, N., Wang, J., and Hintze, T. H. (1994) Chronic exercise in dogs increases coronary vascular nitric oxide production and endothelial cell nitric oxide synthase gene expression. *Circ. Res.* **74,** 349–353.

131. Ornish, D., Scherwitz, L. W., Billings, J. H., Brown, S. E., Gould, K. L., Merritt, T. A., et al. (1998) Intensive lifestyle changes for reversal of coronary heart disease. *JAMA* **280,** 2001–2007.

132. Haskell, W. L., Alderman, E. L., Fair, J. M., Maron, D. J., Mackey, S. F., Superko, H. R., et al. (1994) Effects of intensive multiple risk factor reduction on coronary atherosclerosis and clinical cardiac events in men and women with coronary artery disease: The Stanford Coronary Risk Intervention Project (SCRIP) *Circulation* **89,** 975–990.

133. Scheel, K. W., Ingram L. A., and Wilson, J. L. (1981) Effects of exercise on coronary collateral vasculature of beagles with and without coronary occlusion. *Circ. Res.* **48,** 523–530.

134. Cohen, M. V., Yipintsoi, T., and Scheuer, J. (1982) Coronary collateral stimulation by exercise in dogs with stenotic coronary arteries. *J. Appl. Physiol.* **52,** 664–671.

135. Posch, K., Schmidt, K., and Graier, W. F. (1999) Selective stimulation of L-arginine uptake contributes to shear stress-induced formation of nitric oxide. *Life Sci.* **64,** 663–670.

136. Corson, M. A., James, M. L., Latta, S. E., Nerem, R. M., Berk, B. C., and Harrison, D. G. (1996) Phosphorilation of endothelial nitric oxide synthase in response to fluid shear stress. *Circ. Res.* **79,** 984–991.

137. Ranjan, V., Xiao, Z., and Diamond S. L. (1995) Constitutive NOS expression in cultured endothelial cells is elevated by fluid shear stress. *Am. J. Physiol.* **269,** H550–H555.

138. Fukai, T., Siegfried, M. R., Ushio-Fukai, M., Cheng, Y., Kojda, G., and Harrison, D. G. (2000) Regulation of the vascular extracellular superoxide dismutase by nitric oxide and exercise training. *J. Clin. Invest.* **105,** 1631–1639.

139. Stralin, P., Karlsson, K., Johansson, B. O., and Marklund S. L. (1995) The interstitium of the human arterial wall contains very large amounts of extracellular superoxide dismutase. *Arterioscler. Thromb. Vasc. Biol.* **15,** 2032–2036.

140. Omar, H. A., Cherry, P. D., Mortelliti, M. P., Burke-Wolin, T., and Wolin, M. S. (1991) Inhibition of coronary artery superoxide dismutase attenuates endothelium-dependent and independent nitrovasodilator relaxation. *Circ. Res.* **69,** 601–608.

141. DiCarlo, S. E., Blair, R. W., Bishop, V. S., and Stone, H. L. (1989) Daily exercise enhances coronary resistance vessel sensitivity to pharmacological activation. *J. Appl. Physiol.* **66,** 421–428.

142. Wang, J. S., Jen, C. J., and Chen, H. I. (1995) Effects of exercise training and preconditioning on platelet function in men. *Arterioscler. Thromb. Vasc. Biol.* **15**, 1668–1674.

143. Brown, J. M., Grosso, M. A., Terada, L. S., Whitman, G. J., Banerjee, A., White, C. W., et al. (1989) Endotoxin pretreatment increases endogenous myocardial catalase activity and decreases ischemia-reperfusion injury of isolated rat hearts. *Proc. Natl. Acad. Sci. USA* **86**, 2516–2520.

144. Song, W., Furman, B. L., and Parratt, J. R. (1994) Attenuation by dexamethasone of endotoxin protection against ischaemia-induced ventricular arrhythmias. *Br. J. Pharmacol.* **113**, 1083–1084.

145. Parratt, J. R. (1995) Possibilities for the pharmacological exploitation of ischemic preconditioning. *J. Mol. Cell. Cardiol.* **27**, 991–1000.

146. Qureshi, N., Mascagni, P., Ribi, E., and Takayama, K. (1985) Monophosphoryl lipid A obtained from lipopolysaccharide of Salmonella Minnesota R595. *J. Biol. Chem.* **260**, 5271–5278.

147. Elliott, G. T. (1998) Monophosphoryl lipid A induces delayed preconditioning against cardiac ischemia-reperfusion injury. *J. Mol. Cell. Cardiol.* **30**, 3–17.

148. Zhao, L. and Elliott, G. T. (1999) Pharmacologic enhancement of tolerance to ischemic cardiac stress using monophosphoryl lipid A. A comparation with antecedent ischemia. *Ann. N. Y. Acad. Sci.* **874**, 222–235.

149. Mei, D. A., Elliot, G. T., and Gross, G. J. (1996) K_{ATP} channels mediate late preconditioning against infarction produced by monophosphoryl lipid A. *Am. J. Physiol.* **271**, H2723–H2729.

150. He, S. Y., Deng, H. W., and Li, Y. J. (2001) Monophosphoryl lipid A-induced delayed preconditioning is mediated by calcitonin gene-related peptide. *Eur. J. Pharmacol.* **420**, 143–149.

151. Song, W., Furman, B. L., and Parrat, J. R. (1998) Monophosphoryl lipid A reduces both arrhytmia severity and infarct size in a rat model of ischemia. *Eur. J. Pharmacol.* **345**, 285–287.

152. Tosaki, A., Maulik, N., Elliott, G. T., Blasig, I. E., Engelman, R. M., and Das, D. K. (1998) Preconditioning of rat heart with monophosphoryl lipid A: A role for nitric oxide. *J. Pharmacol. Exp. Ther.* **285**, 1274–1279.

153. Janin, Y., Qian, Y. Z., Hoag, J. V., Elliott, G. T., and Kukreja, R. C. (1998) Pharmacologic preconditioning with monophosphoryl lipid A is abolished by 5-hydroxydecanoate, a specific inhibitor of the K(ATP) channel. *J. Cardiovasc. Pharmacol.* **32**, 337–342.

154. Peng, J., Lu, R., Deng, H. W., and Li, Y. J. (2002) Involvement of [alpha]-calcitonin gene-related peptide in monophosphoryl lipid A-induced delayed preconditioning in rat hearts. *Eur. J. Pharmacol.* **436**, 89–96.

155. Zhou, F. W., Li, Y. J., and Deng, H. W. (1999) Early and delayed protection by capsaicin against reperfusion injury in rat hearts. *Acta Pharmacol. Sin.* **20**, 912–916.

156. Ferdinandy, P., Csont, T., Csouka, C., Torok, M., Dax, M., Nemth, J., et al. (1997) Capsaicin-sensitive local sensory innervation is involved in pacing-induced preconditioning in rat hearts: Role of nitric oxide and CGRP? *Naunyn Schmiedeberg's Arch. Pharmacol.* **356**, 356–363.

157. Lu, R., Li, Y. J., and Deng, H. W. (1999) Evidence for calcitonin gene-related peptide-mediated ischemic preconditioning in the rat heart. *Regul. Pept.* **82**, 53–57.

158. Hu, C. P., Li, Y. J., and Deng, H. W. (1999) The cardioprotective effects of nitroglycerin-induced preconditioning are mediated by calcitonin gene-related peptide in isolated rat hearts. *Eur. J. Pharmacol.* **369**, 189–194.

159. Zhao, L., Weber, P. A., Smith, J. R., Comerford, M. L., and Elliot, G. T. (1997) Role of inducible nitric oxide synthase in pharmacological "preconditioning" with monophosphoryl lipid A. *J. Mol. Cell. Cardiol.* **29**, 1567–1576.

160. Johnson, D. A., Sowell, C. G., Keegan, D. S., and Livesay, M. T. (1998) Chemical synthesis of the major constituents of *Salmonella minnesota* monophosphoryl lipid A. *Carbohydr. Chem.* **17,** 1421–1426.
161. Xi, L., Sallom, F., Tekin, D., Jarrett, N. C., and Kukreja, R. C. (1999) Glycolipid RC-552 induces delayed preconditioning-like effect via iNOS-dependent pathway in mice. *Am. J. Physiol.* **277,** H2418–H2424.

III

FUNCTIONAL ENDPOINTS EVALUATING CARDIAC DRUG ACTIVITY

9

Ionic Mechanisms of Atrial Fibrillation

J. Christian Hesketh and David Fedida

1. CLINICAL PREVALENCE, COMPLICATIONS, AND ASSOCIATED CONDITIONS

Atrial fibrillation (AF) is the most common cardiac dysrhythmia and involves irregular and extremely rapid activation of the atria (approx 400 beats per min [bpm]; ref. *1*). The prevalence of AF increases with age, with an incidence of 0.5% in patients less than 50 yr of age and an incidence of more than 5% in patients greater than 65 yr of age *(2,3)*. AF is associated with an increased risk of death and is an important cause of stroke in the elderly population *(2,4)*. Stroke is more common in the AF population as a result of the high atrial activation rate that compromises contractility and the increased likelihood that thrombus will form in the relatively static pool of atrial blood. Emboli can then break away and travel to the brain.

The etiology of AF is varied, and many diseases can contribute to the emergence of AF, including congestive heart failure (CHF; ref. *5*), hypertension *(6)*, coronary artery disease *(7)*, and mitral valve disease *(8)*. The suspected cause of AF from these co-morbid conditions is thought to be atrial dilatation as a result of the increased atrial pressure. Some of these conditions (especially CHF) cause marked interstitial fibrosis that acts as a substrate for AF because of the creation of localized conduction disturbances *(9)*. In addition, there are cases of AF in which there is no known cause (termed lone AF) that may be caused by a genetic predisposition or unknown environmental factors. Most importantly, the presence of AF seems to be a self-perpetuating phenomenon such that AF creates a substrate that both lengthens the duration of AF and increases the likelihood of recurrence in both animal models *(10)* and humans *(11,12)*. This self-perpetuation of AF will be discussed in more detail in the remodeling section of this review.

From: *Cardiac Drug Development Guide*
Edited by: M. K. Pugsley © Humana Press Inc., Totowa, NJ

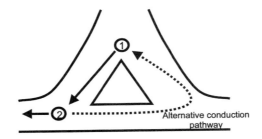

Fig. 1. Schematic diagram of a reentrant circuit created by an alternative conduction pathway between zone 2 and zone 1 (dashed line). Action potentials originating from zone 2 are able to reactivate zone 1 as long as the pathlength of the conduction pathway is less than the wavelength of the tissue.

2. MECHANISMS OF AF

2.1. General Mechanisms

The study of fibrillatory conduction in the heart has a long history, and the first attempt to delineate a mechanism of AF was Cushny *(13)*, who suggested that AF was the result of highly disorganized rhythms that he termed delirium cordis. Over a decade later, Mines *(14)* refined this mechanism, suggesting that the disorganized rhythms were the result of multiple reentrant circuits that could support AF provided that the wavelength of the circuit is shorter than the column of muscle supporting the fibrillatory activity. This was the first suggestion that the electrophysiological parameters of the fibrillatory circuit were related to the maintenance of AF. These studies led to the leading theory for the etiology of AF: multiple circuit reentry.

Mines' multiple circuit reentry was further refined by Gordon Moe *(15)* in 1962 with his multiple wavelet hypothesis. Moe suggested that during AF, the fibrillatory activity was a manifestation of multiple and independent wavelets, each circulating around refractory heart tissue. The maintenance of AF depends on the presence of a sufficient number of wavelets and, therefore, assigns the duration of AF to a probability function. If the trajectory of any given wavelet causes it to encounter refractory tissue, it will be extinguished. This probability function has been described to be proportional to the wavelength of the reentrant circuit. The wavelength concept was first conceptualized by Mines *(14)*. The wavelength of a reentrant circuit is the product of the conduction velocity and the refractory period *(16)*. It defines the smallest size of a circuit required to maintain reentry and, therefore, shorter wavelengths favor maintenance of fibrillatory activity. Reentrant arrhythmias result from abnormal impulse conduction between two separate areas of tissue (Fig. 1). Back propagation of impulses are unlikely in normal tissue due to the fact that sodium channels remain inactivated during much of the action potential and only become available again when the cell has repolarized to about –60 mV. If there is an accessory pathway whereby one zone of tissue can reactivate another previously active zone of tissue, reentrant activity may result. Specifically, the amount of time it takes this aberrant impulse to reactivate the second zone of tissue must be greater than the refractory period of the circuit. Therefore, longer refractory periods reduce the probability of a reentrant circuit sustaining itself. As long as the refractory period is sufficiently short, these two zones may con-

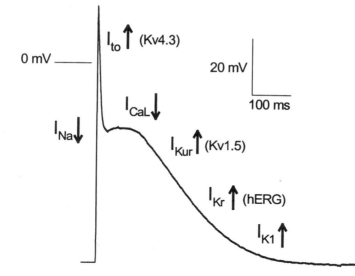

Fig. 2. A schematic of the main ionic currents involved in depolarization and repolarization of human atrial tissue. The currents involved in each phase are indicated next to the phase of the action potential in which they participate. Upward arrows indicate outward current and downward arrows indicate inward current. The ion channel nomenclature in parentheses indicated the suspected molecular determinant of the current.

tinually reactivate each other, creating reentrant arrhythmias. Conduction velocity also plays an important role because more rapidly traveling impulses are more likely to reach the second zone during the refractory period and be extinguished. The refractory period component of the wavelength has been successfully modified pharmacologically to terminate AF and will be discussed in more detail in the current treatment options section of this review.

Control of the refractory period in atrial tissue is mediated by a variety of ionic channels that allow the passage of either inward or outward current at various membrane potentials (Fig. 2). Cells in the sinoatrial node develop slow diastolic depolarizations that depolarize neighboring atrial cells, which in turn generates an action potential when this slow depolarization reaches a threshold potential. The upstroke of the action potential is mediated by rapidly activating and rapidly inactivating inward sodium current (I_{Na}) through hHNa1 channels in the atrial tissue. The membrane potential overshoots 0 mV and is then quickly repolarized by the opening of the transient outward current (I_{to}), which is carried by Kv4.3 channels in human atrium. The I_{to} current quickly inactivates (creating a notch) and the membrane potential is brought to more positive potentials through the opening of L-type calcium channels (I_{CaL}), which carry an inward current and is responsible for the plateau phase of the action potential. During this plateau phase, calcium ions are being released from intracellular stores, generating contraction of the atrial muscle. Although the L-type calcium channels are open, the ultrarapid delayed rectifier potassium current is activated and is mediated by the voltage-gated ion channel, Kv1.5. This results in the repolarization of the action potential and its activity coincides with calcium extrusion and relaxation of the atrial muscle. Later outward currents that activate and act to complete repolarization include the rapid

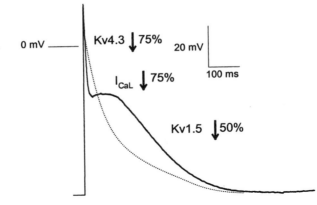

Fig. 3. A representation of an action potential from normal atrial tissue (solid lines) and from a patient with chronic AF (dashed line). Kv4.3, I_{CaL}, and Kv1.5 are believed to be downregulated by the amounts indicated.

delayed rectifier (I_{Kr}), carried by hERG channels, the slow potassium current (I_{Ks}) carried by the heteromultimer, KvLQT1/minK. The inward rectifier (I_{K1}) acts to complete repolarization and maintain the negative resting membrane potential of the atrial cells.

Occasionally, cells outside the nodes exhibit automaticity, and this is termed an ectopic focus. Reentrant circuits can be generated by ectopic activity in which spontaneous depolarizations develop in non-nodal tissue. These ectopic foci can be especially important in the generation of reentrant circuits and result from increased inward current during the diastolic phase of the action potential. This is especially common after myocardial ischemia and explains why AF often accompanies coronary artery disease. Ectopic foci can also result from delayed-after-depolarizations in which inward current during extrusion of Ca^{2+} entering the cell during the systolic phase of the action potential results in the cell prematurely reaching the threshold potential. During Ca^{2+} extrusion, the Na^+/Ca^{2+} exchanger (NCX) transports 3 Na^+ ions into the cell for every one Ca^{2+} ion transported out of the cell, this electrogenicity generates a net inward current that is thought to contribute to after depolarizations *(17)*.

2.2. Structural Remodeling

Of course, ectopic foci are not absolutely necessary for the generation of reentrant arrhythmias, and localized conduction abnormalities may also cause this activity if the wavelength of the circuit is short enough. This is why conditions that cause atrial stretch and/or fibrosis create a substrate for AF. As mentioned earlier, CHF is a strongly associated with AF *(5)* and this may be caused by the extensive fibrosis in atrial tissue found in patients with dilated cardiomyopathy *(18)*. This fibrosis can create local conduction disturbances that can promote reentry. Interestingly, in experimental CHF in dogs, the mechanism of AF is single circuit reentry rather than multiple circuit reentry, suggesting a different etiology from AF in the absence of CHF, which typically involves multiple reentry circuits *(19,20)*. Atrial stretch also seems to create an appropriate substrate for AF as AF often accompanies mitral valve disease *(8)* as well as hypertension *(6)*. The region of the atrium thought to be most vulnerable to stretch is the region around the pulmonary vein, which has a stretch activated nonselective cation current that will depolarize the cell from its resting potential when activated. This may generate ectopic activity and lead to the establishment of reentrant circuits. Isolated pulmonary vein tissue from the guinea pig has been shown to generate slow spontaneous activity *(21)*. Haissaguerre and colleagues *(22)* showed that ectopic beats originating in the pulmonary veins can be the cause of many cases of spontaneous AF in patients. Although the exact mechanisms by which this spontaneous activity occurs are not known, the stretch-activated nonselective cation current may be an interesting drug target. The tarantula toxin GsMtx-4 is a 32 amino acid peptide that blocks this stretch-activated channel and is effective is preventing stretch-activated AF in rabbit hearts *(23)*.

2.3. Ionic Remodeling

In addition to structurally induced AF, the presence of AF causes changes in the expression of various ion channels and other proteins that creates an additional substrate to promote the maintenance of AF. Wijffels et al. *(10)* elegantly showed that goats implanted with a pacemaker that burst paced their hearts into AF whenever sinus rhythm is detected showed a gradual increase between the intervals of spontaneous reversion to sinus rhythm. Initially, the interval between spontaneous reversion was only a few seconds, but this interval quickly increased until AF was maintained for over 24 h after 2 wk of burst pacing. These changes were accompanied by a progressive reduction in the atrial effective refractory period (ERP) and the AF cycle length, an index of refractoriness. These observations are supportive of the theory that reductions in wavelength favor maintenance of reentry. In a later study, Wijffels et al. *(24)* showed that these changes were a result of the high rate of atrial activation and not neurohormonal changes or atrial stretch.

These initial studies in goats led to more detailed examinations of the specific changes in ionic currents, which lead to the AF promoting substrate. Atrial myocytes isolated from patients with chronic AF exhibit a shorter action potential duration (APD) (Fig. 3) as well as a reduced adaption to rate changes *(25,26)*. Similar changes are observed in dogs with experimental AF that is induced by rapid (400 bpm) pacing of the atria for several weeks *(27)*. One possible interpretation is that repolarizing currents, such as I_{Kur}, I_{Kr}, and I_{to} are upregulated during chronic AF, as this would lead to a gradual reduction in ERP and a concomitant reduction in the wavelength. However, detailed molecular studies have demonstrated that I_{to} is actually downregulated by approx 75% during chronic AF *(25,27,28)*. I_{Kur} mRNA may also be downregulated during chronic AF, as shown in isolated myocytes from dogs subjected to chronic atrial pacing. In addition to the reduction in mRNA for I_{to} and I_{Kur}, a reduction in peak and sustained outward K^+ current (I_{to} and I_{Kur}) was demonstrated *(28)*. Pharmacological inhibition of these currents with 4-AP does not produce a large decrease in the action potential duration and, as expected, prolongs the action potential duration *(27)*.

The other possible explanation for the observed shortening of refractoriness and the reduction in APD is a downregulation of the inward calcium current. Indeed, mRNA of the alpha subunit of the L-type calcium channel and inward L-type calcium current is reduced in atrial myocytes from patients with chronic AF *(25,29)* as well as those from dogs with experimentally induced AF (approx 75% reduction in both cases; ref. *27*). Pharmacological block of L-type calcium current with 10 μ*M* nifedipine in myocytes from normal dogs shows a similar reduction in APD as that seen in myocytes from dogs with experimentally induced AF. In addition, when the calcium channel opener, Bay K8644, is applied to myocytes from dogs with AF, the action potential duration is restored *(27)*. These observations have suggested that the precipitating cause of AF is calcium overload resulting from the high atrial activation rate *(17,29,30)*. In response to this assault, there is a downregulation of I_{CaL} and a subsequent reduction in APD and a shortening of ERP. However, this ionic remodeling results in a reduction in the wavelength, a loss of rate adaption, and therefore a promotion of AF maintenance. Perhaps, in an attempt to restore the ionic balance, outward potassium currents are downregulated, but this downregulation is overshadowed by the sharp reduction in L-type Ca^{2+} current, the main inward current responsible for the action potential plateau and rate adaption.

There is some evidence that prevention of calcium overload can prevent ionic remodeling. A study in dogs pretreated with the T-type calcium channel blocker mibefradil showed that the duration of AF was significantly reduced when compared with placebo or the L-type calcium channel blocker, diltiazem. In addition to the reduction in AF duration, mibefradil also greatly reduced the vulnerability to AF induced by extra stimuli *(31)*. T-type calcium channels are not downregulated in AF and they may present a novel therapeutic target for the prevention of electrical remodeling. Despite the inability of L-type calcium channel blockers to prevent remodeling during long-standing AF, it appears that pretreatment with verapamil prevents short-term remodeling *(32)*. The roles of the L-type and T-type calcium channels in long- and short-term remodeling will require further investigation.

As mentioned earlier, CHF often results in concomitant AF and is thought to be largely caused by extensive atrial fibrosis that can create local conduction abnormalities. In addition, the dominant reentry circuit is a single reentry circuit rather than a multiple reentry circuit *(17)*. This evidence suggests that AF in the presence of CHF may be a very different condition than AF in the absence of CHF. Electrophysiological remodeling during CHF-induced AF also strongly differs from the remodeling mentioned previously. Electrophysiological remodeling induced by CHF does not in itself seem to promote AF because atrial myocytes from dogs with experimentally induced AF exhibit longer APDs, a change that would increase the wavelength and therefore increase the minimum circuit size required to maintain reentry. Unlike in atrial tachycardia-induced remodeling, atrial myocytes from dogs with CHF show smaller reductions in Ito (50 vs 70%) and I_{CaL} (30 vs 70%). In addition, these myocytes also showed a reduction in IKs and an increase in inward NCX current *(33)*. In humans with dilated atria, decreases in I_{CaL} *(34,35)* and I_{to} *(35)* have been noted. Other studies have shown variable effects on other important ionic currents in patients with cardiomyopathies, including decreased I_{K1} in some patients *(35)* and no change in others with more severe symptoms *(36)*. Observations in patients with varying degrees of CHF and atrial dilatation likely contribute to the variability in protein expression.

2.4. Neurohormonal Modulators

The autonomic nervous system is known to play an important role in AF. The AF-promoting effects of the parasympathetic nervous system have been known for some time. In fact, bilateral vagal stimulation or acetylcholine administration has been used to induce AF in animal models *(37,38)*. Vagal stimulation activates the I_{Kach} channel, resulting in a strong reduction in atrial action potential refractoriness. However, this

reduction is very heterogeneous because of patchy distribution of vagal nerve terminals in the atrium *(20)*. Refractoriness heterogeneity is an important cause of reentrant
circuits and vagal stimulation can permit AF to be sustained indefinitely *(39)*. Whereas
there is a large spatially heterogenous effect upon atrial refractoriness caused by vagal
stimulation, bilateral sympathetic stimulation seems to produce a much less heterogenous effect, as it has a much less AF-promoting effect. When the degree of sympathetic and parasympathetic stimulation required to produce a similar reduction in
wavelength in dogs was given, the duration of AF was not changed by sympathetic
stimulation nor was the refractoriness heterogeneity *(40)*. Sympathetic induction of AF
is thought to be particularly important after cardiac surgery and patients with robust
calcium currents are unusually prone to postoperative AF *(41)*. Cellular overload caused
by β adrenoceptor stimulation may favor arrhythmogenic mechanisms such as after
depolarizations *(20)*.

3. CURRENT PHARMACOLOGICAL TREATMENT OPTIONS

There are many drugs used to treat AF, including anticoagulants, rate-control drugs,
cardiac glycosides, and calcium antagonists, but this review focuses on the class I and
class III agents, which act directly on ionic channels to terminate or prevent AF. The
first description of a drug that was effective in the termination of AF was Lewis' *(42)*
description of quinidine in 1922. Class I agents primarily block sodium channels, and
their effectiveness is interesting because it does not fit into the wavelength prolonging
approach. In fact, class I agents reduce conduction velocity and may also partially
shorten the refractory period because of blockade of inward sodium window current.
Regardless of these issues, class I agents are extremely potent terminators of AF. Quinidine exhibits conversion rates of 50–92% *(42,43)*, whereas flecainide has been shown
to terminate AF in 74% *(44)* and 86% *(45)* of patients with AF of less than 24 h. However, Crijns et al. *(44)* demonstrated that in patients with AF of more than 24 h in
duration, flecainide was unable to terminate the arrhythmia in any of these patients.
Another class I agent, propafenone, also has a similar profile such that it was effective
in 71% of patients with AF lasting less than 48 h but achieved only 26% efficacy in the
termination of longer-standing AF *(46)*. Clearly, more effective class I agents need to
be developed for longer standing AF.

These class I drugs may reduce ectopic activity by increasing the threshold for the
generation of an action potential. Recently, Pertsov et al. *(47)* described a possible
model of arrhythmia generation called spiral wave reentry. In this model, the core of
the reentry is excitable and maintenance of this spiral wave reentry is dependent upon
the curvature of the wavefronts and this can be modulated by sodium channel blockade. This model is very complex and difficult to demonstrate experimentally but may
partially explain the effectiveness of class I agents. Another controversy surrounding
the use of class I agents was brought about by the Cardiac Arrhythmia Suppression
Trial (CAST), in which 4.5% of patients receiving flecainide for postsurgical ventricular premature depolarizations died as a result of ventricular arrhythmias (compared
with 1.2% placebo; ref. *48*). Flecainide, by shortening the refractory period or slowing
conduction velocity, appears to have proarrhythmic side effects. Clearly, with the
reduced efficacy of class I agents on long-standing AF and with their proarrhythmic
liability, more effective and safer agents need to be developed.

Class III agents act through a different mechanism, and their mode of action is much clearer. These agents prolong refractoriness by selectively blocking I_{Kr} current (hERG). Blockade of this important repolarizing current leads to increases in atrial (and ventricular) refractoriness and therefore an increased wavelength. The increased wavelength leads to a much larger circuit required to maintain reentry and, therefore, many of the reentry waves extinguish. Evidence suggests that sotalol and dofetilide are less effective than class I agents in terminating AF *(49,50)*. In addition, these drugs tend to exhibit reverse-use-dependence, a phenomenon where their I_{Kr} blocking activity is reduced at higher rates, thus rendering them less effective in fibrillating atria *(37)*. Finally, as with class I agents there are significant proarrhythmic effects. These drugs are known to cause torsade de pointes, which can degrade into fatal ventricular fibrillation. In the Survival With ORal D-sotalol (SWORD) trial, 5% of patients died, compared with 3.1% of placebo patients, presumably partially because of fatal ventricular fibrillation *(51)*. The Food and Drug Administration now requires that all new investigational compounds be screened against the hERG channel in cloned channel assays or an in vitro screen of action potential prolonging effects in rabbit or canine Purkinje fibers, which are very sensitive to hERG blockade. New and safer treatments need to be developed to treat AF that do not involve hERG blockade.

4. FUTURE PHARMACOLOGICAL TREATMENT OPTIONS

There are many new and exciting ion channel targets that have shown effectiveness in preliminary preclinical studies. Some of these new compounds prolong the refractory period in an atrially selective manner or block both sodium and potassium channels with fewer ventricular side effects or prevent remodeling through either calcium channel blockade or antioxidant actions. Atrial selectivity is an important feature of a drug used to treat AF because it avoids the proarrhythmic ventricular side effects of current treatments (class I and III agents). An important repolarization current that is present in human atrium but not human ventricle is I_{Kur} *(52,53)*, which is caused by the activity of the delayed rectifier potassium channel, Kv1.5 *(52)*. Blockade of this channel strongly prolongs atrial refractoriness in human myocytes (unpublished data) and has been shown to reduce left atrial vulnerability to AF in pigs as well as selectively prolong the pig atrial ERP but not the ventricular ERP *(54)*. This ion channel target may provide a unique way to prevent AF without ventricular side effects. Another set of ion channel targets includes the mixed sodium–potassium channel blockers. Amiodarone is a commonly used mixed channel blocker for the prevention and termination of AF, but it has an extremely long half-life and can cause significant tissue toxicity. New mixed-channel blockers are being developed that exhibit highly use-dependent sodium channel block with a modest amount of potassium channel block that can impart atrial selectivity to a fibrillating atria. RSD1235 is one such drug being developed by Cardiome Pharma Corp, which shows highly use dependent sodium channel block and selectively prolongs atrial ERP in dogs with experimentally induced AF.

Prevention of remodeling is another potential therapeutic target that may aid in the maintenance of normal sinus rhythm after cardioversion. There are two approaches being developed, one of which is blockade of L-type *(32)* or T-type *(31)* calcium channels. L-type blockade is effective in preventing short-term remodeling whereas T-type blockade is effective in preventing longer-term remodeling. Another treatment area being investigated is the role of free radicals in both structural and ionic remodeling during AF. There is strong biochemical evidence for increased oxidative stress in patients with long-standing AF *(55)*. Patients who receive the antioxidant ascorbate before cardiac surgery experience a 16.3% incidence in postoperative AF compared with 34.9% of control subjects. In dogs with atria paced chronically at 400 bpm, pre-treatment with ascorbate prevented the atrial ERP shortening seen with control dogs *(56)*. The role of these oxidative pathways in the etiology of AF requires further investigation to assess whether or not they can be used to modify progression of the disease.

5. CONCLUSIONS

AF is an extremely common cardiac arrhythmia and is a strong independent predictor of stroke. The ionic mechanisms of AF involve many different ion channels that can contribute to ectopic activity, decreased refractory periods, and subsequent maintenance of AF. Current drug treatments are inadequate because they show significant proarrhythmic liability, but newer drug targets are being evaluated and further research will hopefully lead to safer and more effective drugs in the future.

REFERENCES

1. Waktare, J. E. and Camm, A. J. (1998) Acute treatment of atrial fibrillation: Why and when to maintain sinus rhythm. *Am. J. Cardiol.* **81,** 3C–15C.
2. Benjamin, E. J., Wolf, P. A., D'Agostino, R. B., Silbershatz, H., Kannel, W. B., and Levy D. (1998) Impact of atrial fibrillation on the risk of death: The Framingham Heart Study. *Circulation* **98,** 946–952.
3. Ho, K. K., Pinsky, J. L., Kannel, W. B., and Levy, D. (1993) Related articles The epidemiology of heart failure: The Framingham Study. *J. Am. Coll. Cardiol.* **22,** 6A–13A.
4. Hart, R. G. and Halperin, J. L. (2001) Atrial fibrillation and stroke: Concepts and controversies. *Stroke* **32,** 803–808.
5. Vaziri, S. M., Larson, M. G., Benjamin, E. J., and Levy, D. (1994) Echocardiographic predictors of nonrheumatic atrial fibrillation. The Framingham Heart Study. *Circulation* **89,** 724–730.
6. Vaziri, S. M., Larson, M. G., Lauer, M. S., Benjamin, E. J., and Levy D. (1995) Influence of blood pressure on left atrial size. The Framingham Heart Study. *Hypertension* **25,** 1155–1160.
7. Levy, S. (1998) Epidemiology and classification of atrial fibrillation. *J. Cardiovasc. Electrophysiol.* **9,** S78–S82.
8. Gosselink, A. T., Crijns, H. J., Hamer, H. P., Hillege, H., and Lie, K. I. (1993) Changes in left and right atrial size after cardioversion of atrial fibrillation: Role of mitral valve disease. *J. Am. Coll. Cardiol.* **22,** 1666–1672.
9. Li, D., Fareh, S., Leung, T. K., and Nattel S. (1999) Promotion of atrial fibrillation by heart failure in dogs: Atrial remodeling of a different sort. *Circulation* **100,** 87–95.
10. Wijffels, M. C., Kirchhof, C. J., Dorland, R., and Allessie M. A. (1995) Atrial fibrillation begets atrial fibrillation. A study in awake chronically instrumented goats. *Circulation* **92,** 1954–1968.
11. Yu, W. C., Lee, S. H., Tai, C. T., Tsai, C. F., Hsieh, M. H., Chen, C. C., et al. (1999) Related Articles—Reversal of atrial electrical remodeling following cardioversion of long-standing atrial fibrillation in man. *Cardiovasc. Res.* **42,** 470–476.
12. Tieleman, R. G., Van Gelder, I. C., Crijns, H. J., De Kam, P. J., Van Den Berg, M. P., Haaksma, J., et al. (1998) Early recurrences of atrial fibrillation after electrical cardio-

version: A result of fibrillation-induced electrical remodeling of the atria? *J. Am. Coll. Cardiol.* **31,** 167–173.

13. Cushny, A. R. (1899) On the interpretation of pulse-tracings. *J. Exp. Med.* **4,** 327–347.

14. Mines, G. R. (1913) On dynamic equilibrium in the heart. *J. Physiol.* **46,** 349–382.

15. Moe, G. K. (1962) On the multiple wavelet hypothesis of atrial fibrillation. *Arch. Int. Pharmacodyn. Ther.* **140,** 183–188.

16. Wiener, N. and Rosenblueth, A. (1946) The mathematical formulation of the problem of conduction of impulses in a network of connected excitable elements, specifically in cardiac muscle. *Arch. Inst. Cardiol. Mex.* **16,** 205–265.

17. Nattel, S. (2002) New ideas about atrial fibrillation 50 years on. *Nature* **415,** 219–226.

18. Ohtani, K., Yutani, C., Nagata, S., Koretsune, Y., Hori, M., and Kamada, T. (1995) High prevalence of atrial fibrosis in patients with dilated cardiomyopathy. *J. Am. Coll. Cardiol.* **25,** 1162–1169.

19. Derakhchan, K., Li, D., Courtemanche, M., Smith, B., Brouillette, J., Page, P. L., Nattel, S. (2001) Method for simultaneous epicardial and endocardial mapping of in vivo canine heart: Application to atrial conduction properties and arrhythmia mechanisms. *J. Cardiovasc. Electrophysiol.* **12,** 548–555.

20. Nattel, S., Li, D., and Yue, L. (2000) Basic mechanisms of atrial fibrillation—very new insights into very old ideas. *Annu. Rev. Physiol.* **62,** 51–77.

21. Cheung, D. W. (1981) Electrical activity of the pulmonary vein and its interaction with the right atrium in the guinea-pig. *J. Physiol.* **314,** 445–456.

22. Haissaguerre, M., Jais, P., Shah, D. C., Takahashi, A., Hocini, M., Quiniou, G., et al. (1998) Spontaneous initiation of atrial fibrillation by ectopic beats originating in the pulmonary veins. *N. Engl. J. Med.* **339,** 659–666.

23. Bode, F., Sachs, F., and Franz, M. R. (2001) Tarantula peptide inhibits atrial fibrillation. *Nature* **409,** 35–36.

24. Wijffels, M. C., Kirchhof, C. J., Dorland, R., Power, J., and Allessie, M. A. (1997) Electrical remodeling due to atrial fibrillation in chronically instrumented conscious goats: Roles of neurohumoral changes, ischemia, atrial stretch, and high rate of electrical activation. *Circulation* **96,** 3710–3720.

25. Bosch, R. F., Zeng, X., Grammer, J. B., Popovic, K., Mewis, C., and Kuhlkamp, V. (1999) Ionic mechanisms of electrical remodeling in human atrial fibrillation. *Cardiovasc. Res.* **44,** 121–31.

26. Boutjdir, M., Le Heuzey, J. Y., Lavergne, T., Chauvaud, S., Guize, L., Carpentier, A., Peronneau P. (1986) Inhomogeneity of cellular refractoriness in human atrium: Factor of arrhythmia? *Pacing Clin. Electrophysiol.* **9,** 1095–1100.

27. Yue, L., Feng, J., Gaspo, R., Li, G. R., Wang, Z., and Nattel, S. (1997) Ionic remodeling underlying action potential changes in a canine model of atrial fibrillation. *Circ. Res.* **81,** 512–525.

28. Van Wagoner, D. R., Pond, A. L., McCarthy, P. M., Trimmer, J. S., and Nerbonne, J. M. (1997) Outward K+ current densities and Kv1.5 expression are reduced in chronic human atrial fibrillation. *Circ. Res.* **80,** 772–781.

29. Van Wagoner, D. R., Pond, A. L., Lamorgese, M., Rossie, S. S., McCarthy, P. M., and Nerbonne, J. M. (1999) Atrial L-type Ca2+ currents and human atrial fibrillation. *Circ. Res.* **85,** 428–436.

30. Sun, H., Chartier, D., Leblanc, N., and Nattel, S. (2001) Intracellular calcium changes and tachycardia-induced contractile dysfunction in canine atrial myocytes. *Cardiovasc. Res.* **49,** 751–761.

31. Fareh, S., Benardeau, A., and Nattel S. (2001) Differential efficacy of L- and T-type calcium channel blockers in preventing tachycardia-induced atrial remodeling in dogs. *Cardiovasc. Res.* **49,** 762–770.

32. Tieleman, R. G., De Langen, C., Van Gelder, I. C., de Kam, P. J., Grandjean, J., Bel, K. J., et al. (1997) Verapamil reduces tachycardia-induced electrical remodeling of the atria. *Circulation* **95,** 1945–1953.

33. Li, D., Melnyk, P., Feng, J., Wang, Z., Petrecca, K., Shrier, A., Nattel S. (2000) Effects of experimental heart failure on atrial cellular and ionic electrophysiology. *Circulation* **101,** 2631–2638.

34. Ouadid, H., Albat, B., and Nargeot, J. (1995) Calcium currents in diseased human cardiac cells. *J. Cardiovasc. Pharmacol.* **25,** 282–291.

35. Le Grand, B. L., Hatem, S., Deroubaix, E., Couetil, J. P., and Coraboeuf, E. (1994) Depressed transient outward and calcium currents in dilated human atria. *Cardiovasc. Res.* **28,** 548–556.

36. Koumi, S., Arentzen, C. E., Backer, C. L., and Wasserstrom J. A. (1994) Alterations in muscarinic K+ channel response to acetylcholine and to G protein-mediated activation in atrial myocytes isolated from failing human hearts. *Circulation* **90,** 2213–2224.

37. Wang, J., Bourne, G. W., Wang, Z., Villemaire, C., Talajic, M., and Nattel S. (1993) Comparative mechanisms of antiarrhythmic drug action in experimental atrial fibrillation. Importance of use-dependent effects on refractoriness. *Circulation* **88,** 1030–1044.

38. Nattel, S., Bourne, G., and Talajic, M. (1997) Insights into mechanisms of antiarrhythmic drug action from experimental models of atrial fibrillation. *J. Cardiovasc. Electrophysiol.* **8,** 469–480.

39. Wang, J., Liu, L., Feng, J., and Nattel S. (1996) Regional and functional factors determining induction and maintenance of atrial fibrillation in dogs. *Am. J. Physiol.* **271,** H148–H158.

40. Liu, L. and Nattel S. (1997) Differing sympathetic and vagal effects on atrial fibrillation in dogs: Role of refractoriness heterogeneity. *Am. J. Physiol.* **273,** H805–H816.

41. Kirian, M. A., Lamorgese, M., and Van Wagoner, D. R. (1998) Calcium current density in human atrial myocytes is inversely correlated with the occurrence of post-operative atrial fibrillation. *Circ. Suppl.* I–334.

42. Lewis, T. (1922). The value of quinidine in cases of auricular fibrillation and methods of studying the clinical reaction. *Am. J. Med. Sci.* **163,** 781–794.

43. Parkinson, J. and Campbell, M. (1929) The quinidine treatment of auricular fibrillation. *Quart. J. Med.* **22,** 281–303.

44. Crijns, H. J., van Wijk, L. M., van Gilst, W. H., Kingma, J. H., van Gelder, I. C., and Lie, K. I. (1988) Acute conversion of atrial fibrillation to sinus rhythm: Clinical efficacy of flecainide acetate. Comparison of two regimens. *Eur. Heart J.* **9,** 634–638.

45. Suttorp, M. J., Kingma, J. H., Lie-A-Huen, L., and Mast E. G. (1989) Intravenous flecainide versus verapamil for acute conversion of paroxysmal atrial fibrillation or flutter to sinus rhythm. *Am. J. Cardiol.* **63,** 693–696.

46. Bianconi, L., Boccadamo, R., Pappalardo, A., Gentili, C., and Pistolese M. (1989) Effectiveness of intravenous propafenone for conversion of atrial fibrillation and flutter of recent onset. *Am. J. Cardiol.* **64,** 335–338.

47. Pertsov, A. M., Davidenko, J. M., Salomonsz, R., Baxter, W. T., and Jalife J. (1993) Spiral waves of excitation underlie reentrant activity in isolated cardiac muscle. *Circ. Res.* **72,** 631–650.

48. The Cardiac Arrhythmia Suppression Trial (CAST) Investigators. (1989) Preliminary report: Effect of encainide and flecainide on mortality in a randomized trial of arrhythmia suppression after myocardial infarction. *N. Engl. J. Med.* **321,** 406–412.

49. Singh, B. N. and Nademanee, K. (1987) Sotalol: A beta blocker with unique antiarrhythmic properties. *Am. Heart J.* **114,** 121–139.

50. Suttorp, M. J., Polak, P. E., van 't Hof, A., Rasmussen, H. S., Dunselman, P. H., and Kingma, J. H. (1992) Efficacy and safety of a new selective class III antiarrhythmic agent dofetilide in paroxysmal atrial fibrillation or atrial flutter. *Am. J. Cardiol.* **69,** 417–419.

51. Waldo, A. L., Camm, A. J., deRuyter, H., Friedman, P. L., MacNeil, D. J., Pauls, J. F., et al. (1996) Effect of d-sotalol on mortality in patients with left ventricular dysfunction after recent and remote myocardial infarction. The SWORD Investigators. Survival With Oral d-Sotalol. *Lancet* **348,** 7–12.

52. Fedida, D., Wible, B., Wang, Z., Fermini, B., Faust, F., Nattel, S., Brown A. M. (1993) Identity of a novel delayed rectifier current from human heart with a cloned K+ channel current. *Circ. Res.* **73,** 210–216.

53. Wang, Z., Fermini, B., and Nattel, S. (1993) Sustained depolarization-induced outward current in human atrial myocytes. Evidence for a novel delayed rectifier K+ current similar to Kv1.5 cloned channel currents. *Circ. Res.* **73,** 1061–1076.

54. Knobloch, K., Brendel, J., Busch, A. E., and Wirth, K. J. (2002) Electrophysiological and antiarrhythmic effects of the novel I_{kur} channel blockers S9947 and S20951, on left vs. right pig atrium in vivo in comparison with the I_{kr} blockers dofetilide, azimilide, D,L-sotalol and ibutilide. *Naunym Schmiedebergs Arch. Pharmacol.* **365,** 482–487.

55. Mihm, M. J., Yu, F., Carnes, C. A., Reiser, P. J., McCarthy, P. M., Van Wagoner, D. R., Bauer J. A. (2001) Impaired myofibrillar energetics and oxidative injury during human atrial fibrillation. *Circulation* **104,** 174–180.

56. Carnes, C. A., Chung, M. K., Nakayama, T., Nakayama, H., Baliga, R. S., Piao, S., et al. (2001) Ascorbate attenuates atrial pacing-induced peroxynitrite formation and electrical remodeling and decreases the incidence of postoperative atrial fibrillation. *Circ. Res.* **89,** E32–E38.

10

Targeting Ischemic Ventricular Arrhythmias

Michael J. A. Walker and Leon J. Guppy

1. INTRODUCTION

The purpose of this chapter is to ask why there has been so little success in developing new antiarrhythmic drugs and what can we do to increase our chances of success. Failure has been a fairly common theme in attempts to produce new antiarrhythmic drugs, particularly for lethal ventricular arrhythmias. The chapter considers old and new ways of finding novel drugs for lethal ventricular arrhythmias as a result of myocardial ischemia and infarction and describes new compounds selective for ischemia-induced ventricular tachycardia and fibrillation.

2. GENERAL CONSIDERATIONS

It is possible that the continued invention and application of increasingly intelligent electrical devices for controlling and reverting both ventricular and atrial arrhythmias will obviate the need for newer and better antiarrhythmic drugs. However, such a view is probably simplistic in that devices are costly, invasive, and cannot provide antiarrhythmic coverage for all of the population at risk. In addition, patient preference tends towards drugs rather than devices. All things considered, the need for antiarrhythmic drugs capable of terminating or preventing lethal arrhythmias remains important. This being so, the most important other truism is that a prophylactic drug only has therapeu-

From: *Cardiac Drug Development Guide*
Edited by: M. K. Pugsley © Humana Press Inc., Totowa, NJ

tic value if it reduces or prevents the occurrence or reoccurrence or symptoms of a disease and more importantly reduces mortality. Thus, the goal in developing new antiarrhythmic drugs is especially clear; to reduce or prevent arrhythmias without increasing mortality or adding disproportionate morbidity in terms of drug toxicity. In the history of antiarrhythmic drug development, we have not been very successful in achieving this goal, but that is not to suppose this will always be the case. Previous lack of success may reflect the failure to properly target particular arrhythmias.

2.1. Lethal Ventricular Arrhythmias

The need for better drugs to prevent lethal ventricular arrhythmias is self-evident because, despite all advances, such arrhythmias are still the largest single cause of death in richer countries. Over 300,000 of these deaths occur per year in the United States alone (1). When such deaths occur out of hospital, there is little chance of using electrical defibrillation. Undoubtedly, if an effective and safe prophylactic drug existed for lethal arrhythmias, it would have wide use. Ideally, such a drug would be safe, effective, and given on a prophylactic basis to all those at risk of lethal ventricular arrhythmias—potentially a large number. Some might argue that this ideal is not attainable, but medical science is all about making the impossible, possible. Currently, ventricular defibrillators are implanted in those patients at very high risk of ventricular fibrillation (2); it is hard to imagine their use being expanded to all patients at risk. A safe drug effective against ventricular fibrillation would also be useful in coronary care units, where it would reduce the need for the somewhat-frightening (to patient and doctor) electrical defibrillation. Similarly, such a drug might even be of value in those already fitted with an implanted automatic defibrillator to lessen the risk of the device being activated, again a somewhat distressing event (3).

If the above logic is correct, one has to ask why there is currently so little interest in trying to develop a safe and effective drug for ventricular fibrillation? The easiest answer to this question is the adage, "Once bitten, twice shy." Thus, the pharmaceutical industry has tried before to produce better antiarrhythmic drugs only to fail because of unacceptable drug toxicity and limited effectiveness. This was the case with more potent and selective sodium channel blockers (4) and more recently with highly selective delayed rectifier blockers (5). As a result of their cardiac toxicity, such drugs only have a very limited utility, much less than originally envisioned. Thus, previous attempts to produce better antiarrhythmics for the prevention of lethal ventricular arrhythmias have failed. Why was this? Some of the reasons for failure are discussed below so as to assess whether the particular problem of adequate drug treatment of lethal arrhythmias is insurmountable, or whether there is still hope. It is humbling to realize that the only drug (amiodarone) unequivocally shown to prevent lethal arrhythmias is over 40 yr old. It came very slowly into common use because of its toxicity, and confusing mechanism of action (6,7).

3. GENERAL DIFFICULTIES IN TRYING TO DEVELOP BETTER ANTIARRHYTHMIC DRUGS

The relative lack of success in developing better antiarrhythmic drugs for lethal ventricular arrhythmias, as well as other arrhythmias, probably has many reasons. They all tend to relate to basic deficiencies in our understanding of: (1) normal cardiac electrophysiology; (2) arrhythmic electrophysiology; (3) arrhythmic electropathology; and (4) arrhythmogenic substances released in ischemia.

We continue to add to our understanding of cardiac electrophysiology and arrhythmias, but our knowledge is still not complete enough that we can identify completely rational routes to better antiarrhythmics. We are similar to the person in the dark looking for lost car keys under a street lamp. The keys may have been lost elsewhere, but only the lamp provides sufficient light to warrant a search. In the past, our lamps were sodium channels, and more recently, IK_r blockers and Kv1.5 channels for atrial arrhythmias (*see* refs. *8* and *9* for review). Maybe what we need is to redefine the problem. The following attempts to do this for lethal ventricular arrhythmias. For this, we require a brief review of what is known and what is not known with respect to the problems identified above.

3.1. Current Understanding of Normal Electrophysiology

Ever since the recording of the first electrocardiogram (EKG), there have been continual advances in our understanding of cardiac electrophysiology.

However, we still have far to go before we have a complete understanding of electrogenesis from its molecular basis to the cellular levels and on up to the whole functioning heart in health and in disease. There has been considerable success in producing algorithms as to how the heart generates its normal electrical activity while there are also good models for arrhythmogenesis (*see* refs. *10–12* for reviews). Such models are elegant and intellectually satisfying, but it is not certain as to how complete they are, and more importantly, how predictive. After all, we have still to complete gene and expression maps for the heart, let alone determine the functional significance of such maps. Although we know much about the different ion channels found in the heart, we still do not know just how many types of voltage-dependent and ligand-gated channels there are, or their relative functional importance (*see* ref. *13* for a review on cardiac ion channels). At a functional pharmacological level, we are unsure as to just how blockade or activation of each of the known channels influences the electrical activity in the normal heart, let alone the arrhythmic heart.

3.2. Current Understanding of Arrhythmic Cardiac Electrophysiology

If it is true that our knowledge of normal electrophysiology is incomplete, it is even more so for the abnormal electrophysiology that underlies arrhythmias. Our current models of arrhythmogenesis, such as re-entry and pathological automaticity, are useful both at clinical and experimental levels, but the models are far from complete. Similarly, at the channel level we have incomplete information as to the channel events that underlie arrhythmogenesis. In the absence of complete knowledge, it is hard to identify a specific molecular target whose modulation by drugs will prevent and/or terminate arrhythmias.

3.3. Current Understanding of the Overall Pathology of Arrhythmias

Although we know a great deal about the pathology of some arrhythmias, and less about others, we are a long way from a complete understanding of any one single type of arrhythmia. Thus, there is not one single type of arrhythmia whose pathology we understand so completely that we can use that understanding to rationally create an antiarrhythmic drug for any particular arrhythmia. For example, we understand how changes in the atrium initiate and maintain atrial arrhythmias; how some arrhythmias are dependent upon stimulation of beta adrenoceptors; how ischemia rapidly produces changes in extracellular potassium and hydrogen ions, which relate directly to arrhythmias; and how myocardial scarring contributes to arrhythmogenesis (*see* refs. *11* and *14* for reviews). Even when the pathology is well understood, as for example with certain types of paroxysmal supraventricular reentry tachycardias, we still have not produced the ideal drug. For the acute termination of some of these arrhythmias, adenosine might appear close to the ideal, but only because of its favorable pharmacokinetic profile.

3.4. Current Understanding of the Arrhythmogens Responsible for Arrhythmias

Over the years, many exogenous small molecules have been proposed as the arrhythmogens that give rise to arrhythmias. If this were so, drugs that block the production, or action, of such molecules would be expected to be effective antiarrhythmics. Classic examples of arrhythmogens are norepinephrine and epinephrine (the transmitter molecules responsible for the arrhythmogenic actions of the sympathetic system) and the beta blockers used as antiarrhythmics. However, in this prototypical situation beta blockers have only moderate effectiveness, a fact that speaks directly to the question as to whether norepinephrine and epinephrine are important arrhythmogens. The reality may be more complex in that some of the antiarrhythmic effects of beta blockers may be secondary to their ability to elevate serum potassium concentrations (*see* Sections 6.2.4.2. and 6.2.5.).

Extensive experimentation with a large number of potential arrhythmogens, such as prostaglandins, thromboxanes, endothelins, amines (e.g., 5-HT), and platelet-activating factor have failed to show that they are indispensable for any ischemia-related arrhythmia *(15)*.

Attempts to prevent arrhythmias by blocking the actions or production of such substances have generally met with limited success. Thus, a simple model in which a pathological change, such as ischemia, induces the release of a single arrhythmogen is not very plausible although the synergistic interaction of a number of agents may occur. If the latter is the case, then treatment will require a whole collection of blocking drugs.

4. THE NEED TO TARGET PARTICULAR ARRHYTHMIAS

It is reasonable to draw the conclusion that there can be no universal antiarrhythmic and that the genesis for arrhythmias can be tissue, condition and even time dependent. It was thought that relatively simple classifications of antiarrhythmics, on the basis of their principal ion channel mode of action, would give clear directions as to their use. This is not the case. In view of the limitations to the Vaughan Williams/Harrison classification, the Sicilian Gambit *(16,17)* was created in an attempt to offer another approach to guiding antiarrhythmic therapy on the basis of choosing particular drugs for particular pathologies. However, the incompleteness of our knowledge of arrhythmias and its underlying complexity does not make this classification particularly useful. Current antiarrhythmic classifications are not reliable guides to developing better antiarrhythmic drugs, but they do predict some toxicities.

In considering the above, what is the most rational approach for developing more efficacious and less toxic antiarrhythmic drugs? The reductionist approach would be to identify a particular molecular drug target and, using all of the techniques of high throughput screening and combinatorial chemistry, hit the target potently and selectively. Such an approach would, and does, lead to very potent and selective ion channel blockers, but its weakness lies in the correct choice of target. We often have insufficient functional knowledge to allow us to clearly identify the appropriate molecular target and its functional ramifications. For example, it is encouraging to witness the discovery of tissue-selective channels that offer a chance of selectivity of action. The Kv1.5 channel (*see* Section 6.3.) appears to occur only in atrial tissue. Thus, drugs blocking only this channel would have an atrial tissue selective action and only prolong action potentials in this tissue. However, this begs the question as to whether action potential prolongation occurs in normal and/or diseased atrial tissue, and whether such an action is an effective mechanism for preventing or terminating atrial arrhythmias.

If channel targeting does not always provide a fruitful approach, what other approaches are possible? One is to target specific arrhythmias, as is done for supraventricular nodal reentry tachycardia where slowing calcium-dependent conduction terminates the reentry circuit. If the above is the current general situation regarding arrhythmias, what is the position regarding particular arrhythmias such as the fatal ones induced by myocardial ischemia?

5. ATTEMPTS TO DEVELOP BETTER ANTIARRHYTHMIC DRUGS FOR THE PREVENTION OF ISCHEMIA/INFARCTION-INDUCED FATAL VENTRICULAR ARRHYTHMIAS

In considering drugs designed to treat arrhythmias induced by myocardial ischemia and infarction, it is important to decide whether to consider them one entity, with a common mechanism, or to divide them on some basis. We consider, for the reasons discussed below, that the arrhythmic stimuli resulting from ischemia–infarction fall into three temporal categories: during ischemia, during the process of infarction, and when the infarcting process is complete. The main purpose of this chapter is to discuss possible ways of inventing drugs capable of selectively preventing ischemia-induced arrhythmias.

5.1. The Pathology Associated with Ischemia-Induced Ventricular Arrhythmias

Two distinct stimuli for ischemia-induced arrhythmias occur in the period before infarction develops. Whereas one stimulus is the maintenance of ischemia, the other is reperfusion, after a critical period of ischemia. Because the former is the probably the most common and important in clinical practice (*18–20*), it is only considered here.

In experiments where arrhythmias are induced by ischemia (by occluding a coronary artery), they occur in very distinct temporal phases. The most severe phase occurs within less than 1 h of induction of ischemia. The exact time frame depends upon the size of the species being studied; in smaller species it occurs earlier (15 min in the rat). A later phase occurs hours afterwards, during that time when ischemic tissue is dying and becoming infarcted (*21,22*). Thereafter, the mature and involuting infarct continues to be a lesser source of arrhythmias. In the case of humans, there is an increased risk of cardiac sudden death post infarction, and this risk declines exponentially to reach baseline 4–5 yr after the initial infarct, if reinfarction does not occur.

Overall, we interpret the evidence as showing that the first phase of arrhythmias is the most malignant in animals. Possibly is the most important cause of cardiac-related sudden death in man. Thus, the following discussion concentrates on the early arrhythmias associated with ischemia, rather than infarction although it is recognized that the latter (infarcting and infarcted) phases cannot be ignored. We suppose that the three periods, that is, ischemic, infarcting, and infarcted periods, represent three different arrhythmic stimuli and therefore should be considered independently.

If we accept that most lethal arrhythmias occur relatively early after the onset of ischemia, and before the infarction process is well underway, it is rational to ask what are the changes in ischemic tissue that cause arrhythmias. Changes that temporally relate to the occurrence of arrhythmias include S-T segment elevation of the EKG, falls in extracellular and intracellular pH (to pH 6.4), and corresponding rises in extracellular potassium (to approx 10 mM). The EKG changes relate to, but are not necessarily completely explained by, changes in intracellular potentials *(22,23)*. Changes in intracellular potentials temporally related to arrhythmias include a fall in resting membrane potential, reduced action potential height, and accelerated repolarization; events that result in changes in conduction and refractoriness, respectively. Within the ischemic zone this results in changes from the normal ordered process of conduction and refractoriness. The changes in conduction and refractoriness are sufficient to cause re-entry, the dominant arrhythmic mechanism believed to operate in the early period of ischemic arrhythmias *(24)*. Furthermore, the interaction between disordered ischemic electrophysiology and normal electrophysiology across the border zone is another, and possibly a more important, cause of reentry.

The temporal relationship between the above changes and arrhythmias argues for a causal relationship although the time window for ischemia-induced arrhythmias does not coincide exactly with EKG, pH, or K changes. Although it is possible to argue that the prevention of the changes in potassium and pH might prevent arrhythmias from occurring, the only way to achieve this with certainty is to reperfuse the ischemic area, a different treatment modality from that involving antiarrhythmic drugs. One question that can be asked is, can one take advantage of such changes to create antiarrhythmic drugs selective for ischemia-induced arrhythmias? To concentrate on the changes that appear to induce arrhythmias is to accept the argument that ischemia-induced arrhythmias arise from the ischemic zone, a not unreasonable argument because there would be no arrhythmias without ischemia. One alternative hypothesis is that ischemic arrhythmias arise from the border zone between ischemic and normal tissue, but this could not exist without the ischemic zone.

6. PREVIOUS ATTEMPTS TO TARGET ISCHEMIA-INDUCED ARRHYTHMIAS

The need to target ischemia-induced arrhythmias has been recognized for many years, and there have been many attempts to achieve this. In the following list, we consider various ways for trying to achieve selectivity, so as to increase efficacy and reduced toxicity. Thus, there are drugs that:

1. Target the high frequency arrhythmias, e.g., tachycardias and fibrillation;
2. Target the ion channels and other cellular systems activated by conditions of ischemia, and believed to be responsible for arrhythmias; and
3. Target the production or action of the arrhythmogens released by ischemia that cause arrhythmias.

6.1. Targeting High-Frequency Arrhythmias: State-Dependent Targeting

Tachyarrhythmias, especially ventricular, are the most common cause of morbidity and mortality among all arrhythmias. The rapid rates of such arrhythmias provide a clear drug target because drugs that act only at the rapid rates of tachyarrhythmias would be selective for these arrhythmias. Frequency-dependence is therefore a potentially useful attribute for any drug designed to prevent ischemia-induced tachyarrhythmias, regardless of the molecular target the drug is acting upon. The classic frequency-dependent antiarrhythmics are the class Ib antiarrhythmics, such as lidocaine and mexiletine. These sodium channel blockers act in a frequency-dependent manner and have potential antiarrhythmic actions by reducing excitability (automaticity) and conduction velocity (reentry) in normal and ischemic tissue. Frequency-dependence is important with the current IK_r (human ether a go-go–related gene channel) blockers. Generally, these drugs demonstrate negative frequency-dependence because their actions become more pronounced at slower heart rates. This results in proarrhythmic actions, such as torsade de pointes *(25)*. It therefore appears that positive frequency-dependence is preferred for antiarrhythmics.

One fundamental question is how well does positive frequency-dependent sodium channel blockade translate into antiarrhythmic actions against ischemia-induced arrhythmias? The classic answer is with the drug lidocaine. The evidence obtained in the clinic appears reasonably clear in that lidocaine is now rarely used to treat ventricular fibrillation, despite a long history of its use for this purpose. Thus, although there is evidence that lidocaine lowers the incidence of ventricular fibrillation in patients with an ongoing myocardial infarction, it has limited efficacy and excessive toxicity (cardiac and otherwise; refs. *26* and *27*). A similar situation occurs experimentally with lidocaine where efficacy is limited against ventricular fibrillation, and toxicity is common *(28,29)*. This is exemplified by studies with class Ib drugs in which doses that reduce ischemia-induced ventricular fibrillation cause convulsions in conscious animals *(30,31)*. Such a situation is not unexpected from basic pharmacological knowledge. Thus, frequency-dependent sodium channel blockers have low molecular weights and are lipid soluble. Thus, they easily penetrate the central nervous system (CNS), where high-frequency sodium-dependent action potentials are very common. The block of sodium channels in the CNS at first blocks inhibitory action potentials, and then all action potentials, resulting in initial, and apparently paradoxical, convulsions before coma and death *(31)*.

Because the frequency-dependent blocking action of class Ib drugs depends, at least in part, on binding to the inactive state of the sodium channel, it is difficult to separate an action dependent on channel inactivation from that involving blockade of open channels. Ischemia-induced depolarization would itself potentiate the sodium channel blocking actions of class Ib in the ischemic zone, but despite this, class Ib drugs still do not have highly selective actions against ischemia-induced arrhythmias because CNS and cardiovascular toxicity is always limiting.

None of the currently available potassium channel blocking drugs has marked positive frequency-dependent actions. In fact, the converse occurs with iK_r blockers (*see* Section 6.2.5.).

As a result, we do not know whether positive frequency-dependence for potassium channel blockade confers selectivity for ischemia-induced arrhythmias.

6.2. Targeting Ion Channels and Other Cellular Systems Activated by Conditions of Ischemia and Believed to be Responsible for Arrhythmia

The nature and type of biochemical changes induced by ischemia are well known. They include changes in intra- and extracellular ion concentrations, disturbances in lipid metabolism, production of free radicals, cellular volume changes and changes in the metabolism, as well as the production of many biologically active substances *(14)*. The question as to which of these are specifically activated by ischemia, participate in arrhythmogenesis, and therefore provide suitable targets for antiarrhythmic drugs is considered below. The role of possible arrhythmogens has been thoroughly discussed before and not one single one of them provides a suitable target. Other possible molecular targets for antiarrhythmic drugs include the following: (1) [H$^+$] exchangers; (2) Ca^{2+} channels and calcium handling; and (3) K$^+$ channels, especially those activated by ischemia. These are all considered individually below.

6.2.1. [H$^+$] Exchangers

One process markedly influenced by ischemia is proton regulation. During ischemia both intracellular ([H$^+$]$_i$) and extracellular ([H$^+$]$_o$) increase by three mechanisms: (1) lack of washout of CO_2 and lactate, (2) Na$^+$-dependent extrusion of protons via the Na$^+$/H$^+$ exchanger; and (3) by the Na$^+$/HCO$_3^-$ exchangers. The Na$^+$/H$^+$ exchanger (NHE) plays a minor role in recovery of pH *(32,33)*. However, the influence on [Na$^+$]$_i$ on the exchanger should be taken into account because this influences [Ca^{2+}]$_i$ *(34)* and may explain the improved recovery of contractile function *(35)* and reduction in arrhythmias *(35–38)* that is seen when the exchanger is blocked.

Preclinical experiments have shown some promise with specific blockers of the NHE *(39)*. Cariporide is the most advanced example of drugs that uses this approach *(40–43)*. It has antiarrhythmic efficacy in a number of ischemia models *(37)*. However, the large GUARDIAN clinical trial, involving approx 11,000 patients, showed that cariporide did not decrease mortality in patients with coronary artery disease. *(44)*.

Eniporide, another specific NHE-1 inhibitor, was found to lack clinical benefit when tested in the 1389-patient ESCAMI trial *(45)*. Other NHE inhibitors are in various stages of development *(46–48)*, but the potential utility of these drugs remains to be proven clinically. One difficulty when testing these drugs is the absence of suitable surrogate measures, that is, EKG changes, from which to gauge whether the drug is being given at an effective dose. The general usefulness of this approach to ischemia-induced arrhythmias appears to be mainly in the treatment of reperfusion arrhythmias (ref. *36; see* ref. *49* for review) and not ischemia-induced arrhythmias. Further evidence is required to clarify a role for proton regulation as a target for ischemic antiarrhythmic drugs.

6.2.2. Ca^{2+} Channels and Calcium Handling

The intracellular concentration of calcium, [Ca^{2+}]$_i$, increases during ischemia *(50)* via various possible mechanisms, including T and L-type calcium channel opening, reduced sarcoplasmic reticulum uptake and displacement of bound calcium *(51)* and decreased Na$^+$/Ca^{2+} exchanger activity *(52,53)* secondary to increased [Na$^+$]$_i$ (after Na$^+$/K$^+$ ATPase inhibition). Increases in [Ca^{2+}]$_i$ are considered a trigger for arrhythmias *(54)*. Increased [Na$^+$]$_i$ can result in reversal of the Na$^+$/Ca^{2+} exchanger, resulting in elevation of [Ca^{2+}]$_i$. Under normal circumstances, the Na$^+$/Ca^{2+} exchanger is responsible for approx 77% of the extrusion of Ca^{2+} from the cell *(55,56)*; thus, any reduction in the efficiency of this system could drastically influence $[Ca^{2+}]_i$. The efficiency of the exchanger is further reduced by acidosis *(57)* and free radicals *(58)*. Mitochondria act as a buffer for increased $[Ca^{2+}]_i$, by holding massive mounts of Ca^{2+} *(59)*, but they do not contribute to $[Ca^{2+}]_i$ in ischemia.

A strategy to reduce the increase in $[Ca^{2+}]_i$ with ischemia would be to target the Na^+/Ca^{2+} exchanger. This molecular strategy has been used to treat heart failure, and reverse-mode Na^+/Ca^{2+} exchanger inhibitors, such as KB-R7943, have been reported to have antiarrhythmic actions in preclinical ischemia–reperfusion models *(60–62)*. There are no data available from clinical trials to determine whether Na^+/Ca^{2+} exchanger inhibitors are effective in humans. Although there are changes in systolic Ca^{2+} transients within 18 min of the onset of ischemia, diastolic Ca^{2+} does not change until after 1 h *(63)* of ischemia. Changes in $[Ca^{2+}]_i$ may not occur rapidly enough to play a major role in the early arrhythmias because of ischemia *(64)*. However, variations in the rate of rise in $[Ca^{2+}]$ with ischemia have been reported *(65,66)*. Manipulation of sarcoplasmic calcium by ryanodine has been shown to be antiarrhythmic *(67)*, but overall a role for calcium as a mandatory ischemic arrhythmogen is not clear.

Although a role for $[Ca^{2+}]_i$ as an arrhythmogen in myocardial ischemia is unclear, a number of reports have detailed the antiarrhythmic properties of calcium channel antagonists in ischemia *(68–71)*, albeit only at doses that depress cardiovascular function. A suggestion was made many years ago *(68)* that selective calcium channel blockade in the ischemic zone would confer selectivity for ischemic arrhythmias, but this idea has still to be fully tested.

6.2.3. K+ Channels, Particularly Those Activated by Ischemia

During ischemia there must be a greatly increased permeability for K^+ to account for the rapid increase in extracellular potassium in ischemic tissue that occurs within minutes of the onset of ischemia. Several of the known K^+ channels, including K_{ACh}, K_{ATP}, K_{AA} and K_{Na}, appear to increase their K^+ conductance in response to the metabolic changes induced by ischemia. The K_{ATP} channel is the most likely candidate for a channel specifically activated by ischemia. K_{ATP} channels occur in many tissues, in various isoforms, but all are regulated in a similar fashion. The channels are closed when there are adequate intracellular concentrations of ATP (free ATP or Mg^{2+} bound; ref. *72*). Channel states also depend on levels of nucleotide diphosphates and are regulated by blockers, such as sulphonylureas (e.g., glibenclamide) and K^+ channel openers (e.g., pinacidil). Glibenclamide blocks the K_{ATP} channel in the heart and thereby is expected to cause an increase in action potential duration and decreased K^+ loss in ischemia whereas drugs, such as pinacidil, would have the opposite action.

It appears that the K_{ATP} channel is a good candidate for being a major contributor to the observed increase in K^+ conductance during ischemia. Although some of the evidence is equivocal *(73)*, there is evidence that K_{ATP} channels contribute, in part, to action potential duration shortening under appropriate circumstances. Agents, such as cyanide and dinitrophenol *(74,75)*, which mimic ischemia, cause K_{ATP} channel opening. There is a correlation between channel activation and shortening of the action potential. In addition intracellular application of ATP can reverse shortening. If activation of K_{ATP} channels causes a reduction in refractory period, then this makes the myocardium more vulnerable to arrhythmias *(76)*. With respect to direct evidence using

K_{ATP} channel blockers, some studies have shown them to be antiarrhythmic in ischemia *(77–79)*, whereas other studies show only limited efficacy *(79)* or no antiarrhythmic activity *(80,81)*.

There are two aspects to consider when studying K_{ATP} channels in the heart. One aspect is the activity of K_{ATP} channels in cardiomyocytes in normal and ischemic conditions. The other aspect is K_{ATP} channels in the coronary vasculature which, when activated, mediate vasodilation. This latter effect is blocked by glibenclamide *(82)*. Additionally, glibenclamide reverses the outward current induced by hypoxia as well as the DNP-induced shortening of the action potential *(83,84)*. K_{ATP} channels are also found in both the sarcolemmal and mitochondrial membranes *(85)*, and the latter may protect against ischemia-induced arrhythmias during hypoxia adaptation at high altitudes *(86)*.

Evidence against a role for K_{ATP} channels in ischemia is that the channel is highly sensitive to block by ATP and $[ATP]_I$ levels do not drop sufficiently during early ischemia to open K_{ATP} channels *(87)*. This fact, however, does not negate a role for the K_{ATP} channel in increasing $[K^+]_o$ since ischemia does decrease $[ADP]_i$ *(88)*. However, lactate *(89)*, acidosis *(90)*, oxygen-free radicals *(91)* extracellular adenosine *(92)*, decreased taurine *(93)* and stretch (caused by cell swelling; ref. *94*) all change the sensitivity of the channel to $[ATP]_i$. Further, subsarcolemmal ATP concentrations may be different from total ATP concentrations, that is, compartmentalization of ATP may be important. Such findings confound the problem of determining the exact role of K_{ATP} channels in genesis of ischemic arrhythmias.

Where modulation of the K_{ATP} channel with drugs results in antiarrhythmic activity the mechanism is not always clear. Both openers *(95)* and blockers *(79,96)* have been shown to produce antiarrhythmic actions. However, in the latter case, action potential duration increases were not seen with glibenclamide, making it unlikely that the antiarrhythmic effect is caused by a class III action. One possible mechanism for glibenclamide's actions is a reduction in electrophysiological dispersion between activation and recovery in the ischemic zone *(96)*, possibly by decreasing the rate of increase of $[K^+]_o$ and therefore decreasing heterogeneity. In conclusion, the overall evidence is not strong that K_{ATP} channels are the best targets for potent and selective antiarrhythmic actions in ischemia.

6.2.4. Targeting Arrhythmogens Produced During Ischemia

During acute ischemia, there is an almost immediate increase in $[K^+]_o$, accompanied by increased $[H^+]_i$, $[H^+]_o$, $[Na^+]_i$, $[Ca^{2+}]_i$, and depletion of intracellular $[Mg^{2+}]_o$ plus the accumulation of a host of metabolic breakdown products. The complexity of the interactions between these factors makes it impossible to say with certainty that any combination of factors, or any individual factor, is more or less important in ischemic arrhythmogenesis. The possible nonelemental chemical mediators of arrhythmogenesis include catecholamines, histamine, 5-HT, amphiphiles (e.g., lysophatidylcholine), prostaglandins, thromboxanes, leukotrienes, angiotensin, endothelin, opioids, protons, and free radicals. Inhibition of the release and/or action of such agents is a potential target for ischemia-selective antiarrhythmic drugs. As indicated previously, Curtis et al. *(15)* have provided a comprehensive review of the arrhythmogenic potential of these chemical mediators produced during ischemia.

The particular role of potassium and catecholamines is discussed below in relation to providing a possible basis for developing ischemia-selectivity antiarrhythmic drugs.

6.2.4.1. POTASSIUM

A number of factors could contribute to the increased $[K^+]_o$ in addition to activation of K^+ channels described above (*see* ref. *14* for review), but regardless of this, what is the role $[K^+]_o$ in ischemic arrhythmogenesis and what is its possible use in developing ischemia-selective drugs? The evidence that exists for a role of increased $[K^+]_o$ includes the correlation between the time course of changes in $[K^+]_o$ and the early phase of ischemic arrhythmias. When $[K^+]_o$ is elevated in a region of the nonischemic heart, it produces ischemia-like electrophysiological changes and arrhythmias *(97–100)*.

Extracellular potassium can have pro- or antiarrhythmic actions, depending on concentration. In the absence or presence of ischemic myocardium, both hypo- and hyperkalemia can induce arrhythmias. Within the physiological range of $[K^+]_o$, arrhythmias are five times more likely to occur at lower than at higher $[K^+]_o$ *(101)*. Overall in isolated hearts $[K^+]_o$ displays a U-shaped curve for its effect on the incidence of arrhythmias *(98)*. The incidence of arrhythmias decreases with increasing $[K^+]_o$ then starts to increase again beyond a certain $[K^+]_o$. This situation readily gives rise to confusion in analyzing results obtained in intact animals subject to myocardial ischemia. In intact animals there are two separate questions; one is, what is the arrhythmic effect of raised $[K^+]_o$ in the ischemic tissue; the second is, what are the effects of raised plasma $[K^+]_o$ in the rest of the heart on ischemic arrhythmias? Because the elevated K^+ cannot be readily lowered in the ischemic zone and because it is difficult to modulate plasma $[K^+]_o$ to an optimal antiarrhythmic level, changing $[K^+]_o$ to prevent arrhythmias would be difficult in acute myocardial ischemia. However, it is possible that the moderate elevations in serum K^+ associated with beta blocker or angiotensin-converting enzyme inhibitors therapy might, in part, be responsible, for the limited but very real effect such drugs have on mortality in post myocardial infarction patients.

6.2.4.2. CATECHOLAMINES AND cAMP

Beta blockers are well known antiarrhythmics, albeit of limited efficacy. They undoubtedly reduce, but do not abolish, mortality after a myocardial infarct. Indeed, most of the literature supports a role for catecholamines in the genesis of ischemic arrhythmias (e.g., refs. *102,103*). However, although catecholamines are released in ischemic tissue *(104,105)*, it is not certain that this release is causally related to ischemic arrhythmias. In studies reporting positive correlations between catecholamine concentrations in ischemia and arrhythmias, other pharmacological effects of these drugs (metabolic effects on glycogen metabolism, induction of bradycardia, alterations of serum potassium) could explain their antiarrhythmic actions. Beta blockers are ineffective against acute ischemia-induced arrhythmias in conscious rats *(106,107)*. Other studies support the idea that catecholamines may be indirectly arrhythmic in this situation via a secondary action on serum potassium *(108–111)*. On the other hand, some reports even suggest a cardioprotective role for catecholamines during ischemia *(112)*.

The evidence for cyclic AMP (cAMP), the second messenger for the functional response to β receptor activation, having a role *(113)* in arrhythmogenesis in acute ischemia is not overwhelming. Although cAMP has been shown to produce arrhythmias in some studies *(113,114)*, this appears to be dependent on $[K^+]_o$ with elevated $[K^+]_o$

antagonizing the effect *(115)*. In addition to this, although some studies have shown a correlation in the time–course of increases in cAMP and the severity of ischemia *(116)*, others have not *(117)*. As a result of such studies, it is difficult to conclude that cAMP is a major arrhythmogen in the setting of ischemia.

6.2.5. Targeting Ion Channels in Ischemia

Determination of how the ion channels of normal cardiac electrogenesis are involved in ischemic arrhythmogenesis is potentially confused because most of the evidence comes from the use of ion channel–blocking drugs. Obviously, the behavior of normal channels is altered by ischemia. Thus, on its own, the raised extracellular potassium as the result of ischemia will lower resting membrane potential and thereby inactivate sodium channels, resulting in slower conduction and reduced excitability. Similarly, raised potassium will activate some potassium channels, hastening repolarization and adding to $[K^+]_o$ in ischemic tissue. In addition to sodium and potassium channels, the channels for Ca^{2+} and Cl^- are also influenced by ischemia. However, unless we can clearly differentiate whether ion channel–blocking drugs exert their antiarrhythmic actions on ischemic and/or normal tissue, such drugs may tell us little about the importance of any one channel in ischemia. This is of importance because drugs that are antiarrhythmic by virtue of acting on normal cells, are proarrhythmic.

Current and previous approaches to treating ischemic arrhythmias have been to target ion channels. The Vaughan–Williams scheme presents a popular way of categorizing antiarrhythmic drugs based on the primary ion channel or receptor blocking actions *(16)*: class I for sodium channel blockers, class II for β adrenoceptor blockers, class III for potassium channel blockers, and class IV for calcium channel blockers. This classification will be used in the following discussion.

Class I drugs have been used for many years as general atrial and ventricular antiarrhythmics, and although many are useful, under certain conditions they are not safe *(31,118,119)*. The CAST study highlighted the potential dangers of some members of this class, particularly class I_c *(4)*, with the patients at most risk of drug-related sudden death being those with recurrent myocardial ischemia *(120)*. It is possible that these drugs, such as flecainide, by slowing conduction in ischemic, infarcted or normal myocardium increase the likelihood of reentry *(121)*. Alternatively, they may increase the heterogeneity of action potentials (e.g., between pericardial and endocardial cells), resulting in re-entry *(122,123)*.

Ischemia decreases the amplitude and rate of rise of the action potential and decreases excitability, most probably as a result of the elevated $[K^+]_o$ and consequent inactivation of a greater proportion of Na^+ channels. Despite this inactivation, there may be a transient increase in excitability as the membrane potential (E_m) approaches the threshold potential, resulting in less current being required to reach threshold *(124)*. In infarcted tissue, there is a shift of steady-state Na^+ channel availability to negative potentials that reduces Na^+ channel availability in the action potential *(125)*. Additionally, there is prolongation of postdepolarization refractoriness *(126)*. Increasing, $[K^+]_o$, besides reducing conduction velocity, also shortens action potential duration. The effect on duration is probably due to an increase in potassium conductance *(127,128)*, rather than a decrease in Na^+ conductance. It is against this setting that the actions of antiarrhythmic drugs in ischemia are discussed.

Although class I drugs can suppress some types of arrhythmias *(129–131)*, their efficacy against sudden cardiac death is poor *(132,133)*. This may imply that perhaps one of the contributing types of ventricular fibrillation (ischemic phase 1 and 2 arrhythmias, or reperfusion) in sudden cardiac death is not influenced by these drugs. Even in the isolated hearts, lidocaine, quinidine, and flecainide at peak unbound therapeutic plasma levels failed to suppress ischemia-induced arrhythmias *(27)*.

The previous discussion provides a limited view of the available evidence regarding the efficacy of class I antiarrhythmics against ischemia-induced arrhythmias. If all the experimental evidence is taken in concert, a picture remains of drugs with limited selectivity for ischemic arrhythmias and poor therapeutic ratios for antiarrhythmic actions versus toxicity. Clinically the picture is even more depressing in that the more the issue is investigated the more it becomes apparent that all class I drugs cause as many, or more, deaths than they save.

Class II antiarrhythmics (sympatholytics, especially beta blockers) have been previously discussed. As mentioned some of the effects against ischemic arrhythmias may not be due to direct blockade of myocardial β adrenoceptors *(111, 134)*. The limited antiarrhythmic effects of beta blockers in acutely prepared anesthetized rats subject to regional myocardial ischemia relates to their actions on serum $[K^+]$ *(100,109,110)*. Beta blockers do not protect against ischemia-induced arrhythmias in conscious rats, where there have no effect on serum $[K^+]$ *(106,110)*. The rise in serum $[K^+]$ with beta blockade in anesthetized rats is secondary to acute surgery, increased sympathetic activity, and barbiturate anesthesia. In keeping with this view, blockade of sympathetic activity with tetrodotoxin does not influence ischemic arrhythmias in vitro or in vivo *(135,136)* whereas transplanted hearts (which lack nerves) showed no difference in ischemic arrhythmia incidence compared with normally innervated hearts *(111)*. Although beta-blockers, like other antiarrhythmics, can cause arrhythmias (in the sinoatrial and atrioventricular nodes), the benefit of their prophylactic use after a myocardial infarction is limited, but greater than most other drugs *(137,138)*.

Class III drugs are exemplified by IK_r blockers. The human ether a go-go–related gene α subunit appears to be responsible for the IK_r current *(139)*, and there are a number of drugs that are potent and selective blockers of IK_r (e.g., E4031, dofetilide). Unfortunately, most of these drugs exhibit negative frequency-dependence and produce their greatest effect in increasing action potential duration at slower heart rates *(140)*. Bradycardia with action potential (Q-T) widening is the most common cause of torsade de pointes. The interaction of increased $[K^+]_o$ and drugs may be a critical determinant in producing torsade *(141)*. It has been suggested that IK_S inactivation is incomplete at rapid heart rates and therefore there is accumulation of this current *(142)* and IK_r becomes more important to repolarization during bradycardia. Therefore, although IK_r blockers may be effective against ventricular arrhythmias, they may also be proarrhythmic under ischemic conditions.

The IK_1 current plays a role in maintaining resting membrane potential and in final repolarization *(143)*. There have been reports that selective IK_1 blockers are antifibrillatory *(144)*. However, a role for such drugs in the prevention and/or abolition of life-threatening arrhythmias is uncertain. It is a strongly inward rectifying current and this current should become more pronounced in the presence of increased $[Mg^{2+}]_i$, $[Na^+]_i$, and $[Ca^{2+}]_i$. Additionally, IK_1 is decreased in the presence of other ischemic products, such as lysophosphatidylcholine, oxygen-free radicals, and intracellular acidosis.

The class IV antiarrhythmics, or cardiac calcium channel blockers, such as verapamil and diltiazem, have some efficacy in the treatment of supraventricular tachycardias (*see* ref. *64* for review) by virtue of the fact that the nodal tissues have calcium-dependent action potentials. Experimental studies show class IV drugs have efficacy against ischemia-induced arrhythmias in various species *(63,145)*. The antiarrhythmic activity of enantiomers of verapamil was potentiated by a $[K^+]_o$ similar to that in ischemia *(146)*. This may be because of greater antagonism of the calcium channel by verapamil under depolarizing conditions. However, as with other ion channel blockers, calcium channel blockers have proarrhythmic effects (sinus and atrioventricular nodes) whereas their efficacy against ischemic arrhythmias is limited *(138,147,148)*. Toxic actions include depressant effects on contractility that is not confined to the ischemic zone and profound hypotension when given at antiarrhythmic doses. Most standard clinical pharmacology texts list the arrhythmias for which the presently available antiarrhythmic drugs are recommended *(149)* and their contraindications. Ventricular arrhythmias in ischemia are not found as an indication.

A number of drug companies, because of the disappointment with selective ion channel blockers (e.g., CAST, SWORD) and recent evidence favoring the efficacy of drugs. such as amiodarone *(150,151)*, have begun to develop mixed ion channel blockers based upon amiodarone *(152–154)*. There are a number of other mixed ion channel blockers that are not similar to amiodarone in development or in clinical trials *(155–160)*. Overall, it appears that drugs that target ion channels in normal myocardium and show limited or no selectivity for ischemic myocardium have limited utility against ischemia-induced arrhythmias *(26)*.

6.3. Ischemia-Selective Targeting
for Early Ischemia-Induced Arrhythmias

As discussed, the history of drugs targeted for ion channels in normal cardiac tissue is replete with failures. In consequence, it has been recognized that antiarrhythmic drugs need to be targeted to the pathology causing the arrhythmia but most attempts to achieve this, by assuming involvement of ischemia-dependent arrhythmogens or specific ischemia-dependent channels, have been unrewarding. Such a situation has led to different strategies.

One of the oldest strategies is to take advantage of the special characteristics of arrhythmias. Thus, as discussed, there are frequency-dependent drugs but these have limited efficacy against ischemia-induced arrhythmias *(27)*. Similarly, there are drugs with selectivity for particular types of cardiac tissue, such as adenosine for atrioventricular tissue, or the new Kv1.5 (IK_{ur}) blockers, which appear to be atrial selective *(13)* and as a result may not cause torsade. However, with chronic atrial fibrillation Kv1.5 channels are downregulated *(159)* and this may reduce the action of Kv1.5 blockers.

What strategies can be adopted for ventricular arrhythmias? Any strategy for inventing drugs that are selective for ischemia-induced arrhythmias should be founded on acceptable scientific premises. The first is that such a drug should have direct actions on the electrophysiological disorders in the ischemic tissue. These disorders should either be restored to normal or abolished. The strategy of restoration of the disordered electrophysiology to normal appears at first sight to be rational but ignores the fact that ischemic tissue invariably becomes quiet before it dies unless reperfusion occurs. However, such an approach could serve to keep the heart attack victim alive until reperfusion can be performed.

The latter strategy, that is, making the ischemic zone quiescent, appears counterintuitive until one reflects on the fact the most lethal phase for ischemic arrhythmias occurs when the ischemic tissue is still electrically active and that arrhythmias subside as the tissue becomes electrically quiescent before dying. If this is the case, why not hasten the process of quiescence thereby reducing the chance of arrhythmias? There are, however, potential problems with this approach because there is evidence that sodium channel blockers acting upon ischemic tissue can initiate reentry arrhythmias *(160)*. Indeed, this may be one of the mechanisms responsible for increased mortality seen in the CAST study with class I drugs. However, such potential problems might be lessened if potassium channel blockade is combined with sodium channel blockade so that refractoriness is prolonged at the same time that excitability and conduction is being reduced.

It has repeatedly been shown that selective sodium and potassium channel blockers have limited antiarrhythmic efficacy *(161)*, and all have proarrhythmic activity. Mixed channel blockers may not be that much better although the classic multichannel blocker, amiodarone, remains one of the few antiarrhythmic drugs that unequivocally save lives *(150)*. The trouble with the current blockers is that their effects are not selective for ischemic tissue.

How can the actions of an antiarrhythmic be made selective for ischemic tissue, or for ischemia-induced arrhythmias? One possible approach is to take advantage of frequency-dependence, as has been discussed previously; the other is to take advantage of local conditions existing in ischemic tissue *(14)*. An antiarrhythmic drug activated by the conditions found in ischemia would have an ischemia-selective mechanism of action. Thus, a sodium and potassium blocker acting selectively in ischemic tissue would, by a combination of increased refractoriness, reduced conduction and suppression of excitability, be expected to render the ischemic tissue quiet and less capable of participating in ischemic arrhythmogenesis. However, ischemic tissue is still partially polarized, and therefore a source of injury current and there are hypotheses that injury currents act as arrhythmia generators *(12,14)*. Without arguing all of the pros and cons of such a hypothesis, it may be of note that ischemic arrhythmias are rare during the time when ischemic tissue is electrically quiet but still partially polarized *(162,163)*.

If the above rationale is accepted, the question becomes how can the conditions of ischemia be used to achieve a drug that will act selectively in ischemic tissue? There are many examples in pharmacology of drug selectivity being achieved by using tissue selective enzymes to release a drug from its prodrug. However, currently we know of no enzymes that are activated by ischemia that can be used to release an active drug from its prodrug. Another classic approach to site-specific activation of a prodrug is omeprazole that is activated by the acid conditions found in the stomach *(164,165)*.

Many antiarrhythmic drugs are tertiary amines, active in their charged form, making it possible that the acid conditions found in ischemic tissue could be used to ensure higher concentrations of the active species in ischemic tissue *(166)*. In an analogous manner the elevated extracellular potassium ion concentration in ischemic tissue might be used because raised potassium activates some potassium channels, making them more vulnerable to potassium channel blocking drugs. The depolarization caused by elevated K^+ would potentiate sodium channel drugs that bind to the inactivated form of the channel (*see* discussion in Section 6.2.4.1. on increased $[K^+]_o$).

Thus, if one could create a drug whose potency for both sodium and potassium block-ade increased with raised potassium and hydrogen ion concentrations one could expect such drugs to have some selectivity for ischemic arrhythmias.

7. A STRATEGY FOR DEVELOPING ISCHEMIA-SELECTIVE COMPOUNDS

The following describes efforts to produce a drug that meets the above criteria. It describes a classic structure-activity attempt to produce compounds activated by the conditions of lowered pH and elevated $[K^+]$ found in ischemic tissue *(167)*.

7.1. Chemical Approach

7.1.1. Using Lowered pH

As a result of the above considerations, we embarked on a program to create an ischemia-selective antiarrhythmic drug. The first requirement was a suitable lead com-pound that met certain criteria, including sodium-blocking actions, which could be potentiated by the acidic conditions of ischemia. Exploratory work with tetrodotoxin *(168)*, sparteine analogs *(169)*, and arylbenzacetamides *(170–173)* suggested that the latter would provide the most suitable lead compound. As a result of variations on a lead compound, RSD 921, we were able to produce compounds whose potency was increased in acid (pH 6.4) conditions *(29,30,174)*. Patch clamp analysis suggested, but did not prove, an extracellular site of action and a positive frequency (and inactivation) dependence *(174,175)*. When tested against ischemia-induced arrhythmias in anesthe-tized rats, such compounds protected against arrhythmias. However, further study showed the compounds also blocked potassium channels *(30)*.

The basis of this work was to produce compounds whose potential charge on its active nitrogen (its pKa) could be brought close to 6.4, the pH found in ischemic tissue during the period of arrhythmias. In outline, this was achieved in the following man-ner. After identifying that the pyrrole nitrogen was essential for activity, the pKa of this nitrogen was adjusted by substitution on, or next to, the ring. The nonring nitrogen played no part in conferring antiarrhythmic activity and could be replaced by ester or ether oxygen. In an examination of the effect of such changes it was clear that the compounds which were most efficacious (100% antiarrhythmic protection) against ischemia-induced arrhythmias, and were selective for ischemic vs electrically induced arrhythmias in rats, were those compounds in which the pKa of the nitrogen within the ring was about 6.4 *(30)*.

7.1.2. Using Elevated K

We have examined the effects of elevated $[K^+]_o$ on arrhythmias and found that raising $[K^+]_o$ is antiarrhythmic *(109,110)* up to a certain level *(98,99)*. Indeed, evi-dence we presented earlier implicates a role for raised potassium levels in the antiar-rhythmic activity of beta blockers *(100,110)*. We have found that under conditions of increased $[K^+]_o$ that our compounds exhibit increased efficacy against ischemia-induced arrhythmias *(29,30,173)*. Under conditions of high $[K^+]_o$ and low pH (simu-lated ischemic conditions) we found that RSD 1000 was >10 times more potent than reference class I antiarrhythmics *(174)*. Other morpholinocyclohexyl derivatives, such as RSD 1019 and RSD 1030, also exhibit a similar increased efficacy under conditions of high $[K^+]_o$ and low pH *(29,30)*.

7.2. Effects of Biological Screening

The pharmacological effects of compounds produced were assessed in various ways so as to give a profile of activity possibly relevant to effectiveness against ischemia-induced arrhythmias *(30)*. In view of the multitude of channels and processes that may be involved in arrhythmogenesis and the differences in expression in various species (*see* refs. *13,14* for reviews on cardiac ion channels and ischemia), we felt it appropriate to explore the usefulness of various preparations in predicting not only antiarrhythmic efficacy but also morbidity and mortality of potential antiarrhythmic compounds *(176–178)*. We have established ischemia models in the rat *(135)* and methods for assessing them *(179)*.

7.3. Effectiveness Against Ischemia-Induced and Other Arrhythmias

All compounds with the required profile of activity in the above electrophysiological tests were studied with respect to their activity against ischemia-induced arrhythmias. In addition the same compounds were also investigated against electrically induced arrhythmias. The purpose of such studies was to discover whether the compounds had a selective action against the ischemia-induced arrhythmias in that doses required to reduce ischemia-induced arrhythmias were significantly lower than those required to reduce electrically-reduced arrhythmias. The tests also showed whether the compounds had adverse effects on the cardiovascular system. The results of these studies (*see* ref. *167* for a full review) was the development of compounds that are reasonably potent, effective, and selective against ischemia-induced arrhythmias in rats and pigs while having a satisfactory therapeutic ratio (compared with other antiarrhythmics) in terms of having cardiovascular and CNS toxicity.

8. CONCLUSIONS

Consideration of the literature and our own findings suggest the following:

1. Antiarrhythmics have to be specifically targeted for particular arrhythmias using the pathology of that arrhythmia and that the fatal ventricular tachyarrhythmias occurring in the early phase after the onset of regional myocardial ischemia are a suitable target for specifically targeted antiarrhythmics.
2. No specific ion channel, normally present or activated by ischemia, is of such importance in ischemia-dependent ventricular arrhythmias that it offers a suitable drug target. Similarly, no one arrhythmogen is sufficiently important in ischemic arrhythmogenesis to warrant using its production or actions as targets.
3. Abolition of electrical activity in ischemic tissue is an antiarrhythmic mechanism. This can be achieved with mixed (sodium and potassium) blockers selective for ischemic conditions.
4. Conditions found in ischemic tissue, namely acid pH and elevated $[K^+]_o$ can be used to potentiate the actions of some ion channel–blocking drugs conferring a selective action in ischemic tissue. This had led to the discovery of new antiarrhythmic drugs that show selectivity for ischemia-induced arrhythmias.

Finally, there is still an active need for new and better antiarrhythmic drugs. One way of moving forward is to try and use the pathology underlying the arrhythmias as a way of targeting drugs to particular types of arrhythmia arising from a particular cause so as to achieve the required selectivity and freedom from toxicity. The single major cause of mortality remains ventricular fibrillation in the setting of myocardial ischemia and infarction. Surely, we can do something to reduce this mortality with drugs.

ACKNOWLEDGMENTS

Acknowledgments and thanks are offered to the commitment and efforts of all those associated with the ischemia selective antiarrhythmic project conducted by Cardiome Pharma Corp. MJAW is a founder of, and retains a financial interest in, Cardiome. Some of the work reported here was funded by Cardiome.

REFERENCES

1. Fogel, R. I. and Prystowsky, E. N. (2000) Management of malignant ventricular arrhythmias and cardiac arrest. *Crit. Care Med.* **(10 Suppl),** N165–N169.
2. Atlee, J. L. (2001) Cardiac arrhythmias: Drugs and devices. *Curr. Opin. Anaesthesiol.* **14,** 3–9.
3. Steinberg, J. S., Martins, J., Sadanandan, S., et al. and the AVID Investigators. (2001) Antiarrhythmic drug use in the implantable defribillator arm of the Antiarrhythmics Versus Implantable Defibrillators (AVID) Study. *Am. Heart. J.* **142,** 520–529.
4. Echt, D. S., Liebson, P. R., Mitchell, L. B., et al. and the CAST Investigators. (1991) Mortality and morbidity in patients receiving encainide, flecainide, or placebo. The Cardiac Arrhythmia Suppression Trial. *N. Engl. J. Med.* **324,** 781–788.
5. Waldo, A. L., Camm, A. J., deRuyter, H, et al. for the SWORD Investigators (1996) Effect of d-sotolol on mortality in patients with left ventricular dysfunction after recent and remote myocardial infarction. *N. Engl. J. Med.* **348,** 7–12.
6. Cairns, J. A., Connolly, S. J., Roberts. R., and Gent, M. (1997) Randomised trial of outcome after myocardial infarction in patients with frequent or repetitive ventricular premature depolarisations: CAMIAT. Canadian Amiodarone Myocardial Infarction Arrhythmia Trial Investigators. *Lancet* **349,** 675–682.
7. Julian, D. G., Camm, A. J., Frangin G, Janse, M. J., Munoz A, Schwartz, P. J., et al. (1997) Randomised trial of effect of amiodarone on mortality in patients with left-ventricular dysfunction after recent myocardial infarction: EMIAT. European Myocardial Infarct Amiodarone Trial Investigators. *Lancet* **349,** 667–674.
8. Clare, J. J., Tate, S. N., Nobbs, M., and Romanos, M. A. (2000) Voltage gated sodium channels as therapeutic targets. *Drug Dis. Today* **5,** 506–520.
9. Curran, M. (1998) Potassium ion channels and human disease: Phenotypes to drug targets. *Curr. Opin. Biotech.* **9,** 565–572.
10. Jalife, J. (2000) Ventricular fibrillation: Mechanisms of initiation and maintenance. *Annu. Rev. Physiol.* **62,** 25–50
11. Nattel, S., Li. D., and Lue, L. (2000) Basic mechanisms of atrial fibrillation: Very new insights into very old ideas. *Annu. Rev. Physiol.* **62,** 51–77.
12. Ramaswamy, K. and Hamdan, M. H. (2000) Ischemia, metabolic disturbances and arrhythmogenesis: Mechanisms and management. *Crit. Care Med.* **28 (10 Suppl),** N151–N156.
13. Roden, D. M., Balser, J. R., George, Jr, J. L., and Anderson, M. (2002) Cardiac ion Channels. *Annu. Rev. Physiol.* **64,** 431–475.
14. Carmeliet, E. (1999) Cardiac ion currents and acute ischemia: From channels to arrhythmias. *Physiol. Rev.* **79,** 917–1017.
15. Curtis, M. J., Pugsley, M. K., and Walker, M. J. A. (1993) Endogenous chemical mediators of ventricular arrhythmias in ischaemic heart disease. *Circ. Res.* **27,** 703–719.
16. Vaughn-Williams, E. M. (1970) Classification of antiarrhythmic drugs, in *Symposium on Cardiac Arrhythmias* (Sandoe, E., Flenstedt-Johnson, E., and Oleson, K. H., eds), Sodertalje, Sweden, AB Astra, pp. 440–469.
17. Members of the Sicillian Gambit. (1991) The Sicilian gambit: A new approach to classification of antiarrhythmic drugs based on their actions on arrhythmogenic mechanisms. *Circulation* **84,** 1831–1851.

18. Zipes, D. P. and Wellens, H. J. (2000) What have we learned about cardiac arrhythmias? *Circulation* **102(Suppl 4),** 52–57.
19. Huikuri, H. V., Castellanos, A., and Myerburg, R. J. (2001) Sudden death due to cardiac arrhythmias. *N. Engl. J. Med.* **345,** 1473–482.
20. Priori, S. G., Aliot, E., and Blømstrom-Lundqvist, C. (2002) Task Force on Sudden Cardiac Death, European Society of Cardiology: Summary of recommendations. *Europace* **4,** 3–18.
21. Johnson, K. M., MacLeod, B. A., and Walker, M. J. A. (1983) Responses to ligation of a coronary artery in conscious rats and the actions of antiarrhythmics. *Can. J. Physiol.* **61,** 1340–1353.
22. Inoue, F., MacLeod, B. A., and Walker, M. J. A. (1984) Intracellular potential changes following coronary occlusion in isolated perfused rat hearts. *Can. J. Physiol.* **62,** 658–664.
23. Johnson, K. M., MacLeod, B. A., and Walker, M. J. A. (1981) ECG and other responses to ligation of a coronary artery in the conscious rat, in *The Rat Electrocardiogram in Pharmacology and Toxicology* (Budden, R., Detweiler, D. K., and Zbinden, G., eds), Pergammon Press, New York, pp. 243–252.
24. Xie, F., Qu., K, Garfinkel, A., and Weiss, J. N. (2001) Effects of simulated ischemia on spiral wave stability. *Am. J. Physiol.* **280,** H1667–H1673.
25. Chaudhry, G. M., and Haffajee, C. I. (2000) Antiarrhythmic agents and proarrhythmia. *Crit. Care Med.* **28 (Suppl),** N158–N164.
26. Barrett, T. D., Hayes., E. S., and Walker, M. J. A. (1995) Lack of selectivity for ventricular and ischaemic tissue limits the antiarrhythmic actions of lidocaine, quinidine and flecainide against ischaemia induced arrhythmias. *Eur. J. Pharmacol.* **285,** 229–238.
27. Farkas, A. and Curtis, M. J. (2002) Limited antifibrillatory effectiveness of clinically relevant concentrations of class I antiarrhythmics in isolated perfused rat hearts. *J. Cardiovasc. Pharmacol.* **39,** 412–424.
28. Carson, D. L., Cardinal, R., Savard, P., et al. (1986) Relationship between an arrhythmogenic action of lidocaine and its effects of excitation patterns in acutely ischemic porcine myocardium. *J. Cardiovasc. Pharmacol.* **8,** 126–136.
29. Barrett, T. D., MacLeod, B. A., and Walker, M. J. A. (2000) RSD 1019 suppresses ischemia-induced monophasic action potential shortening and arrhythmias in anesthetized rabbits. *Br. J. Pharmacol.* **131,** 405–414.
30. Barrett, T. D., Hayes, E. S., Yong, S. L., et al. (2000) Ischaemia selectivity confers efficacy for suppression of ischaemia-induced arrhythmias in rats. *Eur. J. Pharmacol.* **398,** 365–374.
31. Igwemezie, L. W., Beatch, G. N., McErlane, K. M., and Walker, M. J. A. (1992) Mexilitine's antifibrillatory actions are limited by the occurrence of convulsions in conscious animals. *Eur. J. Pharmacol.* **210,** 271–277.
32. Pike, G. K., Bretag, A. H., and Roberts, M. L. (1993) Modification of the transient outward current of rat atrial myocytes by metabolic inhibition and oxidant stress. *J. Physiol.* **470,** 365–382.
33. Scholz, W., Albus, U., Counillon, L., et al. (1995) Protective effects of HOE642, a selective sodium-hydrogen exchange subtype 1 inhibitor, on cardiac ischaemia and reperfusion. *Cardiovasc. Res.* **29,** 260–268.
34. Eigel, B. N. and Hadley, R. W. (1999) Contribution of the Na^+ channel and Na^+/H^+ exchanger. *Heart Circ. Physiol.* **277,** H1817–H1822.
35. Hendrikx, M., Mubagwa, K. Verdonck, F., et al. (1994) New Na^+/H^+ exchange inhibitor HOE 694 improves postischemic function and high-energy phosphate resynthesis and reduces Ca^{2+} overload in isolated perfused rabbit heart. *Circulation* **89,** 2787–2798.
36. Xue, Y. X., Aye, N. N., and Hashimoto, K. (1996) Antiarrhythmic effects of HOE642, a novel Na^+-H^+ exchange inhibitor, on ventricular arrhythmias in animal hearts. *Eur. J. Pharmacol.* **317,** 309–316.

37. Aye, N. N., Xue, Y. X., and Hashimoto, K. (1997) Antiarrhythmic effects of cariporide, a novel Na+-H+ exchange inhibitor, on reperfusion ventricular arrhythmias in rat hearts. *Eur. J. Pharmacol.* **339,** 121–127.

38. Gumina, R. J., Daemmgen, J., and Gross, G. J. (2000) Inhibition of the Na+/H+ exchanger attenuates phase 1b ischemic arrhythmias and reperfusion-induced ventricular fibrillation. *Eur. J. Pharmacol.* **396,** 119–124.

39. Avkiran, M. (1999) Rational basis for use of sodium-hydrogen exchange inhibitors in myocardial ischemia. *Am. J. Cardiol.* **83,** 10G–17G.

40. Chin, B. and Lip, G. Y. (2000) Cariporide (Aventis). *Curr. Opin. Invest. Drugs* **1,** 340–346.

41. Karmazyn, M. (2000) Pharmacology and clinical assessment of cariporide for the treatment coronary artery diseases. *Expert Opin. Invest. Drugs* **9,** 1099–1108.

42. Wirth, K. J., Maier, T., and Busch, A. E. (2001) NHE1-inhibitor cariporide prevents the transient reperfusion-induced shortening of the monophasic action potential after coronary ischemia in pigs. *Basic Res. Cardiol.* **96,** 192–197.

43. Gazmuri, R. J., Hoffner, E., Kalcheim, J., et al. (2001) Myocardial protection during ventricular fibrillation by reduction of proton-driven sarcolemmal flux. *J. Lab. Clin. Med.* **137,** 43–55.

44. Theroux, P., Chaitman, B. R., Danchin, N., et al. (2000) Inhibition of the sodium-hydrogen exchanger with cariporide to prevent myocardial infarction in high-risk ischemic situations. Main results of the GUARDIAN trial. Guard during ischemia against necrosis (GUARDIAN) Investigators. *Circulation* **102,** 3032–3038.

45. Zeymer, U., Suryapranata, H., Monassier, J. P., et al. (2001) The Na+/H+ exchange inhibitor Eniporide as an adjunct to early reperfusion therapy for acute myocardial infarction. Results of the ESCAMI trial [abstract]. *Eur. Heart J.* **22,** 640.

46. Banno, H., Fujiwara, J., Hosoya, J., Kitamori, T., Mori, H., Yamashita, H., Ikeda, F. (1999) Effects of MS-31–038, a novel Na+/H+ exchange inhibitor, on the myocardial infarct size in rats after postischemic administration. *Arzneimittelforschung* **49,** 304–310.

47. Lorrain, J., Briand, V., Favennec, E., et al. (2000) Pharmacological profile of SL 59.1227, a novel inhibitor of the sodium/hydrogen exchanger. *Br. J. Pharmacol.* **131,** 1188–1194.

48. Aihara, K., Hisa, H., Sato, T., et al. (2000) Cardioprotective effect of TY-12533, a novel Na(+)/H(+) exchange inhibitor, on ischemia/reperfusion injury. *Eur. J. Pharmacol.* **404,** 221–229.

49. Gazmuri, R. J., Ayoub, I. M., Kolarova, J. D., and Karmazyn, M. (2002) Myocardial protection during ventricular fibrillation by inhibition of the sodium-hydrogen exchanger isoform-1. *Crit. Care Med.* **30(Suppl. 4),** S166–S171.

50. Marban, E., Kitakaze, M., Koretsune, Y., et al. (1990) Quantification of $[Ca^{2+}]_I$ in perfused hearts. Critical evaluation of the 5 F-BAPTA and nuclear magnetic resonance method as applied to the study of ischemia and reperfusion. *Circ. Res.* **66,** 1255–1267.

51. Gambassi, G., Hansford, R. G., Sollott, S. J., et al. (1993) Effects of acidosis on resting cytosolic and mitochondrial Ca^{2+} in mammalian myocardium. *J. Gen. Physiol.* **102,** 575–597.

52. Smith, G. L. and Allen, D. G. (1988) Effects of metabolic blockade on intracellular calcium concentration in isolated ferret ventricular muscle. *Circ. Res.* **62,** 1223–1236.

53. Tani, M. and Neely, J. R. (1989) Role of intracellular Na+ in Ca^{2+} overload and depressed recovery of ventricular function of reperfused ischemic rat hearts. Possible involvement of H+-Na+ and Na+-Ca2+ exchange. *Circ. Res.* **65,** 1045–1056.

54. Yashar, P. R., Fransua, M, and Frishman, W. H. (1998) The sodium-calcium ion membrane exchanger: Physiologic significance and pharmacologic implications. *J. Clin. Pharmacol.* **38,** 393–401.

55. Trafford, A. W, Diaz, M. E., Negretti, N., and Eisener, D. A. (1997) Enhanced Ca^{2+} current and decreased Ca^{2+} efflux restore sarcoplasmic reticulum Ca^{2+} content after depletion. *Circ. Res.* **81,** 477–484.

56. Weber, C. R., Piacentino III, V., Ginsburg, K. S., et al. (2002) Na^+-Ca^{2+} exchange current and submembrane $[Ca^{2+}]$ during the cardiac action potential. *Circ. Res.* **90**, 182–189.

57. Philipson, K. D., Bersohn, M. M., and Nishimoto, A. Y. (1982) Effects of pH on Na^+/Ca^{2+} exchange in canine cardiac sarcolemmal vesicles. *Circ. Res.* **50**, 287–293.

58. Coetzee, W. A., Ichihawa, H., and Hearse, D. J. (1994) Oxidant stress inhibits Na-Ca exchange current in cardiac myocytes: mediation by sulfhydryl groups? *Am. J. Physiol.* **266**, H909–H919.

59. Bassani, J. W., Bassani, R. A., and Bers. D. M. (1993) Ca^{2+} cycling between sarcoplasmic reticulum and mitochondria in rabbit cardiac myocytes. *J. Physiol. (Lond.)* **460**, 603–621.

60. Watano, T., Harada, Y., Harada, K., and Nishimura, N. (1999) Effect of Na^+/Ca^{2+} exchange inhibitor, KB-R7943, on ouabain-induced arrhythmias in guinea-pigs. *Br. J. Pharmacol.* **127**, 1846–1850.

61. Mukai, M., Terada, H., Sugiyama, S., et al. (2000) Effects of a selective inhibitor of Na^+/Ca^{2+} exchange, KB-R7943, on reoxygenation-induced injuries in guinea pig papillary muscles. *J. Cardiovasc. Pharmacol.* **35**, 121–128.

62. Elias, C. L., Lukas, A., Shurraw, S., et al. (2001) Inhibition of Na^+/Ca^{2+} exchange by KB-R7943: Transport mode selectivity and antiarrhythmic consequences. *Am. J. Physiol.* **281**, H1334–H1345.

63. Curtis, M. J., MacLeod, B. A., and Walker, M. J. A. (1984) Antiarrhythmic actions of verapamil against ischaemic arrhythmias in the rat. *Br. J. Pharmacol.* **83**, 373–385.

64. Walker, M. J. A. and Chia, S. K. L. (1989) Calcium channel blockers as antiarrhythmics. *Cardiovasc. Drug Rev.* **73**, 265–284.

65. MacLeod, B. A. and Walker, M. J. A. (1990) Rat models for studying arrhythmic and other adverse responses to myocardial ischemia: Beneficial actions of calcium channel blockade, in *Calcium Channel Modulations in Heart and Smooth Muscle: Basic Mechanisms and Pharmacological Aspects* (Abraham, and Amitai, G., eds), Alan, R. Liss Inc, New York, pp. 339–352 .

66. Curtis, M. J. (1990) Calcium antagonists and coronary artery disease: An opportunity missed? *J. Neural. Trans.* **31 (Suppl)**, 17–38.

67. Lee, J. A., and Allen, D. G. (1992) Changes in intracellular free calcium concentration during long exposures to simulated ischemia in isolated mammalian ventricular muscle. *Circ. Res.* **21**, 58–69.

68. Tani, M. and Neely, J. R. (1990) Mechanisms of reduced reperfusion injury by low Ca^{2+} and/or high K^+. *Am. J. Physiol.* **258**, H1025–H1031.

69. Wagner, S., Wu, S. T., Parmley, W. W., and Wikman Coffelt, J. (1990) Influence of ischemia on $[Ca^{2+}]_i$ transients following drug therapy in hearts from aortic constricted rats. *Cell Calcium* **11**, 431–444.

70. Mohabir, R., Lee, H. C., Kurz, R. W., and Clusin, W. T. (1991) Effects of ischemia and hypercarbic acidosis on myocyte calcium transients, contraction, and pHi in perfused rabbit hearts. *Circ. Res.* **69**, 1525–1537.

71. Thandroyen, F. T., McCarthy, J., Burton, K. M., and Opie, L. H. (1988) Ryanodine and caffeine prevent ventricular arrhythmias during acute myocardial ischemia and reperfusion in rat heart. *Circ. Res.* **62**, 306–314.

72. Terzic, A., Jahangir, A., and Kurachi, Y. (1995) Cardiac ATP-sensitive K^+ channels: Regulation by intracellular nucleotides and K^+ channel-opening drugs. *Am. J. Physiol.* **269**, C525–C545.

73. Yan, G. X., Yamada, K. A., Kleber, A. G., et al. (1993) Dissociation between cellular K^+ loss, reduction in repolarization time, and tissue ATP levels during myocardial hypoxia and ischemia. *Circ. Res.* **72**, 560–570.

74. Noma, A. (1983) ATP-regulated K^+ channels in cardiac muscle. *Nature* **305**, 147–148.

75. Trube, G., and Hescheler, D. J. (1984) Inward-rectifying channels in isolated patches of the heart cell membrane: ATP-dependence and comparison with cell-attached patches. *Pflugers Arch.* **401**, 178–184.

76. Wilde, A. A. M. and Janse, M. J. (1994) Electrophysiological effects of ATP sensitive channel modulation: Implications for arrhythmogenesis. *Cardiovasc. Res.* **28**, 16–24.

77. Kantor, P. F., Coetzee, W. A., Carmeliet, E. E., et al. (1990) Reduction of ischemic K⁺ loss and arrhythmias in rat hearts. Effect of glibenclamide, a sulfonylurea. *Circ. Res.* **66**, 478–485.

78. Gwilt, M., Norton, B., and Henderson, C. G. (1993) Pharmacological studies of K⁺ loss from ischaemic myocardium in vitro: Roles of ATP-dependent K⁺ channels and lactate-coupled efflux. *Eur. J. Pharmacol.* **236**, 107–112.

79. Barrett, T. D. and Walker, M. J.A. (1998) Glibenclamide does not prevent action potential shortening induced by ischemia in anesthetized rabbits but reduces ischemia-induced arrhythmias. *J. Mol. Cell. Cardiol.* **30**, 999–1008.

80. Adams, D., Crome, R., Lad, N., et al. (1990) Failure of the ATP-dependent K⁺ channel inhibitor, glibenclamide, to reduce reperfusion-induced or ischaemia arrhythmias in rat hearts. *Br. J. Pharmacol.* **100**, P438.

81. Rees, S. A. and Curtis, M. J. (1995) Pharmacological analysis in rat of the role of the ATP-sensitive potassium channel as a potential target for antifibrillatory intervention in acute myocardial ischemia. *J. Cardiovasc. Pharmacol.* **26**, 280–288.

82. Fujita, A. and Kurachi, Y. (2000) Molecular aspects of ATP-sensitive K⁺ channels in the cardiovascular system and K⁺ channel openers. *Pharmacol. Ther.* **85**, 35–53.

83. Friedrich, M., Benndorf, K.,. Schwalb, M., and Hirche, H. (1990) Effects of anoxia on K and Ca currents in isolated guinea pig cardiocytes. *Pflugers Arch.* **416**, 207–209.

84. Gasser, R. N. and Vaughn-Jones, R. D. (1990) Mechanism of potassium efflux and action potential shortening during ischaemia in isolated mammalian cardiac muscle. *J. Physiol. (Lond.)* **431**, 713–741.

85. Sato T, Sasaki N, Seharaseyon J, O'Rourke B, and Marban, E. (2000) Selective pharmacological agents implicate mitochondrial but not sarcolemmal K(ATP) channels in ischemic cardioprotection. *Circulation* **101**, 2418–2423.

86. Asemu., Papousek, E., Ostadal, B., and Kolar, F. (1999) Adaptation to high altitude hypoxia protects the rat heart against ischemia-induced arrhythmias. Involvement of mitochondrial K⁺ (ATP) channel. *J. Mol. Cell Cardiol.* **31**, 1821–1831.

87. Workman, A. J., MacKenzie, I., and Northover, B. J. (2000) Do K$_{ATP}$ channel channels open as a prominent and early feature during ischaemia in the Langendorff-perfused rat heart. *Basic Res. Cardiol.* **95**, 250–260.

88. Terzic, A., Tung, R. T., and Kurachi, Y. (1994a) Nucleotide regulation of ATP sensitive potassium channels. *Cardiovasc. Res.* **28**, 746–753.

89. Han, J., Kim, E., Lee, S. H., Yoo, S., et al. (1998) cGMP facilitates calcium current via cGMP-dependent protein kinase in isolated rabbit ventricular myocytes. *Pflugers Arch.* **435**, 388–393.

90. Fan, Z. and Makielski. J. C. (1993) Intracellular H⁺ and Ca²⁺ modulation of trypsin-modified ATP-sensitive K⁺ channels in rabbit ventricular myocytes. *Circ. Res.* **72**, 715–722.

91. Jabr, R. I. and Cole, W. C. (1993) Alterations in electrical activity and membrane currents induced by intracellular oxygen-derived free radical stress in guinea pig ventricular myocytes. *Circ. Res.* **72**, 1229–1244.

92. Terzic, A., Tung, R. T., Inanobe, A., et al. (1994b) G proteins activate ATP-sensitive K⁺ channels by antagonizing ATP-dependent gating. *Neuron* **12**, 885–893.

93. Han, J., Kim, E., Ho, W. K., and Earm, Y. E. (1996) Blockade of the ATP-sensitive potassium channel by taurine in rabbit ventricular myocytes. *J. Mol. Cell. Cardiol.* **28**, 2043–2050.

94. Van Wagoner, D. R. (1993) Mechanosensitive gating of atrial ATP-sensitive potassium channels. *Circ. Res.* **72,** 973–983.

95. Vegh. A., Gyorgyi, K., Papp, J. G., et al. (1996) Nicorandil suppressed ventricular arrhythmias in a canine model of myocardial ischemia. *Eur. J. Pharmacol.* **305,** 163–168.

96. Dhein, S., Pejman, P., and Krusemann, K. (2000) Effects of the I(K. ATP) blockers glibenclamide and HMR1883 on cardiac electrophysiology during ischemia and reperfusion. *Eur. J. Pharmacol.* **398,** 273–284.

97. Hirche, H., Franz, C., Bos, L., et al. (1980) Myocardial extracellular K^+ and H^+ increase and noradrenaline release as possible cause of early arrhythmias following acute coronary artery occlusion in pigs. *J. Mol. Cell. Cardiol.* **12,** 579–593.

98. Curtis, M. J. and Hearse, D. J. (1989) Ischaemia-induced and reperfusion-induced arrhythmias differ in their sensitivity to potassium: Implications for mechanisms of initiation and maintenance of ventricular fibrillation. *J. Mol. Cell Cardiol.* **21,** 21–40.

99. Curtis, M. J. (1991) The rabbit dual coronary perfusion model: A new method for assessing the pathological relevance of individual products of the ischaemic milieu: Role of potassium in arrhythmogenesis. *Cardiovasc. Res.* **25,** 1010–1022.

100. Saint, K. M., Abraham, S., MacLeod, B. A., et al. (1992) Ischemic but not reperfusion arrhythmias depend upon serum potassium concentration. *J. Mol. Cell Cardiol.* **24,** 701–709.

101. Naudrehaug, J. E. and Von der Lippe, G., (1983) Hyperkalaemia and ventricular fibrillation in acute myocardial infarction. *Br. Heart J.* **50,** 525–529.

102. Priori, S. and Schwartz, P. J. (1989) Catecholamine-dependent cardiac arrhythmias: mechanisms and implication, in *Adrenergic System and Ventricular Arrhythmias in Myocardial Infarction* (Brachman, J. and Schömig, A., eds). Springer-Verlag, Heidelberg, pp. 239–247.

103. Culling, W., Penny, W. J., Lewis, M. J., et al. (1984) Effects of myocardial catecholamine depletion on cellular electrophysiology and arrhythmias during ischaemia and reperfusion *Cardiovasc. Res.* **18,** 675–682.

104. Schömig, A., Dart, A. M., Dietz, R., et al. (1984) Release of endogenous catecholamines in the ischemic myocardium of the rat. Part, A. Locally mediated release. *Circ. Res.* **55,** 689–701.

105. Lameris, T. W., de Zeeuw, W., Alberts, G., et al. (2000) Time course and mechanism of myocardial catecholamine release during transient ischemia in vivo. *Circulation* **101,** 2645–2650.

106. Botting, J. H., Johnson, K. M., MacLeod, B. A., and Walker, M. J. A. (1983) The effect of modification of sympathetic activity on responses to the ligation of a coronary artery in the conscious rat. *Br. J. Pharmacol.* **79,** 269–271.

107. Daugherty, A., Frayne, K. N., Refern, W. S., and Woodward, B. (1986) The role of catecholamines in the production of ischemia-induced ventricular arrhythmias in the rat in vivo and in vitro. *Br. J. Pharmacol.* **87,** 265–278.

108. Curtis, M. J., MacLeod, B. A., and Walker, M. J. A. (1985) The effects of ablations in the central nervous system on arrythmias induced by coronary occlusion. *Br. J. Pharmacol.* **86,** 663–670.

109. Curtis, M. J., Botting, J. H., Hearse, D. J., and Walker, M. J. A. (1989) The sympathetic nervous system, catecholamines and ischaemia-induced arrhythmias: Dependence on serum potassium concentration, in *Adrenergic System and Ventricular Arrhythmias in Myocardial Infarction* (Brachman, J. and Schömig, A., eds). Springer-Verlag, Heidelberg, pp. 205–219.

110. Paletta, M., Abraham, S., Beatch, G. N., and Walker, M. J. A. (1989) Mechanisms underlying the antiarrhythmic properties of beta adrenoceptor blockade against ischemia-induced arrhythmias in acutely prepared rats. *Br. J. Pharmacol.* **98,** 87–94.

111. Guo, P., Pugsley, M. K., Yong, S. L., and Walker, M. J. A. (1999) Cardiac transplantation does not effect ischaemia-induced arrhythmias. *Cardiovasc. Res.* **43**, 930–938.

112. Chess-Williams, R. and Milton, R. (2001) Arrhythmogenesis in isolated hearts with enhanced alpha-adrenoceptor mediated responsiveness. *J. Auto. Pharamacol.* **21**, 39–45.

113. Strasser, R. H., Marquetant, R., and Kubler, W. (1989) Sensitization of the adrenergic system in early myocardial ischemia: independent regulation of β-adrenergic receptors and adenylate cyclase, in *Adrenergic System and Ventricular Arrhythmias in Myocardial Infarction* (Brachman, J. and Schömig, A., eds). Springer-Verlag, Heidelberg, pp. 298–111.

114. Podzuweit, T., Binz, K. H., Nennsteil, P., and Flaig, W. (1989) The antiarrhythmic effects of myocardial ischemia. Relation to reperfusion arrhythmias? *Cardiovasc. Res.* **23**, 81–90.

115. Saman, S., Coetzee, W. A., and Opie, L. H. (1988) inhibition by simulated ischemia or hypoxia of delayed afterdepolarizations provoked by cyclic AMP: Significance to ischemia and reperfusion arrhythmia. *J. Mol. Cell Cardiol.* **20**, 91–95.

116. Zeigelhoffer, A., Krause, E. G., Fedelesova, M., et al. (1976) Changes of cyclic AMP levels in the non-ischaemic and ischaemic myocardium after coronary artery ligation. *Seventh European Congress of Cardiology*, p. 691.

117. Kane, K. A., Moricillo-Sanchez, E. J., Parratt, J. R., et al. (1985) The relationship between coronary artery occlusion-induced arrhythmias and myocardial cyclic nucleotide levels in the anesthetized rat. *Br. J. Pharmacol.* **84**, 139–145.

118. Morganroth, J. and Goin, J. E. (1991) Quinidine-related mortality in the short-to-medium-term treatment of ventricular arrhythmias. A meta-analysis. *Circulation* **84**, 1977–1983.

119. Hine, L. K., Laird N, Hewitt P, et al. (1989) Meta-analytic evidence against prophylactic use of lidocaine in acute myocardial infarction. *Arch. Intern. Med.* **149**, 2694–2698.

120. Akiyama, T., Pawitan, Y., Greenberg, H., et al. (1991) Increased risk of death and cardiac arrest from encainide and flecainide in patients after non-Q-wave acute myocardial infarction in the Cardiac Arrhythmia Suppression Trial. CAST Investigators. *Am. J. Cardiol.* **68**, 1551–1555.

121. Coromilas, J., Saltman, A. E., Waldecker, B., et al. (1995) Electrophysiological effects of flecainide on anisotropic conduction and reentry in infarcted canine hearts. *Circulation* **91**, 2245–2263.

122. Krishnan, S. C. and Antzelevitch, C. (1993) Flecainide-induced arrhythmia in canine ventricular epicardium. Phase 2 reentry? *Circulation* **87**, 562–572.

123. Lukas, A. and Antzelevitch, C. (1996) Phase 2 reentry as a mechanism of initiation of circus movement reentry in canine epicardium exposed to simulated ischemia. *Cardiovasc. Res.* **32**, 593–603.

124. Dominguez, G. and Fozzard, H. A. (1970) Influence of extracellular K^+ concentration on cable properties and excitability of sheep cardiac Purkinje fibers. *Circ. Res.* **26**, 565–574.

125. Lue, W. M. and Boyden, P. A. (1992) Abnormal electrical properties of myocytes from chronically infarcted canine heart. Alterations in Vmax and the transient outward current. *Circulation* **85**, 1175–1188.

126. Janse, M. J. and Wit, A. L. (1989) Electrophysiological mechanisms of ventricular arrhythmias resulting from myocardial ischemia and infarction. *Physiol. Rev.* **69**, 1049–1169.

127. Carmeliet, E. (1982) Induction and removal of inward-going rectification in sheep cardiac Purkinje fibres. *J. Physiol. (Lond.)* **327**, 285–308.

128. Scamps, F. and Carmeliet. E. (1989) Effect of external K^+ on the delayed K^+ current in single rabbit Purkinje cells. *Pflugers Arch.* **414(Suppl)**, S169–S170.

129. Lie, K. I., Wellens, H. J., van Capelle, F. J., et al. (1974) Lidocaine in the prevention of primary ventricular fibrillation. A double-blind, randomized study of 212 consecutive patients. *N. Engl. J. Med.* **291**, 1324–1326.

130. Woosley, R. L., Siddoway, L. A., Duff, H. J., et al. (1984) Flecainide dose-response relations in stable ventricular arrhythmias. *Am. J. Cardiol.* **53**, 59B–65B.

131. Dinh, H. A., Murphy, M. L., Baker, B. J., et al. (1985) Efficacy of propafenone compared with quinidine in chronic ventricular arrhythmias. *Am. J. Cardiol.* **55**, 1520–1524.

132. Antman, E. M., Lau, J., Kupelnick, B., et al. (1992) A comparison of results of meta-analyses of randomized control trials and recommendations of clinical experts. Treatments for myocardial infarction. *JAMA* **268**, 240–248.

133. Teo, K. K., Yusuf, S., and Furberg, C. D. (1993) Effects of prophylactic antiarrhythmic drug therapy in acute myocardial infarction. An overview of results from randomized controlled trials. *JAMA* **270**, 1589–1595.

134. Pugsley, M. K., Walker, M. J. A., and Yong, S. L. (1999) Are arrhythmias due to myocardial ischaemia and infarction dependent upon the sympathetic system? *Cardiovasc. Res.* **43**, 830–831.

135. Curtis, M. J., MacLeod, B. A., and Walker, M. J.A. (1987) Models for the study of arrhythmias in myocardial ischaemia and infarction: the use of the rat. *J. Mol. Cell. Cardiol.* **19**, 399–419.

136. Schömig, A. (1990) Catecholamines in myocardial ischemia. Systemic and cardiac release. *Circulation* **82(3 Suppl II)**, 13–22.

137. Andrews, T. C., Reimold, S. C., Berlin, J. A., and Antman, E. M. (1991) Prevention of supraventricular arrhythmias after coronary artery bypass surgery. A meta-analysis of randomized control trials. *Circulation* **84(5 Suppl. III)**, 236–244.

138. Kowey, P. R., Taylor, J. E., Rials, S. J., and Marinchak, R. A. (1992) Meta-analysis of the effectiveness of prophylactic drug therapy in preventing supraventricular arrhythmia early after coronary artery bypass grafting. *Am. J. Cardiol.* **69**, 963–965.

139. Veldkamp, M. W., van Ginneken, A. C., Opthof, T., and Bouman, L. N. (1995) Delayed rectifier channels in human ventricular myocytes. *Circulation* **92**, 3497–3504.

140. Bauer, A., Becker, R., Karle, C., et al. (2002) Effects of IKr-blocking agent dofetilide and of the Iks-blocking agent chromanol 293b on regional disparity of left ventricular repolarization in the intact canine heart. *J. Cardiovasc. Pharmacol.* **39**, 460–467.

141. Yang, T. and Roden, D. M. (1996) Extracellular potassium modulation of drug block of IKr. Implications for torsade de pointes and reverse use dependence. *Circulation* **93**, 407–411.

142. Zhibo, L., Kamiya, K., Tobias, O, et al. (2001) Density and Kinetics of IKr and Iks in guinea pig and rabbit ventricular myocytes explain different efficacy of IKs blockade at high heart rate in guinea pig and rabbit. *Circulation* **104**, 951–956.

143. Shimoni, Y., Clark., R. B., and. Giles, W. R. (1992) Role of an inwardly rectifying potassium current in rabbit ventricular action potential. *J. Physiol. (Lond.)* **448**, 709–727.

144. Rees, S. A. and Curtis, M. J. (1993) Specific IK$_1$ blockade: A new antiarrhythmic mechanism? Effect of RP58866 on ventricular arrhythmias in rat, rabbit, and primate. *Circulation* **87**, 1979–1989.

145. Pugsley, M. K., Ries, C. R., Guppy, L. J., et al. (1995) Effects of anipamil, a long acting analog of verapamil, in pigs subjected to myocardial ischemia. *Life Sci.* **57**, 1219–1231.

146. Curtis, M. J. and Walker, M. J. A. (1986) The mechanism of action of the optical isomers of verapamil against ischaemia-induced arrhythmias in the conscious rat. *Br. J. Pharmacol.* **89**, 137–147.

147. Mauritson, D. R., Winniford, M. D., Walker, W. S., et al. (1982) Oral verapamil for paroxysmal supraventricular tachycardia: A long-term, double-blind randomized trial. *Ann. Intern. Med.* **96**, 409–412.

148. Farkas, A., Qureshi, A., and Curtis, M. J. (1999) Inadequate ischaemia-selectivity limits the antiarrhythmic efficacy of mibefradil during regional ischaemia and reperfusion in the rat isolated perfused heart. *Br. J. Pharmacol.* **128**, 41–50.

149. Curruthers, S. G., Hoffman, B. B., Melmon, K. L., and Nierenberg, D. W., eds. (2000) *Melmon and Morrelli's Clinical Pharmacology*, 4th Edition, McGraw-Hill, Medical Publishing Division, New York.

150. Florent, B., Boissel, J-P.,Connolly, S. J., et al. (1999) Amiodarone interaction with
β-blockers: Analysis of the merged EMIAT (European Myocardial Infarct Amiodarone
Trial) and CAMIAT (Canadian Amiodarone Myocardial Infarction Trial) databases.
Circulation **99,** 2268–2275.

151. Connolly, S. J. (1999) Meta-analysis of antiarrhythmic drug trials. *Am. J. Cardiol.* **84,**
90R–93R.

152. Raatikainen, M. J., Napolitano, C. A., Druzgala, P., and Dennis, D. M. (1996). Electrophysiological effects of a novel, short-acting and potent ester derivative of amiodarone,
ATI-2001, in guinea pig isolated heart. *J. Pharmacol. Exp. Ther.* **277,** 1454–1463.

153. Sun, W, Sarma, J. S., and Singh, B. N. (1999) Electrophysiological effects of dronedarone
(SR33589), a noniodinated benzofuran derivative, in the rabbit heart: Comparison with
amiodarone. *Circulation* **100,** 2276–2281.

154. Domanovits, H., Schillinger, M., Lercher, P., et al. (2000) E 047/1: A new class III antiarrhythmic agent. *J. Cardiovasc. Pharmacol.* **35,** 716–722.

155. Kimura, J, Kawahara, M, Sakai, E., et al. (1999) Effects of a novel cardioprotective drug,
JTV-519, on membrane currents of guinea pig ventricular myocytes. *Jpn. J. Pharmacol.*
79, 275–281.

156. Baczko, I., El-Reyani, N. E., Farkas, A., et al. (2000) Antiarrhythmic and electrophysiological effects of GYKI-16638, a novel N-(phenoxyalkyl)-N-phenylalkylamine, in rabbits. *Eur. J. Pharmacol.* **404,** 181–190.

157. Nakaya, H., Furusawa, Y., Ogura, T., et al. (2000) Inhibitory effects of JTV-519, a novel
cardioprotective drug, on potassium currents and experimental atrial fibrillation in guinea-
pig hearts. *Br. J. Pharmacol.* **131,** 1363–1372.

158. Nattel, S., De Blasio, E., Beatch, G. N., and Wang, W. Q. (2001) RSD1235: A novel
antiarrhythmic agent with a unique electrophysiological profile that terminates AF in
dogs [abstract]. *Eur. Heart J.* **22,** 448.

159. Van Wagoner, D. R., Pond, A. L., Mccarthy, P. M., et al. (1997) Outward KC current
densities and Kv1.5 expression are reduced in chronic human atrial fibrillation. *Circ.
Res.* **80,** 772–781.

160. Heisler, B. E. and Ferrier, G. R. (1996) Proarrhythmic actions of flecainide in an isolated
tissue model of ischemia reperfusion. *J. Pharmacol. Exp. Ther.* **279,** 317–324.

161. Xu, R., Abraham, S., McLarnon, J. G., and Walker, M. J. (1997) KC8851, a tedisamil
analogue with mixed channel blockade, exhibits antiarrhythmic properties against
ischemia- and electrically-induced arrhythmias. *Life Sci.* **61,** 237–248.

162. Knopf, H., McDonald, F. M., Bischoff, A., et al. (1988) Effect of propranolol on early
postischemia arrhythmiasand noradrenaline and potassium release of ischemic myocardium in anesthetized pigs. *J. Cardiovasc. Pharmacol.* **12 (Suppl),** S41–S47.

163. Smith, W. T., Fleet, W. F., Johnson, T. A., et al. (1995) The Ib phase of ventricular
arrhythmias in ischemic in situ porcine heart is related to changes in cell-to-cell electrical
coupling. *Circulation* **92,** 3051–3060.

164. McArthur, K. E., Jensen, R. T., and Gardener, J. D. (1986) Treatment of acid-peptic
disease by inhibition of gastric H+, K+-ATPase. *Annu. Rev. Med.* **37,** 97–105.

165. Maton, P. N., Vinayek, R., Frucht, H., et al. (1989) Long-term efficacy and safety of
omeprazole in patients with Zollinger-Ellison syndrome: A prospective study. *Gastroen-
terology* **97,** 827–836.

166. Gintant, G. A., Hoffman, B. F., and Naylor, R. E. (1983) The influence of molecular form
of local anesthetic-type antiarrhythmic agents on reduction of the maximum upstroke
velocity of canine cardiac Purkinje fibers. *Circ. Res.* **52,** 735–746.

167. Beatch, G. N., Barrett, T. D., Plouvier, B., et al. (2002) ventricular fibrillation, an uncontrolled arrhythmia seeking new targets. *Drug Dev. Res.* **55,** 45–52.

168. Abraham, S., Beatch, G. N., MacLeod, B. A., and Walker, M. J. A. (1989) Antiarrythmic
properties of tetrodotoxin against occlusion-induced arrhythmias in the rat: A novel

approach to the study of the antiarrhythmic effects of ventricular sodium channel blockade. *J. Pharmacol. Exp. Ther.* **251,** 1166–1173.

169. Pugsley, M. K., Saint, D. A., Hayes, E., et al. (1995) The cardiac electrophysiological effects of sparteine and its analogue BRB-1-28 in the rat. *Eur. J. Pharmacol.* **294,** 319–327.

170. Pugsley, M. K., Saint, D. A., Penz, W. P., and Walker, M. J. A. (1993) Electrophysiological and antiarrhythmic actions of the kappa agonist PD 129290 and its R,R (+) enantiomer, PD 129289. *Br. J. Pharmacol.* **110,** 1579–1585.

171. Wat, J. Y. K., Groom, A. J., and Walker, M. J. A. (1994) Effects of arylbenzacetamides on neuromuscular preparations. *Proc. West. Pharmacol. Soc.* Abstract no. 54–II.

172. Walker, M. L., Wall, R. A., and Walker, M. J. A. (1996) Determination of an arylacetamide antiarrhythmic in rat blood and tissue using reversed-phase high-performance liquid chromatography. *J. Chromatogr. Biomed. Appl.* **675,** 257–263.

173. Bain, A. I., Barrett, T. D., Beatch, G. N., et al. (1997) Better antiarrhythmics? Development of antiarrhythmic drugs selective for ischaemia-dependent arrhythmias. *Drug. Dev. Res.* **42,** 198–210.

174. Yong, S. L., Xu, R., McLarnon, J. G., et al. (1999) RSD1000: A novel antiarrhythmic agent with increased potency under acidic and high potassium conditions. *J. Pharmacol. Exp. Ther.* **289,** 236–244.

175. Franciosi, S. and McLarnon, J. G. (2001) pH-dependent blocking actions of three novel antiarrhythmic compounds on K+ and Na+ currents in rat ventricular myocytes. *Eur. J. Pharmacol.* **425,** 95–107.

176. Cheung, P. H., Pugsley, M. K., and Walker, M. J. A. (1993) Arrhythmia models in rats. *J. Pharmacol. Methods* **29,** 179–184.

177. Barrett, T. D. and Walker, M. J. A. (1997) In vivo and in vitro cardiac preparations used in antiarrhythmic assays, in *Measurement of Cardiac Function* (McNeill, J. H., ed.), CRC Press, Boca Raton.

178. Barrett, T. D., MacLeod, B. A., and Walker, M. J. A. (1997) A model of myocardial ischemia for the simultaneous assessment of electrophysiological changes and arrhythmias in intact rabbits. *J. Pharmacol. Toxicol. Methods* **37,** 27–36.

179. Walker, M. J. A., Curtis, M. J., Hearse, D. J., et al. (1988) The Lambeth Conventions: Guidelines for the study of arrhythmias in ischaemia infarction, and reperfusion. *Cardiovasc. Res.* **22,** 447–455.

11

Biochemical Mediators of Ventricular Arrhythmias in Ischemic Heart Disease

Hugh Clements-Jewery and Michael J. Curtis

CONTENTS

INTRODUCTION
MECHANISMS OF ARRHYTHMOGENESIS
THE NOTION OF BIOCHEMICAL MEDIATORS OF ARRHYTHMIAS
HOW CAN ONE TELL IF A BIOCHEMICAL IS A MEDIATOR OF ARRHYTHMOGENESIS?
EXAMPLES OF PUTATIVE MEDIATORS OF ARRHYTHMOGENESIS IN ISCHEMIA
   AND INFARCTION
CONCLUSION
ACKNOWLEDGMENTS
REFERENCES

1. INTRODUCTION

Sudden cardiac death is a euphemism for ventricular fibrillation (VF) in the majority of cases of ischemic heart disease. It occurs most commonly during acute (<1 h duration) ischemia. There is a hierarchy of mechanisms that includes electrophysiological dysfunction and the accumulation or depletion of local cardiac biochemicals (mediators). Unfortunately, there are many biochemicals that accumulate or are depleted during ischemia and infarction, so it is not yet clear which are the true mediators. Candidates include potassium, catecholamines, histamine, serotonin, lysophosphatidylcholine, palmitylcarnitine, platelet activating factor, prostaglandins, leukotrienes, thromboxane A_2, angiotensin-II, endothelin, opioids, protons, and thrombin. Mediators may elicit arrhythmias by acting in series (one biochemical or the effects of its depletion determining the arrhythmogenicity of another) or in parallel (biochemicals or their depletion operating independently to cause ventricular arrhythmias). It remains to be determined whether a series or parallel model best decribes arrhythmogenesis during acute ischemia. A better understanding of the relative importance of individual mediators, and the manner in which their effects interact would greatly assist drug development for prevention of VF.

From: *Cardiac Drug Development Guide*
Edited by: M. K. Pugsley © Humana Press Inc., Totowa, NJ

2. MECHANISMS OF ARRHYTHMOGENESIS

VF and other ventricular arrhythmias are patterns of cardiac electrical propagation. They are defined by their electrocardiogram (EKG) appearance.

VF can be induced to occur in a healthy heart by timing an external electrical stimulus to coincide with the terminal phase of repolarization (1). This means that VF initiation does not require an intrinsic cardiac structural or functional deficit. Nevertheless, it is clear from animal research that pathology greatly increases the probability of the occurrence of VF, which is close to zero in an unmolested healthy heart. For example, in a range of animal models, regional ischemia increases the likelihood of VF from zero to close to 100% (2).

Thus, there are links between pathology and the occurrence of VF. The process of the linkage constitutes the global mechanism. Characterizing the components of the links and defining the nature of their connections has, however, proven problematic. In any setting (this includes adverse drug responses and genetic cardiac dysfunction, as well as ischemic heart disease), VF has three types of mechanisms (Table 1). VF always has a syncytial and an electrophysiological mechanism. The third type of mechanism (the initiating event) may be mechanical, biochemical, or genetic (or a combination).

In humans, VF is strongly associated with coronary artery disease, that is, ischemia and infarction (3). There is no primary genetic defect in the myocardium itself (because the primary lesion is coronary) and because a mechanical mechanism is not regarded of major relevance, it has been argued that it is the biochemical changes that occur in the local milieu that represent the primary (necessary) trigger mechanism for VF in ischemic heart disease (4).

This is the focus of the present chapter.

3. THE NOTION OF BIOCHEMICAL MEDIATORS OF ARRHYTHMIAS

One may define a biochemical that, by its actions or the effects of its depletion, evokes a pathological event (such as an arrhythmia) as a mediator. Harris et al. (5) proposed that biochemicals may act as so-called excitants (i.e., mediators) in ischemic heart disease and showed that one of the substances that accumulates in the ischemic milieu, lactate, could elicit ventricular arrhythmias when infused through a coronary artery subserving the infarcting myocardium (6). (Surprisingly, there has been no further work on the arrhythmogenic properties of lactate, so it is not discussed further here.)

In ischemic heart disease, the great challenge is to establish the identity and relative importance of each possible mediator of VF because different biochemicals accumulate or are depleted at different times after the onset of ischemia (7), because the interactions between them may be complex, and because there is a great need to identify new targets for drugs (8).

No drug that has a specific and selective action on a single putative mediator of VF has yet been shown to reduce the chance of death from VF in ischemic heart disease (8). This is intriguing because it may imply that more than one mediator is necessary or sufficient and that the effects of each must be blocked to achieve benefit. However, it may simply imply that the key biochemical has yet to be identified.

Table 1
The Hierarchy of Arrhythmogenic Mechanisms

Mechanism	Definition	Examples
1. Syncitial	Characteristics of electrical initiation and propagation of the arrhythmia *(192)*	Reentry, reflection, flow of injury current between adjacent regions of the heart, abnormal automatically
2. Electrophysiological	Changes in ion channels and movement of ions that evoke the syncytial mechanisms *(193)*	Delayed after-depolarizations, altered activation or inactivation of ion channels, abnormal depolarization or repolarization
3a. Mechanical	Changes in cell shape that evoke some electrophysiological mechanisms *(194)*	Cell swelling in ischemia, cell stretching in heart failure, hypertrophy
3b. Biochemical	Changes in the intracellular or extracellular milieu that evoke some electrophysiological mechanisms *(45)*	Accumulation or depletion of ions and metabolic substrates and products that occurs in ischemia, infarction and reperfusion; arrhythmogenic drugs
3c. Genetic	Abnormal expression of ion channels, pumps, receptors or neurotransmittors that evoke some electrophysiological mechanisms	Long QT syndromes, pheochromocytoma

4. HOW CAN ONE TELL IF A BIOCHEMICAL IS A MEDIATOR OF ARRHYTHMOGENESIS?

A set of criteria for establishing whether a biochemical is a necessary mediator of arrhythmogenesis was proposed in 1993 by Curtis et al. *(4)*. A simplified and updated version of this is shown in Table 2. It is tempting to overelaborate when addressing this issue. Indeed, even the simplified criteria in Table 2 may be reduced further to: 1) is the substance of interest changed by the disease? and 2) does the change cause the arrhythmia?

Owing to the haphazard nature of scientific progress, the reason why individual substances have been proposed as mediators, and the volume and quality of the evidence in favor or against, varies from substance to substance. Some substances have particular relevance to ischemia owing to their proven accumulation in acutely ischemic tissue, whereas other substances are more relevant to infarction (when the process of necrosis is underway). Reperfusion is an additional complication but has been largely

Table 2
Criteria for Establishing the Role of a Putative Biochemical Mediator
of Arrhythmogenesis

1. Identification of elevated or depleted amounts of the biochemical in the local tissue milieu
2. Identification of proarrhythmic effects of pathophysiologically relevant elevations or depletions of the biochemical (achieved by infusing the biochemical itself, or by stimulating or blocking its synthesis, storage, release or removal from the milieu) in the absence of ischemia or infarction, either:
    (i) Alone (indicating that the biochemical or its depletion is sufficient for arrhythmogenesis, but may not be necessary if other biochemicals show similar effects)
    (ii) Or with other putative mediators (indicating that the biochemical or its depletion may be necessary but is not sufficient alone to account for arrhythmogenesis)
3. Identification of antiarrhythmic effects of drugs that selectively and specifically block pathophysiologically relevant elevations or depletions of the biochemical in the presence of ischemia or infarction, either;
    (i) Alone (indicating that the biochemical or its depletion is sufficient for arrhythmogenesis, but may not be necessary if other biochemicals show similar effects)
    (ii) Or with other putative mediators (indicating that the biochemical or its depletion may be necessary, but is not sufficient alone to account for arrhythmogenesis)

disregarded in this article because its clinical relevance to sudden cardiac death is likely to be minimal *(9)*.

5. EXAMPLES OF PUTATIVE MEDIATORS OF ARRHYTHMOGENESIS IN ISCHEMIA AND INFARCTION

5.1. K^+

There is strong evidence that K^+ is a mediator of arrhythmias during acute ischemia and that most of the criteria in Table 2 have been satisfied *(9,10)*. K^+ is released from ischemic myocardium *(11)* and accumulates in the extracellular space *(12)*. Indeed, the biphasic time–course of accumulation of extracellular K^+ ($[K^+]_o$) coincides with the biphasic appearance of early (so-called phase 1) ischemia-induced arrhythmias *(13)*. Infusion of potassium salts into coronary vessels can evoke ventricular arrhythmias in anesthetized dogs *(6)* and in nonischemic isolated rabbit hearts *(14)*.

Additional circumstantial evidence supports the role of K^+ as a mediator. For example, local elevation of $[K^+]_o$ alters conduction, in addition to action potential and EKG configuration in a manner similar (although not identical) to that produced by ischemia *(9,15)*. These changes can be expected to increase the likelihood of arrhythmias *(10,16–18)*. To prove the role of K^+ as a mediator, it would be necessary to show that selective inhibition of extracellular K^+ accumulation during ischemia can inhibit arrhythmia development. Unfortunately, there are no drugs with the ability to totally block extracellular K^+ accumulation. Further work on the importance of K^+ (to determine whether it is a necessary as well as sufficient mediator) is clearly warranted.

5.2. Catecholamines

Since the synthesis of the first β_1 adrenoceptor antagonist by Black et al. *(19)*, the role of catecholamines as mediators of not only VF but also other adverse events in the cardiovascular system has received a considerable amount of attention *(20,21)*.

β_1 Adrenoceptor antagonists reduce mortality in patients with ischemic heart disease *(8)*. On the basis of this, it is seductive to suppose not only that these agents are thus effective in suppressing ischemia-induced VF but also that catecholamines mediate VF in ischemic heart disease. However, this notion is not supported unequivocally by the facts *(21–29)*.

Although norepinephrine accumulates in ischemic tissue *(30)*, the time–course of accumulation and the absolute levels have not been shown to correlate well with the severity of arrhythmias *(20,29)*. Catecholamines have not been dismissed as mediators because of this, however, because many studies have been hampered by the difficulty in estimating catecholamine content of ischemic tissue by the technique used—analysis of samples of coronary effluent (which is derived primarily from nonischemic tissue). To rectify this, Lameris et al. *(31)* recently measured catecholamines in interstitial fluid; they found a large accumulation of norepinephrine and epinephrine within the ischemic region. However, there was no correlation between this and the occurrence of VF or other arrhythmias.

In a different approach, catecholamine replenishment to (denervated) isolated rat hearts failed to evoke VF during infarct evolution, which shows that the effects of sympathetic drive (i.e., the action of catecholamines) are not sufficient to cause infarction-related VF *(32)*.

Part of the reason for the widely held belief that catecholamines cause VF in ischemic heart disease is that there are numerous suggestive drug studies from animal experiments. However, the data can easily be misinterpreted. Many of the drugs that have been used as tools lack selectivity at the concentrations used. For example, antiarrhythmic effects have been demonstrated with antiadrenergic drugs that also possess at the concentrations used, class I effects on excitability, metabolic effects on glycogen metabolism, or excessive bradycardic actions, whereas more selective antiadrenergic drugs often lack antiarrhythmic activity *(27,33)*.

Although the β_1 and α_1 receptors have been the most commonly investigated molecular targets for mediating the arrhythmogenic effects of catecholamines *(4)*, some of the more intriguing recent data has come from studies on the role of β_2 receptors. In a model of regional ischemia in anesthetized dogs with a healed myocardial infarction *(34)*, β_2 antagonists protected against VF in susceptible animals, and in vitro evidence suggested that these animals had enhanced sensitivity to β_2-adrenergic stimulation *(35)*. The role of β_2 agonism is complicated, however, by the fact that anesthetized animals subjected to a moderate level of experimental surgery have a blood K^+ homeostasis that is highly β_2 receptor dependent. β_2 antagonism elevates blood K^+ in such animals, and this may be sufficient to account for the protection seen *(20,36)*.

Thus, the evidence for a role of catecholamines as important mediators of VF is not as consistent or convincing as one might have anticipated from postinfarct mortality studies *(8)*.

5.3. Histamine

The heart contains a variety of sources of histamine *(37–40)*, which is released during experimental hypoxia *(41)*. Exogenously applied histamine can shorten action potential duration (APD) and evoke enhanced normal automaticity in Purkinje fibers *(42)* and abnormal automaticity in ventricular tissue *(43,44)*. These effects are more consistent with typical changes encountered in infarcting tissue *(45)*. Interestingly, exogenous histamine can evoke cardiac arrhythmias in infarcting dog *(46)* and pig *(47)* hearts in vivo.

It would seem reasonable to deduce that if histamine is an important mediator of VF, then patients taking antihistamines (H1 for allergy or H2 for gastric ulcers) should be less susceptible to sudden cardiac death than the rest of the population. Such data ought to be easily available for analysis. However, to our knowledge, nothing in this regard has been published to date.

There are three main types of histamine receptor. In animal studies, a variety of H1 antagonists can inhibit ischemia-induced ventricular arrhythmias *(48)*; however, drug selectivity is problematic, and effects have been attributed to class I actions. H2 antagonists also have been reported to suppress ischemia-induced arrhythmias in some *(49,50)* but not other *(48)* studies, although when effects were observed they were not necessarily attributable to H2 antagonism *(51)*. Adding to the inconsistency of findings, it has been shown that the H2 antagonist, ranitidine, may actually exacerbate experimental ischemia-induced arrhythmias *(52)*. Agonism at H3 receptors can reduce nonexocytotic carrier-mediated norepinephrine release during myocardial ischemia. H3-agonism inhibits Na^+/H^+ exchange in the sympathetic nerve endings of the heart, thus attenuating the build up of Na^+ within the nerve ending that might occur under conditions of low intracellular pH, such as ischemia, and slowing activity of the Na^+-dependent norepinephrine transporter *(53)*. H3 agonism also appears to reduce exocytotic release of norepinephrine via inhibition of N-type Ca^{2+} channels *(54)*. Whether this has real importance to VF depends on whether local release of catecholamines plays any major role in arrhythmogenesis *(see* Section 5.2.*)*. It is difficult to reconcile the conflicting data concerning the role of histamine in arrhythmogenesis, and more work would appear to be warranted.

5.4. 5-HT

In many respects, the actions of 5-HT in the heart and the nature and quality of the evidence linking it to arrhythmogenesis are similar to those for histamine. 5-HT is found in large quantities within the heart *(55,56)* and has been shown to initiate afterdepolarizations in kitten papillary muscle *(57)*. Its role in arrhythmogenesis (and indeed in any pathological event) is difficult to explore by the use of receptor-selective antagonists, however, owing to the large population of receptor subtypes expressed *(58)* and the considerable species dependence of this expression *(59)*. Like histamine, 5-HT may act directly on cardiac receptors *(57)* and indirectly by norepinephrine release (via activation of 5-HT3 receptors located on sympathetic nerve terminals; refs. *60,61)*.

The use of agonists and antagonists has not provided a clear picture of the role of 5-HT as a mediator of ventricular arrhythmias. The 5-HT2A antagonists ketanserin *(62)* and ICI 170,809 *(63)* were found to have no effect on ischemia-induced arrhythmias in rats. However, poor selectivity of some of the drugs used as tools has hindered elucidation of 5-HT's role.

For example, the antagonists ketanserin and ritanserin are now known to have actions in the myocardium indicative of possible sodium or potassium channel blockade *(64)*. The class III-like properties of ketanserin *(65)* and class I-like actions of the 5-HT3 receptor antagonist ICS-205-930 *(66)* may account for their observed antiarrhythmic effects *(65,67)*. Likewise, although the mixed L-type Ca^{2+} antagonist and 5-HT2 antagonist nepoxamil was found to be antiarrhythmic during ischemia, it was no more effective than diltiazem, indicating that its effects may simply be attributable to its Ca^{2+} antagonist action *(68)*. 5-HT is therefore like histamine—a putative arrhythmogenic mediator whose pathophysiological relevance is questionable.

5.5. Amphiphiles

The role of amphiphilic products of lipid metabolism in arrhythmogenesis is intriguing. It was shown many years ago that several amphiphilic biochemicals possess all the appropriate characteristics as mediators of ischemia-induced VF. The 11-point summary of data by Corr and colleagues *(69)* indicates that many of the criteria outlined in Table 2 are satisfied by these substances when considered collectively. Yet, to our knowledge, there has been no fruitful clinical development of amphiphile antagonists as antiarrhythmics. It is uncertain whether this represents a disturbing dichotomy between animal and clinical data or merely the lack of enthusiasm for antiarrhythmic drug development that followed the Cardiac Arrhythmia Suppression Trial (CAST) and Survival with Oral D-Sotalol (SWORD) studies *(70,71)*.

Lysophosphatidylcholine (LPC) accumulation in ischemic tissue correlates well with the onset of susceptibility to ischemia-induced arrhythmias *(72,73)*. In addition, incorporation of LPC (which is produced in endothelial cells and myocytes in response to thrombin) and long-chain acylcarnitines into the sarcolemma causes similar electrophysiological dysfunction to that which occurs during ischemia in vivo *(74)*.

There are several possible mechanisms responsible for the arrhythmogenic effects of LPC. Low concentrations (μM) can inhibit the inwardly rectifying K^+ current and cause depolarization of cardiac tissue *(75)*. Higher concentrations (10–100 μM) reduce the maximum slope of the upstroke of the action potential (dV/dt_{max}; ref. *76*). At high concentrations, LPC can elicit abnormal automaticity *(76)*. At around 100 μM, LPC applied globally to superfused right ventricular free wall can elicit ventricular tachycardia (VT; ref. *77*). 2-[5-(4-chlorophenyl)-pentyl]-oxirane-2-carboxylate inhibits the activity of carnitine acyltransferase-I, the enzyme that catalyses the synthesis of long chain acylcarnitines and consequently disinhibits the lysophospholipase enzyme that degrades LPC *(78)* and was found to abolish LPC accumulation and the appearance of VT and VF during brief ischemia in cats *(69)*.

Palmitylcarnitine (PC; also known as palmitoylcarnitine) accumulates in ischemic tissue *(79)* but has a profile of activity that is less consistent with a role as a mediator of ischemia-induced arrhythmias. At low concentrations (0.1–1 μM), it prolongs APD, whereas at higher concentrations (100 μM) it shortens APD *(78, 80–82)*, yet at intermediate concentrations (1–10 μM) PC has direct irreversible cardiotoxic effects on structure and function *(83)*. This makes it difficult to envisage PC as a relevant mediator of early ischemia-induced VF because early reperfusion studies have shown that the acute phase of ischemia is characterized by reversible shortening of APD *(45)* and by reversible mechanical dysfunction *(84)*.

Platelet-activating factor (PAF) is another amphiphile that has been implicated as a mediator of ischaemia-induce arrhythmias. The role of PAF in cardiovascular pathophysiology has recently been reviewed *(85)*. Importantly, it has been shown to be released during ischemia in humans *(86)* and baboons *(87)*. PAF has several actions that might be regarded as proischemic *(88,89)* and hence indirectly proarrhythmic, but consideration of this is beyond the scope of the present article.

Several PAF antagonists, including BN50739 *(90,91)*, CV-6209 *(92)*, RP59227 *(93,94)*, WEB2086 *(95)*, and TCV309 *(96,97)* inhibit ischemia- or reperfusion-induced arrhythmias. The problem with these data is that it is difficult to link the effects of the drugs on VF with an effect on the actions of endogenous PAF. This difficulty is partly overcome in one study in which BN50739 was found to exert its protective actions only when administered selectively to the ischemic region, implying that its action on VF results from an action on a target specific to the ischemic tissue—necessary if PAF antagonism is the mechanism of antiarrhythmic action *(91)*.

Exogenous PAF can itself shorten APD and evoke ventricular arrhythmias in nonischemic isolated hearts *(98)*. In summary, PAF may have direct actions in the myocardium that promote arrhythmias. However, the ability of PAF to release other chemicals with potentially arrhythmogenic actions and constrict coronary arteries *(85)* means that its role as a direct mediator remains difficult to determine.

5.6. Prostaglandins (PGs), Excluding Thromboxanes

PG synthesis in the heart from plasmalemmal phospholipid *(99)* occurs primarily in the coronary vasculature *(100)*, although synthesis in myocytes can also occur *(101)*. As in the case of PAF, indirect arrhythmogenic actions are possible owing to the ability of some PGs to elicit thrombosis and constriction of coronary vessels *(102)*.

Cardiac hypoxia facilitates PG synthesis *(99,103)*, although the main product is prostacyclin (PGI2), which is a coronary vasodilator with possible antiarrhythmic properties *(104)*. Indeed, many studies have shown this and other PGs to be antiarrhythmic and protective against a range of effects of cardiac ischemia *(105–108)*. Therefore, most PGs are not likely to play a role as mediators of VF.

5.7. Thromboxane

Sulphinpyrazone *(109)*, aspirin, meclofenamate, and indomethacin *(110)* (all cyclooxygenase inhibitors) have been found to inhibit ischemia-induced arrhythmias in animal models. If inhibition of a cyclooxygenase product was responsible for this, then the most likely candidate mediator may be a thromboxane (TX), which, unlike PGI2, has never been implicated as a protective or antiarrhythmic mediator. TXA2 levels are elevated in venous blood-draining ischemic tissue with levels increasing during the appearance of ventricular arrhythmias *(111)*. Blockers of TXA2 synthesis and blockers of TXA2 receptors can suppress ischemia-induced arrhythmias *(112)*, although it is not clear whether this results from block of an arrhythmogenic action or block of the proischemic effects of TXA2 because TXA2, like PAF, can induce platelet aggregation *(113)* and constriction of coronary arteries *(114)*.

A direct role for TXA2 in arrhythmogenesis is suggested by evidence that close coronary arterial administration of stable TXA2 analogs with agonist properties, such as U46619, can evoke arrhythmias in dogs *(115)*, although thrombosis leading to ischemia cannot omitted as the mechanism here.

Better evidence is provided by the observation that the TX synthase blocker UK38485 suppressed arrhythmias during experimental mechanical coronary ligation, in which thrombosis and resultant ischemia and its alleviation are not relevant factors *(116)*. Likewise, another TX synthase blocker, U-63557A, was found to reduce TXB2 levels and reduce the incidence in cats of ischemia-induced VF *(117)*. However, the TX synthase inhibitor, ICI 192,605, has no effect on the incidence of VF or VT during ischemia in anesthetized rats *(63)*. Species differences may explain the inconsistencies. TXs are good candidate mediators of ischemia-induced arrhythmias, with both direct and indirect (proischemic) mechanisms possible. Further study is warranted.

5.8. Leukotrienes (LTs)

LTs are not known to accumulate specifically in ischemic myocardium; however, LTs are present in cells which themselves accumulate during ischemia (including neutrophils and macrophages). LTs elevate the ST segment *(118)*, which is indicative of a proischemic effect, constrict coronary arteries *(118–121)* and, in the case of LTB4, evoke platelet aggregation and chemotaxis *(122)*, but they do not elicit ventricular arrhythmias when applied globally to the heart *(119,123)*. Although the LT antagonists L660711 and L648051 have been shown to attenuate experimental ischemia-induced VF *(124)*, LY-233569 (a 5-lipoxygenase inhibitor that blocks LT synthesis) and LY-255283 (a selective LTB4 antagonist) had no effect *(125)*. Therefore, LTs are not promising candidates as important mediators of ischaemia-induced arrhythmias, although it is too early to dismiss them entirely.

5.9. Angiotensin II (A-II)

There are several independent types of evidence to suggest that A-II plays a role as an arrhythmogenic mediator. Inhibitors of angiotensin-converting enzyme (ACE) appear to possess antiarrhythmic activity. For example, Z13752A, a combined ACE/neutral endopeptidase inhibitor, has been observed to reduce the incidence of ischemia-induced VT and VF in anesthetized dogs *(126)*. Likewise, captopril and perindopril inhibit ischemia-induced arrhythmias in the rat *(127,128)*. At least part of the action of ACE inhibitors on VF is mediated within the involved part of the myocardium *(129)*.

The antiarrhythmic effects of ACE inhibitors are not necessarily attributable to inhibition of A-II synthesis because ACE is also responsible for degrading bradykinin, a putative endogenous antiarrhythmic mediator *(104)*. Shimada and Avkiran *(129)* observed that the effect of ramiprilat on so-called sustained VF (not all VF is sustained in the rat heart) was abolished by the coinfusion of HOE140, a bradykinin B2 receptor antagonist. In contrast, co-infusion of A-II was ineffective, indicating that the action of ramiprilat was caused by the enhanced availability of bradykinin rather than reduced levels of A-II. Infusion of HOE140 alone increased the incidence of sustained VF, and this was independent of its coronary vasoconstrictor properties *(129)*.

Despite this, the antiarrhythmic effects described previously were weak. Moreover, it has yet to be demonstrated that A-II can elicit arrhythmias independently of other components of ischemia or that bradykinin can ameliorate the arrhythmogenicity of A-II. The electrophysiological effects of A-II are not dramatic. A-II appears to reduce junctional conductance in isolated rat myocyte pairs, an effect that appears to be mediated by A1 angiotensin receptors and may contribute to conduction slowing during ischemia *(130)*. Additionally, spontaneous discharges of action potentials have been shown to be elicited by a single stimulus during the relative refractory period in ventricular fibers exposed to A-II (10^{-9} M; ref. *131*).

Most recently the focus on A-II (and bradykinin) has switched from ischemia to reperfusion. Although this topic is not covered specifically by this chapter, it is worth noting that a range of experiments involving heart perfusion with A-II and bradykinin *(132)* the A1 antagonists candesartan *(133)* and A1a receptor knockout mice *(134)* all support a role for A-II as a mediator of reperfusion arrhythmias.

Clinical data on mortality and its causes during therapy for heart failure and hypertension and the effect of ACE inhibitors (which affect bradykinin as well as A-II), compared with A-II receptor antagonists (A-II-selective), will clarify the role of A-II as an endogenous mediator of arrhythmias and the role of bradykinin as an endogenous protectant.

5.10. Endothelin (ET)

ET binds to two receptor subtypes; ET_A receptors, which predominate in myocytes, and ET_B receptors, which are expressed almost exclusively on cardiac fibroblasts and endothelial cells *(135)*. Of the three ET isoforms, ET_1 is the most widely studied, and elevated levels of ET_B have been detected in patients with myocardial infarction *(136)*. In pigs *(137)* and dogs *(138–141)* ET_B administration (especially intracoronary) can elicit VF, although concomitant coronary constriction and ST segment elevation mean that the arrhythmogenic effects may be secondary to ET_B-induced ischemia. The ET_A receptor antagonist LU 135.252 *(142,143)* and the mixed ET_A and ET_B receptor antagonists bosentan *(141)* and SB 209670 *(144)* prevent the arrhythmogenic effects of ET_B. These drugs also prevent the prolongation of QT intervals and widening of monophasic action potentials seen with infusions of ET_B *(141,142,145)*. In addition to its effects on action potential duration, ET_B has been observed to decrease spontaneous firing rate of myocardial cells at low concentrations and produce early afterdepolarizations at higher concentrations *(146)*. The ability of ET_B to increase the inward rectifying potassium current *(147)* would be expected to result in a shortened action potential duration, so it is difficult to reconcile in vivo actions with single cell effects.

In animal models, ischemia-induced VF is suppressed by endothelin antagonists. The ET_A antagonist LU 135252 is effective in pigs *(148)*, and the ET_A receptor antagonist PD161721 and ET_B receptor antagonists BQ123 and sarafotoxin 6c are effective in rats *(149–151)*. However, exogenously applied ET_B was itself found to be protective in rats *(149)*; the protective mechanism is unknown *(152)*.

From these studies it remains a possibility that ET_B may function as a direct or indirect chemical mediator of arrhythmias (a role similar to that suggested above for several other substances), although there are inconsistencies in the data.

5.11. Opioids

β endorphin and dynorphin are two endogenous opioids that have been proposed to function as endogenous arrhythmogenic substances *(153)*. There are numerous opioid receptors that might mediate arrhythmogenesis. The rat heart, used for many arrhythmia studies, expresses κ_1 and δ but not κ_2 or μ opioid receptors *(154–157)*. Despite this, there is no convincing evidence that opioids play an important role in arrhythmogenesis. There are no reports demonstrating that opioids accumulate in the ischemic myocardium. Moreover, opioid agonists and antagonists do not have well demarcated opposing effects on arrhythmogenesis. Selective activation of δ_1 receptors with TAN-67 appears to reduce severity of ischemia-induced arrhythmias in rats, an effect attributed to opening of mitochondrial KATP channels *(158)*. Other investigators have reported protection with κ antagonists *(159–161)*. Furthermore, the opioid partial agonist meptazinol *(162)* and the antagonist naloxone *(163)* have similar protectiveeffects on ischemia-induced VF in rats. It is difficult to interpret some published studies owing to an additional complicating factor; many opioid agonists and antagonists affect the heart via nonopioid receptor mechanisms *(164)*. Several opioid agonists and antagonists (including + and − optical enantiomers of the same drug) have antiarrhythmic effects that appear to result from opioid receptor-independent actions *(165,166)*. Likewise, the *S,S* (−)-enantiomer PD 129290, a κ agonist, and its corresponding inactive, *R,R* (+)-enantiomer PD 129289, are equally effective at reducing ischemia-induced arrhythmias in anesthetized rats, and both dose dependently reduce heart rate and blood pressure while prolonging PR and QRS intervals of the EKG *(167)*, indicating possible class I activity. Furthermore, there are inconsistencies, with naloxone, for example, which has been shown as protective in some studies *(166)* and inactive in others *(168)*. Studies with supposedly more selective agents are also contradictory.

The once-presumed selective κ agonist U-50,488H *(169)* evoked arrhythmias in perfused hearts *(160)* and exacerbated ischemia-induced arrhythmias in rats *(170)*. The proarrhythmic effect of U-50,488H was associated with increased levels of cardiac inositol triphosphate (InsP3; ref. *171)*. However, the same drug, U-50,488H, can also reduce the incidence of ischemia-induced VF in rats, an effect now attributed to sodium channel blockade (class I activity) *(172)*. It is probable, on the basis of these data, that opioids are not involved in arrhythmogenesis in ischemia.

5.12. Protons

Protons (H+) accumulate in the intra- and extracellular space during ischemia *(13,173)*. The extracellular H$^+$ accumulation has been implicated in producing cellular uncoupling, which contributes to the failure of impulse propagation during acute ischemia and which may be the cause of so-called phase 1b VF *(174)*.

The outward H$^+$ flux that underlies ischemia-induced extracellular H$^+$ accumulation *(175)* occurs partly in exchange with an inward Na$^+$ flux via the cardiac Na$^+$/H$^+$ exchanger (NHE1), which is the main regulator of intracellular pH in myocytes under physiological conditions *(176)*. The extent of the contribution made by NHE1 to ischemia-induced H$^+$ flux is questionable, however, because ischemia tends to block NHE1 activity, whereas reperfusion restores it *(177)*. Thus if NHE1 contributes to the arrhythmogenic effects of H$^+$, it is more likely to do so during reperfusion rather than during ischemia. Despite this, cariporide, otherwise known as HOE642, a selective NHE1 inhibitor, reduces ischemia-induced ventricular premature beats (VPBs), VT, and VF in anesthetized rats *(178,179)*.

Other selective NHE1 inhibitors, including BIIB513 *(180)* and SL 59.1227 *(181)*, have similar effect, which is intriguing. Cariporide does not attenuate accumulation of intracellular H$^+$ during ischemia *(182–184)*, presumably because NHE1 is not involved (*see* above). Therefore, the effects of cariporide (and presumably also other NHE1 blocking drugs) on ischemia-induced arrhythmias cannot be the result of NHE1 block or inhibition of H$^+$ accumulation.

In summary, despite strong evidence in favor of a role for H$^+$ washout as a cause of reperfusion-induced arrhythmias *(185)*, the importance of H$^+$ as a mediator of ischemia-induced arrhythmias remains to be established. The selectivity of some of the drugs used as tools appears to be questionable.

5.13. *Thrombin*

Thrombin is an enzyme that is formed at the site of vascular injury and that plays an important role in coagulation *(186)*. In addition to this role, it exerts effects in a variety of cell types, including platelets, endothelial cells, and fibroblasts *(186)* via activation of the G-protein-coupled cell surface thrombin receptor, part of the protease-activated receptor (PAR) superfamily. Cardiac myocytes express PAR1 and PAR2 receptors but only the former is activated by thrombin *(187)*.

Thrombin has been observed to increase InsP3 production in cardiac myocytes consistent with a stimulatory effect on phospholipase C, to prolong action potential duration in canine Purkinje fibers, to increase beating rate in contracting isolated myocytes, and to increase basal and peak systolic Ca^{2+} levels independently of its effects on beating rate *(188)*. Thrombin receptor activation also appears to increase intracellular Na^+ and lysophosphatidylcholine accumulation during ischemia *(189)*. Although there is evidence that reperfusion arrhythmias are associated with an increase in the production of InsP3 *(190)* and that exogenously applied thrombin can enhance InsP3 production and exacerbate arrhythmias during reperfusion *(191)*, it appears unlikely that thrombin exerts arrhythmogenic effects by the same mechanism during ischemia. This is because InsP3 production appears to cease 5 min after the onset of ischemia *(190)*.

In summary, although there is some evidence that thrombin may exacerbate reperfusion arrhythmias, it is not clear whether endogenous thrombin can itself initiate arrhythmias, especially during ischemia. Given that ischemia-induced VF can occur in isolated perfused hearts *(2)*, which are nominally thrombin free, it is probable that thrombin is neither necessary nor sufficient for arrhythmogenesis.

6. CONCLUSION

There are clearly numerous putative endogenous mediators of VF associated with ischemic heart disease. It is also clear that the role of each is uncertain. It would be naive to assume that one substance alone is sufficient to account for all VF (ischemia-induced and infarction-induced).

Therefore, more than one substance is likely to be necessary. The nature of the interaction between these substances is likely to hold the key to arrhythmogenesis and to determine whether specific antagonist drugs will ameliorate VF. The principals behind the complexity and implications of mediator interactions are, in many respects, independent of the condition (ischemia vs infarction) or the identity of the mediators themselves. Any two substances may interact additively, synergistically, or antagonistically, and the net effect may depend on the presence of the full range of substances that accumulate in the milieu. This is a frightening prospect for those interested in developing drugs for prevention of sudden cardiac death; the pathophysiological reserve for VF may be so excessive that a cocktail of antagonists may be the only viable method of achieving therapeutic benefit *(4)*.

ACKNOWLEDGMENTS

Work by the authors which contributed to parts of this review were funded by the British Heart Foundation, the British Pharmacological Society, the British Columbia and Yukon Heart and Stroke Foundation, and the Canadian Heart Foundation.

REFERENCES

1. Tennant, R. and Wiggers, C. J. (1935) The effect of coronary occlusion on myocardial contraction. *Am. J. Physiol.* **112,** 351–361.
2. Curtis, M. J. (1998) Characterisation, utilisation and clinical relevance of isolated perfused heart models of ischaemia-induced ventricular fibrillation. *Cardiovasc. Res.* **39,** 194–215.
3. Campbell, R. W. (1983) Treatment and prophylaxis of ventricular arrhythmias in acute myocardial infarction. *Am. J. Cardiol.* **52,** 55C–59C.
4. Curtis, M. J., Pugsley, M. K., and Walker, M. J. (1993) Endogenous chemical mediators of ventricular arrhythmias in ischaemic heart disease. *Cardiovasc. Res.* **27,** 703–719.
5. Harris, A. S., Bisteni, A., Russell, R. A., Brigham, J. C., and Firestone, J. E. (1954) Excitatory factors in ventricular tachycardia resulting from myocardial ischaemia. Potassium as a major excitant. *Science* **119,** 200–203.
6. Harris, A. S., Toth, L. A., and Hooey, T. E. (1958) Arrhythmic and antiarrhythmic effects of sodium, potassium, and calcium salts and of glucose injected into coronary arteries of infarcted and normal hearts. *Circ. Res.* **6,** 570–579.
7. Hearse, D. J., Humphrey, S. M., Feuvray, D., and De Leiris, J. (1976) A biochemical and ultrastructural study of the species variation in myocardial cell damage. *J. Mol. Cell Cardiol.* **8,** 759–778.
8. Antman, E. M., Lau, J., Kupelnick, B., Mosteller, F., and Chalmers, T. C. (1992) A comparison of results of meta-analyses of randomized control trials and recommendations of clinical experts. Treatments for myocardial infarction. *JAMA* **268,** 240–248.
9. Curtis, M. J. and Hearse, D. J. (1989) Ischaemia-induced and reperfusion-induced arrhythmias differ in their sensitivity to potassium: Implications for mechanisms of initiation and maintenance of ventricular fibrillation. *J. Mol. Cell Cardiol.* **21,** 21–40.
10. Morena, H., Janse, M. J., Fiolet, J. W., Krieger, W. J., Crijns, H., and Durrer, D. (1980) Comparison of the effects of regional ischemia, hypoxia, hyperkalemia, and acidosis on intracellular and extracellular potentials and metabolism in the isolated porcine heart. *Circ. Res.* **46,** 634–646.
11. Dennis, J. and Moore, R. M. (1938) K^+ changes in the functioning heart under conditions of ischaemia and congestion. *Am. J. Physiol.* **123,** 579–593.
12. Hill, J. L. and Gettes, L. S. (1980) Effect of acute coronary artery occlusion on local myocardial extracellular K^+ activity in swine. *Circulation* **61,** 768–778.
13. Hirche, H., Franz, C., Bos, L., Bissig, R., Lang, R., and Schramm, M. (1980) Myocardial extracellular K^+ and H^+ increase and noradrenaline release as possible cause of early arrhythmias following acute coronary artery occlusion in pigs. *J. Mol. Cell Cardiol.* **12,** 579–593.
14. Curtis, M. J. (1991) The rabbit dual coronary perfusion model: A new method for assessing the pathological relevance of individual products of the ischaemic milieu: role of potassium in arrhythmogenesis. *Cardiovasc. Res.* **25,** 1010–1022.
15. Janse, M. J. and Kleber, A. G. (1981) Electrophysiological changes and ventricular arrhythmias in the early phase of regional myocardial ischemia. *Circ. Res.* **49,** 1069–1081.
16. Schmidt, F. O. and Erlanger, J. (1928) Directional differences in the conduction of the impulse through heart muscle and their possible relation to extrasystolic and fibrillatory contractions. *Am. J. Physiol.* **87,** 326–347.
17. Ettinger, P. O., Regan, T. J., Oldewurtel, H. A., and Khan, M. I. (1973) Ventricular conduction delay and arrhythmias during regional hyperkalemia in the dog. Electrical and myocardial ion alterations. *Circ. Res.* **33,** 521–531.
18. Pelleg, A., Mitamura, H., Price, R., Kaplinsky, E., Menduke, H., Dreifus, L. S., and Michelson, E. L. (1989) Extracellular potassium ion dynamics and ventricular arrhythmias in the canine heart. *J. Am. Coll. Cardiol.* **13,** 941–950.

19. Black, J. W., Duncan, W. A., and Shanks, R. G. (1965) Comparison of some properties of pronethalol and propranolol. *Br. J. Pharmacol.* **25,** 577–591.

20. Curtis, M. J., Botting, J. H., Hearse, D. J., and Walker, M. J. A. (1989) The sympathetic nervous system, catecholamines and ischaemia-induced arrhythmias: dependence upon serum potassium concentration, in *Adrenergic System and Ventricular Arrhythmias in Myocardial Infarction* (Brachmann, J. and Schömig, A., eds.), Springer-Verlag, Berlin, pp. 206–219.

21. Priori, S. and Schwartz, P. J. (1989) Catecholamine-dependent cardiac arrhythmias: mechanisms and implication, in *Adrenergic System and Ventricular Arrhythmias in Myocardial Infarction* (Brachmann, J. and Schömig, A., eds.), Springer-Verlag, Berlin, pp. 239–247.

22. Sheridan, D. J., Penkoske, P. A., Sobel, B. E., and Corr, P. B. (1980) Alpha adrenergic contributions to dysrhythmia during myocardial ischemia and reperfusion in cats. *J. Clin. Invest.* **65,** 161–171.

23. Sheridan, D. J. and Culling, W. (1985) Electrophysiological effects of alpha-adrenoceptor stimulation in normal and ischemic myocardium. *J. Cardiovasc. Pharmacol.* **7,** S55–S60.

24. Culling, W., Penny, W. J., Lewis, M. J., Middleton, K. and Sheridan, D. J. (1984) Effects of myocardial catecholamine depletion on cellular electrophysiology and arrhythmias during ischaemia and reperfusion. *Cardiovasc. Res.* **18,** 675–682.

25. Bolli, R., Fisher, D. J., Taylor, A. A., Young, J. B., and Miller, R. R. (1984) Effect of alpha-adrenergic blockade on arrhythmias induced by acute myocardial ischemia and reperfusion in the dog. *J. Mol. Cell Cardiol.* **16,** 1101–1117.

26. Tosaki, A., Szekeres, L., and Hearse, D. J. (1987) Metoprolol reduces reperfusion-induced fibrillation in the isolated rat heart: Protection is secondary to bradycardia. *J. Cardiovasc. Pharmacol.* **10,** 489–497.

27. Daugherty, A., Frayn, K. N., Redfern, W. S., and Woodward, B. (1986) The role of catecholamines in the production of ischaemia-induced ventricular arrhythmias in the rat in vivo and in vitro. *Br. J. Pharmacol.* **87,** 265–277.

28. Botting, J. H., Johnston, K. M., Macleod, B. A., and Walker, M. J. (1983) The effect of modification of sympathetic activity on responses to ligation of a coronary artery in the conscious rat. *Br. J. Pharmacol.* **79,** 265–271.

29. Cinca, J., Bardaji, A., and Salas-Caudevilla, A. (1989) Ventricular arrhythmias and local electrograms after chronic regional denervation of the ischemic area in the pig heart. *J. Am. Coll. Cardiol.* **14,** 225–232.

30. Schomig, A., Dart, A. M., Dietz, R., Mayer, E., and Kubler, W. (1984) Release of endogenous catecholamines in the ischemic myocardium of the rat. Part A: Locally mediated release. *Circ. Res.* **55,** 689–701.

31. Lameris, T. W., de Zeeuw, S., Alberts, G., Boomsma, F., Duncker, D. J., Verdouw, P. D., et al. (2000) Time course and mechanism of myocardial catecholamine release during transient ischemia in vivo. *Circulation* **101,** 2645–2650.

32. Clements-Jewery, H., Hearse, D. J., and Curtis, M. J. (2002) Independent contribution of catecholamines to arrhythmogenesis during evolving infarction in the isolated rat heart. *Br. J. Pharmacol.* **135,** 807–815.

33. Rochette, L., Didier, J. P., Moreau, D., Bralet, J., and Opie, L. H. (1984) Role of beta-adrenoreceptor antagonism in the prevention of reperfusion ventricular arrhythmias: Effects of acebutolol, atenolol, and d-propranolol on isolated working rat hearts subject to myocardial ischemia and reperfusion. *Am. Heart J.* **107,** 1132–1141.

34. Altschuld, R. A. and Billman, G. E. (2000) Beta2-Adrenoceptors and ventricular fibrillation. *Pharmacol. Ther.* **88,** 1–14.

35. Billman, G. E., Castillo, L. C., Hensley, J., Hohl, C. M., and Altschuld, R. A. (1997) Beta2-adrenergic receptor antagonists protect against ventricular fibrillation: In vivo and in vitro evidence for enhanced sensitivity to beta2-adrenergic stimulation in animals susceptible to sudden death. *Circulation* **96,** 1914–1922.

36. Paletta, M. J., Abraham, S., Beatch, G. N., and Walker, M. J. (1989) Mechanisms underlying the antiarrhythmic properties of beta-adrenoceptor blockade against ischaemia-induced arrhythmias in acutely prepared rats. *Br. J. Pharmacol.* **98**, 87–94.

37. Dai, S. and Ogle, C. W. (1990) Ventricular histamine concentrations and mast cell counts in the rat heart during acute ischaemia. *Agents Actions* **29**, 138–143.

38. Mannaioni, P. F. (1985) Physiology and pharmacology of cardiac histamine, revisited, in: *Fontiers in Histamine Research* (Ganellin, C. R. and Schwartz, J. C., eds.), J Wright, London, pp. 236–297.

39. Ryan, M. J. and Brody, M. J. (1970) Distribution of histamine in the canine autonomic nervous system. *J. Pharmacol. Exp. Ther.* **174**, 123–132.

40. Harvey, S. C. (1978) Studies on myocardial histamine. Effects of catecholamine-depleting drugs. *Arch. Int. Pharmacodyn. Ther.* **232**, 141–149.

41. Anrep, G. V., Barsoum, G. S., and Talaat, M. (1936) Liberation of histamine by the heart muscle. *J. Physiol.* **86**, 431–451.

42. Cerbai, E., Amerini, S., and Mugelli, A. (1990) Histamine and abnormal automaticity in barium- and strophanthidin-treated sheep Purkinje fibers. *Agents Actions* **31**, 1–10.

43. Wolff, A. A. and Levi, R. (1986) Histamine and cardiac arrhythmias. *Circ. Res.* **58**, 1–16.

44. Cameron, J. S., Swigart, C. R., Shin, G. S., Katz, D., and Bassett, A. L. (1990) Enhanced susceptibility to histamine-induced cardiac arrhythmias in spontaneously hypertensive rats. *J. Cardiovasc. Pharmacol.* **15**, 626–632.

45. Gettes, L. S. and Cascio, W. E. (1992) Effects of acute ischaemia on cardiac electrophysiology, in *The Heart and Cardiovascular System,* 2nd Ed. (Fozzard, H. A., Haber, E., Jennings, R. B., Katz, A. M., and Morgan, H. E., eds.), Raven Press, New York, pp. 2021–2054.

46. Harris, A. S. (1950) Delayed development of ventricular ectopic rhythms following experimental coronary occlusion. *Circulation* **1**, 1318–1328.

47. Podzuweit, T. (1982) Early arrhythmias resulting from acute myocardial ischaemia: Possible role of cyclic AMP, in *Early Arrhythmias Resulting from Myocardial Ischaemia* (Parratt, J. R., ed.), McMillan, Basingstoke, UK, pp. 171–198..

48. Rochette, L., Yao-Kouame, J., Bralet, J., and Opie, L. H. (1988) Effects of promethazine on ischemic and reperfusion arrhythmias in rat heart. *Fund. Clin. Pharmacol.* **2**, 385–397.

49. Dai, S. (1987) Ventricular histamine concentrations and arrhythmias during acute myocardial ischaemia in rats. *Agents Actions* **21**, 66–71.

50. Dai, S. (1984) Effects of SKandF 93479 on experimentally induced ventricular arrhythmias in dogs, rats and mice. *Agents Actions* **15**, 131–136.

51. Banning, M. M. and Curtis, M. J. (1995) Protection by cimetidine, but not ranitidine, implies that H2 receptors do not mediate arrhythmogenesis in a rat model of regional ischaemia and reperfusion in vitro. *Cardiovasc. Res.* **30**, 705–710.

52. Wolff, A. A., Levi, R., Chenouda, A. A., and Fisher, V. J. (1984) Ventricular arrhythmias parallel cardiac histamine release after coronary artery occlusion in the dog: effects of ranitidine. *Circulation* **70(Suppl II)**, 225.

53. Imamura, M., Lander, H. M., and Levi, R. (1996) Activation of histamine H3-receptors inhibits carrier-mediated norepinephrine release during protracted myocardial ischemia. Comparison with adenosine A1-receptors and alpha2-adrenoceptors. *Circ. Res.* **78**, 475–481.

54. Levi, R. and Smith, N. C. (2000) Histamine H3-receptors: A new frontier in myocardial ischemia. *J. Pharmacol. Exp. Ther.* **292**, 825–830.

55. Berkowitz, B. A., Lee, C. H., and Spector, S. (1974) Disposition of serotonin in the rat blood vessels and heart. *Clin. Exp. Pharmacol. Physiol.* **1**, 397–400.

56. Sole, M. J., Shum, A., and Van Loon, G. R. (1979) Serotonin metabolism in the normal and failing hamster heart. *Circ. Res.* **45**, 629–634.

57. Kaumann, A. J. (1983) A classification of heart serotonin receptors. *Naunyn Schmiedebergs Arch. Pharmacol.* **322(Suppl)**, R42.

58. Bach, T., Syversveen, T., Kvingedal, A. M., Krobert, K. A., Brattelid, T., Kaumann, A. J., and Levy, F. O. (2001) 5HT4(a) and 5-HT4(b) receptors have nearly identical pharmacology and are both expressed in human atrium and ventricle. *Naunyn Schmiedebergs Arch. Pharmacol.* **363,** 146–160.

59. Saxena, P. R. and Villalon, C. M. (1991) 5-Hydroxytryptamine: A chameleon in the heart. *Trends Pharmacol. Sci.* **12,** 223–227.

60. Richardson, B. P., Engel, G., Donatsch, P., and Stadler, P. A. (1985) Identification of serotonin M-receptor subtypes and their specific blockade by a new class of drugs. *Nature* **316,** 126–131.

61. Thandroyen, F. T., Saman, S., and Opie, L. H. (1985) Serotonin and the heart: Pharmacological evaluation with the S2-serotonergic antagonist ketanserin, in *Serotonin and the Cardiovascular System* (Vanhoutte, P. M., ed.), Raven Press, New York, pp. 87–93.

62. Coker, S. J. (1986) Does ketanserin reduce ischaemia and reperfusion-induced arrhythmias in anaesthetised rats? *Br. J. Pharmacol.* **88,** 288P.

63. Shaw, L. A. and Coker, S. J. (1996) Suppression of reperfusion-induced arrhythmias with combined administration of 5-HT2 and thromboxane A2 antagonists. *Br. J. Pharmacol.* **117,** 817–822.

64. Coker, S. J. and Ellis, A. M. (1987) Ketanserin and ritanserin can reduce reperfusion-induced but not ischaemia-induced arrhythmias in anaesthetised rats. *J. Cardiovasc. Pharmacol.* **10,** 479–484.

65. Saman, S., Thandroyen, F. and Opie, L. H. (1985) Serotonin and the heart: Effects of ketanserin on myocardial function, heart rate, and arrhythmias. *J. Cardiovasc. Pharmacol.* **7,** S70–S75.

66. Williams, F. M., Rothaul, A. L., Kane, K. A., and Parratt, J. R. (1985) Antiarrhythmic and electrophysiological effects of ICS 205-930, an antagonist of 5-hydroxytryptamine at peripheral receptors. *J. Cardiovasc. Pharmacol.* **7,** 550–555.

67. Coker, S. J., Dean, H. G., Kane, K. A., and Parratt, J. R. (1986) The effects of ICS 205-930, a 5-HT antagonist, on arrhythmias and catecholamine release during canine myocardial ischaemia and reperfusion. *Eur. J. Pharmacol.* **127,** 211–218.

68. Nearing, B. D., Hutter, J. J., and Verrier, R. L. (1996) Potent antifibrillatory effect of combined blockade of calcium channels and 5-HT2 receptors with nexopamil during myocardial ischemia and reperfusion in dogs: Comparison to diltiazem. *J. Cardiovasc. Pharmacol.* **27,** 777–787.

69. Corr, P. B., Creer, M. H., Yamada, K. A., Saffitz, J. E., and Sobel, B. E. (1989) Prophylaxis of early ventricular fibrillation by inhibition of acylcarnitine accumulation. *J. Clin. Invest.* **83,** 927–936.

70. Waldo, A. L., Camm, A. J., deRuyter, H., Freidman, P. L., MacNeil, D. J., Pitt, B., et al. (1995) Survival with oral d-sotalol in patients with left ventricular dysfunction after myocardial infarction: rationale, design, and methods (the SWORD trial). *Am. J. Cardiol.* **75,** 1023–1027.

71. CAST. (1989) Preliminary report: Effect of encainide and flecainide on mortality in a randomized trial of arrhythmia suppression after myocardial infarction. The Cardiac Arrhythmia Suppression Trial (CAST) Investigators. *N. Engl. J. Med.* **321,** 406–412.

72. Corr, P. B., Gross, R. W., and Sobel, B. E. (1984) Amphipathic metabolites and membrane dysfunction in ischemic myocardium. *Circ. Res.* **55,** 135–154.

73. Corr, P. B., Yamada, K. A., Creer, M. H., Sharma, A. D., and Sobel, B. E. (1987) Lysophosphoglycerides and ventricular fibrillation early after onset of ischemia. *J. Mol. Cell Cardiol.* **19(Suppl 5),** 45–53.

74. Corr, P. B. and Yamada, K. A. (1995) Selected metabolic alterations in the ischemic heart and their contributions to arrhythmogenesis. *Herz* **20,** 156–168.

75. Kiyosue, T. and Arita, M. (1986) Effects of lysophosphatidylcholine on resting potassium conductance of isolated guinea pig ventricular cells. *Pflugers Arch.* **406,** 296–302.

76. Nakaya, H., Kimura, S., and Kanno, M. (1984) Suppression of lysophosphatidylcholine-induced abnormal automaticity by verapamil in canine Purkinje fibers. *Jpn. J. Pharmacol.* **36,** 371–378.

77. Duan, J. and Moffat, M. P. (1991) Protective effects of d,l-carnitine against arrhythmias induced by lysophosphatidylcholine or reperfusion. *Eur. J. Pharmacol.* **192,** 355–363.

78. van der Vusse, G. J., Prinzen, F. W., van Bilsen, M., Engels, W., and Reneman, R. S. (1987) Accumulation of lipids and lipid-intermediates in the heart during ischaemia. *Basic Res. Cardiol.* **82,** 157–167.

79. Sakata, K., Hayashi, H., Kobayashi, A., and Yamazaki, N. (1989) Mechanism of arrhythmias induced by palmitylcarnitine in guinea pig papillary muscle. *Cardiovasc. Res.* **23,** 505–511.

80. Yokota, S., Hironaka, Y., and Ohara, N. (1989) Effects of l-carnitine on membrane potential derangements induced by palmitoylcarnitine and anoxia in isolated superfused guinea-pig papillary muscle. *Res. Commun. Chem. Pathol. Pharmacol.* **66,** 179–190.

81. Meszaros, J. and Pappano, A. J. (1988) Single cell model for l-palmitoylcarnitine-induced ventricular arrhythmias. *Circulation* **78(Suppl II),** 569.

82. Matsui, K., Nakazawa, M., Takeda, K., and Imai, S. (1985) Effect of l-carnitine chloride and its acetyl derivative on the electrophysiological derangement induced by palmityl-L-carnitine in isolated canine ventricular muscle. *Jpn. J. Pharmacol.* **39,** 263–270.

83. Busselen, P., Sercu, D., and Verdonck, F. (1988) Exogenous palmitoyl carnitine and membrane damage in rat hearts. *J. Mol. Cell Cardiol.* **20,** 905–916.

84. Hearse, D. J. (1990) Ischemia, reperfusion, and the determinants of tissue injury. *Cardiovasc. Drugs Ther.* **4(Suppl 4),** 767–776.

85. Montrucchio, G., Alloatti, G., and Camussi, G. (2000) Role of platelet-activating factor in cardiovascular pathophysiology. *Physiol. Rev.* **80,** 1669–1699.

86. Montrucchio, G., Camussi, G., Tetta, C., Emanuelli, G., Orzan, F., Libero, L., and Brusca, A. (1986) Intravascular release of platelet-activating factor during atrial pacing. *Lancet* **2,** 293.

87. Annable, C. R., McManus, L. M., Carey, K. D., and Pinckard, R. N. (1985) Isolation of platelet activating factor (PAF) from ischaemic baboon myocardium. *Fed. Proc.* **44,** 1271.

88. Sybertz, E. J., Watkins, R. W., Baum, T., Pula, K., and Rivelli, M. (1985) Cardiac, coronary and peripheral vascular effects of acetyl glyceryl ether phosphoryl choline in the anesthetized dog. *J. Pharmacol. Exp. Ther.* **232,** 156–162.

89. Pugsley, M. K., Salari, H., and Walker, M. J. (1991) Actions of platelet-activating factor on isolated rat hearts. *Circ. Shock* **35,** 207–214.

90. Koltai, M., Tosaki, A., Hosford, D., Esanu, A., and Braquet, P. (1991) Effect of BN 50739, a new platelet activating factor antagonist, on ischaemia induced ventricular arrhythmias in isolated working rat hearts. *Cardiovasc. Res.* **25,** 391–397.

91. Baker, K. E. and Curtis, M. J. (1999) Protection against ventricular fibrillation by the PAF antagonist, BN-50739, involves an ischaemia-selective mechanism. *J. Cardiovasc. Pharmacol.* **34,** 394–401.

92. Stahl, G. L., Terashita, Z., and Lefer, A. M. (1988) Role of platelet activating factor in propagation of cardiac damage during myocardial ischemia. *J. Pharmacol. Exp. Ther.* **244,** 898–904.

93. Auchampach, J. A., Muruyama, M., Cavero, I., and Gross, G. J. (1991) Blocking platelet activating factor receptors with RP59227 decreases myocardial infarct size and the incidence of ventricular fibrillation. *J. Mol. Cell. Cardiol.* **23(Suppl 3),** S52.

94. Auchampach, J. A., Pieper, G. M., Cavero, I., and Gross, G. J. (1998) Effect of the platelet-activating factor antagonist RP 59227 (Tulopafant) on myocardial ischemia/reperfusion injury and neutrophil function. *Basic Res. Cardiol.* **93,** 361–371.

95. Sariahmetoglu, M., Cakici, I., and Kanzik, I. (1998) Effects of WEB 2086 on the protective role of preconditioning against arrhythmias in rats. *Pharmacol. Res.* **38,** 173–178.

96. Tamura, K., Kimura, Y., Tamura, T., Kitashiro, S., Izuoka, T., Tsuji, H., et al. (1994) The effect of platelet-activating-factor antagonist TCV-309 on arrhythmias and functional recovery during myocardial reperfusion. *Coron. Artery Dis.* **5,** 267–273.

97. Qayumi, A. K., English, J. C., Godin, D. V., Ansley, D. M., Loucks, E. B., Lee, J. U., and Kim, C. W. (1998) The role of platelet-activating factor in regional myocardial ischemia-reperfusion injury. *Ann. Thorac. Surg.* **65,** 1690–1697.

98. Tamargo, J., Delgado, C., Diez, J., and Delpon, E. (1988) Cardiac electrophysiology of PAF-acether antagonists, in *Ginkgolides, Chemistry, Biology, Pharmacology and Clinical Perspectives* (Braquet, P., ed.), Vol. 1, J. R. Prous SciencePubl., Barcelona, pp. 417–431.

99. Karmazyn, M. and Dhalla, N. S. (1983) Physiological and pathophysiological aspects of cardiac prostaglandins. *Can. J. Physiol. Pharmacol.* **61,** 1207–1225.

100. Hsueh, W. and Needleman, P. (1978) Sites of lipase activation and prostaglandin synthesis in isolated perfused rabbit hearts and hydronephrotic kidneys. *Prostaglandins* **16,** 661–681.

101. Bolton, H. S., Chanderbhan, R., Bryant, R. W., Bailey, J. M., Weglicki, W. B., and Vahouny, G. V. (1980) Prostaglandin synthesis by adult heart myocytes. *J. Mol. Cell Cardiol.* **12,** 1287–1298.

102. Karmazyn, M. (1989) Synthesis and relevance of cardiac eicosanoids with particular emphasis on ischemia and reperfusion. *Can. J. Physiol. Pharmacol.* **67,** 912–921.

103. De Deckere, E. A., Nugteren, D. H., and Ten Hoor, F. (1977) Prostacyclin is the major prostaglandin released from the isolated perfused rabbit and rat heart. *Nature* **268,** 160–163.

104. Parratt, J. (1993) Endogenous myocardial protective (antiarrhythmic) substances. *Cardiovasc. Res.* **27,** 693–702.

105. Mest, H. J., Schror, K., and Forster, W. (1972) Antiarrhythmic properties of PGE2. *Adv. Biosci.* **9,** 395–400.

106. Mest, H. J., Mentz, P. and Forster, W. (1974) Effects of prostaglandins on experimental arrhythmias. *Pol. J. Pharmacol. Pharm.* **26,** 151–156.

107. Au, T. L., Collins, G. A., Harvie, C. J., and Walker, M. J. (1979) The actions of prostaglandins I2 and E2 on arrhythmias produced by coronary occlusion in the rat and dog. *Prostaglandins* **18,** 707–720.

108. Hohlfeld, T., Meyer-Kirchrath, J., Vogel, Y. C., and Schror, K. (2000) Reduction of infarct size by selective stimulation of prostaglandin EP3 receptors in the reperfused ischemic pig heart. *J. Mol. Cell Cardiol.* **32,** 285–296.

109. Dix, R. K., Kelliher, G. J., Jurkiewicz, N., and Smith, J. B. (1982) Effect of sulfinpyrazone on ventricular arrhythmia, prostaglandin synthesis, and catecholamine release following coronary artery occlusion in the cat. *J. Cardiovasc. Pharmacol.* **4,** 1068–1076.

110. Fagbemi, S. O. (1984) The effect of aspirin, indomethacin and sodium meclofenamate on coronary artery ligation arrhythmias in anaesthetized rats. *Eur. J. Pharmacol.* **97,** 283–287.

111. Coker, S. J., Parratt, J. R., Ledingham, I. M., and Zeitlin, I. J. (1981) Thromboxane and prostacyclin release from ischaemic myocardium in relation to arrhythmias. *Nature* **291,** 323–324.

112. Coker, S. J. and Parratt, J. R. (1985) AH23848, a thromboxane antagonist, suppresses ischemia and reperfusion-induced arrhythmias in anaesthetized greyhounds. *Br. J. Pharmacol.* **86,** 259–264.

113. Hamberg, M., Svensson, J., and Samuelsson, B. (1975) Thromboxanes: A new group of biologically active compounds derived from prostaglandin endoperoxides. *Proc. Natl. Acad. Sci. USA* **72,** 2994–2998.

114. Ellis, E. F., Oelz, O., Roberts, L. J., II, Payne, N. A., Sweetman, B. J., Nies, A. S., et al. (1976) Coronary arterial smooth muscle contraction by a substance released from platelets: Evidence that it is thromboxane A2. *Science* **193,** 1135–1137.

115. Parratt, J. R. and Wainwright, C. L. (1986) Ventricular arrhythmias induced by local injections of vasoconstrictors following coronary occlusion. *Br. J. Pharmacol.* **88,** 397P.

116. Coker, S. J. (1984) Further evidence that thromboxane exacerbates arrhythmias: Effects of UK38485 during coronary artery occlusion and reperfusion in anaesthetized greyhounds. *J. Mol. Cell Cardiol.* **16,** 633–641.

117. O'Connor, K. M., Friehling, T. D., and Kowey, P. R. (1989) The effect of thromboxane inhibition on vulnerability to ventricular fibrillation in the acute and chronic feline infarction models. *Am. Heart J.* **117,** 848–853.

118. Ezeamuzie, I. C. and Assem, E. S. (1983) Effects of leukotrienes C4 and D4 on guinea-pig heart and the participation of SRS-A in the manifestations of guinea-pig cardiac anaphylaxis. *Agents Actions* **13,** 182–187.

119. Letts, L. G. and Piper, P. J. (1982) The actions of leukotrienes C4 and D4 on guinea-pig isolated hearts. *Br. J. Pharmacol.* **76,** 169–176.

120. Burke, J. A., Levi, R., Guo, Z. G., and Corey, E. J. (1982) Leukotrienes C4, D4 and E4: Effects on human and guinea-pig cardiac preparations in vitro. *J. Pharmacol. Exp. Ther.* **221,** 235–241.

121. Roth, D. M. and Lefer, A. M. (1983) Studies on the mechanism of leukotriene induced coronary artery constriction. *Prostaglandins* **26,** 573–581.

122. Mayer, M. (1988) Leukotrienes and other lipoxygenase metabolites of arachidonic acid: their role in edema, ischemia and demyelination of the central nervous system. *Acta Univ. Palacki Olomuc Fac. Med.* **119,** 181–186.

123. Terashita, Z. I., Fukui, H., Hirata, M., Terao, S., Ohkawa, S., Nishikawa, K., and Kikuchi, S. (1981) Coronary vasoconstriction and PGI2 release by leukotrienes in isolated guinea pig hearts. *Eur. J. Pharmacol.* **73,** 357–361.

124. Beatch, G. N., Courtice, I. D., and Salari, H. (1989) A comparative study of the antiarrhythmic properties of eicosanoid inhibitors, free radical scavengers and potassium channel blockers on reperfusion induced arrhythmias in the rat. *Proc. West Pharmacol. Soc.* **32,** 285–289.

125. Hahn, R. A., MacDonald, B. R., Simpson, P. J., Potts, B. D., and Parli, C. J. (1990) Antagonism of leukotriene B4 receptors does not limit canine myocardial infarct size. *J. Pharmacol. Exp. Ther.* **253,** 58–66.

126. Rastegar, M. A., Marchini, F., Morazzoni, G., Vegh, A., Papp, J. G., and Parratt, J. R. (2000) The effects of Z13752A, a combined ACE/NEP inhibitor, on responses to coronary artery occlusion; A primary protective role for bradykinin. *Br. J. Pharmacol.* **129,** 671–680.

127. Rochette, L., Ribuot, C., Belichard, P., Bril, A., and Devissaguet, M. (1987) Protective effect of angiotensin converting enzyme inhibitors (CEI): Captopril and perindopril on vulnerability to ventricular fibrillation during myocardial ischemia and reperfusion in rat. *Clin. Exp. Hypertens. A* **9,** 365–368.

128. Ribuot, C. and Rochette, L. (1987) Converting enzyme inhibitors (captopril, enalapril, perindopril) prevent early-post infarction ventricular fibrillation in the anaesthetized rat. *Cardiovasc. Drugs. Ther.* **1,** 51–55.

129. Shimada, Y. and Avkiran, M. (1996) Attenuation of reperfusion arrhythmias by selective inhibition of angiotensin-converting enzyme/kininase II in the ischemic zone: Mediated by endogenous bradykinin? *J. Cardiovasc. Pharmacol.* **27,** 428–438.

130. De Mello, W. and Altieri, P. (1992) The role of the renin-angiotensin system in the control of cell communication in the heart: Effects of enalapril and angiotensin II. *J. Cardiovasc. Pharmacol.* **20,** 643–651.

131. De Mello, W. C. and Crespo, M. J. (1999) Correlation between changes in morphology, electrical properties, and angiotensin-converting enzyme activity in the failing heart. *Eur. J. Pharmacol.* **378,** 187–194.

132. Scholkens, B. A., Linz, W., Lindpainter, K., and Ganten, D. (1987) Angiotensin deteriorates but bradykinin improves cardiac function following ischaemia in isolated rat hearts. *J. Hypertens.* **5(Suppl 5),** S7–S9.

133. Hiura, N., Wakatsuki, T., Yamamoto, T., Nishikado, A., Oki, T., and Ito, S. (2001) Effects of angiotensin II type 1 receptor antagonist (candesartan) in preventing fatal ventricular arrhythmias in dogs during acute myocardial ischemia and reperfusion. *J. Cardiovasc. Pharmacol.* **38,** 729–736.

134. Harada, K., Komuro, I., Hayashi, D., Sugaya, T., Murakami, K., and Yazaki, Y. (1998) Angiotensin II type 1a receptor is involved in the occurrence of reperfusion arrhythmias. *Circulation* **97,** 315–317.

135. Modesti, P. A., Vanni, S., Paniccia, R., Bandinelli, B., Bertolozzi, I., Polidori, G., et al. (1999) Characterization of endothelin-1 receptor subtypes in isolated human cardiomyocytes. *J. Cardiovasc. Pharmacol.* **34,** 333–339.

136. Miyauchi, T., Yanagisawa, M., Tomizawa, T., Sugishita, Y., Suzuki, N., Fujino, M., et al. (1989) Increased plasma concentrations of endothelin-1 and big endothelin-1 in acute myocardial infarction. *Lancet* **2,** 53–54.

137. Ezra, D., Goldstein, R. E., Czaja, J. F., and Feuerstein, G. Z. (1989) Lethal ischemia due to intracoronary endothelin in pigs. *Am. J. Physiol.* **257,** H339–H343.

138. Underwood, D. C., Falotico, R., Cheung, W.-M., and Tobia, A. J. (1989) Dissociation of coronary vasoconstrictor and arrhythmogenic properties of endothelin in the dog. *Circulation* **80(Suppl II),** 149.

139. Salvati, P., Chierchia, S., Dho, L., Ferrario, R. G., Parenti, P., Vicedomini, G., et al. (1991) Proarrhythmic activity of intracoronary endothelin in dogs: Relation to the site of administration and to changes in regional flow. *J. Cardiovasc. Pharmacol.* **17,** 1007–1014.

140. Toth, M., Solti, F., Merkely, B., Kekesi, V., Horkay, F., Szokodi, I., et al. (1995) Ventricular tachycardias induced by intracoronary administration of endothelin-1 in dogs. *J. Cardiovasc. Pharmacol.* **26(Suppl 3),** S153–S155.

141. Horkay, F., Geller, L., Kiss, O., Szabo, T., Vago, H., Kekesi, V., et al. (2000) Bosentan the mixed endothelin-A- and -B-receptor antagonist suppresses intrapericardial endothelin-1-induced ventricular arrhythmias. *J. Cardiovasc. Pharmacol.* **36,** S320–S322.

142. Kiss, O., Geller, L., Merkely, B., Szabo, T., Raschack, M., Seres, L., et al. (2000) Endothelin-A-receptor antagonist LU 135.252 inhibits the formation of ventricular arrhythmias caused by intrapericardial infusion of endothelin-1. *J. Cardiovasc. Pharmacol.* **36,** S317–S319.

143. Merkely, B., Szabo, T., Geller, L., Kiss, O., Horkay, F., Raschack, M., et al. (2000) The selective endothelin-A-receptor antagonist LU 135.252 inhibits the direct arrhythmogenic action of endothelin-1. *J. Cardiovasc. Pharmacol.* **36,** S314–S316.

144. Douglas, S. A., Nichols, A. J., Feuerstein, G. Z., Elliott, J. D., and Ohlstein, E. H. (1998) SB 209670 inhibits the arrhythmogenic actions of endothelin-1 in the anesthetized dog. *J. Cardiovasc. Pharmacol.* **31(Suppl 1),** S99–S102.

145. Geller, L., Merkely, B., Szokodi, I., Szabo, T., Vecsey, T., Juhasz-Nagy, A., et al. (1998) Electrophysiological effects of intrapericardial infusion of endothelin-1. *Pacing Clin. Electrophysiol.* **21,** 151–156.

146. Yorikane, R., Shiga, H., Miyake, S., and Koike, H. (1990) Evidence for direct arrhythmogenic action of endothelin. *Biochem. Biophys. Res. Commun.* **173,** 457–462.

147. Kim, D. (1991) Endothelin activation of an inwardly rectifying K^+ current in atrial cells. *Circ. Res.* **69,** 250–255.

148. Raschack, M., Juchelka, F., and Rozek-Schaefer, G. (1998) The endothelin-A antagonist LU 135 252 supresses ischemic ventricular extrasystoles and fibrillation in pigs and prevents hypoxic cellular decoupling. *J. Cardiovasc. Pharmacol.* **31(Suppl 1),** S145–S148.

149. Sharif, I., Kane, K. A., and Wainwright, C. L. (1998) Endothelin and ischaemic arrhythmias-antiarrhythmic or arrhythmogenic? *Cardiovasc. Res.* **39,** 625–32.

150. Crockett, T. R., Sharif, I., Kane, K. A., and Wainwright, C. L. (2000) Sarafotoxin 6c protects against ischaemia-induced cardiac arrhythmias in vivo and in vitro in the rat. *J. Cardiovasc. Pharmacol.* **36,** S297–S299.

151. Crockett, T. R., Scott, G. A., McGowan, N. W., Kane, K. A., and Wainwright, C. L. (2001) Anti-arrhythmic and electrophysiological effects of the endothelin receptor antagonists, BQ-123 and PD161721. *Eur. J. Pharmacol.* **432,** 71–77.

152. Sharif, I., Crockett, T. R., Kane, K. A., and Wainwright, C. L. (2001) The effects of endothelin-1 on ischaemia-induced ventricular arrhythmias in rat isolated hearts. *Eur. J. Pharmacol.* **427,** 235–242.

153. Lee, A. Y. (1990) Endogenous opioid peptides and cardiac arrhythmias. *Int. J. Cardiol.* **27,** 145–151.

154. Jin, W. Q., Tai, K. K., Chan, T. K., and Wong, T. M. (1995) Further characterization of [3H]U69593 binding sites in the rat heart. *J. Mol. Cell. Cardiol.* **27,** 1507–1511.

155. Zimlichman, R., Gefel, D., Eliahou, H., Matas, Z., Rosen, B., Gass, S., et al. (1996) Expression of opioid receptors during heart ontogeny in normotensive and hypertensive rats. *Circulation* **93,** 1020–1025.

156. Krumins, S. A., Faden, A. I., and Feuerstein, G. (1985) Opiate binding in rat hearts: Modulation of binding after hemorrhagic shock. *Biochem. Biophys. Res. Commun.* **127,** 120–128.

157. Ventura, C., Bastagli, L., Bernardi, P., Caldarera, C. M., and Guarnieri, C. (1989) Opioid receptors in rat cardiac sarcolemma: Effect of phenylephrine and isoproterenol. *Biochim. Biophys. Acta* **987,** 69–74.

158. Fryer, R. M., Hsu, A. K., Nagase, H., and Gross, G. J. (2000) Opioid-induced cardioprotection against myocardial infarction and arrhythmias: Mitochondrial versus sarcolemmal ATP-sensitive potassium channels. *J. Pharmacol. Exp. Ther.* **294,** 451–457.

159. Sitsapesan, R. and Parratt, J. R. (1989) The effects of drugs interacting with opioid receptors on the early ventricular arrhythmias arising from myocardial ischaemia. *Br. J. Pharmacol.* **97,** 795–800.

160. Wong, T. M., Lee, A. Y., and Tai, K. K. (1990) Effects of drugs interacting with opioid receptors during normal perfusion or ischemia and reperfusion in the isolated rat heart—an attempt to identify cardiac opioid receptor subtype(s) involved in arrhythmogenesis. *J. Mol. Cell Cardiol.* **22,** 1167–1175.

161. Pugsley, M. K., Penz, W. P., Walker, M. J., and Wong, T. M. (1992) Cardiovascular actions of the kappa-agonist, U-50,488H, in the absence and presence of opioid receptor blockade. *Br. J. Pharmacol.* **105,** 521–526.

162. Fagbemi, O., Kane, K. A., Lepran, I., Parratt, J. R., and Szekeres, L. (1983) Antiarrhythmic actions of meptazinol, a partial agonist at opiate receptors, in acute myocardial ischemia. *Br. J. Pharmacol.* **78,** 455–460.

163. Fagbemi, O., Lepran, I., Parratt, J. R., and Szekeres, L. (1982) Naloxone inhibits early arrhythmias resulting from acute coronary ligation. *Br. J. Pharmacol.* **76,** 504–506.

164. Pugsley, M. K. (2002) The diverse molecular mechanisms responsible for the actions of opioids on the cardiovascular system. *Pharmacol. Ther.* **93,** 51–75.

165. Boachie-Ansah, G., Sitsapesan, R., Kane, K. A., and Parratt, J. R. (1989) The antiarrhythmic and cardiac electrophysiological effects of buprenorphine. *Br. J. Pharmacol.* **97,** 801–808.

166. Sarne, Y., Flitstein, A., and Oppenheimer, E. (1991) Anti-arrhythmic activities of opioid agonists and antagonists and their stereoisomers. *Br. J. Pharmacol.* **102,** 696–698.

167. Pugsley, M. K., Saint, D. A., Penz, M. P., and Walker, M. J. (1993) Electrophysiological and antiarrhythmic actions of the kappa agonist PD 129290, and its R,R (+)-enantiomer, PD 129289. *Br. J. Pharmacol.* **110,** 1579–1585.

168. Pruett, J. K., Blair, J. R., and Adams, R. J. (1991) Cellular and subcellular actions of opioids in the heart, in *Opioids in Anaesthesia* (Estafonous, F. G., ed.), Vol. II, Butterworth-Heinmann, Boston, MA, pp. 61–70.

169. Lahti, R. A., VonVoigtlander, P. F., and Barsuhn, C. (1982) Properties of a selective kappa agonist, U-50,488H. *Life Sci.* **31,** 2257–2260.

170. Lee, A. Y., Chen, Y. T., Kan, M. N., P'Eng F, K., Chai, C. Y., and Kuo, J. S. (1992) Consequences of opiate agonist and antagonist in myocardial ischaemia suggest a role of endogenous opioid peptides in ischaemic heart disease. _Cardiovasc. Res._ **26,** 392–395.

171. Yu, X., Zhang, W., Bian, J., and Wong, T. M. (1999) Pro- and anti-arrhythmic effects of a kappa opioid receptor agonist: A model for the biphasic action of a local hormone in the heart. _Clin. Exp. Pharmacol. Physiol._ **26,** 842–844.

172. Pugsley, M. K., Penz, W. P., Walker, M. J., and Wong, T. M. (1992) Antiarrhythmic effects of U-50,488H in rats subject to coronary artery occlusion. _Eur. J. Pharmacol._ **212,** 15–19.

173. Garlick, P. B., Radda, G. K., and Seeley, P. J. (1979) Studies of acidosis in the ischaemic heart by phosphorus nuclear magnetic resonance. _Biochem. J._ **184,** 547–554.

174. Smith, W. T., Fleet, W. F., Johnson, T. A., Engle, C. L., and Cascio, W. E. (1995) The Ib phase of ventricular arrhythmias in ischemic in situ porcine heart is related to changes in cell-to-cell electrical coupling. Experimental Cardiology Group, University of North Carolina. _Circulation_ **92,** 3051–3060.

175. Yan, G. X. and Kleber, A. G. (1992) Changes in extracellular and intracellular pH in ischemic rabbit papillary muscle. _Circ. Res._ **71,** 460–470.

176. Lagadic-Gossmann, D., Buckler, K. J., and Vaughan-Jones, R. D. (1992) Role of bicarbonate in pH recovery from intracellular acidosis in the guinea-pig ventricular myocyte. _J. Physiol._ **458,** 361–384.

177. Avkiran, M. (2001) Protection of the ischaemic myocardium by Na^+/H^+ exchange inhibitors: Potential mechanisms of action. _Basic Res. Cardiol._ **96,** 306–311.

178. Scholz, W., Albus, U., Counillon, L., Gogelein, H., Lang, H. J., Linz, W., et al. (1995) Protective effects of HOE642, a selective sodium-hydrogen exchange subtype 1 inhibitor, on cardiac ischaemia and reperfusion. _Cardiovasc. Res._ **29,** 260–268.

179. Aye, N. N., Komori, S., and Hashimoto, K. (1999) Effects and interaction, of cariporide and preconditioning on cardiac arrhythmias and infarction in rat in vivo. _Br. J. Pharmacol._ **127,** 1048–1055.

180. Wu, D., Stassen, J. M., Seidler, R., and Doods, H. (2000) Effects of BIIB513 on ischemia-induced arrhythmias and myocardial infarction in anesthetized rats. _Basic Res. Cardiol._ **95,** 449–456.

181. Lorrain, J., Briand, V., Favennec, E., Duval, N., Grosset, A., Janiak, P., et al. (2000) Pharmacological profile of SL 59.1227, a novel inhibitor of the sodium/hydrogen exchanger. _Br. J. Pharmacol._ **131,** 1188–1194.

182. Hartmann, M. and Decking, U. K. (1999) Blocking Na^+/H^+ exchange by cariporide reduces Na^+-overload in ischemia and is cardioprotective. _J. Mol. Cell Cardiol._ **31,** 1985–1995.

183. Stromer, H., de Groot, M. C., Horn, M., Faul, C., Leupold, A., Morgan, J. P., et al. (2000) Na^+/H^+ exchange inhibition with HOE642 improves postischemic recovery due to attenuation of Ca^{2+} overload and prolonged acidosis on reperfusion. _Circulation_ **101,** 2749–2755.

184. Portman, M. A., Panos, A. L., Xiao, Y., Anderson, D. L., and Ning, X. (2001) HOE-642 (cariporide) alters pHi and diastolic function after ischemia during reperfusion in pig hearts in situ. _Am. J. Physiol. Heart Circ. Physiol._ **280,** H830–H834.

185. Ibuki, C., Hearse, D. J., and Avkiran, M. (1993) Mechanisms of antifibrillatory effect of acidic reperfusion: Role of perfusate bicarbonate concentration. _Am. J. Physiol._ **264,** H783–H790.

186. Coughlin, S. R. (2000) Thrombin signalling and protease-activated receptors. _Nature_ **407,** 258–264.

187. Sabri, A., Muske, G., Zhang, H., Pak, E., Darrow, A., Andrade-Gordon, P., et al. (2000) Signaling properties and functions of two distinct cardiomyocyte protease-activated receptors. _Circ. Res._ **86,** 1054–1061.

188. Steinberg, S. F., Robinson, R. B., Lieberman, H. B., Stern, D. M., and Rosen, M. R. (1991) Thrombin modulates phosphoinositide metabolism, cytosolic calcium, and impulse initiation in the heart. *Circ. Res.* **68,** 1216–1229.

189. Yan, G. X., Park, T. H., and Corr, P. B. (1995) Activation of thrombin receptor increases intracellular Na+ during myocardial ischemia. *Am. J. Physiol.* **268,** H1740–H1748.

190. Anderson, K. E., Dart, A. M., and Woodcock, E. A. (1995) Inositol phosphate release and metabolism during myocardial ischemia and reperfusion in rat heart. *Circ. Res.* **76,** 261–268.

191. Jacobsen, A. N., Du, X. J., Lambert, K. A., Dart, A. M., and Woodcock, E. A. (1996) Arrhythmogenic action of thrombin during myocardial reperfusion via release of inositol 1,4,5-triphosphate. *Circulation* **93,** 23–26.

192. Janse, M. J. (1992) Reentrant arrhythmias, in *The Heart and Cardiovascular System* (Fozzard, H. A., Haber, E., Jennings, R. B., Katz, A. M., and Morgan, H. E., eds.), Raven Press, New York, pp. 2055–2094.

193. Parratt, J. R. (1982) *Early Arrhythmias Resulting from Acute Myocardial Ischaemia,* Macmillan, Basingstoke, UK.

194. Lab, M. J. (1982) Contraction-excitation feedback in myocardium. Physiological basis and clinical relevance. *Circ. Res.* **50,** 757–766.

12

Heterologous Expression Systems and Screening Technologies in Ion Channel Drug Discovery

Maurizio Taglialatela

CONTENTS

1. INTRODUCTION

Drugs acting at the cardiac ion channel level, such as antiarrhythmics, have been in clinical use for several decades, well before the understanding that cardiac excitability was indeed a delicate equilibrium among the activity of specific ion channel classes and that the intimate mechanism of action of these congeners was outlined in detail. The recent progress in the molecular and functional characterization of cardiac ion channels has improved our understanding of their pathophysiological role in cardiac dysfunction, furthering the possibilities for the development of novel therapeutic strategies. These advancements, coupled with technical and conceptual improvements in drug-screening procedures, have had, and are likely to have in the future, a profound impact on drug discovery processes. The aim of the present chapter is to summarize the heterologous expression systems and the available screening techniques currently used in the characterization of the effects of specific modulators on cardiac ion channels, with particular emphasis on new technologies for high-throughput drug screening.

2. HETEROGENEITY AND CLASSIFICATION OF ION CHANNELS

Ion channels are integral membrane proteins that allow the regulated transmembrane flux of one or more ion species. On a purely functional basis, ion channels can be broadly divided into two main classes depending on their gating mechanism. In voltage-gated channels the triggering event regulating ion flux is a change in transmem-

From: *Cardiac Drug Development Guide*
Edited by: M. K. Pugsley © Humana Press Inc., Totowa, NJ

brane voltage; on the other hand, changes in the extra- or intracellular concentration of a specific ligand regulate the opening of ligand-gated channels. Of course, this distinction needs to be considered more as a conceptual framework rather than a rigid scheme because the activity of voltage-gated channels can be profoundly influenced by a number of ligands and the ability of several ligands to gate specific ion channels may be affected by voltage. The permeation characteristics of specific ion channel species allow a further distinction based on their ion selectivity (Na^+, K^+, Ca^{2+}, Cl^- channels show the highest degree of ion selectivity) and on their rectification properties (discriminating between channels having inwardly or outwardly rectifying current-to-voltage relationships). Further classification criteria, such as tissue- or cell-specific expression or exquisite pharmacological selectivity (to specific drugs or toxins), may allow a more-specific characterization of distinct ion channel classes.

Although the identification of the genetic and molecular basis for some specific ion currents is still lacking, in the past two decades, the cloning and functional characterization of most of the genes encoding for ion channels has been achieved. Such studies have revealed that the functional diversity that allows ion channels to contribute to a myriad of cell functions is matched by an extraordinary degree of genetic and structural heterogeneity. Although ion channel nomenclature has undergone several changes in an attempt to follow the rapid developments in ion channel discovery and characterization, a novel classification scheme has been recently adopted by the International Union of Pharmacology (IUPHAR) Committee on Receptor Nomenclature and Drug Classification *(1)*. Given that they encompass most of the currently used drug targets in the cardiovascular system, this chapter will deal preferentially with cationic channels, although reference will also be made, when available, to anionic channels.

Voltage-gated Na^+ channels (VGNCs) are responsible for the membrane currents mediating the rising phase of the action potential in most excitable cells *(2,3)*. Electrophysiological studies, biochemical purification, and gene cloning efforts have revealed the existence of a multigene family encoding for VGNCs. In fact, at least nine genes encoding for different pore-forming main Na^+ channel α subunits have been cloned and characterized. These are mainly classified based on their sensitivity (TTX-S) or resistance (TTX-R) to tetrodotoxin (TTX-S) blockade and on their tissue distribution. TTX-S $Na_V 1.1$, $Na_V 1.2$, $Na_V 1.3$, $Na_V 1.6$, and $Na_V 1.7$ VGNCs are blocked by nanomolar TTX concentrations and are mainly located on neuronal membranes; however, $Na_V 1.5$, $Na_V 1.8$, and $Na_V 1.9$ encode for TTX-resistant VGNC, are blocked at high micromolar TTX concentrations, and are located in the heart ($Na_V 1.5$) or in peripheral sensory neurons ($Na_V 1.8$ and $Na_V 1.9$). Finally, $Na_V 1.4$ encodes for the skeletal muscle VGNC. α subunits of VGNCs may interact with three accessory subunits (β_1, β_2, β_3), which are thought to influence gating and cellular distribution of the fully assembled channels.

Voltage-gated Ca^{2+} channels (VGCCs) are heteromeric multiprotein complexes constituted by a pore-forming α_1 subunit together with auxiliary β, γ, and $\alpha_2\delta$ subunits *(4)*. According to pharmacological and biophysical criteria, at least six types of VGCCs have been described: T, L, N, P/Q, and R. L, N, P/Q, and R constitute the subfamily of high-voltage–activated VGCCs that open in response to strong membrane depolarization, whereas T-type channels are activated by small membrane depolarization and therefore are also known as low-voltage–activated VGCCs. Based on primary sequence information and on their relative phylogenetic distance, VGCCs main α_1 subunits can be classified as follows: $Ca_V1.1$, $Ca_V1.2$, $Ca_V1.3$, and $Ca_V1.4$ that give rise to L-type currents in skeletal muscle ($Ca_V1.1$), in neuroendocrine tissues ($Ca_V1.2$, $Ca_V1.3$, and $Ca_V1.4$), and in cardiac cells ($Ca_V1.2$); $Ca_V2.1$, which underlie the N-type Ca^{2+} currents in nerve terminals and dendrites, $Ca_V2.2$ representing the molecular basis for the P/Q-type neuronal channels and $Ca_V2.3$ for the R-type neuronal channels, and finally, $Ca_V3.1$, $Ca_V3.2$, and $Ca_V3.3$ VGCCs α_1 subunits that encode T-type Ca^{2+} currents.

K+ channels are the most ubiquitous and diverse family of ion channels expressed in both excitable and nonexcitable cells *(5)*. More than 70 genes encoding for K+ channels pore-forming α subunit with diverse functions and gating mechanisms have been identified in the mammalian genome; although this large number of genes makes the K+ channel classification a difficult task, the IUPHAR Committee has proposed a distinction among K_V1–K_V6/K_V8–K_V9, the K_V7, and the K_V10–K_V12 subfamilies (classic 6 transmembrane segment voltage-gated K+ channels or VGKCs). Additional subfamilies include the $K_{Ca}1$–$K_{Ca}5$ (the Ca^{2+}-dependent K+ channels), the $K_{2P}1$–$K_{2P}16$ (the four transmembrane segments-two pore channel subunits), and the $K_{ir}1$–$K_{ir}7$ families (inwardly-rectifying two transmembrane segments-one pore subunits; ref. *1*).

3. CARDIAC ION CHANNELS AS DRUG TARGETS

The coordinated contraction of the cardiac muscle is caused by the sequential opening of several classes of ion channels, with a fine equilibrium between inward and outward currents controlling cardiac action potential shape (frequency, amplitude, duration, and so on; refs. *6,7*). In the last decade, the molecular identity of most cardiac ion channel genes has been unveiled, and human molecular genetics has identified ion channel genes involved in human arrhythmogenic diseases, such as the Long QT syndrome and idiopathic ventricular fibrillations (Brugada syndrome, catecholamine-triggered ventricular tachycardia with short QT, familial conduction system disease, among others).

Although in some rare cases the function of the cloned ion channel genes is intrinsic to the cloning effort itself (expression cloning), more often the specific function of the protein encoded by a novel gene has been revealed by the use of heterologous systems in which the gene product has been expressed in isolation. Based on anatomical, functional, and pharmacological characteristics of the expressed protein, it has often been possible to relate this protein to a specific cardiac current; however, it should be underlined that, in addition to the main pore-forming α subunits, accessory β subunits are frequently needed to recapitulate the native cardiac current. The precise positioning of the function of a specific ion channel in the context of the protein network controlling normal and altered cardiac excitability requires an understanding of a higher level of complexity, whereby the cellular mechanisms required for assembly, trafficking, targeting, and regulation are also properly defined. This appears to be relevant for future drug development since novel mechanisms for drug action at this levels are emerging; our canonical view that ion channels may be drug targets only when properly folded, fully assembled, and positioned at their final targeting destination in the plasma membrane has been recently challenged, a result that may have considerable implications for pharmacogenomics and genotype-specific therapies *(8,9)*.

Despite the fact that this level of complexity is now starting to be addressed and intricate proteomic networks are just beginning to be revealed, the use of heterologous expression systems has been a fundamental tool to investigate the functional property of the ion channel of interest.

In addition to the obvious relevance for the understanding of the role of specific ion channel genes in cardiac pathophysiology, heterologous expression systems have also proven to be crucial for the definition of the pharmacological profile of the ion channel itself. This has major implication for human diseases, considering that ion channels are relevant drug targets for human therapeutic intervention. It has been estimated that 5% of all currently available pharmacological therapeutic strategies involve congeners provided of a direct action at the level of ion channels *(10)*. If one considers that receptors and enzymes together encompass more than 70% of the available drug targets and that in several cases drugs acting at these levels exert their therapeutic actions by indirectly modifying the activity of specific ion channels, it seems evident that the pharmacological characterization of ion channels has a tremendous impact on the development of novel therapeutic approaches.

Several tens of drugs are currently available to treat cardiac dysfunction, and antiarrhythmic compounds represent a significant segment of the cardiac drug market *(11)*. All antiarrhythmic drugs exert their therapeutic actions by direct or indirect interference with the function of specific ion channel classes; therefore, preclinical screening for potential effects of drugs at the level of cardiac ion channels is of fundamental relevance for improving the current repertoire of therapeutic agents. However, the blockade of specific ion channels may exert both proarrhythmic and antiarrhythmic effects, depending on the anatomical site of action, of the characteristics of the cardiac rhythm, and of several other concomitant factors. As a matter of fact, cardiac ion channels have been recently given attention not only as targets for pharmacological actions to be exploited in therapeutic intervention but also as mediators of drug-induced life-threatening proarrhythmic effects by both cardiac and noncardiac drugs *(12,13)*. A growing list of drugs has been shown to cause proarrhythmic actions, including, among many others, antiarrhythmics, antihistamines, antipsychotics, antimicrobials, anticonvulsants, prokinetics, lipid-lowering drugs, and antimigraine compounds *(14)*. Thus, the development of preclinical screening tests for potential proarrhythmic effects resulting from interaction with ion channels prompted by older or newly introduced compounds in all therapeutic areas is of paramount importance to allow the introduction into the market of compounds provided with an optimal safety profile with respect to serious cardiovascular side effects. In addition, it should be underlined that, after the discovery of such serious cardiac adverse effects by widely prescribed compounds and in view of the large body of evidence implicating specific classes of cardiac ion channels as molecular targets for this pharmacological action, regulatory agencies worldwide have been recently issuing guidelines recommending all private and public subjects involved in drug development to devise strategies for both preclinical and clinical studies to better characterize the risk of such adverse effects; as an example of such recommendations, the European Committee for Proprietary Medicinal Products has stated that "... every new chemical entity intended for Phase I evaluation should be screened for potential effects on cardiac repolarization" *(15)*. Similarly, the International Conference on Harmonisation of Technical Requirements for Registration of Pharmaceuticals for Human Use (ICH) has released a set of guidelines for the assessment of the risk of cardiac arrhythmia for human pharmaceuticals (ICHS7B; ref. *16*). These examples highlight the relevance of novel and more efficient ion channel screening technologies for safer drug development.

4. HETEROLOGOUS EXPRESSION SYSTEMS OF CARDIAC ION CHANNELS

Modern developments in the fields of human genetics, molecular and cell biology, chemistry, and pharmacology by virtue of a highly reductionist approach have pinpointed the molecular basis of several pathophysiologically relevant biological processes. Intrinsic to this approach is the view that it might be possible to dissect out individual processes leading to specific functions and that the selective interference with such processes may ultimately lead to a specific modification of these functions. Therefore, target selectivity appears a highly desirable property for drugs because it might ensure the achievement of greater therapeutic efficacy without the simultaneous interference with targets that may result in unwanted modification of other biological functions. Despite the fact that many compounds often achieve their therapeutic effects by affecting multiple targets, this revolutionary target-driven approach has already led to a considerable increase in our therapeutic armamentarium to treat cardiovascular diseases *(17)*. Thus, identifying selective effects of drugs at the level of ion channels involved in specific cardiac functions is currently a fundamental effort in drug development.

As mentioned earlier, the cardiac action potential is the point of convergence of the coordinated activity of several classes, possibly over 20, of ion channels. Although in principle it would be preferable to study the effects of drugs on ion channel targets in their native context (cardiac myocytes in vitro or in vivo), this is often impossible because of technical limitations. In fact, in vivo studies do not allow to relate measurable parameters of cardiac function (action potential properties, contractility, cardiac output, and so on) to the activity of individual classes of ion channels. In addition, the available in vitro techniques used to isolate the currents carried by specific ion channels in native tissues are rather sophisticated and time consuming and require highly trained personnel. Thus, although it seems technically feasible to dissect multiple currents in cardiac myocytes with methods that provide highly detailed descriptions of the molecular characteristics of drug–channel interactions *(18)*, these techniques are not yet suitable for full automation, a highly desirable property for high-throughput assays *(3)*. Thus, the use of heterologous expression systems, where the target ion channel can be expressed and studied in isolation to avoid contamination by overlapping currents, offer distinct advantages over native tissues for the purpose of drug discovery.

Although target-driven drug discovery in the ion channel field is far from revealing its full potential, cell-based heterologous expression systems appear today as the means by which its goals will be achieved. In fact, ion channels are highly dynamic transmembrane proteins, with profound conformational changes associated with their activity. The highly lipophilic nature of ion channel limits their use in traditional cell-free assays in vitro such as those routinely performed with proteins having enzymatic function. Furthermore, although structural data on VGKCs *(19)* and VGNCs *(20)* are starting to reveal some aspects of specific channel function, such as gating and selectivity, and the structural basis for the high drug selectivity of specific ion channels are beginning to be clarified *(21–23)*, a complete picture of the structural requirements for complex channel behaviors in different functional states is yet missing.

This implies, therefore, that a structure-based approach for drug designing is not yet practically feasible, and that most if not all of the drug screening efforts directed toward ion channels are nowadays based on functional assays of specific activities performed by distinct ion channels. Thus, cell-based heterologous expression systems coupled to functional assays represent the basis for the drug screening techniques currently available for ion channels.

4.1. Heterologous Expression Systems for In Vitro Studies

The availability of the gene sequences for most ion channel subunits underlying functionally relevant cardiac currents provides a unique opportunity to investigate their pharmacological modulation in vitro using heterologous expression systems. These are mostly represented by *Xenopus oocytes* and by a variety of prokaryotic and eukaryotic cells (yeast, insect, and mammalian cells are the most widely used). Given that the pharmacological profile of selective ion channels, as discussed earlier, is defined by means of functional assays that can be routinely performed in *Xenopus oocytes* or in mammalian cells, but not in prokaryotes or in yeast cells, these two latter expression systems, although widely used in heterologous protein expression studies, will not be discussed in the present chapter.

4.1.1. Xenopus oocytes

Xenopus oocytes synthesize exogenous proteins when injected with foreign mRNA, an ability recognized more than 30 yr ago *(24)*. Thus, oocytes can be injected with RNAs transcribed in vitro from cloned DNAs, and this leads to the expression of large amounts of the protein encoded by these genes. This technique is relatively simple, fast, and inexpensive. The main advantage offered by the *Xenopus oocytes* is their large size (up to 1.3 mm), which allows microdissection of single cells and makes them amenable to a variety of electrophysiological and biochemical techniques *(25)*. Over the last 20 yr, this system has represented a powerful tool to investigate several functional aspects of ion channels, including their pharmacological profile; however, oocyte-based electrophysiological systems can be considered useful for screening a relatively small number of compounds and are not likely to have a major impact for large-scale assays. Also, one of the main disadvantage of *Xenopus oocytes* is their relatively poor membrane permeability, which may affect the results obtained with lipophilic drugs acting on the intracellular side of the channel protein that may become trapped by the egg yolk *(26)*; in fact, a right shift in the dose–response effect of various entities is often found when comparing the effects of drugs having such characteristics on recombinant channels expressed in *Xenopus oocytes* vs mammalian cells. Thus, the intrinsic properties of the expression system should not be neglected and need to be taken in serious consideration, as they may result in lead compounds turning out to be false-positive or, worse still, false-negative *(27)*.

4.1.2. Mammalian Cells

An alternative expression system for ion channels, which is also extensively used for research purposes, is represented by mammalian cells expressing the channel of interest *(28)*. The recombinant cell lines represent a valuable alternative to native cells for several reasons. First, ion channels of known identity carry the signal of interest because the cells used for such assays are virtually devoid of significant amounts of constitutively expressed ion channels, thus minimizing the background noise. Furthermore, in these cells, a combination of ion channel subunits can be expressed to recapitulate more closely the functional properties of a specific native current, thus providing pharmacological results that may be more relevant for human pathophysiology; accessory subunits have in fact been suggested to contribute to the pharmaco-logical profile of pathophysiologically-relevant cardiac ion channels *(29)*. Second, the engineered cells overexpress the protein of interest, further increasing the signal-to-noise ratio. Third, these cells properly perform most of the post-translational modifications such as proteolytic processing of the propeptide, glycosylation, phos-phorylation, as well as correct assembly (a crucial process for ion channels), which are required for proper protein function. Finally, the growth of these cells, which are robust enough to be handled by automatic screening systems, can be achieved in com-mon laboratory environment, requiring standard technical skills and relatively minor investments. In many cases, these cells continue to consistently express the ion chan-nel of interest over an extended period of time, up to several years. In addition to drug discovery, mammalian cell-based heterologous expression systems have been used for various purposes, such as to verify a cloned gene product; to analyze the effect of the protein expression on cell physiology; to produce and isolate genes from cDNA libraries, to produce correctly assembled and folded proteins for assessment of vari-ous biological activities; to produce suitable quantities of proteins for structural char-acterization; and to produce important clinically active viral surface antigens or therapeutic proteins or monoclonal antibodies *(30)*.

These days several techniques are available to achieve heterologous expression of ion channels in recombinant cell lines. The primary factors to successfully accomplish this aim are as follows: (1) the choice of the mammalian cell host; (2) the choice of the expression vector; and (3) the DNA delivery method. Although these factors are strictly related to each other, they will be discussed individually in the following sections.

4.1.2.1. CHOICE OF THE MAMMALIAN CELL HOST

A variety of mammalian cell hosts can be selected for heterologous protein produc-tion; depending on the ultimate goals, the choice depends on whether the expression has to be transient or stable.

Transient expression is preferred in studies on the regulation of gene expression or when results are needed in a short time frame; using transient systems, there is a burst of gene expression between 12 and 72 h after DNA introduction into the cell, followed by rapid cell death or loss of the expression construct. In these systems, the activity of a reporter gene not endogenously expressed and reflecting the protein product synthe-sis (chloramphenicol acetyltransferase, β galactosidase and firefly luciferase or Luc) is commonly used. More recently, the green fluorescent protein and its variants have been also extensively used *(31)*. When transient expression is the preferred method, transformed African green monkey kidney cells (COS-7 cells) or viral systems are preferred. Of course, the amount of protein yield by transient expression is rather lim-ited. By contrast, stable expression systems have several advantages for pharmacologi-cal screenings to be used for cardiac drug development. In fact, larger amounts of proteins are usually achieved; more importantly, the resulting stably transfected clonal cell line allows for more reproducible results. To achieve stable expression, the expres-sion vector can either be integrated into the host genome or remain as an extrachromo-somal element, under conditions of chronic selection (*see* below; ref. *30*). Chinese hamster ovary (CHO) and human embryonic kidney (HEK-293) cells are among those most widely used for this purpose. The main drawbacks associated with stable expres-sion in mammalian cells are the time needed to produce them and the possible integration of the vector in regions of the genome that are crucial for cell survival or replication, resulting in cell lines having altered phenotypes when compared to the original host cells.

4.1.2.2. Choice of the Expression Vector

Mammalian expression vectors, commercially available from various companies (Promega, Clontech, Invitrogen, among many others) can be divided in two categories: viral vectors or plasmid vectors. Plasmid vectors can be further subdivided into those with animal cell replicons, which do not require chromosome integration for gene product expressions and those without such replicons, thus requiring integration *(32)*. Viral vectors are essentially inactivated viruses where genes are cloned. Viruses can be selected that can either result in the lysis of the host cell (lytic viruses such as vaccinia virus, baculovirus, alphavirus) or that can integrate the genetic material into the host chromosome, thus resulting in stable transformation (adenoviruses, adeno-associated viruses, retroviruses). Both vectors are composed of similar basic elements. Expression of the gene of interest is controlled by promoter–enhancer sequences and signal sequences required for proper processing of the transcript. Usually, the promoter–enhancer sequences, more often of viral origin, can allow constitutive or inducible, as well as cell- or tissue-specific expression of the gene. The vectors used more often carry cytomegalovirus sequences (acting as transcriptional enhancer), metallothionein II sequences (inducible by heavy metals, such as cadmium or zinc, glucocorticoid, and phorbol esters), mouse mammary tumor virus sequences (glucocorticoid-inducible), or the fetal (γ) or adult (β) globin sequences (enhances tissues specific for erythroid cells). Another vector element required to allow selection of transfected/infected cells is a gene that confers the cells unique phenotypic properties. These selectable markers are usually represented by enzymes conferring resistance to cytotoxic drugs (e.g., the aminoglycoside phosphotransferase, conferring resistance to kanamycin, neomycin, and geneticin or G418). Thus, the cells are grown in the presence of the cytotoxic drug and only those that have acquired resistance to the drug will be able to survive and proliferate. Other features of the expression vector are the presence of polyadenylation sequences from viral (SV40) or mammalian (bovine human growth hormone) origin to enhance RNA stability and processing and one or more promoter-distal multiple cloning sites where the gene of interest can be placed. All these sequences affect the degree of gene expression achieved because they influence the number of gene copies into the cell, the transcription efficiency, and the position of integration into the host genome.

4.1.2.3. DNA Delivery Method

Once the DNA expression vector has been engineered and has been purified from proteins, RNA, and other contaminants (usually by CsCl gradient centrifugation or ion-exchange chromatography), it needs to be transferred into the host cells. This, of course, only applies to plasmidic vectors because viral expression vectors can be used to infect the cells directly. The uptake of naked DNA molecules is an extremely inefficient process; thus, transfection vehicles are needed. These can be classified as chemical or physical. The choice of transfection method is also dependent on the cell type to be transfected (whether they grow in suspension or attached) and on the desired transfection efficiency. The cells to be transfected need to be in a log phase of growth, an absolute requirement if stable transfection are to be achieved.

The chemical methods most widely used include the calcium phosphate ($CaPO_4$) method and the use of cationic polymers or of liposomes. For the $CaPO_4$ transfection method, the DNA is coprecipitated with $CaPO_4$ at appropriate pH, and the precipitate is applied onto the cells to allow the uptake of the DNA by pinocytosis. Efficiency of the transfection with this method depends on the form of the plasmid (circular or linear), on the addition of agents to facilitate pinocytosis (e.g., glycerol or dimethyl sulfoxide), and on extensive washing of the precipitate after a few hours of incubation. Cationic polymers used for transfection include DEAE–dextran, protamine, and polyethylenimine. Liposomes are artificial membrane vesicles that fuse with the cell membrane and deliver the DNA content (as well as that of proteins or RNA) into the cytoplasm or can engage in the endocytotic pathway. Various lipids have been used for this purpose, with the LipofectAMINE™ being the most widely used nowadays. Crucial factors for optimal cell uptake using this methodology are as follows: the DNA-liposome ratio, the size of the complexes, and the growth state of the cells.

Physical methods for DNA transfer into the host cells or tissues include the following: electroporation, biolistic (gene gun), and microinjection techniques. Electroporation uses current pulses of specific magnitude and duration to reversibly permeabilize the cells and to allow the entry of the DNA into the cell. A variation of this technique has also been used recently to transfect single neuronal cells in their in vivo environment (brain slices; ref. *33*). Various apparatuses have been developed to facilitate electroporation of cells growing in suspension or of adherent cells. The biolistic approach, instead, uses the coating of high-density metal particles (usually gold particles) with the DNA, and the subsequent shooting of these particles onto the cells. The main advantages of this method are the optimal cell viability and the possibility to use it in in vivo studies; limitations are represented by the poor tissue permeability of the particles and by the high initial cost of the instrumentation. Direct delivery of the DNA into the mammalian cell nucleus is also possible by microinjection techniques, although this approach, despite automation, is practically applicable only for a limited number of cells, and is not suited for large-scale operation.

4.2. Heterologous Expression Systems for In Vivo Studies

Although, as previously mentioned, the pharmacological profile of a wide range of drugs with respect to ion channels is generally characterized with cell-based methodologies, the use of genetically engineered animal models (transgenic and gene-deleted knockout animals) provides unique tools to address specific pharmacological questions where potential target molecules have been characterized *(34)*. It is for this main reason that these animal models, although not extensively used in drug-screening programs, are briefly mentioned here. Owing to their better understanding of the genes involved, transgenic animal models of cardiovascular interest are concentrated in the areas of the renin–angiotensin system, of the β adrenergic receptor system, and of lipoprotein metabolism *(35)*. Ion channels are slower to come into this arena, although genetic manipulation of cardiac ion channels in transgenic animals are likely to provide valuable pathophysiological information that may translate into their use for pharmacological research and, possibly, drug screening *(36)*.

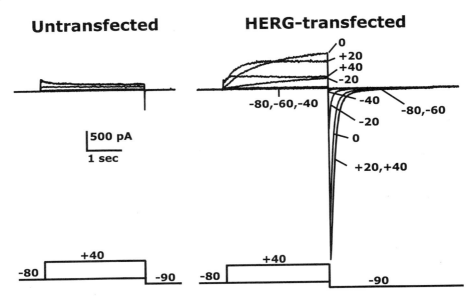

Fig. 1. Heterologous expression of HERG K$^+$ channels in HEK 293 cells. The left panel shows representative current traces recorded in the whole-cell configuration of the patch-clamp technique from a single nontransfected HEK 293 cell. Holding potential was: –80 mV; test potentials were from –80 to +40 mV in 20-mV steps; return potential was –90 mV. In the right panel, the same voltage pulse protocol was applied to an HEK 293 cell stably transfected with HERG cDNA (kindly provided by Dr. Craig January, Section of Cardiology, University of Wisconsin, Madison, WI; ref. 60). A schematic drawing of the voltage protocol is shown on the bottom of the two panels. The extracellular solution contained the following (in mM): 150 NaCl, 10 KCl, 3 CaCl$_2$, 1 MgCl$_2$, 10 HEPES, pH 7.4 with NaOH. The pipets were filled with (in mM): 130 K-Aspartate, 10 NaCl, 4 CaCl$_2$, 2 MgCl$_2$, 10 EGTA, 2 Mg-ATP, 0.25 cAMP, and 10 HEPES, pH 7.4, with NaOH.

5. FUNCTIONAL ASSAYS FOR DRUG DISCOVERY AT THE LEVEL OF ION CHANNELS

5.1. Electrophysiology-Based Assays

The gold standard functional assay for ion channels is electrophysiology. In fact, no other technique is endowed with such high information content as electrophysiology; furthermore, it is the only technique that may provide information on the state dependence of the drug–channel interaction, a major advantage for highly dynamic proteins, such as ion channels. Electrophysiological techniques can be used to record macroscopic or single-channel currents. Macroscopic currents in *Xenopus oocytes* can be recorded with the two-microelectrode voltage-clamp methodology, whereas the various configuration of the patch–clamp techniques are usually used for recording both single-channel and macroscopic currents from smaller (5–20 µm in diameter) mammalian cells (Fig.1). Nevertheless, patch–clamp recordings can also be performed from *Xenopus oocytes*. Despite the fact that electrophysiology remains the gold standard for pharmacological assays aimed at ion channels, it also has drawbacks; dialysis of intracellular compartments during whole-cell recordings using the patch-clamp technique is one of them. This causes the removal of cytosolic factors regulating various aspects of ion channel activity, including their pharmacological profile. Although the electrophysiological techniques allow an highly detailed analysis of ion channel function, even if one considers the recent improvements in liquid-handling technologies for automatic compound delivery, these methodologies are relatively low-output and yield a low number of data points (–100–200/wk per experimenter). Furthermore, they are usually run by highly trained personnel and are not easily amenable to full automation. However, several companies have recently developed multichannel screening devices based on electrophysiological recordings in *Xenopus oocytes* with the aim of increasing the efficiency of drug discovery for ion channels and transporters. Among these devices, the most popular are the Rooboocyte™, now manufactured by the Multi channel Systems (Reutlingen, Germany) and marketed by ALA Instruments (Westbury, NY), or the OpusXpress from Axon Instruments (Foster City, CA). These systems, by using sophisticated mechanics, electronics, and data-analysis tools definitively increase the amount of information generated; nevertheless, despite such technological improvements, their impact for cardiovascular drug primary screening is yet to be demonstrated. It seems more likely that these system will be used in secondary and tertiary screening programs using ion channels as targets. Similarly, attempts are currently made to improve high-throughput screenings (HTS) for ion channels using automated electrophysiological techniques in mammalian cells. These include the NeuroPatch™ robot (marketed under the name Apatchi-1™ by Sophion Bioscience, Ballerup, Denmark) and the AutoPatch™ system developed by the Channelwork division of CeNeS Pharmaceuticals (Cambridge, UK); the latter is a fully automated whole-cell patch–clamp system that can be further miniaturized and scaled up to produce a patch-clamping platform that will enable, in the expectation of the developers, the collection of ≈50,000 data points/wk per experimenter. Also in this case, the impact that this automated technique will have for cardiovascular drug development needs time for proper evaluation.

5.2. Binding Assays

The displacement of radioactivity labeled congeners by the compound(s) of interest has traditionally been one of the means by which the pharmacological actions of drugs were characterized. Binding assays can provide a large number of data points (over 30,000/wk) and are especially suited for HTS. As a matter of fact, these techniques have been recently applied to ion channels of great pathophysiological and pharmacological interest, such as those encoded by the human ether-a-go-go–related gene (HERG) K^+ channels *(37)*. These channels have been implicated in genetically determined and in drug-induced human cardiac arrhythmogenicity and represent one of the most studied cardiac ion channels for drug development *(7,38)*. In a recent study, the pharmacological characteristics of the binding of the class III antiarrhythmic [^{3}H]dofetilide in membranes prepared from HEK-293 cells stably expressing HERG have been investigated. [^{3}H]dofetilide binding was inhibited not only by other class III antiarrhythmic, such as clofilium, E-4031, WAY-123,398, and d-sotalol, but also by the structurally unrelated compounds pimozide, terfenadine, and haloperidol, all of which prolong the QT interval in humans. Based on these observation, the authors suggested that [^{3}H]dofetilide binding assay using membranes from cells stably expressing HERG K^+ channels may help identify compounds that prolong the QT interval.

However, the specificity for HERG of [^{3}H]dofetilide has been questioned by the same authors *(39)*. Furthermore, caution should be exercised when interpreting these data in the context of drug screening; in fact, competition binding assays only give information regarding single binding site and, for most ion channels, multiple drug-binding sites are know to be present, often allosterically coupled *(40)*. Thus, the potential for false-negative data from drug screenings with competition binding techniques against known sites is rather high. In addition, binding studies performed on membranes do not allow to assess state-dependent modification of ion channel activity, a major limitation if one considers the large number of factors that, in intact cells, may influence the activity of the ion channel of interest. Altogether, these considerations make the potential use of these binding techniques rather limited for HTS programs involving cardiac ion channels.

5.3. Flux Assays

Characterization of the pharmacological profile against a possible ion channel target by using flux studies of molecules to which this ion channel is selectively permeable represents another highly automatizable procedure that has been used for HTS. Traditionally, ^{86}Rb$^+$, ^{14}C-guanidine, and ^{45}Ca^{2+} have been used for investigating the activity of K$^+$, Na$^+$, and Ca^{2+} channels; HTS for activity on Cl$^-$ channels can be also performed using ^{125}I$^-$, although the safety considerations as a result of the γ radiation emitted by this isotope impose obvious restrictions on its use *(41)*. Despite the fact that flux studies are especially suited for HTS when coupled to heterologous expression systems of channels of known identity, their use is limited by several considerations *(11)*. The loading procedure with the isotope is laborious and often inefficient; extensive washes are needed to achieve an equilibrium; nonspecific background fluxes are often quite large; and, finally, the flux of the tracer of interest needs to be triggered by toxins, agonists, or other nonphysiological methods, such as gaseous or chemical hypoxia. Recently, by means of atomic absorption spectroscopy, a novel Rb$^+$-detection technique has been developed that does not use radioisotopes and that could be integrated into an HTS platform for drug screening on potassium channels *(42)*.

5.4. Optical Technologies

To overcome some of the limitations imposed by the previously described methods, optical technologies have been implemented to allow detection of ion channel activity in living cells. These techniques, that lend themselves to full miniaturization and automation, can be performed in 96- or 384-well plates for maximal data output. Thus, they may begin to bridge the gap between low-throughput high-information assays (electrophysiological studies) and high-capacity low-information methods (flux and binding studies; ref. *43*).

5.4.1. Membrane Potential Indicators

Small currents carried by few ion channels in the membrane can cause large changes in transmembrane voltage provided that the resistance of the cell is high enough. Therefore, drug-induced changes in the activity of specific classes of ion channels can be inferred from changes in membrane potential. Optical probes are especially suited for membrane potential measurements; in particular, fluorescence intensity of oxonol dyes changes as a function of membrane potential because, by virtue of their lipophilic anionic nature, depolarization of the cells increases their association with the membrane, thereby enhancing their fluorescence *(44,45)*. Among the most widely used dyes is the bis-(1,2-dibuthylbarbituric acid) trimetineoxonol or DiBAC$_4$ *(3)*, whose quantum yield increases on binding to hydrophobic cellular sites. However, the dye redistribution process is much slower that the actual change in membrane potential, making this technique useful only for the detection of slow processes leading to prolonged changes in membrane potential. Another important limitation is that, opposite to what will be described for ion-sensitive fluorescent probes (*see* Section 5.4.2.), the fluorescent signal cannot often be properly calibrated and converted to absolute values of membrane potential. In fact, the valinomycin null-point method, a widely used calibration method, cannot be used because of the formation of complexes between the oxonol dye and the positively charged molecule of valinomycin *(46)*. Finally, the technique is extremely sensitive to temperature changes and the oxonol fluorescence can be quenched by lipophilic compounds under investigation, thus limiting its potential use in large-scale screening procedures.

5.4.2. Ion-Selective Optical Probes

Instead of measuring membrane potential, a function that integrates the activity of several ion channels, it is possible to measure with optical probes the cytosolic concentrations of selective ion species, which reflect the activity of the membrane channel permeable to those ions. In principle, the dye should be provided of a high degree of selectivity for the desired ion, particularly when its concentrations are several orders of magnitude lower that those of other ions. Historically, this degree of selectivity has been established for Ca^{2+}-sensitive probes, which have thus been extensively used to measure cytosolic free Ca^{2+} concentrations; several generations of Ca^{2+}-sensitive optical probes have been used over the years to achieve this aim (Quin-2; Fura-2; Fluo-3; calcium-green; just to mention those that have been most extensively used; ref. *47*), mostly because the low (nanomolar) and highly regulated cytosolic concentrations of this cation allow the development of probes with the required sensitivity and specificity to assess the rapid variations in cytosolic Ca^{2+} concentrations occurring upon activation of channels or transporters. Similar principles have been applied for the development of Na^+- *(48)*, H^+- *(49)*, Cl^-- *(50)*, and K^+- *(51,52)* selective probes, although their application has been much less extensive. Ca^{2+}-sensitive probes are relatively simple to use: The cells can be loaded by incubation in the presence of the nontoxic dye, which usually enters the cell passively and is trapped into the cells by enzymatic reactions. Once the Ca^{2+} concentrations are raised into the cells (via agonist application, membrane potential changes, or other methods), the dye interacts with Ca^{2+} ions, changing its fluorescence intensity or its excitation–emission spectra. Ratiometric or nonratiometric fluorescence signals can thus be converted, by means of appropriate calibration procedures, into the absolute values of cytosolic Ca^{2+} concentrations. Given that variations in cytosolic Ca^{2+} concentrations can be brought about by changes in the activity not only of Ca^{2+}-permeable channels, but also of a number of G-protein–coupled receptors, these assays have the potential to assess the pharmacological profile also of these receptors. Furthermore, the fluorescent signal is usually strong enough to require a rather small number of cells; thus, multiwell microtiter plates are generally used. The use of Fluorometric Image Plate Readers (Molecular Devices, Sunnyvale, CA; ref. *53*) equipped with automated liquid-handling, kinetic detection, and data analysis procedures can be optimized for HTS, allowing the primary screening of up to 10,000 compounds in a single day. Given the prominent role played by VGCCs as pharmacological targets for drugs modifying cardiovascular function, the screening procedures combining the recombinant expression of isolated α_1 VGCC subunits with optical methods for the detection of cytosolic Ca^{2+} changes have already proven to be successful in screening for Ca^{2+} channel blockers and are likely to allow the identification of novel lead compounds to be used as pharmacological tools in further preclinical screenings.

5.4.3. Fluorescence Resonance Energy Transfer (FRET)

As previously mentioned, optical methods using potential-sensitive dyes lack of the resolution required for more sophisticated measurements, particularly to assess rapid changes of membrane potential, such as those associated with the action potential. This limitation has been overcome for the most part by the use of the spectroscopic technique of FRET, which can monitor the dynamic association or dissociation of macromolecular partners in living cells. FRET can be established between the voltage-sensing oxonol dye and a second donor fluorophore (54). Using this method, the donor fluorophore is a coumarin-linked phospholipid (CC2-DMPE) positioned in the outer leaflet of the plasma membrane. When coumarin is excited with a 409-nm light (violet), in the absence of FRET it will fluoresce at 460 nm (blue). If energy is transferred from the donor molecule to the longer wavelength acceptor oxonol DiSBAC$_4$ (3), fluorescence will be emitted at 580 nm (orange). The FRET phenomenon is extremely sensitive to changes in the distance between acceptor and donor molecules; because membrane depolarization causes a preferential redistribution of the mobile oxonol probe toward the intracellular space, this causes a decrease in FRET that can be detected by an orange to blue shift in the peak energy of the emission spectra. The fluorescence change brought about by this electrochromic process is at least 100 times faster than that of conventional oxonol redistribution assays, reaching kinetics in the millisecond timescale. Thus, using FRET-based voltage sensors, a first-generation instrument has been recently generated; this is called VIPR™ (Aurora Bioscience Corp., San Diego, CA) an acronym for Voltage/Ion Probe Reader, specifically designed for HTS. This system integrates an eight-channel liquid handler, a microplate positioning stage, and a fiberoptic illumination and detection system; a xenon arc lamp provides excitation to the samples, which allows the system to adapt to most fluorescent dyes. A second-generation system (VIPR II™) has been recently used to generate a pharmacological fingerprint of voltage-gated Na^+ and K^+ channels constitutively expressed in an astrocytoma cell line (55).

The main advantage of FRET lies in its ability to detect real-time signals, thus allowing to screen for pharmacological modulation of action potentials. This is obviously an highly desired property because it will allow to screen for effect-driven drug actions, such as for their effects on action-potential duration, amplitude, and frequency, bypassing the limitation imposed by the systematic screening of each ion channel involved in the regulation of the cardiac action potential.

Interestingly, when comparing the results obtained from fluorescence screening procedures with potential-sensitive dyes with those of patch–clamp electrophysiology, a good correlation between the results obtained with these two different techniques has been obtained (56).

6. CONCLUSIONS AND FUTURE PROSPECTS

The introduction of the most sophisticated techniques from genetics, organic chemistry, cellular and molecular biology, electrophysiology, and pharmacology, has had a tremendous impact on the drug-discovery process. In fact, the increasing understanding of the functional role played by newly discovered proteins have expanded the array of targets that might be pharmacologically regulated to achieve therapeutic actions or that need to be avoided to prevent possible adverse effects. These consequences are of paramount interest for the field of cardiac ion channels; the cloning of the genes underlying most of the relevant ionic currents of the human heart, a process started in the 1980s, is soon going to be completed. Thus, we have in hand the unique opportunity to evaluate the pharmacological profile of each individual channel class in isolation using heterologous expression systems, a process that, only 20 yr ago, was impossible to foresee for most basic scientists and pharmaceutical companies. Cell-based as well as whole animal-based systems are increasingly becoming available; they will certainly further our comprehension of the pathophysiological roles of individual channels subtypes. However, such target-driven approach might be regarded as highly fragmented; thus, some degree of complementation among the results obtained from different primary, secondary, or tertiary screenings is definitively needed, and highly integrated multidimensional databases need to be established (57) that can be analyzed with reference to targets, diseases, drug classes, and patients. Although these considerations might discourage the undertaking of this approach, it should be highlighted that, whether or not better drugs for human use will result, the intrinsic value of implementing technologies and advancing basic knowledge needs to be reaffirmed. Finally, it seems reasonable to conclude that the times are not ripe yet for a full exploitation of the technical and conceptual advancement that have nevertheless poured at a high speed into the field of ion channel drug screening. For example, in many cases, stable cell lines expressing the channel of interest are difficult to achieve. More sophisticated means of activating FRET signals seem to be needed, such as by means of caged ligands; furthermore, the use of genetically engineered constructs, such as those emerging for cyclic nucleotides or those based on green fluorescent protein variants (58), might further improve our ability to relate the changes in FRET to specific movements of the channel protein, such as those associated with sensors movement, pore opening, and inactivation; this will ensure the design of drugs specifically targeted to interfere with these functions. Also, these genetically designed sensors might be targeted at specific subcellular sites, allowing the study of ion channels that would not be otherwise amenable to conventional flux or electrophysiological techniques. Finally, the future developments in the field of chip-based ion-channel assays (either with patch-clamping or with fluorescence technologies), by eliminating the need for complex electrode micropositioning systems or by reducing the compound consumption, may further improve the achievement of the desired speed required by HTS drug screening yet maintaining adequate temporal resolution (59).

REFERENCES

1. Catterall, W. A., Chandy, K. G., and Gutman, G. A., eds. (2002) International Union of Pharmacology (IUPHAR) Committee on Receptor Nomenclature and Drug Classification. *The IUPHAR Compendium of Voltage-Gated Ion Channels*, IUPHAR Media, Leeds, UK.

2. Catterall, W. A. (2000) From ionic currents to molecular mechanisms: the structure and function of voltage-gated sodium channels. *Neuron* **26,** 13–25.

3. Clare, J. J., Tate, S. N., Nobbs, M., and Romanos, M. A. (2000) Voltage-gated sodium channels as therapeutic targets. *Drug Dis. Today* **5,** 506–520.

4. Catterall, W. A. (2000) Structure and regulation of voltage-gated Ca^{2+} channels. *Annu. Rev. Cell Dev. Biol.* **16,** 521–555.

5. Shieh, C. C., Coghlan, M., Sullivan, J. P., and Gopalakrishnan, M. (2000) Potassium channels: molecular defects, diseases, and therapeutic opportunities. *Pharmacol. Rev.* **52,** 557–594.

6. Carmeliet, E. (1993) Mechanisms and control of repolarization. *Eur. Heart J.* **14,** 3–13.

7. Roden, D. M., Balser, J. R., George, A. L. Jr., and Anderson, M. E. (2002) Cardiac ion channels. *Annu. Rev. Physiol.* **64,** 431–475.

8. Zhou, Z., Gong, Q., and January, C. T. (1999) Correction of defective protein trafficking of a mutant HERG potassium channel in human long QT syndrome. Pharmacological and temperature effects. *J. Biol. Chem.* **274,** 31,123–31,126.

9. Ficker, E., Obejero-Paz, C. A., Zhao, S., and Brown, A. M. (2002) The binding site for channel blockers that rescue misprocessed human long QT syndrome type 2 ether-a-gogo-related gene (HERG) mutations. *J. Biol. Chem.* **277,** 4989–4998.

10. Drews, J. (2000) Drug discovery: A historical perspective. *Science* **287,** 960–964.

11. Numann, R. and Negulescu, P. A. (2001) High-throughput screening strategies for cardiac ion channels. *Trends Cardiovasc. Med.* **11,** 54–59.

12. Yap, Y. G., and Camm, J. (2000) Risk of torsades de pointes with non-cardiac drugs. Doctors need to be aware that many drugs can cause qt prolongation. *Br. Med. J.* **320,** 1158–1159.

13. Taglialatela, M., Timmerman, H., and Annunziato, L. (2000) Cardiotoxic potential and CNS effects of first-generation antihistamines. *Trends Pharmacol. Sci.* **21,** 52–56.

14. http://www.dml.georgetown.edu/depts/pharmacology/torsades.html

15. European Agency for the Evaluation of Medicinal Products. (1997) Committee for Proprietary Medicinal Products. CPMP/986/96.

16. Ebneth, A. (2002) Ion channel screening technologies: Will they revolutionize drug discovery? *Drug Dis. Today* **7,** 227.

17. Timmermans, P. B., Wong, P. C., Chiu, A. T., Herblin, W. F., Benfield, P., Carini, D. J., et al. (1993) Angiotensin II receptors and angiotensin II receptor antagonists. *Pharmacol. Rev.* **45,** 205–251.

18. Spencer, C. I., Uchida, W., Turner, L., and Kozlowski, R. Z. (2000) Signature currents: A patch-clamp method for determining the selectivity of ion-channel blockers in isolated cardiac myocytes. *J. Cardiovasc. Pharmacol. Ther.* **5,** 193–201.

19. Doyle, D. A., Morais Cabral, J., Pfuetzner, R. A., Kuo, A., Gulbis, J. M., Cohen, S. L., et al. (1998) The structure of the potassium channel: Molecular basis of K+ conduction and selectivity. *Science* **280,** 69–77.

20. Sato, C., Ueno, Y., Asai, K., Takahashi, K., Sato, M., et al. (2001) The voltage-sensitive sodium channel is a bell-shaped molecule with several cavities. *Nature* **409,** 1047–1051.

21. Lees-Miller, J. P., Duan, Y., Teng, G. Q., and Duff, H. J. (2000) Molecular determinant of high-affinity dofetilide binding to HERG1 expressed in Xenopus oocytes: Involvement of S6 sites. *Mol. Pharmacol.* **57,** 367–374.

22. Mitcheson, J. S., Chen, J., Lin, M., Culberson, C., and Sanguinetti, M. C. (2000) A structural basis for drug-induced long QT syndrome. *Proc. Natl. Acad. Sci. USA* **97,** 12,329–12,333.

23. Vandenberg, J. I., Walker, B. D., and Campbell, T. J. (2001) HERG K(+) channels: Friend and foe. *Trends Pharmacol. Sci.* **22,** 240–246.

24. Gurdon, J. B., Lane, C. D., Woodland, H. R., and Marbaix, G. (1971) Use of frog eggs and oocytes for the study of messenger RNA and its translation in living cells. *Nature* **233,** 177–182.

25. Soreq, H. and Seidman, S. (1993) Xenopus oocytes microinjection: from gene to protein, in *Methods in Enzymology, Vol. 207: Ion Channels* (Rudy, B., and Iverson, L. E. eds.), Academic Press, New York, pp. 225–265.

26. Taglialatela, M., Vandongen, A. M.J., Drewe, J. A., Joho, R. H., Brown, A. M., and Kirsch, G. E. (1991) Patterns of internal and external tetraehylammonium blockade in four homologous delayed rectifiers K$^+$ channels. *Mol. Pharmacol.* **40,** 229–307.

27. Senior, K. (2000) Higher-throughput automated systems for ion-channel screening. *Drug Dis. Today* **5 (Suppl 12),** S56–S58.

28. Claudio, T. (1993) Stable expression of heterologous multisubunit protein complexes established by calcum-phosphate- or lipid-mediated cotrasnfection, in *Methods in Enzymology*, Vol. 207: Ion Channels (Rudy, B., and Iverson, L. E., eds.), Academic Press, New York, pp. 391–408.

29. Sesti, F., Abbott, G. W., Wei, J., Murray, K. T., Saksena, S., Schwartz, P. J., et al. (2000) A common polymorphism associated with antibiotic-induced cardiac arrhythmia. *Proc. Natl. Acad. Sci. USA* **97,** 10613–10618.

30. Colosimo, A., Goncz, K. K., Holmes, A. R., Kunzelmann, K., Novelli, G., Malone, R. W., et al. (2000) Transfer and expression of foreign genes in mammalian cells. *Biotechniques* **29,** 314–8, 320–2, 324.

31. Cubitt, A. B., Heim, R., Adams, S. R., Boyd, A. E., Gross, L. A., and Tsien, R. Y. (1995) Understanding, improving and using green fluorescent proteins. *Trends Biochem. Sci.* **20,** 448–455.

32. Gray, D. (1997) Overview of protein expression by mammalian cells. *Curr. Protocols Protein Sci.* 5.9.1–5.9.18.

33. Haas, K., Sin, W. C., Javaherian, A., Li, Z., and Cline, H. T. (2001) Single-cell electroporation for gene transfer in vivo. *Neuron* **29,** 583–591.

34. Rudmann, D. G. and Durham, S. K. (1999) Utilization of genetically altered animals in the pharmaceutical industry. *Toxicol. Pathol.* **27,** 111–114.

35. Wei, L-N. (1997) Transgenic animals as new approaches in pharmacological studies. *Annu. Rev. Pharmacol. Toxicol.* **137,** 119–141.

36. Nerbonne, J. M., Nichols, C. G., Schwarz, T. L, and Escande, D. (2001) Genetic manipulation of cardiac K(+) channel function in mice: What have we learned, and where do we go from here? *Circ. Res.* **89,** 944–956.

37. Finlayson, K., Turnbull, L., January, C. T., Sharkey, J., and Kelly, J. S. (2001) [3H]dofetilide binding to HERG transfected membranes: a potential high throughput preclinical screen. *Eur. J. Pharmacol.* **430,** 147–148.

38. Tristani-Firouzi, M., Chen, J., Mitcheson, J. S., and Sanguinetti, M. C. (2001) Molecular biology of K(+) channels and their role in cardiac arrhythmias. *Am. J. Med.* **110,** 50–59.

39. Finlayson, K., Pennington, A. J., and Kelly, J. S. (2001) [3H]dofetilide binding in SHSY5Y and HEK293 cells expressing a HERG-like K+ channel? *Eur. J. Pharmacol.* **412,** 203–212.

40. Striessnig, J., Grabner, M., Mitterdorfer, J., Hering, S., Sinnegger, M. J., and Glossmann, H. (1998) Structural basis of drug binding to L Ca2+ channels. *Trends Pharmacol. Sci.* **19,** 108–115.

41. Mulvaney, A. W., Spencer, C. I., Culliford, S., Borg, J. J., Davies, S. G., and Kozlowski, R. Z. (2000) Cardiac chloride channels: Physiology, pharmacology and approaches for identifying novel modulators of activity. *Drug Dis. Today* **5,** 492–505.

42. Terstappen, G. (1999) Functional analysis of native and recombinant ion channels using a high-capacity non radioactive rubidium efflux assay. *Anal. Biochem.* **272,** 149–155.

43. Gonzalez, J. E., Oades, K., Leychkis, Y., Harootunian, A., and Negulescu, P. A. (1999) Cell-based assays and instrumentation for screening ion-channel targets. *Drug Dis. Today* **4,** 431–439.

44. Taglialatela, M., Canzoniero, L. M.T., Di Renzo, G. F., Yasumoto, T., and Annunziato, L. (1990) Effect of maitotoxin on cytosolic Ca++ levels and membrane potential in purified rat brain synaptosomes. *Biochim. Biophys. Acta* **1026,** 126–132.

45. Zochowski, M., Wachowiak, M., Falk, C. X., Cohen, L. B., Lam, Y. W., Antic, S., and Zecevic, D. (2000) Imaging membrane potential with voltage-sensitive dyes. *Biol. Bull.* **198,** 1–21.

46. Rink, T. J., Montecucco, C., Hesketh, T. R., and Tsien, R. Y. (1980) Lymphocyte membrane potential assessed with fluorescent probes. *Biochim. Biophys. Acta* **595,** 15–30.

47. Grynkiewicz, G., Poenie, M., and Tsien, R. Y. (1985) A new generation of Ca2+ indicators with greatly improved fluorescence properties. *J. Biol. Chem.* **260,** 3440–3450.

48. Minta, A. and Tsien, R. Y. (1989) Fluorescent indicators for cytosolic sodium. *J. Biol. Chem.* **264,** 19,449–19,457.

49. Paradiso, A. M., Tsien, R. Y., and Machen, T. E. (1984) Na+-H+ exchange in gastric glands as measured with a cytoplasmic-trapped, fluorescent pH indicator. *Proc. Natl. Acad. Sci. USA* **81,** 7436–7440.

50. Geddes, C. D., Apperson, K., Karolin, J., and Birch, D. J. (2001) Chloride-sensitive fluorescent indicators. *Anal. Biochem.* **293,** 60–66.

51. Zoeteweij, J. P., van de Water, B., de Bont, H. J., and Nagelkerke, J. F. (1994) Mitochondrial K+ as modulator of Ca(2+)-dependent cytotoxicity in hepatocytes. Novel application of the K(+)-sensitive dye PBFI (K(+)-binding benzofuran isophthalate) to assess free mitochondrial K+ concentrations. *Biochem. J.* **299,** 539–543.

52. Meuwis, K., Boens, N., De Schryver, F. C., Gallay, J., and Vincent, M. (1995) Photophysics of the fluorescent K+ indicator PBFI. *Biophys. J.* **68,** 2469–2473.

53. Sullivan, E., Tucker, E. M., and Dale, I. L. (1999) Measurement of [Ca2+] using the Fluorometric Imaging Plate Reader (FLIPR). *Methods Mol. Biol.* **114,** 125–133.

54. Gonzalez, J. E. and Tsien, R. Y. (1997) Improved indicators of cell membrane potential that use fluorescence resonance energy transfer. *Chem. Biol.* **4,** 269–277.

55. Leychkis, Y., Numann, R., Kansagara, A. G., Oades, K. V., and Gonzalez, J. E. (2001) High-throughput sodium channel assay using FRET-based voltage sensors in a astrocytoma cell line. *Soc. Neurosci. Meeting. Abs* 46.27.

56. Netzer, R., Ebneth. A., Bischoff, U., and Pongs, O. (2001) Screening lead compounds for QT interval prolongation. *Drug Dis. Today* **6,** 78–84.

57. Ahlberg, C. (1999) Visual exploration of HTS databases. *Drug Dis. Today* **4,** 370–376.

58. Sakai, R., Repunte-Canonigo, V., Raj, C.D., and Knopfel, T. (2001) Design and characterization of a DNA-encoded, voltage-sensitive fluorescent protein. *Eur. J. Neurosci.* **13,** 2314–2318.

59. Xu, J., Wang, X., Ensign, B., Li, M., Wu, M., Guia, A., et al. (2001) Ion channel assay technologies: Quo vadis? *Drug Dis. Today* **6,** 1278–1287.

60. Taglialatela, M., Pannaccione, A., Castaldo, P., Giorgio, G., Zhou, Z., January, C. T., et al. (1998) The molecular basis for the lack of HERG K+ channels block-related cardiotoxicity by the H1 receptor blocker cetirizine as compared to other second-generation antihistamines. *Mol. Pharmacol.* **54,** 113–121.

13

Molecular Diversity of Ion Channels in the Mouse Heart

A Suitable Model for Cardiac Drug Development?

Jeanne M. Nerbonne

1. INTRODUCTION

Action potential waveforms in the mammalian myocardium reflect the synchronized activation (and inactivation) of multiple types of membrane ion channels *(1)* contributing inward (depolarizing) or outward (repolarizing) ionic currents (Fig. 1). These (inward and outward) current channels, therefore, are important potential therapeutic targets for controlling the amplitudes and the duration of action potentials in the heart. In addition, it is clear that action potential waveforms change during normal cardiac development *(2,3)* and in a variety of myocardial disease states *(4–6)* owing to changes in the biophysical properties and/or the expression of the underlying ionic channels. Thus, there is considerable interest in defining the molecular correlates of the functional inward and outward current channels expressed in myocardial cells and in delineating the molecular mechanisms controlling the properties and the functional expression of these channels *(1,7)*. Although a variety of experimental models have been exploited in these efforts over the years, the mouse is now being used increasingly owing to the ease with which genetic manipulations can be made in the mouse *(7,8)*.

From: *Cardiac Drug Development Guide*
Edited by: M. K. Pugsley © Humana Press Inc., Totowa, NJ

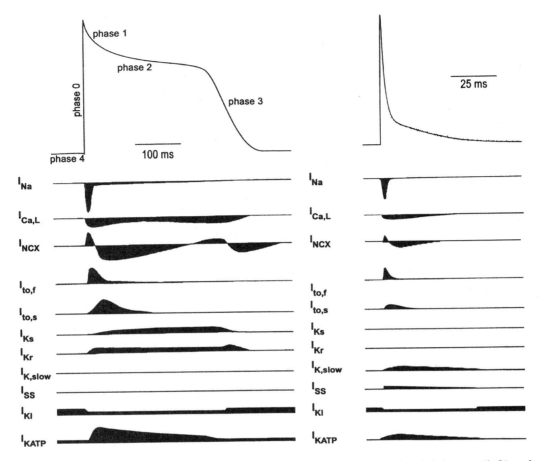

Fig. 1. Schematic of action potentials and underlying ionic currents in adult human (left) and mouse (right) ventricular myocytes. The diversity of outward K$^+$ currents in myocardial cells is greater than for the inward Na$^+$ and Ca^{2+} currents, and the various K$^+$ currents play distinct roles in action potential repolarization in human and mouse ventricular cells.

Importantly, there are marked differences in cardiac action potential waveforms in different species, as well as in myocardial cells in different regions of the heart in the same species *(7,9,10)*. In human and mouse ventricular myocytes, for example, the rapid upstroke of the action potential (phase 0) reflects inward current through voltage-gated Na$^+$ channels. In human ventricular cells, the upstroke is followed by a transient repolarization (phase 1) to a plateau phase (phase 2), reflecting the balance of inward currents through voltage-gated (L-type) Ca^{2+} channels and outward K$^+$ currents through voltage-gated (and other) K$^+$ channels. The driving force for K$^+$ efflux is high during the plateau and, as Ca^{2+} channels inactivate, outward K$^+$ currents predominate, resulting in a second, rapid phase (phase 3) of repolarization back to the resting potential (Fig. 1). In mouse ventricular cells, in contrast, there is no clear plateau phase and the upstroke is followed by rapid repolarization, again reflecting K$^+$ efflux, primarily through voltage-gated K$^+$ channels (Fig. 1).

Electrophysiological studies in myocardial tissues and isolated cells have detailed the distributions and the properties of the major voltage-gated inward Na^+ and Ca^{2+} and outward K^+ channel currents (Table 1) that determine the heights and the durations of cardiac action potentials (*1*). In contrast to the voltage-gated Na^+ and Ca^{2+} channels, there are multiple types of voltage-gated K^+ currents in mammalian cardiac cells (*1,7*). At least two types of transient outward currents, $I_{to,f}$ and $I_{to,s}$, and several components of delayed rectification, including I_{Kr} ($I_{K(rapid)}$) and I_{Ks} ($I_{K(slow)}$), I_{Kur} ($I_{K,ultrarapid}$), $I_{K,slow1}$, I_{Kslow2}, for example, have been distinguished (Table 1). In addition, there are species- and region-specific differences in the expression patterns of the various voltage-gated K^+ channel currents, and these contribute to differences in action potential waveforms observed in different cardiac cell types (*9,10*). Importantly, however, the biophysical properties of the various repolarizing K^+ currents in myocytes isolated from different species and/or from different regions of the heart in the same species are remarkably similar, suggesting that the molecular correlates of the underlying channels are also the same (*7*). A rather large number of pore-forming (α) and accessory (β, γ, and δ) subunits (Fig. 2) encoding Na^+, Ca^{2+} and K^+ channels have been identified, and considerable progress has been made in defining the relationships between these subunits and functional cardiac Na^+, Ca^{2+}, and K^+ channels (*1,7,8*). For cardiac K^+ channels in particular, many of these studies have exploited transgenic (*11–21*) or targeted deletion (*22–43*) strategies in mice *in situ* to allow cardiac specific expression of mutant K^+ channel α subunit transgenes (*11–21*) or to disrupt the expression of individual K^+ channel subunit genes (*22–43*). The in vivo molecular genetic manipulation of K^+ channel expression should facilitate studies focused on exploring the functional roles of specific K^+ channels in the myocardium and allow experimental testing of the predictions of computer models of cardiac action potential waveforms and impulse propagation in the myocardium. Nevertheless, it is important to note that the waveforms of action potentials in mouse cardiac myocytes (Fig. 1), as well as the electrical properties of the intact murine heart, are really quite different from those of larger animals, particularly humans, and it seems reasonable to suggest that the cellular, molecular, and systemic mechanisms underlying these differences could impact the usefulness of the mouse as a model system.

This chapter summarizes our present understanding of the electrophysiological and molecular diversity of the sarcolemmal membrane ion channels contributing to shaping action potential waveforms in the mammalian heart and the progress made in defining the subunits contributing to the formation of these channels. In addition, the phenotypic consequences of manipulating K^+ channel expression in the mouse myocardium *in situ* as well as the advantages, disadvantages, and limitations of the mouse as an experimental tool for cardiac drug development are discussed.

2. VOLTAGE-GATED NA⁺ AND CA²⁺ CURRENTS IN THE MAMMALIAN MYOCARDIUM

Voltage-gated Na^+ channels open rapidly on membrane depolarization and underlie the rapid rising phases of the action potentials in mammalian ventricular (Fig. 1) and atrial myocytes. Although voltage-gated Na^+ channels also inactivate rapidly and, during the action potential plateau, most of the Na^+ channels are inactivated (*44*), there is a finite (albeit small) probability of channel reopening during the plateau. The resulting

Table 1
Ionic Currents Contributing to Action Potential Repolarization

Current	Activation	Inactivation	Recovery	Pharmacology[a]	Tissues	Regional
I_{Na}	fast	fast	fast	TTX	Atria, Ventricles, Purkinje	no
$I_{Ca(L)}$	fast	Ca^{2+}-dep	fast	DHP Cd^{2+}	Atria, Ventricles, Nodal, Purkinje	no
$I_{Ca(T)}$	fast	fast	fast		Atria, Nodal	no
$I_{to,f}$	fast	fast	fast	mM 4-AP Flecainide HaTX HpTX	Atria, Ventricles, Purkinje	yes
$I_{to,s}$	fast	slow	slow	mM 4-AP	Ventricles	yes
I_{Kr}	moderate	fast	slow	E-4031 Dofetilide Lanthanum	Ventricles	yes
I_{Ks}	very slow	no	—	NE-10064 NE-10133 mM 4-AP	Ventricles	yes
I_{Kur}	fast	no	—		Atria	no
I_{Kp}	fast	no	—	Ba^{2+}	Ventricles	??
I_K	slow	slow	slow	mM TEA	Ventricles	??
$I_{K,slow1}$	fast	slow	slow	mM 4-AP	Atria, Ventricles	no
$I_{K,slow2}$	fast	very slow	slow	mM TEA	Atria, Ventricles	no
I_{ss}	slow	no	—	mM TEA	Atria, Ventricles	no
I_{Kl}	—	—	—	Ba^{2+}	Atria, Ventricles	no

[a]TTX, tetrodotoxin; DHP, dihydropyridines; 4-AP, 4-aminopyridine; HaTX, hanatoxin; HpTX, heteropodatoxin; TEA, tetraethylammonium; SUR, sulfonylureas.

248

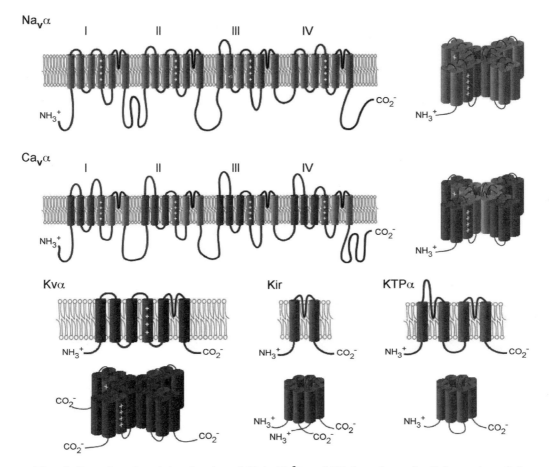

Fig. 2. Pore-forming (α) subunits of Na^+, Ca^{2+} and K^+ ion channels. Schematics of the sequences and the membrane topologies of individual α subunits encoding Na_v, Ca_v, Kv, Kir, and two pore domain (KTP) K^+ channels are illustrated. Adjacent to (for $Na_v\alpha$ and $Ca_v\alpha$) or below (for Kvα, Kirα, and KTPα) the α subunits, schematics of assembled monomeric Na_v and Ca_v channels, tetrameric Kv and K_{ir} channels and dimeric KTP K^+ channels are illustrated.

inward current contributes to maintaining the depolarized state and it does, therefore, also play a role in ventricular action potential repolarization *(1)*. Although the properties and densities of voltage-gated Na^+ channels in atrial and ventricular myocardium are similar, the density of the persistent component of the current is variable in the ventricle *(45)*. Together with the marked differences in voltage-gated K^+ current densities, the variable expression of the persistent Na^+ current may contribute to regional heterogeneity in ventricular action potential amplitudes and durations *(9,10)*.

In the mammalian myocardium, Ca^{2+} entry during the plateau phase of the action potential occurs primarily through high threshold, L-type, voltage-gated Ca^{2+} channels, although in pacemaker cells, low threshold, T-type, channels are also expressed (Table 1). Similar to the voltage-gated Na^+ channels, the densities of the L-type Ca^{2+} channel currents do not vary appreciably in different species and/or in myocytes isolated from different region of the ventricles of the same species *(1)*. These channels require strong depolarization for activation, and channel opening on membrane depolarization is delayed relative to the opening of the voltage-gated Na^+ channels (Fig. 1). Importantly, the Ca^{2+} influx through the L-type Ca^{2+} channels triggers Ca^{2+} release from intracellular Ca^{2+} stores, contributing to excitation–contraction coupling. During the plateau phase of the action potential, the L-type Ca^{2+} channels undergo voltage- and Ca^{2+}-dependent inactivation, contributing to the termination of the action potential plateau and action potential repolarization.

3. VOLTAGE-GATED OUTWARD K+ CURRENTS IN THE MAMMALIAN MYOCARDIUM

In mammalian cardiac cells, two broad classes of voltage-gated K^+ currents have been distinguished: transient outward K^+ currents, I_{to}, and delayed, outwardly rectifying K^+ currents, I_K (Table 1). The transient currents (I_{to}) activate and inactivate rapidly and underlie the early phase (phase 1) of repolarization, whereas the delayed rectifiers (I_K) determine the latter phase (phase 3) of action potential repolarization (Fig. 1). These are broad classifications, however, and multiple types of transient and delayed rectifier K^+ currents are expressed in myocardial cells (Table 1). In addition, there are species and regional differences in the densities, as well as the properties, of these currents, and these differences contribute to the heterogeneity in action potential waveforms recorded in different cell types and species *(7,9,10)*.

Electrophysiological and pharmacological studies on adult mouse ventricular myocytes provided clear evidence that there are two distinct types of cardiac transient outward K^+ currents, now referred to as $I_{to,fast}$ ($I_{to,f}$) and $I_{to,slow}$ ($I_{to,s}$), and that these currents are differentially distributed *(46)*. The rapidly activating and inactivating $I_{to,f}$ is also characterized by rapid recovery from steady-state inactivation *(7,46)*. Importantly, the time- and voltage-dependent properties of $I_{to,f}$ in different species and cell types (Table 1) are similar in that activation, inactivation and recovery from steady-state inactivation are all rapid *(7)*. In addition, $I_{to,f}$ is readily distinguished from other voltage-gated cardiac K^+ currents using the K^+ channel spider toxins, *Heteropoda* toxin-2 or -3 *(47)*. Although $I_{to,f}$ densities vary considerably in right and left ventricles and through the thickness of the ventricular wall *(9,10)*, the fact that the properties of ventricular $I_{to,f}$ in different cell types and species are similar (Table 1) led to the hypothesis that the molecular correlates of functional ventricular $I_{to,f}$ channels in different cell types/species are the same *(7)*, and considerable experimental evidence in support of this hypothesis has now been provided. In electrophysiological studies, mouse ventricular $I_{to,s}$ is readily distinguished from $I_{to,f}$ by the slow rates of inactivation and recovery from inactivation *(46)*, and it has also been demonstrated that the molecular correlates of (mouse ventricular) $I_{to,s}$ and $I_{to,f}$ are distinct *(30)*.

Delayed rectifier K^+ currents, I_K, have been characterized extensively in myocytes isolated from a variety of species and, in most cells, multiple components of I_K (Table 1) are expressed. In canine ventricular myocytes, for example, two prominent components of I_K, I_{Kr} ($I_{K,rapid}$) and I_{Ks} ($I_{K,slow}$), can be distinguished based on differences in time- and voltage-dependent properties and pharmacological sensitivities *(48)*. In human ventricular cells, both I_{Kr} and I_{Ks} are expressed *(49)*. Although neither I_{Kr} nor I_{Ks} appears to be a prominent repolarizing current in adult mouse heart *(46)*, distinct components of I_K, including $I_{K,slow1}$ *(11,17,19,21,39,46,50,51)*, $I_{K,slow2}$ *(15,21,46)*, and I_{ss} *(46)* have been identified (Table 1). In contrast with the differential distribution of $I_{to,f}$ and $I_{to,s}$, $I_{K,slow1}$, $I_{K,slow2}$, and I_{ss} appear to be expressed in all mouse ventricular myocytes *(46)*.

4. OTHER K⁺ CURRENTS IN THE MAMMALIAN MYOCARDIUM

In addition to the voltage-gated K⁺ channels, two types of inwardly rectifying K⁺ channel currents, I_{K1} and the ATP-dependent, I_{KATP} (Table 1), contribute to setting resting membrane potentials and determining the waveforms of cardiac action potentials, and the densities of these currents vary in different regions (atria, ventricles, and conducting tissue) of the heart *(1,52,53)*. In human ventricular myocytes, the strongly inwardly rectifying I_{K1} channels play a role in establishing the resting membrane potential and the plateau potential, in addition to contributing to phase 3 repolarization (Fig. 1). The strong inward rectification evident in these channels is attributed to block by intracellular Mg $^{2+}$ *(54)* and by polyamines *(55,56)*.

The weakly inwardly rectifying ATP-dependent K⁺ channels are inhibited by intracellular ATP and activated by nucleotide diphosphates *(53)*. These channels are thought to provide a link between cellular metabolism and membrane potential. In ventricular myocytes, activation of I_{KATP} channels has been suggested to play a role in the shortening of action potentials and the loss of K⁺ that occurs with ischemia and hypoxia *(57)*. The opening of I_{KATP} channels has also been suggested to contribute to the cardioprotection resulting from ischemic preconditioning *(58,59)*. Unlike voltage-gated K⁺ channels, I_{KATP} channels appear to be distributed uniformly at high density in the right and left ventricles and through the thickness of the ventricular wall.

5. MOLECULAR CORRELATES OF VOLTAGE-GATED CARDIAC NA⁺ AND CA⁺ CURRENTS

Voltage-gated Na⁺ (Na_v) channel pore-forming α subunits (Fig. 2) belong to the S4 superfamily of genes encoding voltage-gated ion channels. Each Na_v α subunit consists of four homologous domains (I to IV), each of which has six α helical transmembrane repeats (S1–S6) and a hydrophilic region between S5 and S6 that contributes to the Na⁺-selective pore (Fig. 2). Although there are multiple members of the Na_v α subunit subfamily, $Na_v1.5$ is the predominant isoform expressed in the mammalian heart *(1)*. Functional voltage-gated cardiac Na⁺ channels appear to be multisubunit complexes (Fig. 3) consisting of a central pore-forming Na_v α subunit (Fig. 2) and one to two auxiliary β subunits *(60)*, although the roles of these subunits in controlling the properties and/or the functional expression of myocardial Na⁺ channels remain to be determined.

Importantly, inherited mutations in the linker between domains III and IV in $Na_v1.5$ that cause one form of Long QT syndrome, LQT3, have been shown to disrupt inactivation, leading to an increase in the relative amplitude of the persistent Na⁺ current *(61,62)*. It is also of interest to note that increased persistent Na⁺ current density also prolongs action potentials in genetically engineered mice *(63)*.

Voltage-gated Ca²⁺ (Ca_v) channel pore-forming (α) subunits (Fig. 2) also belong to the S4 superfamily of voltage-gated ion channel genes. Similar to the Na_v α subunits, $Ca_v\alpha_1$ subunits comprise four homologous domains (domain I–IV), each of

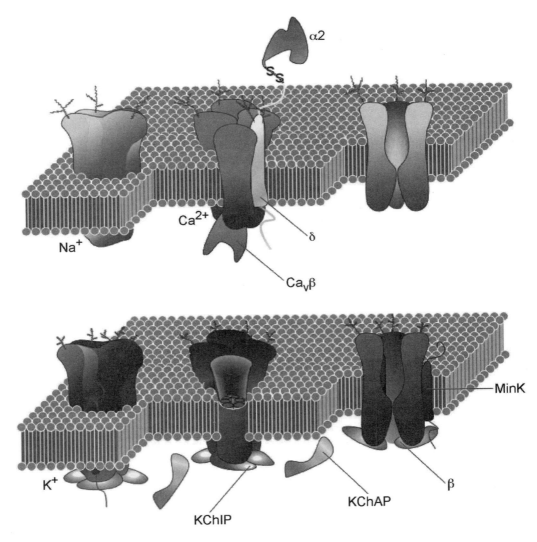

Fig. 3. Molecular composition of cardiac Na⁺, Ca²⁺, and K⁺ channels. Upper panel: The four domains of the Ca_v (or Na_v) α subunit, together with accessory subunits, assemble to produce functional Ca_v (or Na_v) channels. Lower panel: Four Kv (or Kir) α subunits, together with one or more accessory β subunits, co-assemble to produce functional outwardly (or inwardly) rectifying cardiac K⁺ channels.

which is composed of six putative transmembrane segments (S1–S6), including the S4 voltage sensing domain, and a region between S5 and S6 that contributes to the Ca^{2+} selective pore (Fig. 2). Also similar to Na⁺ channels, functional voltage-gated Ca^{2+} (Ca_v) channels are multimeric proteins consisting of a Ca_v $α_1$ subunit and auxiliary, Ca_v β and Ca_v $α_2δ$, subunits (Fig. 3), although the $α_1$ subunit is the primary determinant of channel properties.

Four distinct subfamilies of Ca_v channel pore-forming $α_1$ subunits, Ca_v1, Ca_v2, Ca_v3, and Ca_v4 have been identified *(1)* and a member of the Ca_v1 subfamily, $Ca_v1.2$, encodes

α_{1C} (α_1 1.2), the pore-forming α subunit in voltage-gated cardiac L-type Ca^{2+} channels. There are also multiple $Ca_v\beta$ and $Ca_v\alpha_2\delta$ subunit genes that can co-assemble with Ca_v1 α subunits to increase functional voltage-gated Ca^{2+} channel expression and modify channel properties. The $Ca_v\alpha_2\delta$ subunits are heavily glycosylated proteins that are cleaved post-translationally to yield disulfide-linked α_2-proteins (Fig. 3). The $Ca_v\alpha_2$ domain is located extracellularly, whereas the $Ca_v\delta$ domain has a large hydrophobic region, which inserts into the membrane (Fig. 3) and anchors the channel complex *(64,65)*. Although the molecular compositions of functional voltage-gated Ca^{2+} channels in different cardiac cell types and species remain to be defined, it seems likely that the structures of these channels will be identical based on the similarities in the biophysical properties of the currents (channels) expressed.

6. MOLECULAR DIVERSITY OF SUBUNITS ENCODING VOLTAGE-GATED CARDIAC K⁺ CHANNELS

Voltage-gated K^+ channel (Kv) pore-forming (α) subunits are six transmembrane spanning domain proteins (Fig. 2) with a region between the fifth and sixth transmembrane domains that contributes to the K^+-selective pore. The positively charged fourth transmembrane domain in the Kv α subunits is homologous to the corresponding region in voltage-gated Na^+ and Ca^{2+} channel α subunits, placing them in the S4 superfamily of voltage-gated channels. In contrast with voltage-gated Na^+ and Ca^{2+} channels, however, functional voltage-gated K^+ channels comprise four α subunits (Fig. 2). The identification of several homologous Kv subunit subfamilies, including Kv1.x, Kv2.x, Kv3.x, Kv4.x, many of which are expressed in the heart (Table 2), in combination with alternative splicing of transcripts and/or the formation of heteromultimeric channels between distinct Kv subunit proteins, suggests considerable potential for generating the functional diversity of voltage-gated cardiac K^+ channels (Table 1).

Additional subfamilies of voltage-gated K^+ (Kv) channel (Table 2), as well a large number of inwardly rectifying (Kir) channel (Table 3) α subunit genes have also been identified. The Kv α subunit ERG1 *(66)* is the locus of mutations leading to one form of familial long QT-syndrome, LQT2 *(67)*. Heterologous expression of ERG1 reveals inwardly rectifying voltage-gated, K^+-selective currents *(68,69)* with properties similar to cardiac I_{Kr} (Table 2). Alternatively processed forms of ERG1 have also been cloned from mouse and human heart cDNA libraries and postulated to contribute to cardiac I_{Kr} *(70–72)*. Another subfamily of voltage-gated K^+ channel α subunits was revealed with the cloning of KvLQT1 *(73)*, the loci of mutations in LQT1. Although KvLQT1 expressed alone yields rapidly activating, noninactivating K^+ currents, co-expression with the accessory subunit minK *(74,75)* produces slowly activating K^+ currents that resemble the slow component of cardiac delayed rectification, I_{Ks} *(76,77)*.

A number of other voltage-gated K^+ (Kv) channel accessory subunits have also now been identified (Table 4), and it has been suggested that one of the minK homologs, MiRP1 *(78)*, functions as an accessory subunit of ERG1 to generate cardiac I_{Kr} channels *(79)*. It has also been reported, however, that that MiRP1 assembles with Kv3.4 in mammalian skeletal muscle *(80)* and with Kv4.x α subunits in heterologous expression systems *(81)*. Although these findings suggest that KCNE accessory subunits might contribute to multiple K^+ channels, the functional importance of associa-

Table 2
Voltage-Gated K⁺ Channel Pore-Forming α Subunits

Family	Subfamily	Protein	Gene	Location		Current
				Human	Mouse	
Kv						
	Kv1					
		Kv1.1	KCNA1	12p13	6	
		Kv1.2	KCNA2	1p11	3	$I_{K,slow(rat)}$ ($I_{K,DTX}$)
		Kv1.3	KCNA3	1p21	3	
		Kv1.4	KCNA4	11p14	2	$I_{to,s}$
		Kv1.5	KCNA5	12p13	6	I_{Kur} (human/rat) $I_{K,slow}$ (mouse)
		Kv1.6	KCNA6	12p13	6	
		Kv1.7	KCNA7	19q13	7	
		Kv1.10	KCNA10	1p11		
	Kv2					
		Kv2.1	KCNB1	20q13.1	2	$I_{K,slow}$ (mouse)
		Kv2.2	KCNB2	8q13		??
	Kv3					
		Kv3.1	KCNC1	11p15	7	I_{Kur} (canine)
		Kv3.2	KCNC2			
		Kv3.3	KCNC3	19q13.4	7	
		Kv3.4	KCNC4	1p11		
	Kv4					
		Kv4.1	KCND1	Xp11.2	X	??
		Kv4.2	KCND2	7q32	6	$I_{to,f}$
		Kv4.3	KCND3	1p11	3	$I_{to,f}$
	Kv5					
		Kv5.1	KCNF1	2p25		??
	Kv6					
		Kv6.1	KCNG1	20q13.1		
		Kv6.2	KCNG2	18q23		
	Kv8					
		Kv8.1	KCN?			
	Kv9					
		Kv9.1	KCNS1	20q12	2	
		Kv9.2	KCNS2			
		Kv9.3	KCNS3	2p25		
EAG						
	eag					
		eag	KCNH1	1q32	1	
		erg1	KCNH2	7q36	5	I_{Kr}
		erg2	KCNH3		15	
		erg3	KCNH4	17q21		
		elk				
	KvLQT					
		KvLQT1	KCNQ1	11p15	7	I_{Ks}
		KCNQ2	KCNQ2	20p11.1	2	
		KCNQ3	KCNQ3	8q24.3		
		KCNQ4	KCNQ4	1p34.3		

Table 3
Inward Rectifier and Two-Pore-K⁺ Channel α Subunits

Family	Subfamily	Protein	Gene	Location Human	Location Mouse	Current
Kir						
	Kir1					
		Kir1.1	KCNJ1	11q25		??
	Kir2					
		Kir2.1	KCNJ2	17q23	11	I_{K1}
		Kir2.2	KCNJ12	17p11.2	11	I_{K1}
		Kir2.3	KCNJ4	22U		??
		Kir2.4	KCNJ14	19q13.4		??
	Kir3					
		Kir3.1	KCNJ3		2	I_{KACh}
		Kir3.2	KCNJ6	21q22		
			KCNJ7		16	
		Kir3.3	KCNJ9	1q21	1	
		Kir3.4	KCNJ5	11q25	9	I_{KACh}
	Kir4					
		Kir4.1	KCNJ10	1q21	1	
		Kir4.2	KCNJ15	21q22	16	
	Kir5					
		Kir5.1	KCNJ16	17q25		
	Kir6					
		Kir6.1	KCNJ8	12p11.1	6	
		Kir6.2	KCNJ11	11p15		I_{KATP}
Two-Pore						
	TWIK					
		TWIK-1	KCNK1	1q42	8	??
		TWIK-2	KCNK6	19q11	7	??
		TWIK-3	KCNK7			
		TWIK-4	KCNK8	11q12	19	
	TREK					
		TREK-1	KCNK2		1	??
		TREK-2	KCNK10	14q32		
	TASK					
		TASK-1	KCNK3	2p24		I_{Kp} ??
		TASK-2	KCNK5	6p21.1	14	
		TASK-3	KCNK9	8q24.3		
		TASK-4	KCNK14			
		TASK-5	KCNK15	20q12		
	TRAAK					
		TRAAK-1	KCNK4	11q12	19	
	THIK					
		THIK-1	KCNK13	14q32		
		THIK-2	KCNK12	2p21		??
	TALK					
		TALK-1	KCNK16	6p21		
		TALK-2	KCNK17	6p21		??

Table 4
Accessory Subunits
of Voltage-Gated K+ Channels

Family	Subunit	Gene	Chromosome		Cardiac Current
			Human	Mouse	
Kvβ					
	Kvβ1	*KCNAB1*	3q25	3	??
	Kvβ2	*KCNAB2*		4	??
	Kvβ3	*KCNAB3*	17p13	11	
KCNE					
	Mink	*KCNE1*	21q22	16	I_{Ks}
	MiRP1	*KCNE2*	21q22		I_{Kr} ??, $I_{to,f}$??
	MiRP2	*KCNE3*	11q13		
	MiRP3	*KCNE4*			
KChAP					
	KChAP				$I_{to,f}$??, I_K ??,
KChIP					
	KChIP1	*KCNIP1*	5q35		
	KChIP2	*KCNIP2*	10q25		$I_{to,f}$
	KChIP3	*KCNIP3*			
NCS					
	NCS-1	*FREQ*	9q34		$I_{to,f}$

tions with MiRP subunits in the generation of voltage-gated cardiac K+ channels remains to be determined.

Low molecular cytosolic Kv accessory subunits were first identified in brain *(82)*. Four homologous Kvβ subunits, Kv β1, Kv β2, Kv β3, and Kv β4 (Table 3), as well as alternatively spliced transcripts, have been identified, and both Kv β1 and Kv β2 are expressed in heart *(83)*. Heterologous expression studies suggest that Kv β subunits interact with the intracellular domains of Kv1 subunits and modify the properties and the cell surface expression of Kv1 α subunit-encoded K+ currents *(84,85)*. It has not, however, been demonstrated directly that Kv α and Kv β subunits associate in the myocardium, and the roles of Kv β subunits in the generation of functional cardiac K+ channels remain to be determined. This is also the case for another voltage-gated K+ channel accessory protein, KChAP *(86)*, which has been shown in expression systems to interact with the N termini of Kv α subunits and with the C termini of Kv β subunits.

The Kv channel-interacting proteins, KChIPs (Table 3), identified by An and colleagues *(87)*, belong to the recoverin family of neuronal Ca^{2+}-sensing proteins, which contain multiple EF-hand domains *(88)*. The N termini of the KChIP proteins are unique *(87)*, and only KChIP2 appears to be expressed in heart *(87,89)*. Heterologous expression of α subunits of the Kv4 subfamily with any one of the KChIPs increases the functional cell surface expression of Kv4.x-encoded K+ currents, slows current inactivation, speeds recovery from inactivation, and shifts the voltage-dependence of activation *(87)*. Interestingly, the KChIPs do not affect Kv1.4- or Kv2.1-encoded K+ currents, suggesting that the modulatory effects of the KChIP proteins are specific for Kv4 α subunit-encoded channels *(87)*. Although KChIP binding to Kv4 α subunits is not Ca^{2+}-dependent, mutations in EF hand domains 2, 3, and 4 eliminate the modulatory effects of KChIP1 on Kv4.x-encoded K+ currents *(87)*. It has also been demonstrated that KChIP2 co-immunoprecipitates with Kv4.2 and Kv4.3 α subunits from adult mouse ventricles, consistent with a role for this subunit in the generation of Kv4-encoded mouse ventricular $I_{to,f}$ channels *(90)*. Interestingly, a gradient in KChIP2 message expression is observed through the thickness of the ventricular wall in human heart, suggesting that KChIP2 underlies the differences in $I_{to,f}$ densities in the epicardium and endocardium *(89)*. In rodents, there is no KChIP2 gradient *(89,90)*, and regional variations in Kv4.2 expression underlie differences in $I_{to,f}$ densities *(90,91)*.

7. MOLECULAR CORRELATES OF CARDIAC VOLTAGE-GATED TRANSIENT OUTWARD K⁺ CHANNELS

Considerable evidence has accumulated documenting a role for Kv4 α subunits in the generation of myocardial $I_{to,f}$ channels. In mouse ventricular myocytes exposed to antisense oligodeoxynucleotides targeted against Kv4.2 or Kv4.3, for example, $I_{to,f}$ density is reduced by ~50 % *(90)*. It has also been shown that $I_{to,f}$ is eliminated in atrial and ventricular myocytes isolated from transgenic mice (Table 5) expressing a pore mutant of Kv4.2, Kv4.2W362F, that functions as a dominant negative *(12,14)*. Biochemical studies have also revealed that Kv4.2 and Kv4.3 are associated in mouse ventricles, suggesting that functional mouse ventricular $I_{to,f}$ channels are heteromeric *(90)*. Given the similarities in the properties of $I_{to,f}$ in different species (Table 1), it seems reasonable to suggest that Kv4 α subunits also underlie human $I_{to,f}$ channels. In human heart, however, the candidate subunit is Kv4.3 because Kv4.2 appears not to be expressed *(91)*. Although two splice variants of Kv4.3 have been identified in human *(92)*, the expression levels of the two Kv4.3 proteins and the role(s) of these subunits in the generation of functional cardiac $I_{to,f}$ channels remain to be defined.

The properties of the slow transient outward K⁺ currents, $I_{to,s}$, in ventricular myocytes are distinct from $I_{to,f}$ (Table 1), suggesting that the molecular correlates of ventricular $I_{to,s}$ and $I_{to,f}$ channels are also distinct. Direct experimental support for this hypothesis was provided with the demonstration that $I_{to,s}$ is undetectable in ventricular (septum) myocytes *(30)* from mice with a targeted deletion in Kv1.4, Kv1.4–/– *(23)*. Interestingly, $I_{to,s}$ (and Kv1.4 protein) is upregulated in left ventricular apex and in right ventricular cells in the Kv4.2W362F-expressing transgenics *(33)*. When the Kv4.2W362F transgene is expressed in the Kv1.4–/– null background, however, both $I_{to,f}$ and $I_{to,s}$ are eliminated *(33)*. Indeed, the waveforms of the outward K⁺ currents in all Kv4.2W362F-expressing Kv1.4–/– ventricular cells are indistinguishable *(33)*. Given the similarities in the properties of the slow transient outward K⁺ currents in different species (Table 1), it seems likely that Kv1.4 also encodes $I_{to,s}$ in and human ventricular myocytes, although this has not been demonstrated directly to date.

8. MOLECULAR CORRELATES OF CARDIAC VOLTAGE-GATED DELAYED RECTIFIER K⁺ CHANNELS

Expression of ERG1, the locus of LQT2 *(67)*, reveals voltage-gated K⁺ currents that resemble cardiac I_{Kr} *(68,69)*. The findings that antisense oligodeoxynucleotides targeted against minK attenuate I_{Kr} in AT-1 (an atrial tumor line) cells *(93)* and that heterologously expressed ERG1 and minK co-immunoprecipitate *(94)*, however, suggest that cardiac I_{Kr} channels are multimeric. To date, however, it has not been demonstrated that ERG1 and minK are associated in the mammalian heart. Alternatively processed forms of ERG1 with unique N- and C-termini have also been identified *(70–72)*

Table 5
Genetically Altered Mice with Altered K⁺ Current Expression

Mouse	Type[a]	Strain	Current affected[b]	Cellular phenotype[b]	Whole animal cardiac phenotype[b]	Ref.
Kv4.2W362F	Tg/Point Mutation	C57BL6	$I_{to,f}$ eliminated	↑APD	QT prolongation	12, 14, 33
Kv4.2N	Tg/Truncation	C57BL6	↓$I_{to,f}$; ↓I_{K1}	↑APD	ND	16
Kv4.2-/-	Exon 1 deletion	FVB and C57BL6	$I_{to,f}$ eliminated	↑APD	ND	35
Kv1.4-/-	1.4 deletion	C57BL6	$I_{to,s}$ eliminated	No change	None	26, 30, 33
Kv4.2W362F/ Kv1.4-/-	Tg in Kv1.4-/-	C57BL6	$I_{to,f}$ and $I_{to,s}$ eliminated	↑APD	QT prolongation	33
Kv1.1N206	Tg/Truncation at 216	FVB/N	$I_{K,slow}$ (1) (4-AP) eliminated	↑APD	QT prolongation arrhythmias	11
Kv2.1N216	Tg/Truncation at 206	C57BL6	$I_{K,slow}$ (2) (TEA) eliminated	↑APD	QT prolongation	15
SWAP	Replace mouse Kv1.5 with rat Kv1.1	C57BL6	$I_{K,slow}$ (1) eliminated	None	None	39
Kv1.1N16/ Kv2.1N206	Double Tg	C57BL6/FVB	$I_{K,slow}$ (1) and $I_{K,slow}$ (2) eliminated	↑APD	QT prolongation	19
Kv1.1N216/ Kv4.2W362F	Double Tg	C57BL6/FVB	$I_{to,f}$ eliminated $I_{K,slow}$ (1) eliminated	↑APD	QT prolongation	21
KCNE -/-	KCNE1 deletion	129Sv	ND	ND	None	22, 28
KCNE -/-	Replace KCNE1 with lac Z	129Sv	ND	ND	None	29
KCNQ1 -/-	KCNQ1 exon 1 deletion	C57BL6	ND	ND	None	31
KCNQ1 -/-	KCNQ1 exon 2 deletion	C57BL6	ND	ND	QT prolongation P.T Wave	38
KCNQ1-isoform 2	Tg	FVB/N	↓$I_{to,f}$; ↓I_{K1}	↑APD	QT prolongation bradycardia	18
KCNH2-G628S	Tg	FVB/N	↓K_r	↑APD	None	13
ERG1 -/-	Deletion?	129Sv	ND	ND	ND	23
ERG1B -/-	Exon 1b deletion	Not reported	ND	ND	QT prolongation bradycardia	36
Kir2.1 -/-	Kir2.1 deletion	FVB	I_{K1} eliminated	↑APD	Bradycardia	34, 42
Kir 2.2 -/-	Kir2.2 deletion	FVB	↓I_{K1}	None	None	34, 42
Kir3.4-/-	Exon 1 deletion	129Sv/J	I_{KACh} eliminated	None	Heart rate variability altered	24, 43
Kir 6.2 -/-	Insert at Xho I	129ySv	I_{KATP} eliminated	None	None	25, 37, 40
SUR1 -/-	Exon 1 deletion	129Sv/J	ND	None	None	32
SUR2A-/-	Not described	?	↓K_{ATP}	None	None	41
Kir6.2ΔNK185Q	Tg/N terminal deletion and point mutation	C57BL6	ATP sensitivity of I_{KATP} decreased	None	Heart rate decrease	20

[a]Tg, transgenic. [b]ND, not determined.

and suggested to be important in the generation of functional I_{Kr} channels *(70,71)*. Western blot analysis, however, has revealed that only the full-length ERG1 proteins in human (mouse and rat) heart *(95)*.

Co-expression of KCNQ1, the locus of mutations in LQT1 *(73)*, with minK produces very slowly activating, noninactivating K^+ currents *(76,77)*. These observations, together with biochemical data demonstrating that heterologously expressed KvLQT1 and minK associate *(76)*, have been interpreted as suggesting that minK co-assembles with KvLQT1 to form functional cardiac I_{Ks} channels *(76,77)*. Nevertheless, biochemical evidence demonstrating co-assembly of KvLQT1 and minK in heart has yet to be provided, and the stoichiometry of functional I_{Ks} channels has not been determined. In addition, the functional role of the N terminal splice variant of KvLQT1, which function as dominant negative *(96)*, in the generation of functional cardiac I_{Ks} channels remains to be determined.

Transgenic and targeted deletion strategies in mice have been exploited to define the molecular correlates of several of the other delayed rectifier K^+ currents expressed in the heart (Table 5). Roles for Kv1 and Kv2 α subunits in the generation of mouse ventricular $I_{K,slow}$, for example, were revealed with the demonstration that $I_{K,slow}$ is selectively attenuated in ventricular myocytes isolated from transgenic mice expressing either a truncated Kv1.1 or Kv2.1 α subunit, Kv1.1N206 or Kv2.1N216, that function as dominant negatives *(11,15)*. Further analyses revealed that there are actually two distinct components of wild-type mouse ventricular $I_{K,slow}$: $I_{K,slow1}$, which is sensitive to μ*M* concentrations of 4-aminopyridine and encoded by Kv1 (subunits and $I_{K,slow2}$, that is sensitive to TEA and encoded by Kv2 α subunits *(15)*. Consistent with this hypothesis, both $I_{K,slow1}$ and $I_{K,slow2}$ are eliminated in crossbred mice expressing both the Kv1 and the Kv2 subfamily-specific dominant-negative transgenes *(21)*. In addition, experiments completed on myocytes from mice with a targeted deletion Kv1.5 have shown that Kv1.5 encodes $I_{K,slow1}$ *(39)*. This finding, together with the results obtained on Kv1.4–/– myocytes *(26)*, in which $I_{to,s}$ is eliminated *(30,33)*, suggest that, in contrast to the Kv4 α subunits *(90)*, Kv1 α subunits do not associate in adult mouse ventricles *in situ*. Rather, functional Kv1 α subunit-encoded K^+ channels in mouse ventricular myocytes are homomeric, composed of Kv1.4 ($I_{to,s}$) or Kv1.5 ($I_{K,slow1}$).

Although neither I_{Ks} nor I_{Kr} is a prominent repolarizing K^+ current in adult mouse myocardium *(19,21,30,33,46)*, the functional consequences of the in vivo manipulation of the LQT K^+ channel genes, *KCNQ1*, *KCNH2* (ERG1), and *KCNE1*, encoding these channels *(13,18,22,27–29,31,38)* have been examined. In mice with targeted deletions in *KCNE1* (*KCNE1–/–*) or *KCNQ1* (*KCNQ1–/–*), the most striking phenotype is a *Shaker/Waltzer* behavior *(22,29,31,38)*, attributed to loss of transepithelial K^+ secretion and collapse of the spaces normally containing the K^+-rich endolymph in the inner ear *(22)*, that are reminiscent of the sensorineural deficits observed in Jervell and Lange-Nielsen syndrome patients *(97)*. In one line of *KCNE1–/–* mice *(22)*, baseline electrocardiograms (ECGs) are normal, although the mice display accentuated QT adaptation to heart rate *(98)*. In another *KCNE1–/–* line *(29)*, in contrast, both the baseline ECG and the QT adaptation to rate *(99)* are normal (Table 5). Phenotypic differences were also seen in *KCNQ1–/–* animals *(31,38)*. In exon1-*KCNQ1–/–* mice *(31)*, for example, heart rate, heart rate variability, ventricular repolarization, and AV conduction are normal (Table 5), whereas in exon2-*KCNQ1–/–* animals, QT prolongation, P and T wave abnormalities, and delayed AV conduction are observed *(38)*.

Transgenic mice expressing mutant ERG1 and KvLQT1 proteins in the heart have also been described *(13,18)*. ECG recordings from mice expressing a human ERG1 mutation *(13)* and whole cell recording from myocytes isolated from these animals were indistinguishable from wild-type controls (Table 5), consistent with the suggestion that I_{Kr} is not an important repolarizing K^+ current in adult mouse heart. The phenotype of mice expressing a splice variant of KvLQT1 that functions as a dominant negative, in contrast, is quite dramatic *(18)*. These animals exhibit sinus bradycardia, QT prolongation, abnormal P wave morphology, and intranodal conduction block (Table 5). In addition, electrophysiological recordings from ventricular myocytes from these animals revealed that action potentials are prolonged and that outward (I_{to}) and inward (I_{K1}) K^+ current densities are reduced *(18)*. In addition, the severity of the cardiac phenotype observed in these animal is directly correlated with the amount of the transgenic protein produced *(18)*, raising some concern that at least some of the effects seen in these animals reflect nonspecific effects of overexpression of the truncated protein in vivo.

9. MOLECULAR CORRELATES OF OTHER K+ CURRENTS IN THE MAMMALIAN MYOCARDIUM

Inwardly rectifying K^+ channels are encoded by a subfamily of inward rectifier K^+ (Kir) channel pore-forming α subunit genes, which encode proteins with two transmembrane domains (Fig. 2). Similar to Kv channels, Kir subunits assemble as tetramers to form K^+-selective pores (Fig. 2). The Kir2 α subunits encode the strong inwardly rectifying cardiac I_{K1} channels *(100)* and, several members of the Kir2 subfamily are expressed in the myocardium *(101)*. Direct insights into the role(s) of Kir 2 α subunits in the generation of ventricular I_{K1} channels was provided in studies completed on myocytes isolated from mice with a targeted deletion of the coding region of Kir2.1 (K2.1 –/–) or Kir 2.2 (Kir2.2 –/–) *(34,42)*. Although the Kir2.1–/– mice have cleft palate and die shortly after birth precluding electrophysiological studies on adult animals *(34)*, voltage–clamp recordings from newborn Kir2.1–/– ventricular myocytes reveal that I_{K1} is absent *(42)*. A slowly activating inward rectifier current, distinct from I_{K1}, however, is evident in Kir2.1–/– myocytes *(42)*. Voltage–clamp recordings from adult Kir2.2–/– ventricular myocytes reveal that I_{K1} is reduced (but not eliminated) with deletion of Kir2.2 *(42)*. Taken together, these results suggest that both Kir2.1 and Kir2.2 contribute to mouse ventricular I_{K1} channels and that functional cardiac I_{K1} channels are heteromeric.

In the heart, I_{KATP} channels play a role in myocardial ischemia and preconditioning *(102,103)*. In heterologous systems, I_{KATP} channels can be reconstituted by co-expression of Kir6.x subunits with ATP-binding cassette proteins that encode sulfonylurea receptors, SURx *(102)*. The essential role of the Kir6.2 subunit in the generation of cardiac I_{KATP} channels, however, was revealed with the demonstration that I_{KATP} channel activity is absent in ventricular myocytes isolated from mice with a targeted deletion of the Kir6.2 gene, Kir6.2–/– *(37,40)*. A role for SUR2 is suggested by the finding that I_{KATP} channel density is reduced in myocytes from SUR2–/– animals *(41)*, whereas there are no cardiac effects of deletion of SUR1 *(32)*. The properties of the I_{KATP} channels evident in SUR2–/– myocytes are similar to those produced on co-expression of Kir6.2 and SUR1 *(41)*, suggesting that SUR1 may also co-assemble with Kir6.2.

Although action potentials in wild-type and Kir6.2–/– myocytes are indistinguishable, the action potential shortening observed in wild-type cells during ischemia or metabolic blockade is abolished in the Kir6.2–/– cells *(40)*. Action potential durations are largely unaffected, however, in cells from transgenic animals expressing mutant I_{KATP} channels with markedly (40-fold) reduced ATP sensitivity *(20)*, suggesting that there are additional pathways that regulate cardiac I_{KATP} channel activity in vivo.

Although expression studies suggested that the ACh-regulated current, I_{KACh}, in atrial myocytes reflects heteromeric assembly of Kir3.1 and Kir3.4 *(104)*, the essential role of Kir3.4 was demonstrated in mice with a targeted deletion of the Kir3.4 gene, Kir3.4–/– *(24)*. Recordings from Kir3.4–/– atrial myocytes revealed the absence of (GTPγS-activated) I_{KACh} channels (Table 5) that are prominent in wild-type atrial cells. The observation that Kir3.1 is expressed in Kir3.4–/– atria further suggests that Kir3.1 cannot form functional I_{KACh} channels in the absence of Kir3.4 *(24)*. Although resting heart rates in Kir3.4–/– animals are not significantly different from those recorded in wild-type animals *(24)*, heart rate variability in response to stimulation of the vagus or A1 receptors is reduced (Table 5). Interestingly, atrial fibrillation is not observed in Kir3.4–/– animals challenged with carbachol *(43)*, confirming that I_{KACh} activation is a critical step in the cholinergic induction of atrial fibrillation.

A novel type of K$^+$ channel α subunit with four transmembrane spanning regions and two pore domains (Fig. 2) was identified with the cloning of TWIK-1 *(104)*. Both pore domains contribute to the formation of the K$^+$-selective pore and functional TWIK channels assemble as dimers *(105)*, rather than tetramers as is the case for other K$^+$ channels (Fig. 3). After the identification of TWIK-1, a number of four transmembrane, two-pore domain K$^+$ channel α subunit genes were identified, many of which are expressed in the myocardium (Table 3). Heterologous expression of the various two pore domain subunits gives rise to currents with distinct properties *(105)*, although the physiological roles of these subunits/channels in the myocardium remain to be determined. Both TREK-1 and TASK-1, however, are expressed in the heart and heterologous expression of either of these subunits gives rise to instantaneous, noninactivating K$^+$ currents that display little or no voltage dependence *(105)*. These properties have led to suggestions that these subunits contribute to "background" or "leak" currents in cardiac cells *(106)*. It is interesting to note that the properties of the currents produced on expression of TREK-1 or TASK-1 are similar to those of the current referred to as I_{Kp} identified in guinea pig ventricular myocytes *(107,108)*, as well as to I_{SS} in mouse *(46)*. Clearly, experiments focused on delineating the functional roles of two-pore domain-encoded K$^+$ channels in the mammalian myocardium are needed to test these hypotheses directly.

10. SUMMARY, CONCLUSION, AND FUTURE DIRECTIONS

Electrophysiological studies have clearly identified multiple types of voltage-gated inward and outward currents that contribute to shaping the waveforms of action potentials in the mammalian myocardium (Table 1). Outward K$^+$ currents are more numerous and diverse than inward currents and are largely responsible for the differences in action potential waveforms in different species and in different cardiac cell types. Molecular cloning has revealed an unexpected diversity of voltage-gated ion channel pore-forming α and accessory subunits that contribute to the formation of the various inward and outward current channels. Similar to the electrophysiological diversity of K^+ channels, the molecular analyses has revealed that multiple voltage-gated (Kv; Table 2) and inwardly rectifying (Kir; Table 3) K^+ channel pore-forming α and accessory (Table 4) subunits are expressed in the myocardium.

A variety of experimental approaches have been exploited to probe the relationship(s) between these subunits and functional cardiac K^+ channels, and important insights have been provided through the application of techniques that allow functional channel expression to be manipulated in vitro and in vivo. These efforts have led to the identification of the pore-forming α subunits contributing to the formation of most of the K^+ channels expressed in the mammalian heart. Exploiting dominant negative strategies in transgenic animals, for example, has revealed that distinct Kv subfamilies encode $I_{to,f}$ (Kv4; refs. *12,14,19,33*) and $I_{K,slow}$ (Kv1 and Kv2; refs. *11,15,19,21*) and has led to the identification of two, molecularly distinct (i.e., Kv1- and Kv2-encoded) components of $I_{K,slow}$ *(15,21)* that could not be distinguished unequivocally using conventional approaches *(46)*. The targeted deletion of individual α subunits has revealed the essential subunits required for $I_{to,s}$(Kv1.4; refs. *30,33*), $I_{K,slow1}$ (Kv1.5; ref. *39*), I_{K1} (Kir2.1; refs. *34,42*), I_{KACh} (Kir3.4; ref. *24*), and I_{KATP} (Kir6.2; refs. *25,40*). Based on the fact that the properties of the various K^+ currents in human cardiac myocytes are similar to those in the mouse, it seems reasonable to speculate that these Kv α subunits encode the corresponding K^+ channels in human heart. Although little is presently known about the roles of most of the Kv accessory subunits (Table 3) in the generation and/or the functioning of myocardial K^+ channels, it seems certain that this will be an important area for future studies and that the mouse will also be the model of choice for these studies.

The in vivo molecular genetic analysis of cardiac K^+ channels has also provided insights into the functional roles of these channels in the mouse myocardium. The results obtained with the Kv4.2W362F animals, for example, reveal a prominent role for $I_{to,f}$ in action potential repolarization in mouse atrial and ventricular myocytes *(12,14)*. This contrasts markedly with human, in which $I_{to,f}$ contributes primarily to phase 1 repolarization (Fig. 1). Although QT prolongation is seen in animals lacking $I_{to,f}$, action potential repolarization remains fast even in animals lacking $I_{to,f}$and $I_{to,s}$ *(12,33)*. The lack of pronounced electrophysiological effects of deletion of either *KCNE1 (22,29)* or *KCNQ1 (31,38)* is consistent with the suggestion that, in contrast with large mammals, I_{Ks} does not play a major role in repolarization in the adult mouse *(46)*. Although this clearly limits the usefulness of the mouse as an experimental model system to evaluate the efficacy of drugs targeting I_{Ks}, the absence of measurable I_{Ks} (and I_{Kr}) could make the mouse a suitable model to assay the pharmacological effects of putative I_{Ks} (and I_{Kr}) blockers on other cardiac outward and inward currents.

In several of the mouse models developed to date, remodeling of cardiac K^+ currents is evident (Table 5). In Kv4.2W362F animals, for example, $I_{to,s}$ is selectively upregulated in (right and left) ventricular myocytes that do not normally express this current *(33)*. In addition, no changes in $I_{K,slow}$ and/or I_{SS} densities are evident in Kv4.2W362F × Kv1.4–/– cells, which lack both $I_{to,f}$ and $I_{to,s}$ *(33)*. Remodeling is also seen in Kv1.1N216- and Kv2.1N206- expressing ventricular cells, in which one component of $I_{K,slow}$ is selectively attenuated *(11,15,21)*. In both cases, the density of the component of $I_{K,slow}$ remaining is increased, whereas $I_{to,f}$ and I_{SS} are unaffected *(11,15,21)*. These observations suggest that the mouse might be useful as a model system to probe the molecular mechanism underlying cardiac remodeling and to test the efficacy of drugs targeted to these mechanisms. In this context, it would clearly be of interest to control the level, as well perhaps as the timing, of transgene expression. It seems reasonable to suggest that in the future, transgenic and targeted deletion animals should be generated using inducible (and cardiac-specific) promoters to allow transgene expression levels to be tightly controlled *(109–111)*. This would make the mouse an important experimental tool in studies aimed at detailing the molecular mechanisms involved in controlling the expression and the properties of functional cardiac K^+ channels in the normal and diseased myocardium, as well as in the preclinical evaluation of pharmaceutical approaches to regulating these mechanisms.

REFERENCES

1. Nerbonne, J. M. and Kass, R. S. (2002) Physiology and molecular biology of ion channels contributing to ventricular repolarization, in *Cardiac Repolarization.Bridging Basic and Clinical Science* (I. B. Gussak, C. Antzelevitch, eds.), Humana Press, New Jersey, pp. 25–62.
2. Wetzel, G. T. and Klitzner, T. S. (1996) Developmental cardiac electrophysiology recent advances in cellular physiology. *Cardiovasc. Res.* **31,** E52–E60.
3. Nerbonne, J. M. (1998) Regulation of voltage-gated K^+ channel expression in the developing mammalian myocardium. *J. Neurobiol.* **37,**O 37–59.
4. Nabauer, M. and Kaab, S. (1998) Potassium channel down-regulation in heart failure. *Cardiovasc. Res.* **37,** 324–334.
5. Bolli, R. and Marban, E. (1999) Molecular and cellular mechanisms of myocardial stunning. *Physiol. Rev.* **79,** 609–634.
6. Tomaselli, G. F. and Marban, E. (1999) Electrophysiological remodeling in hypertrophy and heart failure. *Cardiovasc. Res.* **42,** 270–283.
7. Nerbonne, J. M. (2002) Molecular analysis of voltage-gated K^+ channel diversity and functioning in the mammalian heart, in *Handbook of Physiology, Vol. 1* (E. Page, H. A. Fozzard, and R. J. Solaro, eds.), Oxford Press, New York, pp. 568–594.
8. Nerbonne, J. M., Nichols, C. G., Schwarz, T. L, and Escande, D. (2001) Genetic manipulations of cardiac K+ channel function in mice. What have we learned and where do we go from here? *Circ. Res.* **89,** 944–956.
9. Antzelevitch, C. and Dumaine, R. (2002) Electrical heterogeneity in the heart: Physiological, pharmacological and clinical implications, in *Handbook of Physiology, Vol. 1* (E. Page, H. A. Fozzard, and R. J. Solaro, eds.), Oxford Press, New York, pp. 654–692.
10. Nerbonne, J. M. and Guo, W. (2002) Heterogeneous expression of voltage-gated potassium channels in the heart: Roles in normal excitation and arrhythmias. *J. Cardiovasc. Electrophysiol.* **13,** 406–409.
11. London, B., Jeron, A., Zhou, J., Buckett, P., Han, X., Mitchell, G. F., and Koren, G. (1998) Long QT and ventricular arrhythmias in transgenic mice expressing the N terminus and first transmembrane segment of a voltage-gated potassium channel. *Proc. Natl. Acad. Sci. USA* **95,** 2926–2931.
12. Barry, D. M., Xu, H., Schuessler, R. B., and Nerbonne, J. M. (1998) Functional knockout of the transient outward current, long-QT syndrome, and cardiac remodeling in mice expressing a dominant-negative Kv4 alpha subunit. *Circ. Res.* **83,** 560–567.
13. Babij, P., Askew, G. R., Nieuwenhuijsen, B., Su, C. M., Bridal, T. R., Jow, B., et al. (1998) Inhibition of cardiac delayed rectifier K+ current by overexpression of the long-QT syndrome HERG G628S mutation in transgenic mice. *Circ. Res.* **83,** 668–678.
14. Xu, H., Li, H., and Nerbonne, J. M. (1999) Elimination of the transient outward current and action potential prolongation in mouse atrial myocytes expressing a dominant negative Kv4 a subunit. *J. Physiol. (Lond).* **519,** 11–21.

15. Xu, H., Barry, D. M., Li, H., Brunet, S., Guo, W., and Nerbonne, J. M. (1999) Attenuation of the slow component of delayed rectification, action potential prolongation, and triggered activity in mice expressing a dominant-negative Kv2 alpha subunit. *Circ. Res.* **85,** 623–633.

16. Wickenden, A. D., Lee, P., Sah, R., Huang, Q., Fishman, G. I., and Backx, P. H. (1999) Targeted expression of a dominant negative Kv4.2 K+ channel subunit in mouse heart. *Circ. Res.* **85,** 1067–1076.

17. Jeron, A., Mitchell, G. F., Zhou, J., Murata, M., London, B., Buckett, P., et al. (2000) Inducible polymorphic ventricular tachyarrhythmias in a transgenic mouse model with a long Q-T phenotype. *Am. J. Physiol.* **278,** H1891–H1898.

18. Demolombe, S., Lande, G., Charpentier, F., van Roon, M. A., van den Hoff, M. J., Toumaniantz, G., et al. (2001) Transgenic mice overexpressing human KvLQT1 dominant-negative isoform. Part I: Phenotypic characterisation. *Cardiovasc. Res.* **50,** 314–327.

19. Brunner, M., Guo, W., Mitchell, G. F., Buckett, P. D., Nerbonne, J. M., and Koren, G. (2001) Characterization of mice with a combined suppression of I(to) and I(K,slow). *Am. J. Physiol.* **281,** H1201–H1209.

20. Koster, J. C., Knopp, A., Markova, K. P., Sha, Q., Enkvetchakul, D., Betsuyaku, T., et al. (2001). Tolerance for reduced ATP-sensitivity of KATP channels in transgenic mice. *Circ. Res.* **89,** 1022–1029.

21. Zhou, J., Kodirov, S., Murata, M., Buckett, P. D., Nerbonne, J. M., and Koren, G. (2003) Regional upregulation of Kv2.1-encoded current, $I_{K,slow2}$, in Kv1DN mice is abolished by crossbreeding with Kv2DN mice. *Am. J. Physiol.* **284,** H491–H500.

22. Vetter, D. E., Mann, J. R., Wangemann, P., Liu, J., McLaughlin, K. J., Lesage, F., et al. (1996) Inner ear defects induced by null mutation of the isk gene. *Neuron* **17,** 1251–1264.

23. London, B., Pan, X-H., Lewarchik, C. M., and Lee, C. S. (1998) QT interval prolongation and arrhythmias in heterozygous Merg1-targeted mice. *Circulation* **98,** I–56.

24. Wickman, K., Nemec, J., Gendler, S. J., and Clapham, D. E. (1998) Abnormal heart rate regulation in GIRK4 knockout mice. *Neuron* **20,** 103–114.

25. Miki, T., Nagashima, K., Tashiro, F., Kotake, K., Yoshitomi, H., Tamamoto, A., et al. (1998) Defective insulin secretion and enhanced insulin action in KATP channel-deficient mice. *Proc. Natl. Acad. Sci. USA* **95,** 10,402–10,406.

26. London, B., Wang, D. W., Hill, J. A., and Bennett, P. B. (1998) The transient outward current in mice lacking the potassium channel gene Kv1.4. *J. Physiol. (Lond.)* **509,** 171–182.

27. Charpentier, F., Merot, J., Riochet, D., Le Marec, H., and Escande, D. (1998) Adult KCNE1-knockout mice exhibit a mild cardiac cellular phenotype. *Biochem. Biophys. Res. Commun.* **29,** 251:806–810.

28. Drici, M. D., Arrighi, I., Chouabe, C., Mann, J. R., Lazdunski, M., Romey, G., et al. (1998) Involvement of IsK-associated K+ channel in heart rate control of repolarization in a murine engineered model of Jervell and Lange-Nielsen syndrome. *Circ. Res.* **83,** 95–102.

29. Kupershmidt, S., Yang, T., Anderson, M. E., Wessels, A., Niswender, K. D., Magnuson, M. A., and Roden, D. M. (1999) Replacement by homologous recombination of the minK gene with lacZ reveals restriction of minK expression to the mouse cardiac conduction system. *Circ. Res.* **84,** 146–152.

30. Guo, W., Xu, H., London, B., and Nerbonne, J. M. (1999) Molecular basis of transient outward K+ current diversity in mouse ventricular myocytes. *J. Physiol. (Lond.)* **521,** 587–599.

31. Lee, M. P., Ravenel, J. D., Hu, R. J., Lustig, L. R., Tomaselli, G., Berger, R. D., et al. (2000) Targeted disruption of the KvLQT1 gene causes deafness and gastric hyperplasia in mice. *J. Clin. Invest.* **106,** 1447–1455.

32. Seghers, V., Nakazaki, M., DeMayo, F., Aguilar-Bryan, L., and Bryan, J. (2000) SUR1 knockout mice. A model for K(ATP) channel-independent regulation of insulin secretion. *J. Biol. Chem.* **275,** 9270–9277.

33. Guo, W., Li, H., London, B., and Nerbonne, J. M. (2000). Functional consequences of elimination of $I_{to,f}$ and $I_{to,s}$: Early afterdepolarizations, atrioventricular block, and ventricular arrhythmia in mice lacking Kv1.4 and expressing a dominant-negative Kv4 alpha subunit. *Circ. Res.* **87** 73–79.

34. Zaritsky, J. J., Eckman, D. M., Wellman, G. C., Nelson, M. T., and Schwarz, T. L. (2000) Targeted disruption of Kir2.1 and Kir2.2 genes reveals the essential role of the inwardly rectifying K^+ current in K^+- mediated vasodilation. *Circ. Res.* **87,** 160–167.

35. Guo, W., Jung, W. E., Schwarz, T. L., and Nerbonne, J. M. (2000) $I_{to,f}$ is eliminated in mouse ventricular myocytes isolated from mice lacking Kv4.2; so what is the role of Kv4.3? [abstract] *Biophys. J.* **78,** 451a.

36. Lees-Miller, J. P., Swirp, S. L., Schade, K. J., Thorstad, K., Rancourt, D. E., and Duff, H. J. (2000) Selective knock-out of the ERG1 B potassium channel: A mouse model for the long QT syndrome. [abstract] *Circulation* **102,** II–285.

37. Li, R. A., Leppo, M., Miki, T., Seino, S., and Marban, E. (2000) Molecular basis of electrocardiographic ST-segment elevation. *Circ. Res.* **87,** 837–839.

38. Casimiro, M. C., Knollmann, B. C., Ebert, S. N., Vary, J. C. Jr., Greene, A. E., Franz, M. R., et al. (2001) Targeted disruption of the Kcnq1 gene produces a mouse model of Jervell and Lange- Nielsen Syndrome. *Proc. Natl. Acad. Sci. USA* **98,** 2526–2531.

39. London, B., Guo, W., Pan, X. H., Lee, J. S., Shusterman, V., Logothetis, D.A, et al. (2001) Targeted replacement of Kv1.5 in the mouse leads to loss of the 4-aminopyridine-sensitive component of $I_{K,slow}$ and resistance to drug-induced QT prolongation. *Circ. Res.* **88,** 940–946.

40. Suzuki, M., Li, R. A., Miki, T., Uemura, H., Sakamoto, N., Ohmoto-Sekine, Y., et al. (2001) Functional roles of cardiac and vascular ATP-sensitive potassium channels clarified by Kir6.2-knockout mice. *Circ. Res.* **88,** 570–577.

41. Pu, J., Wada, T., Valdivia, C., Chutkow, W. A., Burant, C. F., and Makielski, J. C. (2001) Evidence of KATP channels in native cardiac cells without SUR. [abstract] *Biophys. J.* **80,** 625a–626a.

42. Zaritsky, J. J., Redell, J. B., Tempel, B. L., and Schwarz, T. L. (2001) The consequences of disrupting cardiac inwardly rectifying K^+ current (I_{K1}) as revealed by the targeted deletion of the murine *Kir2.1* and *Kir2.2* genes. *J. Physiol. (Lond.)* **533,** 697–710.

43. Kovoor, P., Wickman, K., Maguire, C. T., Pu, W., Gehrmann, J., Berul, C. I., and Clapham, D. E. (2001) Evaluation of the role of I(KACh) in atrial fibrillation using a mouse knockout model. *J. Am. Coll. Cardiol.* **37,** 2136–2143.

44. Catterall, W. A. (2000) From ionic currents to molecular mechanisms: The structure and function of voltage-gated sodium channels. *Neuron* **26,** 13–25.

45. Sakmann, B. F., Spindler, A. J., Bryant, S. M., Linz, K. W., and Noble, D. (2000) Distribution of a persistent sodium current across the ventricular wall in guinea pigs. *Circ. Res.* **87,** 910–914.

46. Xu, H., Guo, W., and Nerbonne, J. M. (1999) Four kinetically distinct depolarization-activated K^+ currents in adult mouse ventricular myocytes. *J. Gen. Physiol.* **113,** 661–678.

47. Sanguinetti, M. C., Johnson, J. H., Hammerland, L. G., Kelbaugh, P. R., Volkmann, R. A., Saccomano, N. A., and Mueller, A. L. (1997) Heteropodatoxins: Peptides isolated from spider venom that block Kv4.2 potassium channels. *Mol. Pharmacol.* **51,** 491–498.

48. Liu, D. W. and Antzelevitch, C. (1995) Characteristics of the delayed rectifier current (IKr and IKs) in canine ventricular epicardial, midmyocardial, and endocardial myocytes. A weaker I_{Ks} contributes to the longer action potential of the M cell. *Circ. Res.* **76,** 351–365.

49. Li, G. R., Feng, J., Yue, L., Carrier, M., and Nattel, S. (1996) Evidence for two components of delayed rectifier K^+ current in human ventricular myocytes. *Circ. Res..* **78,** 689–696.

50. Fiset, C., Clark, R. B., Larsen, T. S., and Giles, W. R. (1997) A rapidly activating sustained K^+ current modulates repolarization and excitation-contraction coupling in adult mouse ventricle. *J. Physiol.* **504,** 557–563.

51. Zhou, J., Jeron, A., London, B., Han, X., and Koren, G. (1998) Characterization of a slowly inactivating outward current in adult mouse ventricular myocytes. *Circ. Res.* **83,** 806–814.

52. Nichols, C. G. and Lopatin, A. N. (1997) Inward rectifier potassium channels. *Annu. Rev. Physiol.* **59,** 171–191.

53. Noma, A. (1983) ATP-regulated K$^+$ channels in cardiac muscle. *Nature* **305,** 147–148.

54. Vandenberg, C. A. (1987) Inward rectification of a potassium channel in cardiac ventricular cells depends on internal magnesium ions. *Proc. Natl. Acad. Sci. USA* **84,** 2560–2564.

55. Lopatin, A. N., Makhina, E. N., and Nichols, C. G. (1994) Potassium channel block by cytoplasmic polyamines as the mechanism of intrinsic rectification. *Nature* **372,** 366–369.

56. Ficker, E., Taglialatela, M., Wible, B. A., Henley, C. M., and Brown, A. M. (1994) Spermine and spermidine as gating molecules for inward rectifier K$^+$ channels. *Science* **266,** 1068–1072.

57. Findlay, I. (1994) The ATP sensitive potassium channel of cardiac muscle and action potential shortening during metabolic stress. *Cardiovasc. Res.* **28,** 760–761.

58. Downey, J. M. (1992) Ischemic preconditioning: Nature's own cardio-protective intervention. *Trends Cardiovasc. Med.* **2,** 170–176.

59. Grover, G. J. and Garlid, K. D. (2000) ATP-sensitive potassium channels: A review of their cardioprotective pharmacology. *J. Mol. Cell. Cardiol.* **32,** 677–695.

60. Isom, L. L., De Jongh, K. S., and Catterall, W. A. (1994) Auxiliary subunits of voltage-gated ion channels. *Neuron.* **12,** 1183–1194.

61. Bennett, P. B., Yazawa, K., Makita, N., and George, A. L. Jr. (1995) Molecular mechanism for an inherited cardiac arrhthymia. *Nature* 376:683–685.

62. Balser, J. R. (2002) Inherited sodium channelopathies: Models for acquire arrhythmias? *Am. J. Physiol.* **282,** H1175–1180.

63. Nuyens, D., Stengl, M., Dugarmaa, S., Rossenbacker, T., Compernolle, V., Rudy, Y., et al. (2001) Abrupt rate accelerations or premature beats cause life-threatening arrhythmias in mice with long-QT3 syndrome. *Nat. Med.* **7,** 1021–1027.

64. Gurnett, C. A., De Waard, M., and Campbell, K. P. (1996) Dual function of the voltage-dependent Ca^{2+} channel alpha 2 delta subunit in current stimulation and subunit interaction. *Neuron.* **16,** 431–440.

65. Gurnett, C. A., Felix, R., and Campbell, K. P. (1997) Extracellular interaction of the voltage-dependent Ca^{2+} channel alpha2delta and alpha1 subunits. *J. Biol. Chem.* **272,** 18,508–18,512.

66. Warmke, J. W. and Ganetzky, B. (1994) A family of potassium channel genes related to eag in Drosophila and mammals. *Proc. Natl. Acad. Sci. USA* **91,** 3438–3442.

67. Curran, M. E., Splawski, I., Timothy, K. W., Vincent, G. M., Green, E. D., and Keating, M. T. (1995) A molecular basis for cardiac arrhythmia: HERG mutations cause long QT syndrome. *Cell* **80,** 795–803.

68. Sanguinetti, M. C., Jiang, C., Curran, M. E., and Keating, M. T. (1995) A mechanistic link between an inherited and an acquired cardiac arrhythmia: HERG encodes the I$_{Kr}$ potassium channel. *Cell* **81,** 299–307.

69. Trudeau, M. C., Warmke, J. W., Ganetzky, B., and Robertson, G. A. (1995) HERG, a human inward rectifier in the voltage-gated potassium channel family. *Science* **269,** 92–95.

70. Lees-Miller, J. P., Kondo, C., Wang, L., and Duff, H. J. (1997) Electrophysiological characterization of an alternatively processed ERG K$^+$ channel in mouse and human hearts. *Circ. Res.* **81,** 719–726.

71. London, B., Trudeau, M. C., Newton, K. P., Beyer, A. K., Copeland, N. G., Gilbert, D. J., et al. (1997) Two isoforms of the mouse ether-a-go-go-related gene coassemble to form channels with properties similar to the rapidly activating component of the cardiac delayed rectifier K$^+$ current. *Circ. Res.* **81,** 870–878.

72. Kupershmidt, S., Snyders, D. J., Raes, A., and Roden, D. M. (1998) A K$^+$ channel splice variant common in human heart lacks a C-terminal domain required for expression of rapidly activating delayed rectifier current. *J. Biol. Chem.* **273,** 27,231–27,235.

73. Wang, Q., Curran, M. E., Splawski, I., Burn, T. C., Milholland, J. M., VanRaay, T. J., et al. (1996) Positional cloning of a novel potassium channel gene: KVLQT1 mutations cause cardiac arrhythmias. *Nat. Genet.* **12,** 17–23.

74. Murai, T., Kakizuka, A., Takumi, T., Ohkubo, H., and Nakanishi, S. (1989) Molecular cloning and sequence analysis of human genomic DNA encoding a novel membrane protein which exhibits a slowly activating potassium channel activity. *Biochem. Biophys. Res. Commun.* **161,** 176–81.

75. Folander, K., Smith, J. S., Antanavage, J., Bennett, C., Stein, R. B., and Swanson, R. (1990) Cloning and expression of the delayed-rectifier IsK channel from neonatal rat heart and diethylstilbestrol-primed rat uterus. *Proc. Natl. Acad. Sci. USA* **87,** 2975–2979.

76. Barhanin, J., Lesage, F., Guillemare, E., Fink, M., Lazdunski, M., and Romey, G. (1996) K(V)LQT1 and lsK (minK) proteins associate to form the I$_{(Ks)}$ cardiac potassium current. *Nature* **384,** 78–80.

77. Sanguinetti, M. C., Curran, M. E., Zou, A., Shen, J., Spector, P. S., Atkinson, D. L., et al. (1996) Coassembly of KvLQT1 and minK (IsK) proteins to form cardiac I$_{(Ks)}$ potassium channel. *Nature* **384,** 80–83.

78. Abbott, G. W. and Goldstein, S. A. (1998) A superfamily of small potassium channel subunits: form and function of the MinK-related peptides (MiRPs). *Quart. Rev. Biophys.* **31,** 357–398.

79. Abbott, G. W., Sesti, F., Splawski, I., Buck, M. E., Lehmann, M. H., Timothy, K. W., et al. (1999) MiRP1 forms I$_{Kr}$ potassium channels with HERG and is associated with cardiac arrhythmia. *Cell* **97,** 175–187.

80. Abbott, G. W., Butler, M. H., Bendahhou, S., Dalakas, M. C., Ptacek, L. J., and Goldstein, S. A. (2001) MiRP2 forms potassium channels in skeletal muscle with Kv3.4 and is associated with periodic paralysis. *Cell* **104,** 217–231.

81. Zhang, M., Jiang, M., and Tseng, G. N. (2001) minK-related peptide 1 associates with Kv4.2 and modulates its gating function: Potential role as beta subunit of cardiac transient outward channel? *Circ. Res.* **88,** 1012–1019.

82. Rettig, J., Heinemann, S. H., Wunder, F., Lorra, C., Parcej, D. N., Dolly, J. O., and Pongs, O. (1994) Inactivation properties of voltage-gated K$^+$ channels altered by presence of beta-subunit. *Nature* **369,** 289–294.

83. England, S. K., Uebele, V. N., Shear, H., Kodali, J., Bennett, P. B., and Tamkun, M. M. (1995) Characterization of a voltage-gated K$^+$ channel beta subunit expressed in human heart. *Proc. Natl. Acad. Sci. USA* **92,** 6309–6313.

84. Shi, G., Nakahira, K., Hammond, S., Rhodes, K. J., Schechter, L. E., and Trimmer, J. S. (1996) Beta subunits promote K$^+$ channel surface expression through effects early in biosynthesis. *Neuron* **16,** 843–852.

85. Accili, E. A., Kiehn, J., Yang, Q., Wang, Z., Brown, A. M., and Wible, B. A. (1997) Separable Kvbeta subunit domains alter expression and gating of potassium channels. *J. Biol. Chem.* **272,** 25,824–25,831.

86. Wible, B. A., Yang, Q., Kuryshev, Y. A., Accili, E. A., and Brown, A. M. (1998) Cloning and expression of a novel K$^+$ channel regulatory protein, KChAP. *J. Biol. Chem.* **273,** 11,745–11,751.

87. An, W. F., Bowlby, M. R., Betty, M., Cao, J., Ling, H. P., Mendoza, G., et al. (2000) Modulation of A-type potassium channels by a family of calcium sensors. *Nature* **403,** 553–556.

88. Burgoyne, R. D. and Weiss, J. L. (2001) The neuronal calcium sensor family of Ca^{2+}-binding proteins. *Biochem. J.* **353,** 1–12.

89. Rosati, B., Pan, Z., Lypen, S., Wang, H. S., Cohen, I., Dixon, J. E., et al. (2001) Regulation of KChIP2 potassium channel beta subunit gene expression underlies the gradient of transient outward current in canine and human ventricle. *J. Physiol.* **533,** 119–125.

90. Guo, W., Li, H., Aimond, F., Johns, D. C., Rhodes, K. J., Trimmer, J. S., and Nerbonne, J. M. (2002) Role of heteromultimers in the generation of myocardial transient outward K+ currents. *Circ. Res.* **90,** 586–593.

91. Dixon, J. E., Shi, W., Wang, H. S., McDonald, C., Yu, H., Wymore, R. S., et al. (1996). Role of the Kv4.3 K+ channel in ventricular muscle. A molecular correlate for the transient outward current. *Circ. Res.* **79,** 659–668.

92. Kong, W., Po, S., Yamagishi, T., Ashen, M. D., Stetten, G., and Tomaselli, G. F. (1998) Isolation and characterization of the human gene encoding Ito: Further diversity by alternative mRNA splicing. *Am. J. Physiol.* **275,** H1963–H1970.

93. Yang, T., Kupershmidt, S., and Roden, D. M. (1995) Anti-minK antisense decreases the amplitude of the rapidly activating cardiac delayed rectifier K+ current. *Circ. Res.* **77,** 1246–1253.

94. McDonald, T. V., Yu, Z., Ming, Z., et al. (1997) A minK-HERG complex regulates the cardiac potassium current I(Kr). *Nature* **388,** 289–292.

95. Pond, A. L., Scheve, B. K., Benedict, A. T., Petrecca, K., Van Wagoner, D. R., Shrier, A., et al. (2000) Expression of distinct ERG proteins in rat, mouse, and human heart. Relation to functional I(Kr) channels. *J. Biol. Chem.* **275,** 5997–6006.

96. Jiang, M., Tseng-Crank, J., and Tseng, G. N. (1997) Suppression of slow delayed rectifier current by a truncated isoform of KvLQT1 cloned from normal human heart. *J. Biol. Chem.* **272,** 24,109–24,112.

97. Neyroud, N., Tesson, F., Denjoy, I., Leibovici, M., Donger, C., Barhanin, J., et al. (1997) A novel mutation in the potassium channel gene KVLQT1 causes the Jervell and Lange-Nielsen cardioauditory syndrome. *Nat. Genet.* **15,** 186–189.

98. Demolombe, S., Franco, D., de Boer, P., Kuperschmidt, S., Roden, D., Pereon, Y., et al. (2001) Differential expression of KvLQT1 and its regulator IsK in mouse epithelia. *Am. J. Physiol.* **280,** C359–C372.

99. Lande, G., Kyndt, F., Baro, I., Chabannes, D., Boisseau, P., Pony, J. C., et al. (2001) Dynamic analysis of the QT interval in long QT1 syndrome patients with a normal phenotype. *Eur. Heart J.* **22,** 410–422.

100. Takahashi, N., Morishige, K., Jahangir, A., Yamada, M., Findlay, I., Koyama, H., et al. (1994) Molecular cloning and functional expression of cDNA encoding a second class of inward rectifier potassium channels in the mouse brain. *J. Biol. Chem.* **269,** 23,274–23,279.

101. Liu, G. X., Derst, C., Schlichthorl, G., Heined, S., Seebohm, G., Bruggemann, A., et al. (2001) Comparison of cloned Kir2 channels with native inward rectifier K+ channels from guinea-pig cardiomyocytes. *J. Physiol.* **532,** 115–126.

102. Babenko, A. P., Aguilar-Bryan, L., and Bryan, J. (1998) A view of sur/KIR6.X, KATP channels. *Annu. Rev. Physiol.* **60,** 667–87.

103. Pountney, D. J., Sun, Z. Q., Porter, L. M., Nitabach, M. N., Nakamura, T. Y., Holmes, D., et al. (2001) Is the molecular composition of K(ATP) channels more complex than originally thought? *J. Mol. Cell Cardiol.* **33,** 1541–1546.

104. Lesage, F., Guillemare, E., Fink, M., Duprat, F., Lazdunski, M., Romey, G., and Barhanin, J. (1996) TWIK-1, a ubiquitous human weakly inward rectifying K+ channel with a novel structure. *EMBO J.* **15,** 1004–1011.

105. Lesage, F. and Lazdunski, M. (1999) Potassium channels with two P domains, in *Current Topics in Membranes* (L. Y. Jan, ed), Academic Press, San Diego, CA, pp. 199–222.

106. Goldstein, S. A., Bockenhauer, D., O'Kelly, I., and Zilberberg, N. (2001) Potassium leak channels and the KCNK family of two-P-domain subunits. *Nat. Rev. Neurosci.* **2,** 175–184.

107. Yue, D. T. and Marban, E. (1988) A novel cardiac potassium channel that is active and conductive at depolarized potentials. *Pflugers Arch.* **413,** 127–133.

108. Backx, P. H. and Marban, E. (1993) Background potassium current active during the plateau of the action potential in guinea pig ventricular myocytes. *Circ. Res.* **72,** 890–900.

109. Yu, Z., Redfern, C. S., and Fishman, G. I. (1996) Conditional transgene expression in the heart. *Circ. Res.* **79,** 691–697.

110. Redfern, C. H., Degtyarev, M. Y., Kwa, A. T., Salomonis, N., Cotte, N., Nanevicz, T., et al. (2000) Conditional expression of a Gi-coupled receptor causes ventricular conduction delay and a lethal cardiomyopathy. *Proc. Natl. Acad. Sci. USA* **97,** 4826–4831.

111. Chien, K. R. (2001) To Cre or not to Cre: The next generation of mouse models of human cardiac diseases. *Circ. Res.* **88,** 546–549.

14

Delayed Protection of the Myocardium
A Novel Therapeutic Window for Cardiac Drug Development

László Szekeres and James Parratt

CONTENTS

1. INTRODUCTION

It is known that the administration of drugs can relieve or prevent many of the consequences of myocardial ischemia; this is the basis for the current therapy of angina of effort by, for example, organic nitrites and nitrates and β adrenoceptor-blocking drugs. These are effective in the short term; protection is lost soon after the cessation of the treatment. More recently the emphasis, in experimental situations, of alleviating the consequences of ischaemia in a variety of organs has shifted to the prolonged and delayed protection by adaptation induced by a variety of stimuli, many of which involve some form of cellular stress. It is well known that adaptation to changing conditions is a basic function of living organisms that enables the individual and the species to survive. This phenomenon is effective in different organs and organ systems, and a variety of mechanisms are able to induce it. Delayed cardioprotection induced by adaptation appears to be a universal response. Although some metabolic changes underlie all types of adaptive mechanisms, the metabolic adaptation of an organ to stressful situations is characterized by the predominance of metabolic changes even in the absence of other adaptive alterations.

The aim of the present review is to summarize this delayed cellular adaptation, stressing in particular the heart and especially those procedures that have clinical relevance,

From: *Cardiac Drug Development Guide*
Edited by: M. K. Pugsley © Humana Press Inc., Totowa, NJ

such as cardiac pacing, exercise, and the administration of various substances that evoke delayed and prolonged protection of the myocardium.

2. STAGES IN THE HISTORY OF DELAYED CARDIAC PROTECTION BY ADAPTATION; DELAYED PROTECTION BY CHEMICAL SUBSTANCES

Historically, the use of chemical substances represents the earliest examples of delayed and prolonged protection of the heart against ischemia or chemically induced cellular damage. For example, studies in rats showed that myocardial resistance develops against toxic doses of isoprenaline if they were pretreated with smaller doses of isoprenaline *(1–3)* and also that coronary artery ligation protects against the toxic effects of isoprenaline *(4)*. This phenomenon, referred to by Rona as myocardial resistance or protection *(1)*, was not associated with β adrenoceptor downregulation and lasted several days or even weeks *(5)*. Poupa and his colleagues *(6)* also demonstrated that catecholamine administration resulted in delayed protection of the heart against both anoxia and ischemia, but only in doses that themselves produced necrotic changes *(5)*.

In 1984, Szekeres et al. *(7,8)* showed that prostacyclin, or its stable analog 7-oxo-PgI$_2$, in doses that produced only transient and fully reversible falls in blood pressure and only a moderate inhibition of platelet aggregation, could induce a late-appearing, prolonged cardiac protection and could attenuate the harmful influence of a subsequent intensive stimulus, even 24–48 h after treatment *(7,8)*. These experiments demonstrated for the first time that a single drug-induced noninjurious stimulus (a minor stress) may trigger adaptive processes in the heart, which protected it against the consequences of a severe ischemic insult.

In 1993, it was shown independently in three laboratories, using different forms of stress to induce a cardioprotective adaptive process, that protection resulting from frequency loading *(9)*, repeated brief coronary occlusions *(10)*, and heat stress *(11)* was evident 24–48 h later. A prerequisite of such delayed cardioprotection is that the intensity of the inducing stress should reach a certain threshold level *(12)*. The event became known as the second window phenomenon *(13)*.

In 1994 Parratt's group *(14)* showed that hearts removed from rats previously treated with low doses of *Escherichia coli* endotoxin and then perfused and subjected to coronary artery occlusion several hours later had a lower incidence of ventricular fibrillation during ischemia than hearts taken from vehicle-treated rats. Thus, nontoxic doses of endotoxin are also able to evoke delayed cardioprotection

2.1. Delayed Cardiac Protection by Catecholamines

As mentioned above, the earliest observations of delayed cardiac protection followed isoprenaline administration *(1–3,5)*. Later, Beckman and his colleagues *(15)* showed that dogs that developed long-term tolerance to intravenously administered adrenaline were also resistant to coronary embolization with microspheres. For example, only one of 14 tolerant dogs fibrillated on coronary artery occlusion compared with 11 of 32 in the control group; all the deaths occurred early, that is, within the first 15 min of occlusion. More recently, the administration of noradrenaline to rats 24 h, but not 4 h, before ischemia induced by coronary artery occlusion resulted in enhanced recovery of contractile function in isolated hearts subjected to ischemia and reperfusion *(16)* and also in a markedly reduced arrhythmia severity *(17)*. Under these conditions, there were marked increases in c-*fos* and c-*jun* mRNA levels and in heat shock protein (hsp) 70 gene expression *(16)*. This β adrenoceptor-mediated cardiac oncogene and stress protein gene expression was believed to be responsible for the delayed protection.

There is evidence that not only α but also β adrenoceptor stimulation is able to induce delayed cardiac protection. In chronically instrumented conscious rabbits, repeated β adrenergic stress by low doses of isoprenaline evoked cardiac adaptive processes, resulting in a significant reduction of those harmful ischemic changes that resulted from rapid pacing 24 and 48 h later *(18)*. It was also found that at least five intravenous administrations of isoprenaline, repeated at 10-min intervals, were necessary to induce this delayed cardioprotection *(18)*. These results suggest that a well-defined threshold level of this particular stress is needed to trigger induction of the metabolic changes that lead to delayed and long-term cardiac adaptation to stress.

2.2. Delayed Cardioprotection by Prostacyclin and Stable Analogs

In the early 1980s, the effects were described of a stable derivative of prostacyclin, 7-oxo-prostacyclin (7-oxo-PgI$_2$). As mentioned previously, administration of low doses of prostacyclin or 7-oxo-PgI$_2$ to a variety of species (dogs, rabbits, rats) resulted in a late appearing and long-lasting cardioprotection (reviewed by Szekeres in ref. *12*) that had a time course similar to that described several years later for the delayed effects of ischemic preconditioning and of cardiac pacing *(9,10)*.

This protection of the heart was manifested in a number of ways. It was shown that this more prolonged form of cardiac adaptation to stress (delayed cardioprotection) protects for 24–48 h against the consequences of a more severe stress, such as myocardial ischemia *(8)*. These consequences included the myocardial loss of ATP, creatine phosphokinase (CP), and K$^+$, increased lactate *(19,21)* and accumulation of Na$^+$ and Ca^{2+} *(19,20)*, as well as the early ultrastructural changes that are secondary to ischemia and reperfusion *(19–21)* and early *(22–24)* and late postocclusion and reperfusion arrhythmias *(25,26)*. This form of delayed cardioprotection also increased tolerance to isoprenaline-induced tachycardia *(19)* and to the toxic effects of cardiac glycosides *(27–29)*. For example, in hearts removed from rats given 50 µg/kg of 7-oxo-PgI$_2$ 48 h previously and then perfused and subjected to ischemia and reperfusion, there was enhanced recovery of contractile function and a reduced accumulation of lactate *(21)*. Particularly interesting were the effects on coronary occlusion-induced ischemia and reperfusion-induced ventricular arrhythmias in dogs *(23,25)*. The maximum protection was at 48 h, although there was some evidence of protection even 72 h after the injection. The protection against arrhythmias seemed to result from reduced ischemia severity (less pronounced ST-segment changes) after coronary artery occlusion as well as to a prolongation of action potential duration and an increase in effective refractory period *(30,31)*.

There has been a good deal of interest lately in the possibility of renewing, or prolonging, cardiac protection against the consequences of coronary artery occlusion by repeating the preconditioning stimulus at times when the protection afforded by the initial stimulus has faded. Udvary et al. *(25)* were the first to show that the late protection resulting from 7-oxo-PgI$_2$ against the consequences of coronary artery occlusion (epicardial ST-segment elevation, postischemic ventricular, and reperfusion arrhythmias) could be prolonged if the initial dose was renewed by a maintenance dose

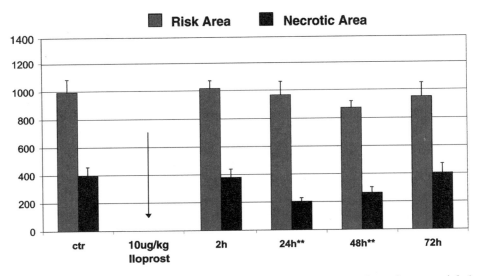

Fig. 1. Effect of the stable prostacyclin analog iloprost on extension of area at risk (white bars) and necrotic area (black bars) of the myocardium after 25-min coronary ligation and 90-min reperfusion in rabbits at different times after drug administration. Values are mean of six animals ± SEM. *$p < 0.001$ vs control. Adapted from ref. *98*.

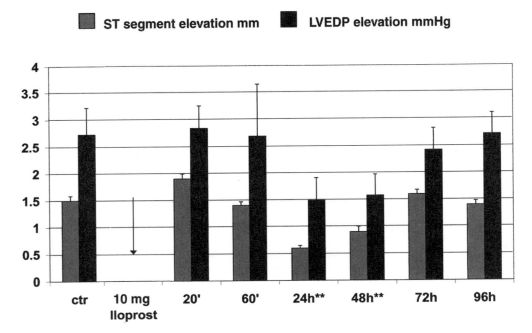

Fig. 2. Effect of the stable prostacyclin analog iloprost on ST-segment elevation (white bars) recorded from an endocardial electrogram, and on the increase of left ventricular end-diastolic pressure (black bars) induced by cardiac pacing (500 beats/min for 5 min) in the chronically instrumented conscious rabbit. Values are mean of six animals ± SEM. *$p < 0.001$ vs control. Adapted from ref. *98*.

of 25 µg/kg every third day. In these experiments, the protection was present even 2 wk later. Theoretically, this late protection could be prolonged indefinitely.

This is an impressive array of beneficial effects. There was morphological protection (also seen with another prostacyclin analog, iloprost, Fig. 1), metabolic protection, (Fig. 2), electrophysiological changes supporting suppression of life-threatening ventricular arrhythmias, and an enhanced recovery of contractile function following a period of ischemia and reperfusion.

An exploration of possible mechanisms has shown that 7-oxo-PgI$_2$ induces a delayed, indirect antiadrenergic and cytoprotective effect on the myocardium, the mechanism of which is still unclear. To demonstrate that a single dose of 7-oxo-PgI$_2$ (50 µg/kg i.m.) given 48 h previously attenuates isoprenaline inotropic responses and the subsequent accumulation of cyclic adenosine monophosphate (cAMP), isolated hearts of pretreated rats were perfused in the Langendorff mode with and without isoprenaline. The late antiadrenergic effects of the drug were manifested by a significant attenuation in the elevation of myocardial cAMP levels as well as in contractile force development. This effect was not caused by changes in cAMP generation because there were identical β_1 adrenoceptor densities and affinities (as calculated from [^{3}H]-CGP binding studies), Gi and Gs alpha protein patterns (as shown by Western blots), as well as adenylyl cyclase activity measurements in the hearts studied. The antiadrenergic potency of 7-oxo-PgI$_2$, however, was found to be related to a significant rise in cyclic nucleotide hydrolysis by phosphodiesterase (PDE). Using fast-performance liquid chromatographic separation for the PDE isoforms, a significant increase in the activity of PDE isoforms I and IV was found in the solubilized fraction of cardiac membranes in comparison with untreated controls; PDE IV activity was also increased in the cytosolic fraction. The hypothesis that the delayed antiadrenergic effect of 7-oxo-PgI$_2$ is initiated by an induction and accelerated synthesis of PDE I and IV in the heart is underlined by the fact that cycloheximide suppressed completely both the rise in PDE activities and the antiadrenergic effects studied. It was suggested that an inducible predominance of cAMP degradation over its generation might be of relevance in processes related to heart protection *(32)*. In another study *(33)*, 50 µg/kg 7-oxo-PgI$_2$ administered intramuscularly significantly stimulated the activity of Na$^+$/K$^+$ ATPase in rat heart sarcolemma 24 and 48 h after application. These results show that protein synthesis is involved in the mechanism of the increase in enzyme activity.

2.3. Delayed Cardiac Protection by Bacterial Endotoxin and by Nontoxic Derivatives of Lipid A

Under normal circumstances and in all species (although there is a marked difference in sensitivity), the administration of bacterial endotoxin results in severe respiratory, hemodynamic, and hematologic changes that ultimately result in death. These changes result from the release of a large number of mediators (reviewed recently in ref. *34*), leading to pulmonary dysfunction, elevated body temperature, and reduced tissue perfusion, terminating in a shock-like state and death. The sustained decrease in vascular resistance that precedes shock is characterized by a reduced responsiveness to sympathetic nerve stimulation and to exogenous catecholamines. It is the result of the induction, by cytokines released by endotoxin, of an enzyme (inducable nitric oxide synthase, iNOS) capable of producing large amounts of nitric oxide within the vascular wall and the heart (reviewed by Parratt and Stoclet in ref. *35*).

However, small doses of endotoxin result in an increased tolerance to the toxic effects of the subsequent administration of much larger doses of endotoxin. This may be related to the paradoxical finding that sublethal doses of endotoxin result in a delayed protection of the heart against other forms of injury, such as ischemia. This phenomenon is known as cross-tolerance. As with the cardioprotective effects of ischemic preconditioning (*see* Section 3.), bacterial endotoxin protects the heart against ischemia-induced cellular necrosis *(36)*, the depressed myocardial contractility that follows a period of ischemia and reperfusion *(37,38)*, and the life-threatening arrhythmias that occur both during ischemia and reperfusion *(14,36)*. For example, hearts removed from rats previously given *E. coli* endotoxin and then perfused through the aorta and subjected to coronary artery occlusion had a lower incidence of ventricular fibrillation during ischemia than those taken from vehicle-treated rats *(14)*. This protection against ischemia-induced arrhythmias is also seen when the coronary artery is occluded in vivo several hours after endotoxin administration *(36)*, and the time course (Fig. 3) closely follows that for inducing NOS. The most pronounced effect is seen when the coronary artery is occluded 8 h after endotoxin administration, although it is still pronounced at 24 h. It is lost if ischemia is induced 48 h after administration. All indices of arrhythmia severity are reduced (ventricular fibrillation, ventricular tachycardia, ventricular ectopic, i.e., premature beats), and the protection against ventricular fibrillation is particularly remarkable. Thus, no rat given endotoxin 4 or 8 h before coronary artery occlusion fibrillated or died during the occlusion period *(36)*. Both the antiarrhythmic effects of endotoxin and its ability to reduce myocardial infarct size were abolished by the prior administration of dexamethasone *(14,36)*. This suggests that the protection is to the result of the induction of, for example, cyclooxygenase-2 (COX-2) or NOS. To further explore which pathways are primarily involved, experiments were performed in which selective inhibition of these pathways was attempted with, for example, aminoguanidine (fairly selective for iNOS), indomethacin (which inhibits both COX-1 and COX-2, and a combination of L-nitroarginine and indomethacin, which should inhibit both NOS and COX. None of these procedures was as effective as dexamethasone at counteracting the cardioprotection afforded by endotoxin, although a combination of L-nitro-arginine methyl ester and indomethacin, albeit in very high doses, was almost as effective. The conclusion reached was that there may be other substances, apart from those derived from COX (perhaps prostacyclin) and the NOS pathway that participates in the cardioprotection induced by bacterial endotoxin.

There have been a number of interesting attempts to modify the active lipid A component of the endotoxin molecule to detoxify it and yet retain some other helpful properties of bacterial lipopolysaccharide, for example, its ability to regress tumors. These attempts have been successful. For example, monophosphoryl lipid A *(39,40)*, which differs structurally from lipid A by the absence of a phosphoester at the reducing end of the diglucosamine residue, is about a thousand times less toxic than the parent endotoxin molecule yet retains an ability to induce tolerance to endotoxin itself and to regress tumors. Monophosphoryl lipid A also retains the anti-ischemic and cardioprotective properties of bacterial endotoxin. Thus, it reduces myocardial ischemic damage in dogs *(41)*, rabbits *(42)*, and rats *(43)* and also markedly reduces arrhythmia severity after coronary artery occlusion in dogs *(44)* and rats *(43)*. This is illustrated for a canine model of myocardial ischemia and reperfusion in Fig. 4.

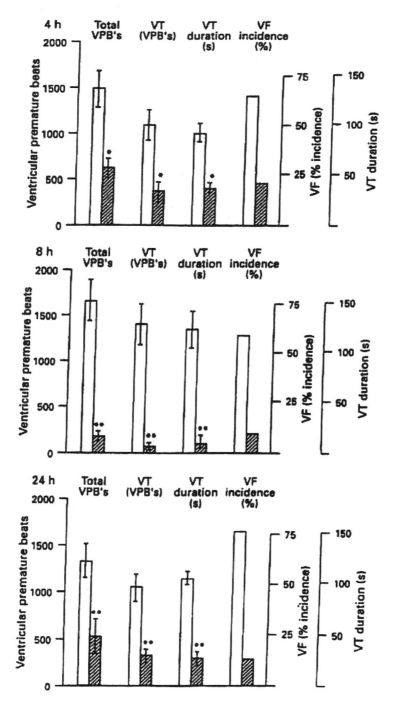

Fig. 3. The time course of the antiarrhythmic effects of bacterial endotoxin in rats. The animals were sacrificed and the hearts removed at different times after endotoxin administration and were perfused by the Langendorff technique. Arrhythmias were assessed after left coronary artery occlusion. The time course follows almost precisely that for the induction of nitric oxide synthase by endotoxin. Reproduced from ref. *36* with permission from Nature Publishing Group.

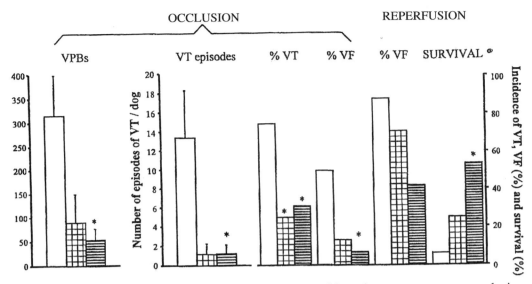

Fig. 4. Ventricular arrhythmias in anesthetized dogs subjected to coronary artery occlusion after treatment with monophosphoryl lipid A 10 µg/kg (shaded histograms), 100 µg/kg (vertically shaded histograms), or the appropriate vehicle (open histograms). VPBs are the total number of ventricular premature beats during the occlusion period. VT, ventricular tachycardia; VF, ventricular fibrillation. Also shown is the survival from the combined ischemia–reperfusion insult. *$p < 0.05$ compared with the vehicle controls. Reprinted from ref. *44* with permission from Elsevier Science.

We do not yet know whether the cardioprotection afforded by monophosphoryl lipid A is dexamethasone sensitive as the cardioprotection by endotoxin certainly is. However, the most likely explanation for the mechanism of this protection is the induction of enzymes capable of producing so-called endogenous myocardial protective substances *(45)*, such as nitric oxide and prostacyclin. In our own studies with monophosphoryl lipid A in a canine model of ischemia and reperfusion, we were unable to demonstrate the presence of iNOS on the day after the administration of the lipid A derivative, a time when there was marked protection against ischemia-induced ventricular arrhythmias. However, Zhao et al. *(46)* have reported augmented iNOS activity in the hearts of rabbits treated with monophosphoryl lipid A and then subjected to coronary artery occlusion; the levels were elevated, although not markedly so, after ischemia but not in the normally perfused left ventricular wall. This is perhaps surprising; one would expect, as with endotoxin, elevated iNOS levels of activity prior to ischemia. In support of a possible role of iNOS in mediating the protective effects of monophosphoryl lipid A was the finding that aminoguanidine, which is fairly selective for iNOS, prevented the infarct-limiting effect of monophosphoryl lipid A in the rabbit model when given 1 h before ischaemia *(46)*. The hypothesis for the mechanism of action would then be that there is an increased generation of nitric oxide during ischemia in animals treated with monophosphoryl lipid A and that this would open K_{ATP} channels (there is direct evidence, using patch–clamp techniques, that nitric oxide enhances cardiomyocyte K_{ATP} channel activity) and it is this opening of K_{ATP} channels that mediates the cardioprotection. There is evidence that drugs that block K_{ATP} channels, such as glibenclamide, reverse the ability of monophosphoryl lipid A to reduce myocardial infarct size *(47)*. There are thus close similarities between the effects of ischemic preconditioning *(see* Section 5.) and those of monophosphoryl lipid A in reducing myocardial ischemic damage.

Both involve the generation of endogenous myocardial protective substances leading ultimately, perhaps through protein kinase C translocation, to the opening of K_{ATP} channels, almost certainly in mitochondria. However, this mechanism is unlikely to explain the pronounced antiarrhythmic effects of monophosphoryl lipid A because, in the canine model, it is doubtful if these channels, at least those in the sarcolemma, are involved in the antiarrhythmic effects of ischemic preconditioning *(48)*.

3. DELAYED ADAPTATION OF THE HEART BY ISCHEMIA

When a coronary artery is occluded the consequences, which may well be life-threatening, include the generation of ventricular arrhythmias, depressed cardiac function, and ultimately necrotic cell death. Murry and his colleagues *(49)* showed that these effects of ischemia can be markedly reduced by a process of cardiac adaptation termed ischemic preconditioning. This means that the effects of a prolonged period of myocardial ischemia can be reduced by brief periods of the same ischemic stimulus given some time earlier. For example, one or more brief (e.g., 5 min) periods of coronary artery occlusion can adapt the heart to a more prolonged period of ischemia (e.g., 1 h). Under these conditions, the detrimental effects of prolonged ischemia are much less marked than in virgin (unadapted) myocardium. The area and severity of ischemic damage (infarct size) and the severity of ventricular arrhythmias are much reduced by ischemic preconditioning. This subject has been reviewed many times (e.g., refs. *50,51*).

In the early studies on ischemic preconditioning, it was shown that brief periods of coronary occlusion (or global hypoxia or anoxia in isolated hearts) protected the heart in the short term, that is, the protective effects were seen if the interval between the preconditioning stimulus and the period of prolonged ischemia was not too long. However, if the time interval between the stimulus and the prolonged occlusion was increased (e.g., to 1 h) most of the protection was lost. It seemed, therefore, that the myocardium was adapted to ischemia only for a short period of time. Somewhat surprisingly, the Japanese group of Kuzuya et al. *(10)* examined the effects of brief periods of coronary occlusion on myocardial infarct size when the reperfusion interval was increased to several hours. They found that four brief repeated episodes of 5-min coronary artery occlusion resulted in a reduction in infarct size both when the coronary artery was reoccluded immediately after the preconditioning stimulus and also 24 h later; no protection was observed when the artery was reoccluded 3 or 12 h after the preconditioning stimulus. These experiments demonstrated, for the first time, that there are two phases of myocardial protection elicited by brief periods of ischemia. There is thus what Yellon and his colleagues subsequently described as a second window of protection *(11,52)* and recently reviewed in ref. *53*. This is illustrated from the studies of the Kuzuya et al. *(10)* in Fig. 5. It also seems that the antiarrhythmic effects of ischemic preconditioning, which are marked when a coronary artery is occluded soon after the preconditioning stimulus *(54–58)* and which then fade with a similar time course to that described for infarct size reduction, returns 20–24 h after the preconditioning stimulus *(59)*.

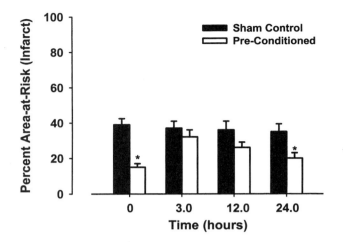

Fig. 5. Depicts the time interval between sublethal and sustained ischemia in relation to the infarcted area (expressed as a percentage of the area-at-risk) in sham control (open columns) and preconditioned (filled columns) dogs. All hearts were subjected to 90 min of regional ischemia followed by 5 h of reperfusion. Data values are the means ± SEM for *n* = 10 animals per group. Note that there is a marked reduction in infarct area when the prolonged occlusion is induced immediately after the preconditioning protocol (*see* 0 h data), but this protection is lacking when there is either a 3- or 12-h interval between the preconditioning stimulus and the period of prolonged occlusion. Examination of the 24-h data shows that the observed protection returns, which corresponds to the delayed or second window of myocardial protection. **p* < 0.05 when data are compared with sham controls. Adapted from ref. *10*.

4. DELAYED MYOCARDIAL PROTECTION BY CARDIAC PACING

In 1991 Vegh et al. *(60)* described the protective effects against coronary artery occlusion induced arrhythmias when the preconditioning stimulus was not brief and complete periods of occlusion but brief periods of rapid cardiac pacing. It is likely, as with pacing-induced cardiac failure, that this degree of heart rate increase (300 beats/min in the studies of Vegh et al., ref. *20*; 220 beats/min in the later studies of Kaszala et al., ref. *59*) is sufficient to cause myocardial ischemia. The evidence comes from recordings from the endocardium of the right ventricle immediately after cessation of the pacing stimulus, when there is an increase in ST-segment elevation, and from recordings using needle electrodes in the subendocardium of the left ventricle, which demonstrate more marked post-pacing electrocardiographic ischemic changes. The method was based on earlier findings of Szekeres et al. *(61)* in which pacing of dog hearts with coronary artery constriction (around twice the spontaneous heart rate) evoked ischemic changes, a model that was used to screen for potential antianginal activity. We think then that the pacing stimulus used results in a form of ischemic preconditioning and that this ischemia induced as a result of pacing can be explained by the increased myocardial oxygen demands resulting from the increase in heart rate, together with the concurrent hemodynamic changes (decrease in coronary artery perfusion pressure; increase in left ventricle end-diastolic pressure). These would markedly reduce both the time for endocardial perfusion and the perfusion pressure of those deeper, highly susceptible regions of the left ventricular wall. This is because tachycar-

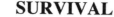

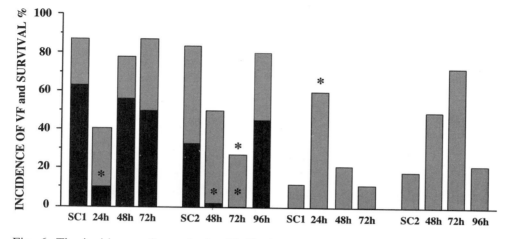

Fig. 6. The incidence of ventricular fibrillation (VF) and survival from the combined ischemia–reperfusion insult in control dogs (SC1; data taken from ref. *59*, and SC2; present experiments *n* = 21), in dogs subjected to a single pacing stimulus (left hand columns; data taken from ref. *59*) or to a repeat pacing stimulus and then subjected to coronary artery occlusion either 24, 48, 72, or 96 h after the end of the pacing stimulus. The results show that a single period of pacing protects dogs 24 h after the stimulus but that this protection is lost after 48 h. However, repeat pacing prolongs the protection for at least 72 h. The filled columns show VF during occlusion and the shaded columns VF during reperfusion. *$p < 0.05$ vs controls. Adapted from ref. *59* with permission from Elsevier Science.

dia would reduce diastolic filling time. Further, calculations of subendocardial driving pressure *(62)* reveal a reduction from around 90 mmHg under control conditions to below 50 mmHg during pacing.

Such a pacing stimulus markedly reduces the severity of arrhythmias, which result when the left anterior descending coronary artery is occluded 24 h later *(59)*. The time course of this protection, both early (classic) and delayed (second window of protection) is illustrated in Fig. 6. The protocol for these studies was to place (under light pentobarbitone anesthesia) a pacing electrode into the lumen of the right ventricle and against the endocardial surface. The dogs were then paced at the rate of 220 beats/min for four 5-min periods with a 5-min resting (reperfusion) period between. At different times after this pacing stimulus (5, 15, 60 min), the left anterior descending branch of the coronary artery was occluded for a 25-min period and ventricular arrhythmias assessed. It is important to remember that this was the first time the coronary artery had been occluded; this is therefore different from the ischemic preconditioning induced by brief periods of coronary artery occlusion described previously. Some of the dogs were allowed to recover for varying periods of time (6, 24, 48, and 72 h) and were then reanesthetized and subjected to coronary artery occlusion. The antiarrhythmic effects of the ischemic (pacing) stimulus that were marked immediately after cessation of the pacing stimulus were lost as soon as 15 min after the stimulus but then returned 24 h later. The time course is thus somewhat different from that achieved after precondi-

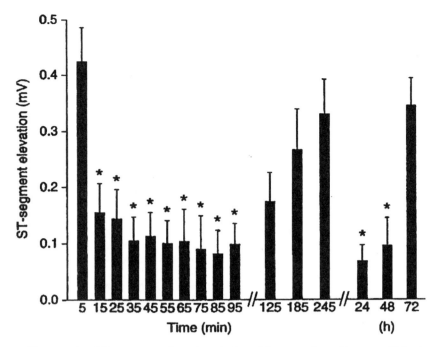

Fig. 7. Changes in ST-segment elevation induced by a series of preconditioning pacing stimuli on transient ischemic ST-segment elevation (recorded from an intracavital electrogram) in conscious rabbits. Ten pacings at a rate of 500 beats/min for 5 min were delivered with 5-min intervals between the pacing periods. Note the marked decline in ST-segment elevation during serial pacing; this protection gradually disappears (e.g., at 185 and 245 min) but reappears after 24 and 48 h after the preconditioning pacing stimulus. The protection is not seen after 72 h. This time course is similar to that seen by preconditioning with brief coronary artery occlusions and also by endotoxin and monophosphoryl lipid A. *$p < 0.05$ compared to ST-segment elevation before preconditioning. Reprinted from ref. *9* with permission from Elsevier Science.

tioning by brief coronary artery occlusions when the protection is most apparent 15–20 min after the end of the preconditioning stimulus. This could be explained by the much more severe ischemia achieved during preconditioning by coronary artery occlusions compared with that achieved during, or after, cardiac pacing. That the reduced arrhythmia severity results from a less marked severity of ischemia during occlusion in paced dogs is suggested by the results of epicardial ST-segment mapping.

There is other evidence that rapid cardiac pacing induces ischemia and protects the myocardium. This is clear from the growing number of studies in which conscious rabbits have been subjected to rapid ventricular pacing (e.g., refs. *9,63*) and recently reviewed *(12)*. This model uses the technique of ventricular overpacing in conscious rabbits with implanted right ventricular electrodes and a permanent catheter in the left ventricular cavity. When rabbits were paced at a rate of 500 beats/min for 5 min, there was a resultant ST-segment elevation recorded from the intracavital electrogram and an increase in left ventricular end-diastolic pressure. This pacing stimulus was then repeated later at different times. Second, and subsequent, overpacings resulted in less marked ST-segment elevation and increases in left ventricular end-diastolic pressure than with the initial (first) overpacing stimulus. It is interesting that there were two distinct phases in protection against ischemic changes resulting from rapid cardiac pacing. The first phase lasted for up to 1.5 h, was lost at 2–3 h after the initial preconditioning rapid pacing stimulus, but returned 24 and 48 h later (Fig. 7; ref. 9). This time course is remarkably similar to that for ischemic preconditioning induced by brief periods of coronary artery occlusion such as revealed in the Kuzuya et al. *(10)* study and illustrated in Fig. 4.

There has been a good deal of interest lately in the possibility of renewing or prolonging protection against coronary artery occlusion by repeating the preconditioning stimulus at times when the protection afforded by the initial stimulus has faded. For example, Kis et al. *(64)* showed that when the pacing stimulus was repeated 48 h after the initial stimulus, a time when protection from the initial stimulus has already faded, then protection against coronary artery occlusion induced ventricular arrhythmias was apparent even 72 h after the second pacing stimulus *(65)*. It is possible, then, that repeated cardiac pacing can keep the heart in an almost permanent state of protection against ischemia-induced ventricular arrhythmias, an intriguing possibility discussed by Parratt and Vegh *(65)*. The analogy with exercise is clear, especially as the increase in heart rate required to induce cardioprotection is just over twice the normal heart rate in resting conscious dogs and only 30–40% above that of anesthetized dogs.

5. DELAYED MYOCARDIAL PROTECTION BY EXERCISE

Although heavy physical exercise and psychological stress that produces similar physiological responses may trigger a cardiac event in the immediate (within 1 h) postexercise period *(66,67)* there is prospective evidence that the relative risk of sudden cardiac death and nonfatal myocardial infarction occurring during this period is reduced in individuals who exercise regularly *(67,68)*. The intensity of the exercise required to induce this protection, as well as the time course, are subjects of ongoing debate *(68)*. The conclusion that the protective effect of exercise requires continued exertion *(68)* implies that the duration of the protection is relatively short-lived. The mechanisms of this risk reduction remain unclear but include an increase in baroreflex sensitivity (increased vagal activity is antifibrillatory) and favorable effects on other risk factors.

Very little has been done to examine the relationship between the intensity and duration of exercise and protection of the heart. Perhaps the most relevant investigations in this regard are those using trained and conscious dogs *(69,70)* showing that in dogs with an healed anterior wall infarct, daily exercise for 6 wk protected against the effects of coronary artery occlusion when this was induced at the end of a further exercise period. This was attributed to a shift in the autonomic balance favoring increased cardiac vagal activity and to the preservation of baroreflex sensitivity *(70)*.

Studies in the Szeged department began with the effects of cardiac pacing, the results of which are summarized previously. This protection could be extended to several days if the pacing stimulus was repeated *(65,71)*. Because the pacing rate in these studies was 220 beats/min, we exercised untrained dogs acclimatized to the laboratory conditions on a treadmill for a 20-min period, which allowed the heart rate to increase to that in the pacing studies. The initial aim was to examine the time course between such a single exercise stimulus and the effects of a subsequent coronary artery occlusion. The results *(72,73)* demonstrated that the severity of ventricular arrhythmias which occurred

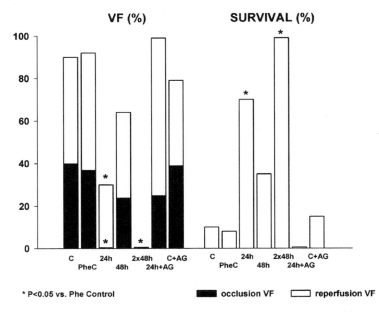

Fig. 8. VF during coronary artery occlusion and reperfusion. The incidence of VF during coronary artery occlusion (filled bars) and after reperfusion (open bars) is shown for control (C) and phenylephrine control (PheC) dogs for dogs exercised 24 h (Ex24 h) or 48 h (Ex48 h) previously, for exercised dogs given aminoguanidine (Ex24 h + AG), and for nonexercised dogs given aminoguanidine (AG). Also shown in the right-hand panel (open bars) is survival after the combined ischemia/reperfusion insult. *$p < 0.05$ compared with Phe controls; *$p < 0.05$ compared with exercised (Ex24 h) dogs. Modified from ref. *73* with permission from the Biochemical Society and the Medical Research Society.

during a 25-min coronary artery occlusion, induced 24 h after the exercise protocol, was significantly less than in the controls. This is illustrated in Fig. 8. Other indices of ischemia severity were also reduced by even a single period of exercise; baroreflex sensitivity, which is markedly reduced under conditions of ischemia, was maintained during coronary occlusion only in the exercised dogs. This protection, which was still apparent 48 h after the exercise stimulus, was not due to the result of changes in myocardial blood flow and was attributed to induction of NOS; iNOS measurements showed a threefold increase in inducible NOS in homogenized pieces of the left ventricular wall taken from exercised dogs. Constitutive NOS was not significantly changed, and neither iNOS nor constitutive NOS were significantly upregulated by exercise in noncardiac tissue *(73)*.

The involvement of nitric oxide in the cardioprotective effects of exercise bears a marked similarity to the protection afforded by cardiac pacing and by bacterial endotoxin. In all three instances, the protection is largely abolished by inhibitors of NOS, such as aminoguanidine and *S*-(2-aminoethyl)-methylisothiuorea or by dexamethasone, which inhibits the formation both of prostanoids and of nitric oxide. Thus, the protective effects of exercise are prevented by either of these two inhibitors *(73)* as are the protective effects of cardiac pacing *(71,74,75)*; as discussed previously, the protective effects of endotoxin and of monophosphoryl lipid are also prevented by these treatments.

6. DELAYED MYOCARDIAL PROTECTION VIA HEAT STRESS AND BY CHRONIC HYPOXIA

As outlined previously, many tissues and individual cells respond to a variety of stresses in ways that enable them to withstand a subsequent period of the same stress several hours later. This phenomenon has been reviewed on a number of occasions (e.g., refs. *76,77*). A good example is the response to hyperthermia; this is presumed to be mediated by the generation of a series of highly protective proteins known as heat shock or stress proteins. The fact that animals subjected to hyperthermia are also able to tolerate other forms of stress, such as myocardial ischemia (another example of cross-tolerance) was first reported by Currie et al. *(78)* in 1988. They showed that whole body hyperthermia in rats (42°C for 15 min) resulted in an increased tolerance to ischemia (reduced creatine kinase efflux; enhanced post-ischemia contractile recovery) and that this was associated with elevation of heart levels of catalase and also of hsp 70. These proteins are part of a family of constitutively expressed and/or stress-induced proteins that differ according to their molecular weight (e.g., 27 kDa, or hsp 27); these have a variety of functions basically concerned with cellular integrity. Thus, animals subjected to heat stress are also resistant to manifestations of ischemic injury, such as cell death; again, this protection is delayed, being maximal 24 or 48 h after the initial heat stress stimulus. Further, it seems that the degree of the increase in hsp correlates with both the degree of hyperthermia and the extent of ischemic tolerance *(79,80)*. Such cardiac protection by heat stress has been documented in a variety of animal models and in several species. The whole area has been extensively reviewed (e.g., refs. *80–82*).

A perhaps similar form of protection to that achieved by brief periods of local or global ischemia is that resulting from chronic hypoxia. It has been known for many years that the resistance of the heart to injury can be increased by long-term adaptive processes resulting from chronic hypoxia. A good example of this is the chronic high-altitude hypoxia encountered naturally in a mountain environment or simulated under laboratory conditions in a hypobaric chamber *(83)*. Thus, intermittent exposure to simulated high altitude (equivalent to about 7000 m) increases the tolerance of hearts to the consequences of ischemia and reperfusion, such as life-threatening ventricular arrhythmias; this protection persists long after removal of the animals from the chronic hypoxic environment. In hearts of rats subjected to intermittent high altitude and acclimatized, the activities of sarcolemmal Na*K-ATPase, Mg-ATPase, and Ca-ATPase decreased, a sign of adaptation to hypoxia at the enzyme level. Moreover the affinity of these enzymes to ATP increased. Treatment of such rats with 7-oxoPgI_2 resulted in an increase of sarcolemmal activities of these enzymes and enhanced tolerance of the heart to anoxia *(84)*. The cardioprotective effects of chronic hypoxia have been recently reviewed by Kolar *(85)*.

7. POSSIBLE MECHANISMS OF DELAYED MYOCARDIAL PROTECTION

The discussed findings suggest that the mechanism of delayed cardioprotection is based on the fact that the impulse evoking adaptation may stimulate the adenylate-cyclase cAMP system (PgI_2, isoprenaline) as well as the phosphatidyl-inositol/diacylglycerol pathway. In addition, calcium is released, acting as an intracellular sec-

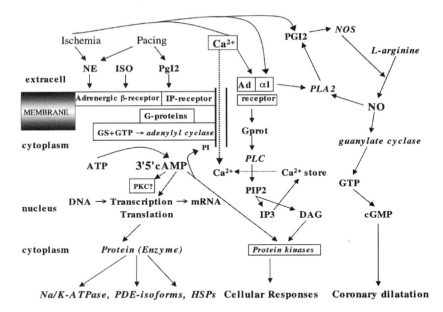

Fig. 9. Possible mechanism of delayed cardioprotection. For explanation, *see* text. NE, nore-pinephrine; ISO, isoprenaline; PgI₂, prostacyclin; GS, stimulatory G-protein complex; GTP, guanosine triphosphate; IP receptor, prostacyclin receptor; cAMP, cyclic adenosine monophosphate; cGMP, cyclic guanosine monophosphate; PKC, protein kinase C; PDE, phosphodiesterase; HSP, heat shock proteins; AD, adenosine receptor; α-1, alpha-1 adrenoceptor; PL, phospholipase; PLA2, phopholipase A2; PLC, phospholipase C; NO, nitric oxide; NOS, nitric oxide synthase; PIP2, phosphatidyl-inositol 4,5-biphosphate; IP3, triphospho-inositol; DAG, 1,2-diacylglycerol.

ond messenger (Fig. 9). Such initiating stresses are ischemia, pacing, α and β adrenoceptor agonists (noradrenaline, isoprenaline), prostacyclin, nitric oxide, adenosine, and according to a recent review *(86)*, opioids and reactive oxygen species may be also involved. In case of prostacyclin and isoprenaline, the resulting elevation of cardiac cAMP level triggers the induction of some key enzymes, such as Na/K-ATPase *(33)* and PDE isoforms I and IV *(26,32)*. The increased amount and activity of Na/K-AT-Pase may account for preservation of the normal membrane function, moderation of ischemic loss of potassium, and accumulation of sodium and calcium in the myocardium, as well as for reduced ouabain toxicity. The detrimental consequences of heavy stress-induced accumulation of cAMP in the heart are mitigated by hydrolysis of the latter, carried out by an enhanced amount and activity of PDE isoforms (Fig. 9).

There is a good deal of evidence, some of which is outlined above, that one of the key mediators of this cardioprotection is nitric oxide. This is true both of classic ischemic preconditioning (that protection arises shortly after the preconditioning stimulus; ref. *56*) and of the delayed protection afforded by exercise, cardiac pacing, and the administration of bacterial endotoxin (*see* Sections 2., 4., and 5.).

This is interesting in view of the fact that donors of nitric oxide have been used extensively for more than 120 yr in the treatment of acute coronary episodes, implying that this replaces endogenous nitric oxide produced, for example, from coronary vascular endothelial cells. It is known both that there is endothelial dysfunction in patients with coronary artery disease and that it is not possible to protect the myocardium with preconditioning if the endothelial cells have been damaged by chemical means *(87)*. The precise mechanisms of this increased nitric oxide production and release are presently unclear. There is some evidence that initial nitric oxide release involves bradykinin acting on endothelial cell receptors and that prostanoids (perhaps prostacyclin) are also released under these conditions. This hypothesis has been summarized, for example, by Parratt and Vegh *(65)*. An additional pathway probably involves protein kinase C activation. Although these pathways have been reasonably well worked out in relation to classic ischemic preconditioning, the precise pathways involved, e.g., after exercise are unknown.

8. POSSIBLE ROLE OF DELAYED CARDIOPROTECTION IN THERAPY

The overwhelming majority of data on delayed cardioprotection by adaptation to stress is based on animal experiments. Whether the phenomenon might represent a novel therapeutic window for cardiac drug development depends on the demonstration that it is active in clinical situations. Because delayed cardioprotection is a universal phenomenon and can be demonstrated in experimental animals (even by ischemia in distant parts of the body, ref. *88*) it is reasonable to conclude that it can also occur in humans. In cultured human ventricular myocytes, delayed cardioprotection is mimicked by adenosine *(89)*. Human right atrial appendages obtained during coronary bypass surgery, preconditioned by exposure to brief ischemic and reperfusion periods, have shown both the first (2 h or less) and the second window (24 h) of cardiac protection *(90)*.

We should also take into consideration that investigations on ischemic and delayed preconditioning were performed in healthy animals or organs or tissues taken from such animals. Therefore, it is of great importance to demonstrate that delayed cardiac protection based on cardiac adaptation to stress is effective even under pathological conditions. It has been shown that delayed cardioprotection, although not classic short-lived ischemic preconditioning, operates in rabbits who were made hypercholesterolemic and atherosclerotic by feeding them for 2 mo with a cholesterol-rich diet *(91)*.

There is some clinical evidence that delayed cardioprotection induced by adaptation may occur in cardiac patients. For example, a beneficial effect of preinfarction angina on the ventricular wall motion has been described *(92)*. It was also found that postinfarction, short-term exercise training increases exercise tolerance; decreases heart rate, systolic blood pressure, and responses to exercise; and improves the ischemic threshold *(93)*. Patients with a previous history of angina before a myocardial infarction sustain smaller infarcts and have an improved survival *(94)*. However, a number of preconditioning stresses used in animal experiments, such as repeated coronary occlusions, heat stress, or immobilization cannot be applied in human patients. The heart rate can be increased for brief periods by frequency loading, an easily controllable method, or by gradually intensified exercise. Its value as an intervention to reach fitness is well known. However, its application depends closely on the patient's actual state of health. The use of moderate global cardiac ischemia by rapid pacing, exercise-induced tachycardia, or thermal stress is limited by the risk of arrhythmias or heart failure in patients with some cardiac disease. Confirming the pioneer work with prostacyclin and its stable analogs *(7,8)*, there is increasing recognition that adaptation induced by drugs seems to be most suitable for clinical application. Administration of a drug is the most convenient form of stimulus because the dose needed to evoke delayed adaptation can be determined fairly precisely; furthermore, its effect is nearly the same in all animal species used. An essential requirement is that the use of the drug as a trigger should involve minimal, if any, side effects Another fundamental problem is the timing of the drug administrations to maintain protection for a longer period, as the protective effect usually fades after 72 to 96 h. As mentioned above, in 1991 it was shown that the duration of protection can be prolonged at will by periodic (every third day) use of a lower maintenance dose *(25,26)*. This was later confirmed using other substances *(95)*. The next question is which type of drugs could serve to trigger adaptive processes resulting in delayed cardioprotection in patients? Possible candidates may be monophosphoryl lipid A or the selective adenosine Al receptor agonist 2-chloro-*N*6-cyclopentyl-adenosine *(95)*, prostacyclin derivatives, or prostacyclin releasers. If possible, the drug should be available in an orally administered form. Certainly, further studies are needed to find a drug suitable for inducing delayed cardioprotection in patients. The problem has been recently repeatedly reviewed *(96–98)*. We conclude that the use of drug-induced delayed cardiac adaptation to stress could be an important future trend in the prevention of life-threatening cardiac events.

ACKNOWLEDGMENTS

Most of our own studies were undertaken in collaboration with Professor Zoltán Szilvássy, Dr. Éva Udvary, and Professor Ágnes Végh in the Szeged department supported, at various times, with grants from the European Union, from the Hungarian Scientific Research Foundation, and Ministry of Culture and Education and by the British Council. Professor Parratt is at present a Leverhulme Emeritus Research Fellow and the recipient of an Albert Szent-Györgi Fellowship from the Hungarian State Government.

REFERENCES

1. Rona, G. and Dusek, J. (1972) Studies on the mechanism of increased myocardial resistance, in *Recent Advances in Studies on Cardiac Structure and Metabolism* Vol. 1, Myocardiology (Bajusz, E. E. and Rona G., eds.), University Park Press, Baltimore, MD, pp. 422–429.
2. Dusek, J., Rona, G., and Kahn D. S. (1970) Myocardial resistance: A study of its development against toxic doses of isoproterenol. *Arch. Pathol.* **89,** 79–83.
3. Balazs, T. (1972) Cardiotoxicity of isoproterenol in experimental animals. Influence of stress, obesity, and repeated dosing, in *Myocardiology–Recent Advances in Studies on Cardiac Structure and Metabolism* (Bajusz, E. E. and Rona G., eds.), University Park Press, Baltimore, MD, pp. 770–778.
4. Selye, H., Veilleux, R., and Grasso, S. (1960) Protection by coronary ligature against isoproterenol-induced myocardial necroses. *Proc. Soc. Exp. Biol. Med.* **104,** 343–345.
5. Joseph, X., Bloom, S., Pledger, G., and Balázs, T. (1983) Determinants of resistance to the cardiotoxicity of isoproterenol in rats. *Toxicol. Appl. Pharmacol.* **69,** 199–205.
6. Poupa, O., Turek, Z., Pelouch, V., Prochazka, J., and Krofta, K. (1965) Increased resistance of the myocardium to anoxia in vitro after repeated application to isoprenalíne. *Physiol. Bohemoslov.* **14,** 536–541.
7. Szekeres, L., Koltai, M., Pataricza, J., Takáts I., and Udvary É. (1984) On the late antiischemic action of the stable PgI$_2$ analogue: 7-oxo-PgI2-Na and its possible mode of action. *Biomed. Biochim. Acta* **43,** 135–142.

8. Szekeres, L., Krassói, I., Pataricza, J., and Udvary, É. (1985) Delayed antiischemic effect of prostaglandin I2 and of a new stable prostaglandin I_2 analogue, 7-oxo-prostacyclin-Na, in experimental model angina in dogs, in *Advances in Myocardiology*, Vol. 6. (Dhalla, N. S. and Hearse, D. J., eds.) Plenum Press, New York, pp. 607–618.

9. Szekeres, L., Papp, J. Gy. Szilvássy, Z., Udvary, É., and Végh, Á. (1993) Moderate stress by cardiac pacing may induce both short term and long term cardioprotection. *Cardiovasc. Res.* **27,** 593–596.

10. Kuzuya, T., Hoshida, S., Yamashita, N., Fuji, H., Oe, H., Hori, M., et al. (1993) Delayed effects of sublethal ischemia on the acquisition of tolerance to ischemia. *Circ. Res.* **72,** 1293–1299.

11. Marber, M. S., Latchman, D. S., Walker, J. M., and Yellon, D. M. (1993) Cardiac stress protein elevation 24 hours after brief ischemia or heat stress is associated with resistance to myocardial infarction. *Circulation* **88,** 1264–1272.

12. Szekeres, L. (1996) On the mechanism and possible therapeutic application of delayed cardiac adaptation to stress. *Can. J. Cardiol.* **12,** 177–185.

13. Yellon, D. (1994) Delayed myocardial preconditioning: The role of stress proteins, in *Cardiac Preconditioning,* William Harvey Research Conferences (Parratt, J. and Thiemermann, C., eds.) William Harvey Research Institute, London, p. 12.

14. Wu, S., Furman, B. L., and Parratt, J. R. (1994) Attenuation by dexamethasone of endotoxin protection against ischaemia-induced ventricular arrhythmias. *Br. J. Pharmacol.* **113,** 1083–1084.

15. Beckman, C. B., Niazi, Z., Dietzman, R. H., and Lillehi, R. C. (1981) Protective effects of epinephrine tolerance in experimental cardiogenic shock. *Circ. Shock* **8,** 137–149.

16. Meng, X., Brown, J. M., Ao, L., Mitchell, M. B., Banerjee, A., and Harken, A. H. (1993) Norepinephrine induces late cardiac protection preceded by oncogene and heat shock protein gene overexpression. [abstr 3407] *Circulation* **88(Suppl),** I633.

17. Ravingerova, T., Song, W., Pancza, D., Dzurba, A., Ziegelhoeffer, A., and Parratt, J. R. (1997) Pretreatment with catecholamines can suppress severe ventricular arrhythmias in rats: Relevance to ischemic preconditioning. *Exp. Clin. Cardiol.* **2,** 19–24.

18. Kovanecz, I., Papp, J. G., and Szekeres L. (1996) Long-term ischemic preconditioning of the heart induced by repeated beta-adrenergic stress. *Acta Phys. Hung.* **84,** 297–298.

19. Szekeres, L., Nemeth, M., Szilvassy, Z., Tosaki, A., Udvary, E., and Vegh, A. (1988) On the nature and molecular basis of prostacyclin induced late cardiac changes. *Biomed. Biochim. Acta* **47,** 6–11.

20. Szekeres, L., Bálint, Zs., Karcsú, S., and Tósaki, Á. (1990) Delayed protection by 7-oxo-PgI_2 against cardiac transmembrane ion shifts and early morphological changes due to ischemia and reperfusion. *Cardioscience* **1,** 280–286.

21. Ravingerova, T., Tribulova, N., Ziegelhöffer, A., Dzurba, A., and Szekeres, L. (1991) 7-oxo-PgI_2 prevents partially the postischemic reperfusion injury of the rat heart. *J. Mol. Cell. Cardiol.* **23(Suppl.V),** 104.

22. Udvary, É. and Szekeres, L. (1986) Prostacyclin: antiischemic or cardioprotective?, in *Advances in Pharmacological Research and Practice*, Vol. 3., Section 7. Prostanoids (Kecskeméti, V., Gyires, K., and Kovács, G., eds.). Akadémiai Kiadó, Budapest, pp. 333–338.

23. Szekeres, L., Németh, M., Papp, J. Gy., Udvary, É., Végh, Á., and Virág L. (1998) Neue Entwicklungen der antiarrhythmischen Therapie, in *Perspektiven der Arrhythmiebehandlung* (Lüderitz, B. and Antoni, B., eds.), Springer, Berlin, pp. 24–34.

24. Ravingerová, T., Tribulová, N., Ziegelhöffer, A., Styk, J., and Szekeres, L. (1993) Suppression of reperfusion induced arrhythmias in the isolated rat heart: Pretreatment with 7-oxo prostacyclin in vivo. *Cardiovasc. Res.* **27,** 1051–1055.

25. Udvary, É., Végh, Á., and Szekeres, L. (1991) 7-oxo-PgI2 induced late protective action from arrhythmias due to local myocardial ischaemia. *Bratysl. Lek. Listy* **92,** 146–149.

26. Krause, E. G. and Szekeres, L. (1995) On the mechanism and possible therapeutic application of delayed adaptation of the heart to stress situations. *Mol. Cell. Biochem.* **147,** 115–122.

27. Szekeres, L., Szilvássy, Z., Udvary, É., and Végh Á. (1988) 7-oxo-PgI$_2$ induced late appearing protection against ouabain induced cardiac arrhythmias in anesthetized guinea pigs. *Pharmacol. Res. Commun.* **20,** 77–78.

28. Szilvássy, Z., Szekeres, L., Udvary, É., and Végh, Á. (1988) On the 7-oxo-PgI$_2$ induced lasting protection against ouabain arrhythmias in anesthetized guinea pigs. *Biomed. Biochim. Acta* **47(Suppl.),** 35–38.

29. Szilvássy, Z., Szekeres, L., Udvary, É., Karcsú, S., and Végh, Á. (1991) 7-oxo-PgI2 dramatically increases the safety margin of digitalis. *Bratisl. Lek. Listy* **92,** 134–137.

30. Szekeres, L., Szilvássy, Z., Udvary, É., and Végh, Á. (1989) 7-oxo-PgI2 induced late appearing and long-lasting electrophysiological changes in the heart in situ of the rabbit, guinea pig, dog and cat. *J. Mol. Cell. Cardiol.* **21,** 545–554.

31. Szekeres, L., Németh, M., Papp, J. Gy., and Udvary, É. (1990) Short incubation with 7-oxo-prostacyclin induces long lasting prolongation of repolarisation time and effective refractory period in rabbit papillary muscle preparation. *Cardiovasc. Res.* **24,** 37–41.

32. Borchert, G., Bartel, S., Beyerdorfer, I., Kuttner, I., Szekeres, L., and Krause, E. G. (1994) Long lasting anti-adrenergic effect of 7-oxo-prostacyclin in the heart: A cycloheximide sensitive increase of phosphodiesterase isoform I and IV activities. *Mol. Cell. Biochem.* **132,** 57–67.

33. Dzurba, A., Ziegelhoeffer, A., Breier, A., Vrbjar, N., and Szekeres, L. (1991) Increased activity of sarcolemmal (Na+K+)-ATPase is involved in the late cardioprotective action of 7-oxo-prostacyclin. *Cardioscience* **2,** 105–108.

34. Neugebauer, E. A. and Holaday, J. W., eds. (1993) *Handbook of Mediators in Septic Shock.* CRC Press, Boca Raton, FL.

35. Parratt, J. R. and Stoclet, J. C. (1995) Vascular smooth muscle functionunder conditions of sepsis and endotoxaemia, in *Role of Nitric Oxide in Sepsis and ARDS* (Fink, M. P. and Payen, D., eds.), Springer, Berlin, pp. 44–61.

36. Wu, S., Song W., Furman, B. L., and Parratt, J. R. (1996) Delayed protection against ischaemia-induced ventricular arrhythmias and infarct size limitation by the prior administration of Escherichia coli endotoxin. *Br. J. Pharmacol.* **118,** 2157–2163.

37. Brown, J. M., Grosso, M. A., Terada, L. S., Whitman, G. J. R., Banerjee, A., White, C. W., et al. (1989) Endotoxin pretreatment increases endogenous myocardial catalase activity and decreases ischemia-reperfusion injury of isolated rat hearts. *Proc. Natl. Acad. Sci. USA* **86,** 2526–2530.

38. McDonough, K. H. and Causey, K. M. (1994) Effects of sepsis on recovery of the heart from 50 min ischemia. *Shock* **1,** 432–437.

39. Qureshi, N., Takayama, K., and Ribi, E. (1982) Purification and structural determination of nontoxic lipid A obtained from the lipopolysaccharide of Salmonella typhimurium. *J. Biol. Chem.* **257,** 11,808–11,815.

40. Takayama, K., Qureshi, N., Ribi, E., and Cantrell, J. L. (1984) Separation and characterization of toxic and nontoxic forms of lipid A. *Rev. Infect. Dis.* **6,** 439–443.

41. Yao, Z., Elliott, G. T., and Gross, G. J. (1994) Monophosphoryl lipid A: A new approach for cardioprotection. *Drug News Perspect.* **7,** 96–102.

42. Baxter, G. F., Goodwin R. W., Wright, M. J., Kerac, M., Heads, R. J., and Yellon, D. M. (1996) Myocardial protection after monophosphoryl lipid A: Studies of delayed anti-ischaemic properties in rabbit heart. *Br. J. Pharmacol.* **117,** 1685–1692

43. Song, W., Furman, B. L., and Parratt, J. R. (1997) Monophosphoryl lipid A reduces both arrhythmia severity and infarct size in a rat model of ischaemia. *Eur. J. Pharmacol.* **345,** 285–287.

44. Vegh, A., Györgyi, K., Rastegar, M. A., Papp, J. Gy., and Parratt, J. R. (1999) Delayed protection against ventricular arrhythmias by monophosphoryl lipid-A in a canine model of ischaemia and reperfusion. *Eur. J. Pharmacol.* **382,** 81–90.

45. Parratt, J. R. (1993) Endogenous myocardial protective (antiarrhythmic) substances. *Cardiovasc. Res.* **27,** 693–702.

46. Zhao, L., Weber, P. A., Smith, J. R., Comerford, M. L., and Elliott, G. T. (1997) Role of inducible nitric oxide synthase in pharmacological "preconditioning" with monophosphoryl lipid A. *J. Mol. Cell. Cardiol.* **29,** 1567–1576.

47. Mei, D. A., Elliott, G. T., and Gross, G. J. (1996) KATP channels mediate late preconditioning against infarction produced by monophosphoryl lipid A. *Am. J. Physiol.* **271,** H2723–H2729.

48. Vegh, A., Papp. J. Gy., Szekeres, L., and Parratt, J. R. (1993) Are ATP sensitive potassium channels involved in the pronounced antiarrhythmic effects of preconditioning? *Cardiovasc. Res.* **27,** 38–643.

49. Murry, C. E., Jennings, R. B., and Reimer, K. A. (1986) Preconditioning with ischemia: A delay of lethal cell injury in ischemic myocardium. *Circulation* **74,** 1124–1126.

50. Marber, M. S. and Yellon, D. M., eds. (1996) *Ischaemia: Preconditioning and Adaptation*, BIOS Scientific, Oxford, UK.

51. Wainwright, C. L. and Parratt, J. R., eds. (1996) *Myocardial Preconditioning*, Springer-Verlag, New York.

52. Baxter, G. F., Marber, M. S., Patel, V. C., and Yellon, D. M. (1994) Adenosine receptor involvement in a delayed phase of myocardial protection 24 hours after ischemic preconditioning. *Circulation* **90,** 2993–3000.

53. Baxter, G. F. and Yellon, D. M. (1996) Delayed myocardial protection following ischemic preconditioning. *Basic Res. Cardiol.* **91,** 53–56.

54. Komori, S., Fujimaki, S., Ijili, H., Asakawa, T., Watanabe, Y., Tamura, Y., et al. (1990) Inhibitory effect of ischemic preconditioning on ischemic arrhythmia using a rat coronary artery ligation model. *Jpn. J. Electrocardiol.* **10,** 774–782.

55. Vegh, A., Szekeres, L., and Parratt, J. R. (1990) Protective effects of preconditioning of the ischaemic myocardium involve cyclo-oxygenase products. *Cardiovasc. Res.* **24,** 1020–1023.

56. Vegh, A., Komori, S., Szekeres, L. and Parratt, J. R. (1992) Antiarrhythmic effects of preconditioning in anaesthetised dogs and rats. *Cardiovasc. Res.* **26,** 487–495.

57. Lawson, C. S., Coltart, D. J., and Hearse, D. J. (1993) "Dose"-dependency and temporal characteristics of protection by ischemic preconditioning against ischemia-induced arrhythmias in rat hearts. *J. Mol. Cell. Cardiol.* **25,** 1391–1402.

58. Piacentini, L., Wainwright, C. L., and Parratt, J. R. (1993) The antiarrhythmic effect of ischemic preconditioning in isolated rat heart involves a pertussis toxin sensitive mechanism. *Cardiovasc. Res.* **27,** 674–680.

59. Kaszala, K., Vegh, A., Papp, J. Gy., and Parratt, J. R. (1996) Time course of the protection against ischemia and reperfusion-induced ventricular arrhythmias resulting from brief periods of cardiac pacing. *J. Mol. Cell. Cardiol.* **28,** 2085–2095.

60. Vegh, A., Szekeres, L., and Parratt, J. R. (1991) Transient ischaemia induced by rapid cardiac pacing results in myocardial preconditioning. *Cardiovasc. Res.* **25,** 1051–1053.

61. Szekeres, L., Csik, V., and Udvary, E. (1976) Nitroglycerin and dipyridamole on cardiac metabolism and dynamics in a new experimental model of angina pectoris. *J. Pharmacol. Exp. Ther.* **196,** 15–28.

62. Marshall, R. J. and Parratt, J. R. (1974) Drug-induced changes in blood flow in the acutely ischaemic canine myocardium; relationship to subendocardial driving pressure. *Clin. Exp. Pharmacol. Physiol.* **1,** 97–112.

63. Szilvassy, Z., Ferdinandy, P., Bor, P., Jakab, I., Lonovics, K., and Koltai, M. (1994) Ventricular overdrive pacing-induced anti-ischemic effect: A conscious rabbit model of preconditioning. *Am. J. Physiol.* **266,** H2033–H2041.

64. Kis, A., Vegh, A., Papp, J. Gy., and Parratt, J. R. (1996) Repeated pacing widens the time window of delayed protection against ventricular arrhythmias in dogs *J. Mol. Cell. Cardiol.* **28,** A229.

65. Parratt, J. R. and Vegh, A. (1997) Delayed protection against ventricular arrhythmias by cardiac pacing. *Heart* **78,** 423–425.

66. Willich, S. N., Lewis, M., Löwel, H., Arntz, H-R., Schubert, F., and Schröder, R. (1993) Physical exertion as a trigger of acute myocardial infarction. Triggers and Mechanisms of Myocardial Infarction Study Group. *N. Engl. J. Med.* **329,** 1684–1690.
67. Mittleman, M. A., Maclurf, M., Toffler, G. H., Sherwood, J. B., Goldberg, R. J., and Muller, J. E. (1993) Triggering of acute myocardial infarction by heavy physical exertion. Protection against triggering by regular exertion. Determinants of Myocardial Infarction Onset Study Investigators. *N. Engl. J. Med.* **329,** 1677–1683.
68. Tofler, G. H., Mittleman, M. A., and Muller, J. E. (1996) Physical activity and the triggering of myocardial infarction: the case for regular exercise. *Heart* **75,** 323–325.
69. Billman, G. E. W., Schwartz, P. J., and Stone, H. L. (1984) The effects of daily exercise on susceptibility to sudden cardiac death. *Circulation* **69,** 1182–1189.
70. Hull, S. S., Vanoli, E., Adamson, P. B., Verrier, R. L., Foreman, R. D., and Schwartz, P. J. (1994) Exercise training confers anticipatory protection from sudden death during acute myocardial ischemia. *Circulation* **89,** 548–552.
71. Kis, A., Vegh, A., Papp, J. Gy., and Parratt, J. R. (1999) Repeated cardiac pacing extends the time during which canine hearts are protected against ischaemia-induced arrhythmias: role of nitric oxide. *J. Mol. Cell. Cardiol.* **31,** 1229–1241.
72. Vegh, A., Babai, L., Kovacs, S. K., Papp, J. Gy., and Parratt, J. R. (2000) Exercise 24 h prior to coronary artery occlusion reduces arrhythmia severity in dogs: Role of nitric oxide. *J. Physiol.* **525,** 14P.
73. Babai, L., Szigeti, Z., Parratt, J. R., and Vegh, A. (2002) Delayed cardioprotective effects of exercise in dogs are aminoguanidine sensitive: Possible involvement of nitric oxide. *Clin. Sci.* **102,** 435–445.
74. Kis, A., Vegh, A., Papp, J. Gy., and Parratt, J. R. (1999) Pacing-induced delayed protection against arrhythmias is attenuated by aminoguanidine, an inhibitor of nitric oxide synthase. *Br. J. Pharmacol.* **127,** 1545–1550.
75. Kis, A., Vegh, A., Papp, J. Gy., and Parratt, J. R. (2000) Cardiac pacing-induced delayed protection against ventricular arrhythmias: Evidence for the role of nitric oxide protection. *Exp. Clin. Cardiol.* **5,** 17–24.
76. Lindquist, S. C. (1986) The heat-shock response. Annu. Rev.Biochem. 55, 1151–1191.
77. Minowada, G. and Welch, W. J. (1995) Clinical implications of the stress response. *J. Clin. Invest.* **95,** 3–12.
78. Currie, R. W., Karmazyn, M., Kloc, M., and Mailer, K. (1988) Heat-shock response is associated with enhanced postischemic ventricular recovery. *Circ. Res.* **63,** 543–549.
79. Hutter, M. E., Sievers, R. E., Barbosa, V., and Wolfe, C. L. (1994) Heat-shock protein induction in rat hearts. A direct correlation between the amount of heat-shock protein induced and the degree of myocardial protection. *Circulation* **89,** 355–360.
80. Marber, M. S., Walker, J. M., Latchman, D. S., and Yellon, D. M. (1994) Myocardial protection after whole body heat stress in the rabbit is dependent on metabolic substrate and is related to the amount of the inducible 70-kD heat stress protein. *J. Clin. Invest.* **93,** 1087–1094.
81. Steare, S. E. and Yellon, D. M. (1993) The protective effect of heat stress against reperfusion arrhythmias in the rat. *J. Mol. Cell. Cardiol.* **25,** 1471–1481.
82. Walker, D. M., Pasini, A., Kuckukoglu, S., Marber, M. S., Iliodromitis, E., Ferrari, R., et al. (1993) Heat stress limits infarct size in the isolated perfused rabbit heart. *Cardiovasc. Res.* **27,** 962–967.
83. Poupa, O., Krofta, K., Prochazka, J. (1966) Acclimation to simulated high altitude and acute cardiac necrosis. *Fed. Proc.* **25,** 1243–1246.
84. Ziegelhöffer, A., Grünermel, J., Dzurba, A., Procházka, J., Kolár, F., Vrbjar, N., et al. (1993) Sarcolemmal cation transport systems in rat hearts acclimatised to high altitude hypoxia: Influence of 7-oxo-prostacyclin, in *Heart Function in Health and Disease* (Ostádal, B. and Dhalla, N. S., eds.), Kluwer Academic Publishers, Boston/Dordrecht/London, pp. 219–228.

85. Kolar, F. (1996) Cardioprotective effects of chronic hypoxia: Relation to preconditioning, in *Myocardial Preconditioning* (Wainwright, C. L. and Parratt, J. R., Eds.), Springer-Verlag, New York, pp. 261–275.

86. Bolli, R. (2000) The late phase of preconditioning. *Circ. Res.* **87,** 972–983.

87. Hassanabad, Z. F., Furman, B. L., Parratt, J. R., and Aughey, E. (1998) Coronary endothelial dysfunction increases the severity of ischaemia-induced ventricular arrhythmias in rat isolated perfused hearts. *Basic Res. Cardiol.* **93,** 241–249.

88. Oxman, T., Arad, M., Klein, R., Avazov, N., and Rabinowitz, B. (1997) Limb ischemia preconditions the heart against reperfusion tachyarrhythmia. *Am. J. Physiol.* **273,** H1707–1712.

89. Carroll, R. and Yellon, D. M. (2000) Delayed cardioprotection in a human cardiomyocyte-derived cell line: the role of adenosine, p38MAP kinase and mitochondrial KATP. *Basic Res. Cardiol.* **95,** 243–249.

90. Ghosh, S., Standen, N. B., and Galinanes M. (2000) Preconditioning the human myocardium by simulated ischemia; Studies on the early and delayed protection. *Cardiovasc. Res.* **45,** 339–50.

91. Szekeres, L., Szilvássy, Z., Ferdinándy, P., Nagy, I., Karcsu, S., and Csáti S. (1997) Delayed cardiac protection against harmful consequences of stress can be induced in experimental atherosclerosis in rabbits. *J. Mol. Cell. Cardiol.* **29,** 1977–1983.

92. Noda, T., Minaloguchi, S., Fuji, K., Hori, M., Ito, T., Kanmatsuse, K., et al. (1999) Evidence for the delayed effect in human ischemic preconditioning: Prospective multicenter study for preconditioning in acute myocardial infarction. *J. Am. Coll. Cardiol.* **34,** 1966–1974.

93. Tsoukas, A., Andonakoudis, H., and Christakos, S. (1995) Short-term exercise training effect after myocardial infarction on myocardial oxygen consumption indices and ischemic threshold. *Arch. Phys. Med. Rehabil.* **76,** 262–265.

94. Carrol, R. and Yellon D. M. (1999) Myocardial adaptation to ischaemia—the preconditioning phenomenon. *Int. J. Cardiol.* **68(Suppl 1),** S93–S101.

95. Dana, A., Baxter, G. F., Walker, J. M., and Yellon, D. M. (1998) Prolonging the delayed phase of myocardial protection. repetitive adenosine A1 receptor activation maintains rabbit myocardium in a preconditioned state. *J. Am. Coll. Cardiol.* **31,** 1112–1119.

96. Parratt, J. R. (1995) Possibilities for the pharmacological exploitation of ischaemic preconditioning. *J. Mol. Cell. Cardiol.* **27,** 991–1000.

97. Parratt, J. R. and Szekeres, L. (1995) Delayed protection of the heart against ischemia. *Trends Pharmacol. Sci.* **16,** 351–355.

98. Szekeres L. (2000) Delayed adaptation to stress—A clinically useful form of cardiac protection. *Exp. Clin. Cardiol.* **5,** 116–121.

IV

CLINICAL ASPECTS
IN CARDIAC DRUG DEVELOPMENT

15

Cardiac Troponin Testing for Detection of Myocardial Infarction

Clinical Utility and Analytical Issues

Fred S. Apple

CONTENTS

INTRODUCTION
PATHOPHYSIOLOGY OF MYOCARDIAL INJURY
MI REDEFINED
CHEST PAIN EVALUATION
ASSAYS FOR MARKERS OF MYOCARDIAL INJURY
CONCLUSIONS
REFERENCES

1. INTRODUCTION

Assessment of patients with acute coronary syndromes (ACS), including chest pain, is often a diagnostic challenge to physicians. Biochemical markers of myocardial injury have become routine in assisting clinicians in confirming the diagnosis of acute myocardial infarction (AMI) in both patients with and without a diagnostic electrocardiogram (EKG; refs. *1–3*).

In patients with ACS where the EKG fails to provide conclusive diagnostic information, biochemical markers have also become risk predictors of adverse short- and long-term outcomes *(1–3)*. Improvements in technology and the implementation of monoclonal antibodies in immunoassays have lead to an explosion of new instrumentation designed for rapid turnaround time (TAT). Instrumentation has been developed that allows for quantitative detection of multiple markers of myocardial injury in whole blood, serum, or plasma. Systems have been designed to provide testing in either the central laboratory, in satellite laboratories, or closer to the bedside, designated as point-of-care (POC) testing.

Numerous patient groups with varying clinical needs are optimal targets for rapid TAT testing of markers of myocardial injury, including (1) high-risk, EKG-diagnosed AMI patients qualifying for thrombolytic therapy; (2) high-risk non-ST-segment elevation AMI patients; (3) moderate risk ACS patients; and (4) low-risk noncardiac, chest pain patients. The goal of this chapter will be to address the clinical and analyti-

From: *Cardiac Drug Development Guide*
Edited by: M. K. Pugsley © Humana Press Inc., Totowa, NJ

cal aspects of testing of biochemical markers of myocardial injury. First, the patho-physiology of myocardial injury and implications of its diagnosis regarding use of markers will be addressed. Second, the recently published guidelines and consensus documents (1) redefining the definition of AMI and (2) reclassifying ACS patients as either non-ST-segment myocardial infarction (MI) or unstable angina (UA; both heavily predicated on cardiac biomarkers) will be discussed. Third, the goal and ratio-nale for chest pain evaluation using clinical studies will address the role of testing of markers of myocardial injury. The urgency to obtain results and how results impact patient care, triage, management, and therapy will be addressed. Clinical pathways will be proposed that use multiple measurements of a single cardiac marker. The appropri-ate use of this pathway will be discussed with regard to optimizing medical and eco-nomic outcomes. Fourth, potential differences in standardization for selected markers between testing devices and instrumentation used in the central laboratory and near the bedside will be addressed.

2. PATHOPHYSIOLOGY OF MYOCARDIAL INJURY

The major course of AMI is atherosclerotic coronary artery disease (CAD), which contributes to narrowing of coronary arteries, plaque disruption, and thrombus forma-tion (4–6). Myocardial ischemia and subsequent MI usually begins in the endocardium and spreads to the epicardium. Irreversible injury has been documented if occlusion is complete for 15–20 min. However, restoration of blood flow within 6 h is associated with myocardial salvage. A major determination of morbidity is the extent of myocar-dial damage.

The clinical history remains of substantial value in establishing an AMI diagnosis. The first symptom is usually angina at rest or with minimal activity and can be found in up to 50% of patients with AMI. Chest pain can be variable in intensity, is pro-longed, and usually lasts for more than 30 min. In some patients, particularly the eld-erly, AMI is manifested not by chest pain but rather by chest tightness, weakness, congestion, nausea, or fainting. Studies show that between 40% and 50% of nonfatal AMIs are unrecognized by the patient and are found only on subsequent routine EKG.

The EKG changes of an AMI are those of ischemia. Myocardial cell injury and death are reflected by T-wave changes, ST-segment changes, and the appearance of Q waves. The ST-segment is elevated after myocardial injury. The diagnostic specificity of the EKG is 100%. If the EKG pattern is equivocal, then the clinician must depend on markers of myocardial injury. In approx 15–20% of AMIs, there are no changes on the initial EKG. The EKG diagnosis of an old infarct is often difficult, especially without a tracing from the initial acute episode.

The precipitating factors in most patients are different to identify. The terminology of ACS has been defined to encompass a broad spectrum of ischemic heart disease symptoms, including unstable angina and non-ST-segment elevation AMI. Vascular injury and thrombus formation are key events in the initiation and progression of CAD and in the pathogenesis of ACS. Pathophysiologically, the classification of vascular damage has been based on three stages consisting of (1) functional alterations of endot-helial cells without substantial morphologic changes, (2) endothelial denudation and critical damage with intact internal elastic lamina, and (3) endothelial denudation with damage to both intima and media.

Most AMIs result from coronary atherosclerosis, which evolve from coronary thrombosis. Numerous factors contribute to the evaluation of atherosclerotic plaques that may rupture acutely, releasing thrombogenic substances that mediate platelet activation, thrombin generation, and fibrinolytic deficit. Newly formed thrombi interrupts blood flow and cause ischemic myocardial injury, leading to myocardial necrosis. The process of plaque rupture has both immunologic and thrombotic activation. Enzymes, such as collagenases and gelatinase, which mediate plasma disruption, usually are released by the intracellular components of the plaque. In AMI, the primary activation of the coagulation process is through the activation of factor VII, initiated by tissue factor from the ruptured plaque.

In patients with stable CAD, angina often results from increases in myocardial oxygen demands that overwhelm the ability of an occluded coronary artery to increase its delivery. In contrast, unstable angina, non-ST-segment elevation AMI, and ST-segment elevation AMI present a continuation of the disease process characterized by abrupt decreases in coronary flow. In UA, episodes of thrombotic occlusion at a site of plaque disruption may lead to angina at rest. This labile thrombus may only occlude a vessel for 10–20 min. In non-ST-segment elevation AMI, the morphology of the lesion is often similar to that observed in UA, with one-quarter of non-ST-segment elevation patients demonstrating a completely occluded artery at angiography. Often this complete coronary occlusion is followed by spontaneous reperfusion within the first 2 h. In non-ST-segment elevation AMIs, the plaque damage is usually worse than in UA, resulting from a more persistent thrombotic occlusion, that is, more myocardial injury. In ST-segment elevation AMI, plaque disruption can be associated with ulceration and deep arterial damage, with high thrombogenic risk. This results in the formation of a fixed and persistent thrombus, which are occlusive and lead to abrupt cessation of myocardial perfusion and necrosis of the involved myocardial tissue. Some thrombus formation appears to be an important factor in the progression of CAD and in the conversion of chronic to acute events after plaque disruption.

3. MI REDEFINED

A consensus document authored by a joint committee of the European Society of Cardiology (ESC) and the American College of Cardiology (ACC) recently described that MI should be redefined as any amount of myocardial necrosis, as indicated by an increase in cardiac biomarkers (cardiac troponin I [cTnI] or T [cTnT] or creatine kinase MB (CKMB) in the setting of clinical ischemia *(7,8)*. In addition, the ACC and American Heart Association (AHA) also recently published guidelines for the reclassification of patients with ACS, for which patients presenting with an increased cardiac marker (cTn) are classified as non-ST-segment elevation MI and those with a normal troponin as UA *(9)*. Both documents stress that any concentration of cardiac troponin exceeding the decision limit (99th percentile of the values) for a reference (normal) population on at least one occasion during the first 24 h after the index clinical event (ischemia) is defined as an MI. This redefinition is significant because an individual who was previously diagnosed as having UA would now be classified as an MI if positive for troponin. Several key issues regarding the document should be noted by both clinicians and laboratorians. First, the criteria for acute, evolving, or recent MI includes the typical rise or fall of cardiac troponin (or CKMB) with at least one of the following: ischemia symptoms, development of Q waves on the EKG, EKG changes indicative of ischemia (ST-segment elevation or depression), or coronary artery intervention. Second, detectable increases in cardiac troponin (or CKMB) are indicative of myocardial injury but are not synonymous with an ischemic mechanism. Third, increases in cardiac troponin likely reflect irreversible injury. Fourth, the diversity of cardiac troponin assays, specifically for cTnI, has led to misunderstandings by clinicians and laboratories because of lack of standardization of assays. Therefore, clinical and analytical information for each cardiac troponin method should be validated through publication in the peer-reviewed literature. Fifth, for patients with an ischemic mechanism of injury, cTn increases are related to prognosis. Sixth, blood sampling should be obtained 6–9 h after onset of symptoms before a patient is ruled out for myocardial injury. Seventh, manufacturers of cTn assays should clarify sources of interferences, including heterophile antibodies, clot issues, serum vs plasma variability, and antibody epitope recognition diversity for free, complex, degraded, phosphorylated, and oxidized forms of cTnI. Eighth, the acceptable imprecision at the 99th percentile of normal, the revised recommended medical decision cutpoint, should be ≤10% coefficient of variation (CV). Manufacturers need to document at what concentrations their assay demonstrates a 10% CV. Finally, classification of patients with increases in cardiac troponins who undergo interventional procedures, such as angioplasty, should be classified as MI if increased troponins are found post-procedure. No markers should be used to determine MI in cardiac surgery patients, such as in coronary artery bypass grafting.

4. CHEST PAIN EVALUATION

4.1. Strategies for Ruling In and Ruling Out Acute Myocardial Infarction

The evaluation of patients presenting to the emergency department (ED) with chest pain continues to be a diagnostic challenge to clinicians. Both new and traditional biochemical markers for myocardial cell injury have become important in helping clinicians to (1) avoid sending home non-EKG diagnostic AMIs (estimated to be 30,000/yr in the United States); (2) assist in the triage of both high-risk and moderate-risk ACS patients into appropriate monitored and intensive care unit beds; and (3) confidently discharge patients with low risk of cardiac etiology. New strategies of cardiac marker use have also provided clinicians with strong, independent information on the short- and long-term risk of cardiac events both in hospital and after hospital discharge.

Internationally, hospitals continue to use total creatine kinase (CK) because of economics to rule in and rule out AMI in patients presenting with chest pain *(10)*, despite the limitations that total CK and its isoenzyme CKMB present. These include lack of absolute myocardial specificity, with the influence of muscle mass, exercise, sex, race, and age *(11,12)*. Cost constraints often limit the use of the more expensive testing for CKMB mass. However, the new redefinition of MI *(7,8)* and reclassification of UA guidelines *(9)* strongly support the equivalence of cTnI and cTnT (with CKMB mass as an acceptable alternative if troponin testing is not available) for the detection of AMI. The 100% cardiac specificity of cardiac troponins also support these conclusions *(13,14)*. Because it is recognized that CKMB as well as both cTnI and cTnT are not early markers of myocardial injury (it takes 3–8 h after onset of chest pain to document increases above their respective upper reference limits; refs. *15,16*) early markers, such as myoglobin and CKMB isoforms have been investigated (and recommended in the new guidelines) to assist in the sensitive earlier detection and early triage of ACS patients. Figure 1 demonstrates using receiver operator characteristic (ROC) curves that both clinical sensitivity and specificity of myoglobin, CKMB, cTnI, and cTnT improve over time after presentation to the ED *(16)*. The ROC curves display myoglobin as the most sensitive early marker at <6 h, with CKMB, cTnI, and cTnT >90% sensitivity and specificity 6–12 h after presentation. Clinicians must acknowledge the lack of cardiac tissue specificity and lack of outcome studies regarding these myoglobin *(17,18)*.

Rule-in and rule-out AMI protocols have been published to assist in the triage of chest pain patients within 12 h of presentation *(19–27)*. It should be noted that throughout this discussion, the decision trees used for early diagnosis of AMI in the ED are based on the timing of presentation to the hospital being 0 hour (h), and not the onset of chest pain as 0 h. It is so designated because the only reliable time is the time when the patient physically presents to the hospital. Unfortunately, the onset of chest pain taken during the patient's history is often unreliable, with greater than 50% of the chest pain onset times being inaccurate.

The strategy established by the Heart ER Program for rapidly evaluating chest pain patients with low to intermediate probability of AMI (nondiagnostic EKG at presentation) appears to be the model most often used in clinical studies *(27)*. A patient with chest pain or discomfort clinically consistent with acute myocardial ischemia or AMI are evaluated over a 9–12-h period. Based on the Heart ER Program findings, serial CKMB mass monitoring every 3 h up to 9 h has consistently demonstrated >98% sensitivity and >98% specificity for ruling in and ruling out AMI at 9 h after admission compared with <50% sensitivities for serial EKG monitoring, echocardiography, and graded exercise testing.

Similar studies enrolling low to intermediate probability of AMI patients with nondiagnostic EKGs that have monitored cTns have also followed the guidelines established by the Heart ER protocol (monitoring markers of myocardial injury up to 12 after presentation; refs. *23,26*). Other studies have used the strategy of following markers up to 24 h after presentation *(16,22)*. For both cTnI and cTnT, the most widely cited study examined over 700 patients with acute chest pain for less than 12 h presenting with a nondiagnostic (no ST-segment elevations) EKG *(28)*. Blood was tested (qualitatively for both cTnI and cTnT) at admission (onset of chest pain was ≤2 h after presentation) and one sample taken at least 6 h after the onset of chest pain. Of the 6% of patients with AMI, clinical sensitivity of a positive cTnT was 94% and sensitivity for cTnI was 100% (no statistical difference). Further, during 30 d of follow-up among patients with UA, increases in cTnI or cTnT were shown to be independent predictors of AMI or cardiac related death. Negative cTnI or cTnT test results were associated with low risk and allowed the rapid and safe discharge of patients.

In chest pain evaluation, protocols that have used quantitative cTnT and cTnI assays similar clinical sensitivities and specificities of >90% at >12 h after presentation have been documented. One of several representative studies to compare cTnI and cTnT with CK MB using serial 0-, 1-, 3-, 6-, 9-, and 12–24-h sample draws demonstrated that both cardiac troponins were equivalent to CKMB mass at >6 h, with sensitivities and specificities >90% by 12 h *(16)*. Neither cTn assisted in the early (2 h) screening for AMI, as expected.

Studies have also used combined marker approaches using both quantitative and qualitative POC testing devices for cTnI, cTnT, myoglobin, and CKMB mass measure-

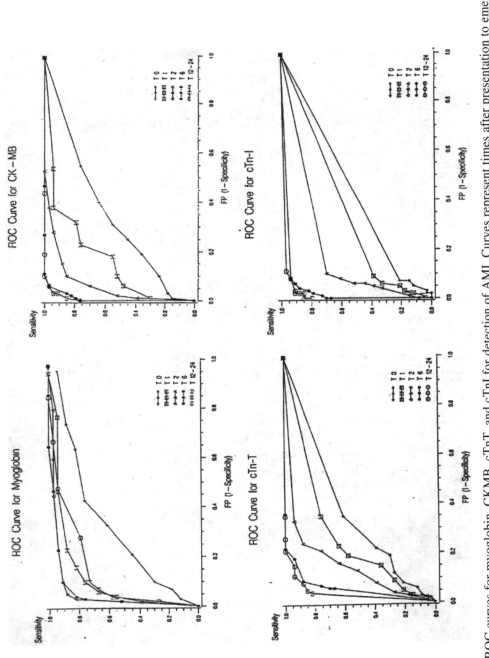

Fig. 1. ROC curves for myoglobin, CKMB, cTnT, and cTnI for detection of AMI. Curves represent times after presentation to emergency department at 0, 1, 2, 6, and 12–24 h for each marker. Myoglobin, CKMB, and cTnI were all measured by the Dade Stratus analyzer and cTnT on the ES300 analyzer (Roche-BM). Adapted from ref. *16.*

ments in chest pain evaluation protocols (16,20,22). Several trials have demonstrated that myoglobin is the most sensitive, early marker of these, with >90% sensitivity by 0–3 h after presentation (29,30). No published study to date, however, has convincingly demonstrated that the added cost of testing for myoglobin assists in improving patient therapies, or outcomes. However, it has been shown that myoglobin is an excellent negative predictor of muscle injury, as demonstrated by two early successive (usually separate by 1–3 h) negative results (whether qualitative or quantitative) with >95% confidence for ruling out AMI (31). This type of testing approach may be beneficial in rural hospitals or clinics that may need to transport patients with more critical illnesses to larger medical complexes for appropriate care. However, at larger medical centers, a 6–12-h blood draw window, with monitoring of cTns, have gained considerable favor.

Using CKMB isoforms as a proposed early marker, Puleo et al. (32) have shown that the CKMB1/MB2 ratio could be used to diagnosis or rule out AMI at 6 h after presentation, with a sensitivity of 95.7% when compared with 48% sensitivity for CKMB activity (32). A multicenter trial of patients who presented to the ED with chest pain recently directly compared diagnostic sensitivity and specificity for CKMB mass, CKMB isoforms, cTnI, cTnT, and myoglobin (33). The findings suggested that CKMB isoforms and myoglobin were more efficient for the early diagnosis (within 6 h) of MI, whereas cTnI and cTnT were highly cardiac specific and were particularly efficient after 6 h. However, no statistical analysis of data at any time point was described. The Helena REP (electrophoresis) system appears to be the only technology currently available for reliable isoform measurement and has not been readily accepted by laboratories as a ASAP, 24-h technology that could be adapted inside or outside the central laboratory.

Regarding clinical studies that use quantitative and qualitative whole blood POC testing systems, which incorporate multiple markers in one device or side by side using multiple devices, data have been generated demonstrating consistent findings compared with central laboratory instrumentation for clinical sensitivity and specificity for CKMB mass, cTnI, and cTnT, with >90% sensitivity and specificity 9 to 12 h after admission in chest pain evaluation patients (34–39). In a study evaluating the Biosite Triage (38), measures cTnI, CKMB, and myoglobin, simultaneously, cTnI demonstrated 93% sensitivity at 12 h after presentation, which was comparable with parallel determinations of either CKMB, myoglobin, or cTnI, which gave a sensitivity of 97% (no statistical differences). Similar clinical sensitivities were demonstrated in the evaluation of the First Medical Alpha Dx, (a POC testing system that simultaneously measures CKMB, cTnI, myoglobin, and total CK (39), which showed >90% sensitivity at 12 h after admission using either cTnI or CK MB. Neither the Biosite nor First Medical study was designed to appropriately address the role of multiple markers.

Several studies have now evaluated the Dade-Behring Stratus CS whole blood POC testing system for cTnI (CKMB and myoglobin are also available on this platform; refs. 40,41). Based on ROC curve analysis, a decision cutpoint of 0.15 µg/L was calculated for the detection of MI. In ACS patients 4 h after arrival in the ED, at the 0.15 µg/L cutpoint, MI sensitivity was 98%, compared with the older-generation central laboratory Stratus II assay sensitivity of 85%. The 97.5% percentile in a healthy population was 0.08 µg/L. In 42% of patients with UA, cTnI was 0.08 µg/L. Performing a 30-d outcomes analysis, death or MI occurred in 25% of cTnI-positive vs 3% cTnI-negative patients. Thus, this second-generation POC cTnI testing system demonstrated accurate, analytically sensitive, and clinically reliable information.

A quantitative whole blood bedside cTnT assay that complements the central laboratory Elecsys cTnT assay has recently been evaluated *(42)*. In a method comparison of 140 samples, the cTnT POC test correlated well with the cTnT ELISA assay ($r = 0.98$). After 4–8 h in patients with MI, 91% of all samples were positive. Areas under the ROC curves for detection of MI at the 0.1 µg/L cutpoint were comparable between the POC testing and enzyme-linked immunosorbent assay methods. The 99th percentile for healthy individuals was <0.05 µg/L. Thus, accurate, analytically sensitive and clinically reliable bedside cTnT testing, within 15 min, is now possible in suspected ACS patients.

In summarizing the rapidly growing literature involving rapid evaluation protocols used in EDs that use markers of myocardial injury, one can conclude that a fast-track protocol can assist in accurately triaging patients at high, intermediate, and low risk of cardiac pathology to appropriate levels of care and management by clinicians *(43)*. However, an essential component of any protocol involves the timing of blood draws following presentation. Figure 2 is a proposed schematic pertaining to how cardiac markers could be used to assist in patient triage. Either cTnI or cTnT is used instead of CKMB mass, and myoglobin (as an early marker) is not recommended unless appropriate documentation becomes available to support the additional expense. Further, total CK, total lactate dehydrogenase, and lactate dehydrogenase isoenzymes (which are not discussed in this chapter) are never recommended as part of any strategy *(44)*. This schematic supports the recently published ESC/ACC/AHA guidelines *(7–9)*.

4.2. Strategies for the Role of Cardiac Markers for Risk Assessment

Numerous prospective and retrospective clinical studies have evaluated and compared the utility of measurements of cTnI, cTnT, and CKMB for risk stratification or outcomes assessment of ACS patients with possible myocardial ischemia *(28,45–54)*. Patients presenting with a complaint of chest pain or other symptoms suggesting ACS have been assigned to blood sampling protocols, including only a single draw at presentation to several serial draws over a 12–24-h period after presentation. A large proportion of this heterogeneous ACS group are patients presenting with unstable angina. It is within this group that up to 50% progress to AMI or cardiac death within the first year.

Studies have demonstrated prognostic similarities between unstable angina patients and those with ST-segment elevation infarction. The use of markers is not just simply one of rapidly ruling in or ruling out AMI but also is important for the medical management of patients who are undergoing an acute coronary process (high to moderate risk) from those with chronic or stable coronary disease (low risk). Therefore, the goal of monitoring cardiac markers in ACS patients without AMI would be to identify possible unstable coronary disease and triage to an appropriate therapy regimen. This might allow the clinician to offer the patient, assuming an abnormal cardiac marker test is identified, alternative medical and procedural options, such as antiplatelet or antithrombotic therapies, a coronary angiogram, an echocardiography, a radionuclide scan, or exercise stress test to possibly identify the pathologic etiology responsible for the tissue release of markers of myocardial injury.

One quarter to one third of ACS patients in whom AMI has been ruled out have shown increased cTnI and or cTnT. Figure 3 summarizes data from a recent meta-analysis on this subject *(55)*. Increases in cTnT or cTnI are predicative of adverse outcomes in ACS patients. Twenty-one studies were evaluated, and odds ratios (ORs;

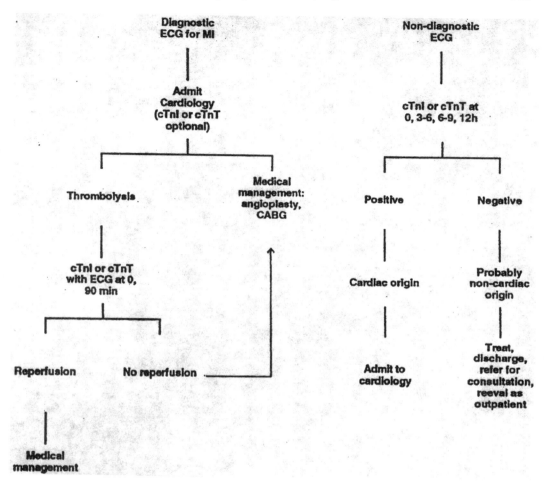

Fig. 2. Schematic for chest pain evaluation using cTnI or T as a single marker to assist clinicians in ruling in and ruling out AMI.

endpoint death or nonfatal MI) were calculated for both short-term (30 d) and long-term (5 mo to 3 yr) outcomes in patients with and without ST-segment elevation and in UA patients. Overall, in the approx 18,000 patients included, at 30 d the OR for an adverse outcome was 3.4 for an increased troponin. For patients with a positive troponin, the OR to have an adverse outcome in patients with UA was higher (9.3) compared with patients with ST-segment elevation (4.9) for both short- and long-term outcomes. Therefore, both cTnT and cTnI offer the best risk assessment, and their testing needs to be eased into current practice guidelines regarding diagnosis and management of ACS patients as useful risk stratification tools. This approach is supported in the new ESC/ACC/AHA guidelines. It is recommended to draw two samples (for either cTnI or cTnT) on ACS patients who do not rule in for AMI; one at presentation and one at 9 h after presentation. This will allow for an increase in either cardiac troponin to occur above baseline in a patient presenting with a very recent acute coronary lesion *(54)*. It should not be overlooked, however, that a normal cardiac troponin does not remove all

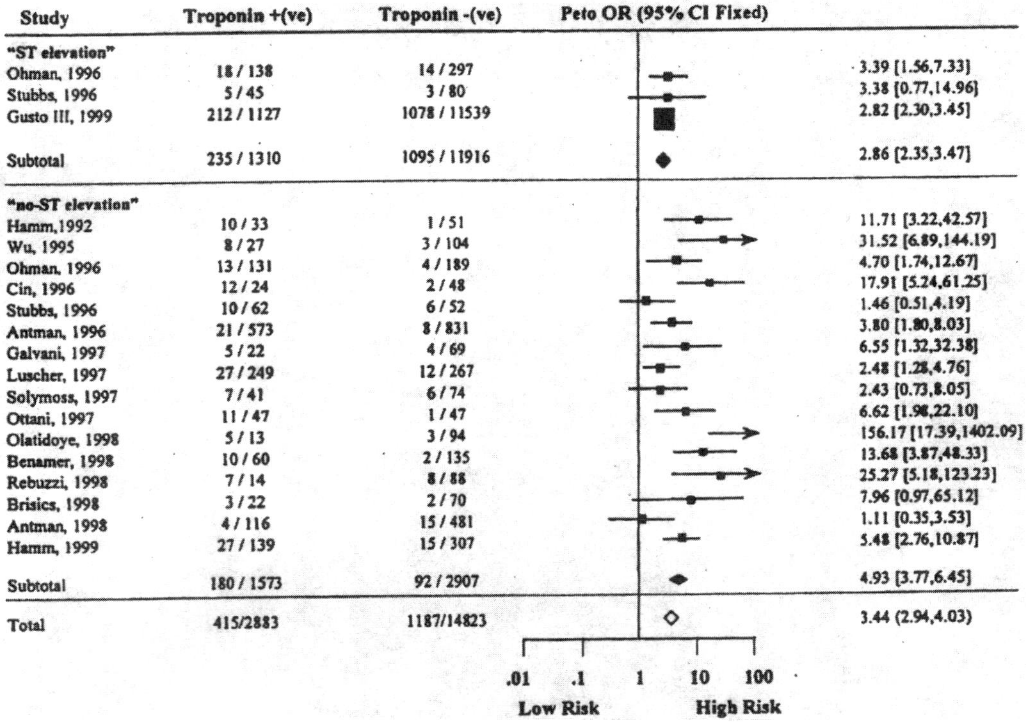

Study	Troponin +(ve)	Troponin -(ve)	Peto OR (95% CI Fixed)	
"ST elevation"				
Ohman, 1996	18 / 138	14 / 297		· 3.39 [1.56,7.33]
Stubbs, 1996	5 / 45	3 / 80		3.38 [0.77,14.96]
Gusto III, 1999	212 / 1127	1078 / 11539		2.82 [2.30,3.45]
Subtotal	235 / 1310	1095 / 11916		2.86 [2.35,3.47]
"no-ST elevation"				
Hamm,1992	10 / 33	1 / 51		11.71 [3.22,42.57]
Wu, 1995	8 / 27	3 / 104		31.52 [6.89,144.19]
Ohman, 1996	13 / 131	4 / 189		4.70 [1.74,12.67]
Cin, 1996	12 / 24	2 / 48		17.91 [5.24,61.25]
Stubbs, 1996	10 / 62	6 / 52		1.46 [0.51,4.19]
Antman, 1996	21 / 573	8 / 831		3.80 [1.80,8.03]
Galvani, 1997	5 / 22	4 / 69		6.55 [1.32,32.38]
Luscher, 1997	27 / 249	12 / 267		2.48 [1.28,4.76]
Solymoss, 1997	7 / 41	6 / 74		2.43 [0.73,8.05]
Ottani, 1997	11 / 47	1 / 47		6.62 [1.98,22.10]
Olatidoye, 1998	5 / 13	3 / 94		156.17 [17.39,1402.09]
Benamer, 1998	10 / 60	2 / 135		13.68 [3.87,48.33]
Rebuzzi, 1998	7 / 14	8 / 88		25.27 [5.18,123.23]
Brisics, 1998	3 / 22	2 / 70		7.96 [0.97,65.12]
Antman, 1998	4 / 116	15 / 481		1.11 [0.35,3.53]
Hamm, 1999	27 / 139	15 / 307		5.48 [2.76,10.87]
Subtotal	180 / 1573	92 / 2907		4.93 [3.77,6.45]
Total	415/2883	1187/14823		3.44 (2.94,4.03)

.01   .1   1   10   100   ·

Low Risk   High Risk

Fig. 3. ORs and 95% confidence intervals for risk of cardiac death and reinfarction at 30-d follow-up in patients with ACS. Pooled OR for overall group of patients with ACS was 3.44, $p < 0.00001$. Troponin + (ve) = troponin positive; troponin – (ve) = troponin negative. Reprinted from ref. *55* with permission from Elsevier Science.

risk *(55)*. It is highly recommended that cardiac marker results be provided to clinicians within 60 min either by using POC testing or central laboratory instrumentation.

4.3. Strategies for the Noninvasive Assessment of Reperfusion

Biochemical markers of myocardial injury are not needed for the diagnosis of AMI in patients with diagnostic EKG evidence of AMI but are useful for confirmation. Further, markers do not serve as an indication of which patients do or do not receive thrombolytic therapy. However, in patients who are indicated for and receive thrombolytic therapy, there is a growing body of evidence that early monitoring of markers may be useful in the noninvasive assessment of reperfusion success *(56–59)*. Early and complete patency of infarct-related arteries are an important therapeutic goal during the early hours after the onset of AMI, and markers may assist clinicians in patient management strategies. It is accepted that the kinetics of myocardial protein appearance in the circulation after AMI depends on the infarct area perfusion status. Early, successful reperfusion is characterized by a rapid increase of markers and an early peak. It is difficult to assess the amount of irreversible injury by biochemical infarct sizing because of the variability in amount of protein washout that appears in the circulation after reperfusion. The laboratory can best be used to assess reperfusion status after thrombolytic therapy when early, frequent blood sampling is combined with rapid analysis of a marker of myocardial injury. Several studies *(56–59)*, all retrospective, have demonstrated that the use of one of three criteria, using the rate of increase of markers from pretherapy to 60–120 min posttherapy to determine the (1) slope, (2) an absolute increase, or (3) the ratio of the 90 to 0 min values, will, with a high degree of accuracy, predict the success or failure of reperfusion. Studies that show the rapid increase of serum CKMB, myoglobin, cTnT, and cTnI have all demonstrated high sensitivities (>75%) to predict successful TIMI 3 reflow.

4.4. Summary

AMI is now managed in a systemic, stepwise manner, where the use of anticoagulant, antiplatelet, and thrombolytic drugs all play pivotal roles. Thus, although the emphasis of this chapter is on the monitoring of biochemical markers of myocardial injury, such as cardiac troponins, CKMB, and myoglobin, the profile of activation analytes of coagulation and platelets, along with vascular distress markers, may provide important information in the management of patients in the near future. Improvements in therapies for unstable angina and non-ST-segment elevation MI are rapidly progressing. Glycoprotein IIb/IIIa platelet inhibitiors have recently been shown in several clinical trials to improve outcomes in unstable angina patients *(60)*. Management has thus been directed at preventing progression of unstable angina to AMI because of the poorer prognosis such patients carry. However, thrombolytic therapy in unstable angina is not indicated. Therefore to be able to distinguish between unstable angina from infarction in patients as soon possible after presentation to the ED becomes important. The clinical studies discussed in this chapter strongly support the use of cardiac troponins to assist clinicians with their differential diagnosis. However, clinicians continue to order multiple serial markers in AMI documented patients, with the explanation that they are looking for a peak concentration to occur or to assist in sizing of the infarction. At present, it is not clear whether the expense of measuring several markers are justified based or whether patient management or therapy will be altered by the timing of the peak value of a biochemical marker.

5. ASSAYS FOR MARKERS OF MYOCARDIAL INJURY

5.1. Central Laboratory Assays

With the development of numerous central laboratory biomarker (cardiac troponin) assays (Table 1), as well as rapid whole-blood POC testing devices (Table 2), for measurement of cTnT and cTnI and CKMB and myoglobin, it is important to briefly discuss how absolute concentrations from the same marker may or may not differ between instruments. Selection of antibodies for the epitopes they recognize as well as how an assay is standardized may affect results among assays from different manufacturers. Currently, there is not an internationally accepted standard reference material for myoglobin, CKMB, or cTnI. Because only one manufacturer markets cTnT assays, independent of the qualitative or quantitative platform used, whole blood, serum, or plasma, within-sample cTnT results should be highly concordant *(42)*. For myoglobin, although there currently is no accepted reference standard material, concentrations between assays do not vary widely, likely because of common epitopes recognized by commer-

Table 1
cTn Assay Characteristics as Stated by Manufacturers

Manufacturer	Assay	Generation	LLD	99%	10% CV con	AMI ROC	10% CV/99th ratio
Abbott	AxSYM	1st	0.14	0.5	0.8	2	1.6
Bayer	Immuno 1	1st	0.1	0.1	0.35	0.9	3.5
	ACS: 180	1st	0.03	0.1	0.35	1	3.5
	Centaur	1st	0.02	0.1	0.35	1	3.5
Beckman-Coulter	Access	2nd	0.01	0.04	0.06	0.5	1.5
Biosite	Triage	1st	0.19	<0.19	0.5	0.4	2.6
Dade Behring	Dimension RxL	2nd	0.04	0.07	0.14	0.6–1.5	2
	Stratus CS	2nd	0.03	0.04	0.06	0.6–1.5	1.5
	Opus/Opus Plus	1st	0.1	0.1	0.3	0.6–1.5	3
DPC	Immulite	1st	0.2	0.2	0.6	1	3
	Immulite Turbo	1st	0.5	0.48	0.6	1	1.2
First Medical	Alpha Dx	1st	0.017	0.15	0.3	0.4	2.5
Ortho	Vitros ECi	1st	0.038	0.08	0.12	0.4	1.5
Roche	Elecsys	3rd	0.01	0.01	0.035	0.1	3.5
Tosoh	AIA	2nd	0.06	<0.06	0.06	0.31–0.64	1.2

LLD, lower limit of detection; 99th, 99th percentile of the reference range; 10% CV conc, concentration with ≤10% precision; AMI ROC, AMI cut-off value determined by ROC analysis, usually using a CKMB standard; centration values expressed as µg/L; DPC, Diagnostics Products Corporation.

Table 2
Whole Blood POC Testing Platforms and Cardiac Marker Assays

Manufacturer	Platform	Markers	Volume (μL)	TAT (min)	Detection limit (μg/L)	URL (μg/L)
Quantitative						
Dade Behring	Stratus CS	Myoglobin	200	13[b]	1.0	82.0
Glasgow, DE		CK MB	200		0.3	3.5
		cTnI	200		0.03	0.6
First Medical[a]	Alpha DX	Myoglobin	250	20	5.0	180.0
Mountain View, CA		CK MB			0.5	7.0
		cTnI			0.9	0.4
		Total CK			10.0	190.0
Biosite[a]	Triage	Myoglobin	250	10	2.7	107.0
San Diego, CA		CK MB			0.75	4.3
		cTnI			0.19	0.4
Roche-BM	CARDIAC	cTnT	150	12	0.1	0.1
Indianapolis, IN		Myoglobin	150		30.0	70.0
Qualitative						
Spectral[a]	Cardiac	cTnI	200	15	1.5	1.5
Toronto, Canada	STATus	Myoglobin	200	15	100.0	100.0
		MB	200	15	5.0	5.0
Roche-BM	Rapid assay	cTnT	150	20	0.18	0.18
Indianapolis, IN						
Investigational						
i-STAT	i-STAT	cTnI	25	10	0.02	0.08
Princeton, NJ	meter					
Response Biomedical		Myoglobin[c]	70	10	2.4	100
Vancouver, BC,		CKMB	70	10	4.0	NA
Canada		cTnI	70	10	0.04	NA

[a] Panel of tests obtained with each analysis.
[b] Additional test results are obtained every 4 min.
[c] FDA approved.
TAT, turnaround time; URL, upper reference limit; ROC curve derived.

cial antimyoglobin antibodies. An IFCC Scientific Committee is in the process of developing a standard material for myoglobin. For CKMB mass, an American Association for Clinical Chemistry (AACC) standard subcommittee has been successful in developing a primary reference material that eliminates the 40–60% differences currently experienced among the more than 10 commercial immunoassays *(61)*. For cTnI, the AACC, with assistance from the IFCC committee, has established a standards subcommittee to develop a primary standard. Preliminary findings indicate that three materials (IC or TIC complexes) have been identified, and round-robin validation studies are underway with the manufacturers of all cTnI immunoassays *(62)*.

5.2. POC Assays

As shown in Table 2, two qualitative and four quantitative, rapid (≤ 20-min TAT), whole-blood POC testing devices have been evaluated and Food and Drug Administration (FDA) approved for one or more of the following markers *(28,34–41)*: myoglobin, CKMB mass, cTnI, cTnT, and total CK. In addition, two quantitative investigational devices are also noted. Numerous other platforms (normally found in the central laboratory as noted previously) are also available for the (rapid) quantitative measurement of these markers in serum and plasma *(3)*.

These also provide analytical TATs within 20 min of placing a specimen on the instrument. However, the focus of this section will mainly be on the whole blood devices. At present, approx 10% of laboratories report using POC testing devices, determined from the 2000 College of American Pathology Survey CAR-C. With the recent FDA approval and release of quantitative, whole blood POC testing devices, it will be noteworthy to follow the changing trends.

Currently, for cTnI, only Dade Behring has both a whole blood POC testing device (Stratus CS) and a central laboratory instrument (Dimension RxL) measuring cTnI, both of which that give equivalent results. Among all other cTnI methods, published slopes of regression equations compared against the Dade Behring Stratus II range from 0.10–3.50 *(3,63)*. The wide variation in slopes are partially explained by the multiple forms of cTnI found in the blood, by the multiple epitope regions recognized by the many different anti-cTnI-antibodies used, as well as by lack of standardization *(64)*. The development of clinical databases for each cTnI assay becomes mandatory, although clinical trends between assays are comparable. For cTnT, Roche now has both an FDA-approved POC testing method (Cardiac Reader) and a central laboratory method (Elecsys) that give equivalent results. A description of the whole blood POC testing devices follows.

5.3. POC Testing Assay Evaluation

The analytical and clinical evaluation of POC testing assays and devices should be conducted along similar processes used to evaluate instrumentation evaluated for the central laboratory. Precision and accuracy should be held to the same standards as the central laboratory technology. Furthermore, clinical sensitivity and specificity determinations should be assessed using appropriate patient populations needed to establish decision cutoffs for ruling in and ruling out AMI (using ROC curves over time after presentation to the hospital) as well as for establishing risk stratification decision cutoffs in ACS patients. However, the new ESC/ACC/AHA guidelines support the use of the 99th percentile of a reference population as the desired upper cutpoint for detection of AMI. Both the laboratory and cardiology communities support this new cut point, emphasizing that the imprecision at this cutpoint be ≤10%. At present, few manufacturer's assays approach this imprecision goal. As an example, Fig. 4 demonstrates the type of data analysis that manufacturers should present regarding imprecision calculations at 20% CV, 10% CV, and where these imprecision values relates to the assay's 99th percentile cutpoint. Current protocols used for submission to the FDA for 510K approval do not appear to satisfy these needs. Both the laboratory and clinical communities are lobbying the FDA to revise the imprecision standards required for troponin (and CKMB mass) immunoassays prior to 510K approval.

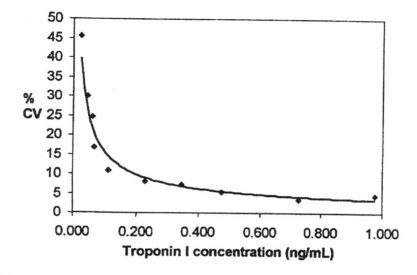

Fig. 4. Sensitivity data for Ortho Vitros ECi cTnI assay for ten pools, ranging from 0.025 to 0.97 μg/L, analyzed over 28 d. The concentrations at 10% CV and 20% CV were 0.194 μg/L and 0.070 μg/L, respectively.

Selecting the most appropriate POC testing device for a specific hospital or clinic setting will highly depend on the numerous clinical and analytical issues addressed in this chapter, including need for rapid test TATs, cost issues, impact on clinician's patient management, comparability of POC testing results with central laboratory results, and so on. All issues essentially must be tied into the clinician's needs to evaluate AMI, risk assessments and medical management in ACS patients, reperfusion assessment, and laboratory and hospital economics. Two recent publications using POC testing assays attempt to address the role of near bedside testing using a single marker vs a multiple marker strategy for ruling in or out AMI and risk assessment in ACS patients (Stratus CS; ref. *65*; Biosite Triage; ref. *66*). Upon careful review of their methods, both works still fail to validate the analytical issues between central laboratory and POC testing pertaining to assay imprecision at medical decision cutpoints as discussed and highlighted in this chapter.

6. CONCLUSIONS

Advancements in technology and the incorporation of monoclonal antibodies into POC testing and central laboratory instrumentation now allows for the detection of several biochemical markers of myocardial injury.

1. The new ESC/ACC/AHA guideline have redefined the definition of MI and is predicated on an increased cardiac troponin (cTnI or cTnT) in the clinical setting of ischemic symptoms.
2. POC testing devices provide both whole blood qualitative and quantitative results in less than 20 min, comparable to the central laboratory systems, which use serum and plasma. This alleviates lost time in specimen processing, transport and result reporting, which in some situations may take as long as 2–4 h, diminishing the value of the test in real time decision making.

3. Rapid turnaround times of cardiac markers, within 30–60 min to clinicians, need to be the standard to allow for optimal patient care.

4. In chest pain patients who present to the ED with an equivocal EKG for MI, markers of myocardial injury are critically important in the assessment of myocardial injury. Specifically cTnI and cTnT, evaluated over a 12-h period from presentation to the ED, demonstrates >90% clinical sensitivity and specificity for ruling in and ruling out a myocardial infarction.

5. Either cTnI or cTnT should replace CKMB and total CK.

6. An early marker, such as myoglobin, may not be necessary unless a rapid triage protocol (<6 h) is implemented and demonstrated to improve patient management.

7. Further, cTns provide information to clinicians improving their ability to appropriately risk stratify (assist in predicting clinical outcomes) ACS patients, make therapeutic decisions, monitor reperfusion success, and differentiate skeletal muscle from heart muscle injury.

REFERENCES

1. Wu, A. H. B., ed. (1998) *Cardiac Markers*, 1st Edition, Humana Press, Totowa, NJ.

2. Kaski J. C. and Holt, D. W., eds. (1998) *Myocardial Damage: Early Detection by Novel Biochemical Markers*, 1st Edition, Kluwer Academic Publishers, London, UK.

3. Adams J. E. II., Apple, F. S., Jaffe, A.., and Wu, A. H. B., eds. (2001) *Markers in Cardiology: Current and Future Clinical Applications. AHA Monograph Series*, Futura Publishing Co, Armonk, New York.

4. Apple, F. S. and Henderson, A. R. (1998) Cardiac function, in *Tietz Textbook of Clinical Chemistry* (Burtis, C. A. and Ashwood, E. R., eds.), 3rd Edition, W. B. Saunders Co., Philadelphia, pp. 1178–1203.

5. Braunwald, E. (1997) *Heart Disease: A Textbook of Cardiovascular Medicine,* 5th Edition, W. B. Saunders Co, Philadelphia, PA, pp. 1900.

6. Roberts, R., Morris, D., Pratt, C. M., and Alexander, R. W. (1994) *The Heart: Pathophysiology, Recognition, and Treatment of Acute Myocardial Infarction and its Complications* (Schlant, R. C. and Alexander, R. W., eds.), McGraw-Hill Inc, New York, pp. 1107–1184.

7. Joint European Society of Cardiology/American College of Cardiology. (2000) Myocardial infarction redefined-a consensus document of the Joint European Society of Cardiology/American College of Cardiology Committee for the redefinition of myocardial infarction. *J. Am. Coll. Cardiol.* **36,** 959–969.

8. Jaffe, A. S., Ravkilde, J., Roberts, R., Naslund, U., Apple, F. S., Galvani, M., et al. (2002) It's time for a change to troponin standard. *Circulation* **102,** 1216–1220.

9. Braunwald, E., Antman, E. M., Beasley, J. W., Califf, R. M., Cheitlin, M. D., Hochman, J. S., et al. (2000) ACC/AHA guidelines for the management of patients with unstable angina and non-ST-segment elevation myocardial infarction. *J. Am. Coll. Cardiol.* **36,** 970–1062.

10. De Leon, A., Farmer, C. A., King, G., Manternach, J., and Ritter, D. (1989) Chest pain evaluation unit: A cost effective approach for ruling out acute myocardial infarction. *South Med. J.* **82,** 1083–1089.

11. Silverman, L. M., Mendell, J. R., Sahenk, Z., and Fontana, M. B. (1976) Significance of creatine phosphokinase isoenzymes in Duchenne dystrophy. *Neurology* **26,** 561–564.

12. Apple, F. S., Rogers, M. A., Casal, D., Sherman, W., and Ivy, J. L. (1985) Creatine kinase MB isoenzyme adaptations in stressed human skeletal muscle obtained from marathon runners. *J. Appl. Physiol.* **59,** 149–153.

13. Bodor, G. S., Porterfield, D., Voss, E. M., Smith, S., and Apple, F. S. (1995) Cardiac troponin I is not expressed in fetal and healthy or diseased adult human skeletal tissue. *Clin. Chem.* **41,** 1710–1715.

14. Ricchiuti, V., Voss, E. M., Ney, A., Odland, M., Anderson, P. A. W., and Apple, F. S. (1998) Cardiac troponin T isoforms expressed in renal diseased skeletal muscle will not cause false-positive results by the second generation cardiac troponin T assay by Boehringer Mannheim. *Clin. Chem.* **44,** 1919–1924.

15. Wu, A. H. B., Valdes, R. Jr., Apple, F. S., Gornet, T., Stone, M. A., Mayfield-Stokes, S., et al. (1994) Cardiac troponin T immunoassay for diagnosis of acute myocardial infarction and detection of minor myocardial injury. *Clin. Chem.* **40,** 900–907.

16. Tucker, J. F., Collins, R. A., Anderson, A. J., Hauser, J., Kalas J, and Apple, F. S. (1997) Early diagnostic efficiency of cardiac troponin I and troponin T for acute myocardial infarction. *Acad. Emerg. Med.* **4,** 13–21.

17. Vaidya, H. C. (1994) Myoglobin: An early biochemical marker for the diagnosis of acute myocardial infarction. *J. Clin. Immunoassay* **17,** 35–39 .

18. Wu, A. H. B., Wang, X. M., Gornet, T. G., and Ordonez-Llanos, J. (1992) Creatine kinase MB isoforms in patients with myocardial infarction and skeletal muscle injury. *Clin. Chem.* **38,** 2396–2400.

19. Lee, T. H., Juarex, G., Cook, E. F., Weisberg, M. C., Rouan, G. W., Brand, D. A., et al. (1991) Ruling out acute myocardial infarction: A prospective multicenter validation of a 12 hour strategy for patients at low risk. *N. Engl. J. Med.* **324,** 1239–1246.

20. Levitt, M. A., Promes, S. B., Bullock, S., Disano, M., Young, E. P., Gee, G., et al. (1996) Combined cardiac marker approach with adjunct two-dimensional echocardiography to diagnose acute myocardial infarction in the emergency department. *Ann. Emerg. Med.* **27,** 1–7.

21. Fesmire, F. M., Percy, R. F., Bardoner, J. B., Wharton, D. R., and Calhoun, F. B. (1998) Serial creatine kinase MB testing during the emergency department evaluation of chest pain: utility of a 2 hour delta CK MB of +1.6 ng/mL. *Am. Heart J.* **136,** 237–244.

22. Kost, G. J., Kirk, J. D., and Omand, K. (1998) A strategy for the use of cardiac injury markers (troponin I and T, creatine kinase MB mass and isoforms, and myoglobin) in the diagnosis of acute myocardial infarction *Arch. Pathol. Lab. Med.* **122,** 245–251.

23. D'Costa, M., Fleming, E., and Patterson, M. C. (1997) Cardiac troponin I for the diagnosis of acute myocardial infarction in the emergency department. *Am. J. Clin. Pathol.* **108,** 550–555.

24. Chang, C. C., Ip, M. P. C., Hsu, R. M., and Vrobel, T. (1998) Evaluation of a proposed panel of cardiac markers for diagnosis of acute myocardial infarction in patients with atraumatic chest pain. *Arch. Pathol. Lab. Med.* **122,** 320–324.

25. Gomez, M. A., Anderson, J. L., Karagounis, L. A., Muhlestein, J. B., and Mooers, F. B. for the ROMIO Study Group. (1996) An emergency department based protocol for rapidly ruling out myocardial ischemia reduces hospital time and expense: Results of a randomized study (ROMIO). *J. Am. Coll. Cardiol.* **28,** 25–33.

26. Pervaiz, S., Anderson, F. P., Lohmann, T. P., Lawson, C. J., Feng, Y. J., Wasiewicz, D., et al. (1997) Comparative analysis of cardiac troponin I and creatine kinase MB as markers of acute myocardial infarction. *Clin. Cardiol.* **20,** 269–271.

27. Gibler, W. B., Runyon, J. P., Levy, R. C., Sayre, M. R., Kacich, R., Hattemer, C. R., et al. (1995) A rapid diagnostic and treatment center for patients with chest pain in the emergency department. *Ann. Emerg. Med.* **25,** 1–8 .

28. Hamm, C. V., Goldmann, B. U., Heeschen, C., Kreymann, G., Berger, J., and Meinertz, T. (1997) Emergency room triage of patients with acute chest pain by means of rapid testing for cardiac troponin I or troponin T. *N. Engl. J. Med.* **337,** 1648–1653.

29. Gibler, W. B., Gibler, C. D., Weinshenker, E., Abbottsmith, C., Hedges, J. R., Barsan, W. G., et al. (1987) Myoglobin as an early indicator of acute myocardial infarction. *Ann. Emerg. Med.* **16,** 851–856.

30. Tucker, J. F., Collins, R. A., Anderson, A. J., Hess, M., Farley, I. M., Hagemann, D. A., et al. (1994) Value of serial myoglobin levels in the early diagnosis of patients admitted for acute myocardial infarction. *Ann. Emerg. Med.* **24,**704–708.

31. Montague, C. and Kircher, T. (1995) Myoglobin on the early evaluation of acute chest pain. *Am. J. Clin. Pathol.* **104,** 472–476.

32. Puleo, P. R., Meyer, D., Wathen, C., Tawa, C. B., Wheeler, S., Hamburg, R. J., et al. (1994) Use of a rapid assay of subforms of creatine kinase MB to diagnose or rule out acute myocardial infarction. *N. Engl. J. Med.* **331,** 561–566.

33. Zimmerman, J., Fromm, R., Meyer, D., Boudreaux, A., Wun, C. C., Smalling, R., et al. (1999) Diagnostic marker cooperative study for diagnosis of myocardial infarction. *Circulation* **99,** 1671–1677.

34. Panteghini, M., Cuccia, C., Pagani, F., and Turla, C. (1998) Comparison of the diagnostic performance of two rapid beside biochemical assays on the early detection of acute myocardial infarction. *Clin. Cardiol.* **21,** 394–398.

35. Sylven, C., Lindahl, S., Hellkvist, K., Nyguist, O., and Rasmanis, G. (1998) Excellent reliability of nurse-based bedside diagnosis of acute myocardial infarction by rapid dry-strip creatine kinase MB, myoglobin, and troponin T. *Am. Heart J.* **135,** 677–683.

36. REACTT Investigators Study Group. (1997) Evaluation of a bedside whole blood rapid troponin T assay in the emergency department. *Acad. Emerg. Med.* **4,** 1083–1089.

37. Gerhardt, W., Ljungdahl, L., Collinson, P. O., Louis C, Sylven, C., Leinberger, R., et al. (1997) An improved rapid troponin T test with a decreased detection limit: A multicenter study of the analytical and clinical performance in suspected myocardial damage. *Scan. J. Clin. Lab. Invest.* **57,** 549–558.

38. Apple, F. S., Christenson, R. H., Valdes, R., Andriak, A. J., Berg, A., Duh, S. H., et.al. (1999) Simultaneous rapid measurement of whole blood myoglobin, CK MB, and cardiac troponin I by the Triage Cardiac Panel for detection of myocardial infarction. *Clin. Chem.* **45,** 199–205.

39. Apple, F. S., Anderson, F. P., Collinson, P., Jesse, R. L., Kontos, M. C., Levitt, M. A., et al. (2000) Clinical evaluation of the First Medical whole blood, point-of-care testing device for detection of myocardial infarction. *Clin. Chem.* **46,** 1604–1609.

40. Heeschen, C., Goldmann, B. V., Langenbrink, L., Matschuck, G., and Hamm, C. W. (1999) Evaluation of a rapid whole blood ELISA for quantification of troponin I in patients with acute chest pain. *Clin. Chem.* **45,** 1789–1796.

41. Heeschen, C., Deu, A., Langenbrink, L., Goldmann, B. U., and Hamm, C. V. (2000) Analytical and diagnostic performance of troponin assays in patients suspicious of acute coronary syndromes. *Clin. Biochem.* **33,** 359–368.

42. Muller-Bardorff, M., Rauscher, T., Kampmann, M., Schoolman, S., Laufenberg, F., Mangold, D., et al. (1999) Quantitative bedside assay for cardiac troponin T: A complimentary method to centralized laboratory testing. *Clin. Chem.* **45,** 1002–1008.

43. Selker, H. P., Zalenski, R. J., Antman, E. M., Aufderheide, T. P., Bernard, S. A., Bonow, R. O., et al. (1997) An evaluation of technologies for identifying acute cardiac ischemia in the emergency department: A report from a national heart attack alert program working group. *Ann. Emerg. Med.* **29,** 13–87.

44. Jaffe, A. S., Landt, Y., Parvin, C. A., Abendschein, D. R., Geltman, E. M., and Ladenson, J. H. (1996) Comparative sensitivity of cardiac troponin I and lactate dehydrogenase isoenzymes from diagnosis of acute myocardial infarction. *Clin. Chem.* **42,** 1770–1776.

45. Green, G. B., Li, D. J., Bessman, E. S., Cox, J. L., Kelen, G. D., and Chan, D. W. (1998) Use of troponin T and creatine kinase MB subunit levels for risk stratification of emergency department patients with possible myocardial ischemia. *Ann. Emerg. Med.* **31,** 19–29.

46. Sayre, M. R., Kaufmann, K. H., Chen, I. W., Sperling, M., Sidman, R. D., Diercks, D. B., et al. (1998) Measurement of cardiac troponin T is an effective method for predicting complications among emergency department patients with chest pain. *Ann. Emerg. Med.* **31,** 539–549.

47. Polanczyk, C. A., Lee, T. H., Cook, E. F., Walls, R., Wybenga, D., Printy-Klein, G., et al. (1998) Cardiac troponin I as a predictor of major cardiac events in emergency department patients with acute chest pain. *J. Am. Coll. Cardiol.* **32**, 8–14.

48. Newby, L. K., Christenson, R. H., Ohman, E. M., Armstrong, P. W., Thompson, T. D., Lee, K. L., et al. (1998) Value of serial troponin T measures for early and late risk stratification in patients with acute coronary syndromes. *Circulation* **98**, 1853–1859.

49. Antman, E. M., Sacks, D. B., Rifai, N., McCabe, C. H., Cannon, C. P., and Braunwald, E. (1998) Time to positivity of a rapid bedside assay for cardiac specific troponin T predicts prognosis in acute coronary syndromes: a thrombolysis in myocardial infarction IIAQ substudy. *J. Am. Coll. Cardiol.* **31**, 326–330.

50. Galvani, M., Ottani, F., Ferrini, D., Ladenson, J. H., Destro, A., Baccos, D., et al. (1997) Prognostic influence of elevated values of cardiac troponin I in patients with unstable angina. *Circulation* **95**, 2053–2059.

51. Wu, A. H. B. (1997) Use of cardiac markers as assessed by outcomes analysis. *Clin. Biochem.* **30**, 339–350.

52. Christenson, R. H., Duh, S. H., Newby, L. K., Ohman, E. M., Califf, R. M., Granger, C. B., et al. (1998) Cardiac troponin T and cardiac troponin I: Relative values in short term risk stratification of patients with acute coronary syndromes. *Clin. Chem.* **44**, 494–501.

53. Olatidoye, A. G., Wu, A. H. B., Feng, Y. J., and Waters, D. (1998) Prognostic role of troponin T versus troponin I in unstable angina pectoris for cardiac events with meta-analysis comparing published studies. *Am. J. Cardiol.* **81**, 1405–1410.

54. Hamm, C. V., Ravkilde, J., Gerhardt, W., Jorgensen, P., Peheim, E., Ljungdahl, L., et al. (1992) The prognostic value of serum troponin T in unstable angina. *N. Engl. J. Med.* **327**, 146–150.

55. Ottani, F., Galvani, M., Nicolini, A., Ferrini, D., Pozzati, A., Di Pasquale, G., et al. (2000) Elevated cardiac troponin levels predict the risk of adverse outcome in patients with acute coronary syndromes. *Am. Heart J.* **140**, 917–927.

56. Apple, F. S., Sharkey, S. W., and Henry, T. D. (1995) Early serum cardiac troponin I and T concentrations after successful thrombolysis for acute myocardial infarction. *Clin. Chem.* **41**, 1197–1198.

57. Christenson, R. H., Ohman, E. M., Topol, E. J., Peck, S., Newby, L. K., Duh, S. H., et al. (1997) Assessment of coronary reperfusion after thrombolysis with a model combining myoglobin, creatine kinase MB and clinical variables. *Circulation* **96**, 1776–1782.

58. Tanasijevic, M. J., Cannon, C. P., Wybenga, D. R., Fischer, G. A., Grudzien, C., Gibson, C. M., et al. (1997) Myoglobin, creatine kinase MB, and cardiac troponin I to assess reperfusion after thrombolysis for acute myocardial infarction: results from TIMI 10A. *Am. Heart J.* **134**, 622–630.

59. Laperche, T., Steg, P. G., Dehoux, M., Benessiano, J., Grollier, G., Aliot, E., et al. (1995) A study of biochemical markers of reperfusion early after thrombolysis for acute myocardial infarction. *Circulation* **92**, 2079–2086.

60. The PURSUIT Trial Investigators. (1998) Inhibition of platelet glycoprotein IIb/IIIa with eptifibatide in patients with acute coronary syndromes. *N. Engl. J. Med.* **339**, 436–443.

61. Christenson, R. H., Vaidya, H., Landt, Y., Bauer, R. S., Green, S. F., Apple, F. A., et al. (1999) Standardization of creatine kinase MB mass assays: The use of recombinant CK MB as reference material. *Clin. Chem.* **45**, 1414–1423.

62. Christenson, R. H., Duh, S. H., Apple, F. S., Bodor, G. S., Bunk, D. M., Dalluge, J., et al. (2001) Standardization of cardiac troponin I assays: round robin of ten candidate reference materials. *Clin. Chem.* **47**, 431–437.

63. Apple, F. S. (1999) Clinical and analytical standardization issues confronting cardiac troponin I. *Clin. Chem.* **45**, 18–20.

64. Wu, A. H. B., Feng, Y. J., Moore, R., Apple, F. S., McPherson, D. H., and Bodor, G. (1998) Characterization of cardiac troponin subunit release into serum after acute myocardial infarction and comparision of assays for troponin T and I. *Clin. Chem.* **44,** 1198–1208.
65. Newby, L. K., Storrow, A. B., Gibler, W. B., Garvey, J. L., Tucker, J. F., Kaplan, A. L., et al. (2001) Bedside multimarker testing for risk stratification in chest pain units: The chest pain evaluation by creatine kinase-MB, myoglobin, and troponin I (CHECKMATE) study. *Circulation* **103,** 1832–1837.
66. Ng, S. M., Krishnaswamy, Morrisey, R., Clopton, P., Fitzgerald, R., and Maisel, A. S. (2001) Mitigation of the clinical significance of spurious elevations of cardiac troponin I in settings of coronary ischemia using serial testing of multiple cardiac markers. *Am. J. Cardiol.* **87,** 994–999.

16

A Genetic Basis for Cardiac Arrhythmias

Current Status and the Future

Jeffrey A. Towbin, Matteo Vatta, Hua Li, and Neil E. Bowles

Contents

1. INTRODUCTION

Cardiac arrhythmias are major causes of morbidity and mortality, including sudden cardiac death. Sudden cardiac death in the United States occurs with a reported incidence of greater than 300,000 persons per year (*1*). Although coronary heart disease is a major cause of death, other etiologies contribute to this problem. In many of these nonischemia-related cases, autopsies are unrevealing. Interest in identifying the underlying cause of the death in these instances has been focused on cases of unexpected arrhythmogenic death, which is estimated to represent 5% of all sudden deaths. In cases in which no structural heart disease can be identified, the long QT syndrome (LQTS; ref. *1*), ventricular preexcitation (Wolff-Parkinson-White syndrome; *2*), and idiopathic ventricular fibrillation or Brugada syndrome (characterized by ST-segment elevation in the right precordial leads with or without right bundle branch block; *3*) are most commonly considered as likely causes. Another important disease in which

From: *Cardiac Drug Development Guide*
Edited by: M. K. Pugsley © Humana Press Inc., Totowa, NJ

arrhythmias are thought to play a central role is sudden infant death syndrome (SIDS; *4*), a disorder with no structural abnormalities. Arrhythmogenic right ventricular dysplasia (ARVD) is also a significant cause of sudden death *(5)* and is considered to be a primary electrical disease despite being associated with fibrosis and fatty infiltration of the right ventricle. The arrhythmias associated with ARVD have also been seen in other disorders in which structurally normal myocardium is seen, such as catecholaminergic ventricular tachycardia *(6)*. The purpose of this chapter is to describe the current understanding of the clinical and molecular genetic aspects of inherited diseases in which arrhythmias are prominent features.

2. LQTS

2.1. Clinical Description

LQTS are inherited or acquired disorders of repolarization identified by the electrocardiographic (EKG) abnormalities of prolongation of the QT interval corrected for heart rate (QTc), usually above 460–480 ms, relative bradycardia, T-wave abnormalities (Fig. 1), and episodic ventricular tachyarrhythmias (7), particularly torsade de pointes (Fig. 2). The inherited form of LQTS is transmitted as an autosomal-dominant or autosomal-recessive trait. Acquired LQTS may be seen as a complication of various drug therapies or electrolyte abnormalities. Whether the abnormality is genetic based or acquired, the clinical presentation is similar *(1,7)*. The initial presentation of LQTS is heterogeneous and most commonly includes syncope, which in many instances is triggered by emotional stress, exercise, or auditory phenomena. Other presenting features include seizures or palpitations. Some individuals have sudden death as their first symptom, whereas others are diagnosed by surface EKG during a family screening evaluation, undertaken because of family history of LQTS or sudden death.

2.2. Clinical Genetics

Two differently inherited forms of familial LQTS have been reported. The Romano–Ward Syndrome is the most common of the inherited forms of LQTS and appears to be transmitted as an autosomal-dominant trait *(8,9)*. In this disorder, the disease gene is transmitted to 50% of the offspring of an affected individual. However, low penetrance has been described and therefore gene carriers may, in fact, have no clinical features of disease *(10)*. Individuals with Romano–Ward syndrome have the pure syndrome of prolonged QT interval on EKG with the associated symptom complex of syncope, sudden death and, in some patients, seizures *(11,12)*. Occasionally, other noncardiac abnormalities, such as diabetes mellitus *(13,14)*, asthma *(15)*, or syndactyly *(16)* may also be associated with QT prolongation. LQTS may also be involved in some cases of SIDS *(5,17,18)* which, in some cases, appears in several family members.

The Jervell and Lange–Nielsen Syndrome (JLNS) is a relatively uncommon inherited form of LQTS. Classically, this disease has been described as having apparent autosomal-recessive transmission *(19–21)*. These patients have the identical clinical presentation as those with Romano–Ward syndrome but also have associated sensorineural deafness. Clinically, patients with JLNS usually have longer QT intervals as compared with individuals with Romano–Ward syndrome and also have a more malignant course. Priori and colleagues *(22)* have reported autosomal-recessive cases of Romano–Ward syndrome as well, thus changing one of the sina qua nons of JLNS.

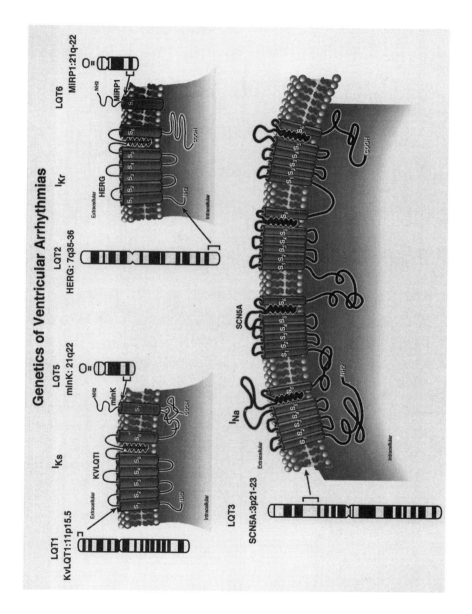

Fig. 1. Genetics of ventricular arrhythmias. The genetic loci and known genes identified for LQTS initially are shown along with the ion channel protein structure. Note that the potassium channel α subunits KvLQT1 and *HERG* require association with β subunits (*minK* and *KVLQT1* and *HERG* = Iks; MiRP1 and *HERG* = Ikr) for normal function.

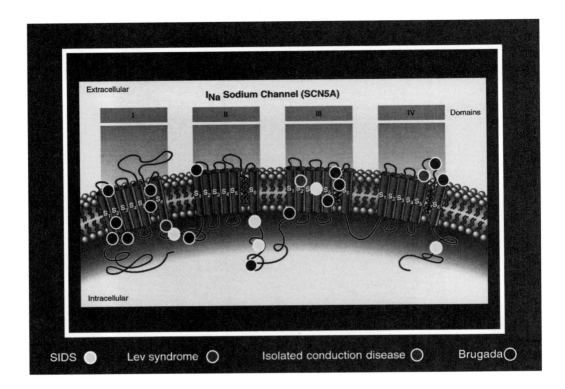

Fig. 2. Cardiac sodium channel (*SCN5A*) gene mutations associated with cardiac arrhythmias and conduction system diseases. Cardiac arrhythmias: SIDS; Brugada syndrome; Conduction System Disease: Lev syndrome; isolated conduction disease. Note that mutations for all the disorders that are scattered throughout the channel protein domains are found within the transmembrane portions and pore regions of the channel, as well as within intracellular and extracellular regions of the protein.

2.3. Gene Identification in Romano–Ward Syndrome

2.3.1. KVLQT1 *or* KCNQ1: *The* LQT1 *Gene*

The first of the genes mapped for LQTS, termed *LQT1*, required 5 yr from the time that mapping to chromosome 11p15.5 was first reported *(23)* to gene cloning. This gene, originally named *KVLQT1*, but more recently called *KCNQ1* (Table 1), is a novel potassium channel gene that consists of 16 exons, spans approx 400 kb, and is widely expressed in human tissues, including heart, inner ear, kidney, lung, placenta, and pancreas, but not in skeletal muscle, liver, or brain *(24)*. Although most of the mutations are "private" (i.e., only seen in one family), there is at least one frequently mutated region (called a "hot-spot") of *KVLQT1 (25–27)*. This gene is the most commonly mutated gene in LQTS.

Table 1
Genetics and Cardiac Arrhythmias

Disease	Rhythm abnormality	Inheritance	Chromosome location	Gene
Ventricular arrhythmias				
Romano-Ward syndrome	TdP, VF	AD	11p15.5, 7q35, 3p21, 4q25, 21q22^a	*KVLQT1* (11p15.5); *HERG* (7q35); *SCN5A* (3p21); *minK* (21q22); *MiRP1* (21q22)
Jervell-Lange-Nielsen syndrome	TdP, VF	AD/AR*	11p15.5, 21q22	*KVLQT1* (11p15.5); *minK* (21q22)
Brugada syndrome	VT, VF	AD	3p21	*SCN5A*
Sudden Infant Death Syndrome	VT/VF	AD	3p21	*SCN5A*
Familial VT	VT	AD	?	?
Familial bidirectional VT	VT	AD	1q42	RYR2
Familial Polymorphic VT	VT	AD	1q42^a	RYR2
Arrhythmogenic RV Dysplasia	VT	AD	1q42	RYR2
Naxos Disease	VT	AR	17q21, 6p24	Plakoglobin (17q21); Desmoplakin (6p24)
Supraventricular arrhythmias				
Familial atrial fibrillation	AF	AD	10q22	?
Familial total atrial standstill	SND, AF	AD	?	?
Familial absence of sinus rhythm	SND, AF	AD	?	?
Wolff-Parkinson-White syndrome	AVRT, AF, VF	AD	7q3	AMPK
Familial PJRT	AVRT	AD	?	?
Conduction abnormalities				
Familial AV block	AVB, AF, SND, VT, SD	AD	19q13	?
Isolated AV block	AVB, AF, SND, VT, SD	AD	3p21	*SCN5A*
Lev-Lengre syndrome	AVB, AF, SND, VT, SD	AD	3p21	*SCN5A*
Familial bundle branch block	RBBB	?	?	?

Abbreviations: AF, atrial fibrillation; AVB, atrioventricular block; AVRT, atrioventricular reciprocating tachycardia; RBBB, right bundle branch block; SD, sudden death; SND, sinus node dysfunction; TdP, torsade de pointes; VT, ventricular tachycardia; VF, ventricular fibrillation; AD, autosomal dominant; AR, autosomal recessive; PJRT, permanent form of junctional reciprocating tachycardia.

^{a}At least one other unknown.

*JLNS: autosomal-dominant rhythm abnormality and autosomal-recessive sensorineural deafness.

Analysis of the predicted amino acid sequence of *KVLQT1* suggests that it encodes a potassium channel α subunit with a conserved potassium-selective pore-signature sequence flanked by six membrane-spanning segments similar to shaker-type channels *(24,27–29)*. A putative voltage sensor is found in the fourth membrane-spanning domain (S4), and the selective pore loop is between the fifth and sixth membrane-spanning domains (S5, S6). Biophysical characterization of the *KVLQT1* protein confirmed that KVLQT1 is a voltage-gated potassium channel protein subunit that requires coassembly with a β subunit called *minK* to function properly *(28,29)*. Expression in either *KVLQT1* or *minK* alone results in either inefficient or no current development. When *minK* and *KVLQT1* are co-expressed in either mammalian cell lines or *Xenopus oocytes*, however, the slowly activating potassium current [I_{Ks}] is developed in cardiac myocytes *(28,29)*. Combination of normal and mutant *KVLQT1* subunits forms abnormal I_{Ks} channels, and these mutations are believed to act through a dominant-negative mechanism (the mutant form of *KVLQT1* interferes with the function of the normal wild-type form through a "poison pill"-type mechanism) or a loss-of-function mechanism (only the mutant form loses activity; ref. *30*).

Because *KVLQT1* and *minK* form a unit, mutations in *minK* could also be expected to cause LQTS, and this fact was subsequently demonstrated (*see* section on LQT5; ref. *31*).

2.3.2. HERG *or* KCNH2: *The* LQT2 *Gene*

The *LQT2* gene was initially mapped to chromosome 7q35-36 by Jiang et al. *(27,32)* and, subsequently, candidate gene screening identified the disease-causing gene human ether-a-go-go-related gene (*HERG*), a cardiac potassium channel gene to be the *LQT2* gene (Table 1). *HERG* was originally cloned from a brain cDNA library *(33)* and found to be expressed in neural-crest–derived neurons *(34)*, microglia *(35)*, a wide variety of tumor cell lines *(36)*, and the heart *(37)*. LQTS-associated mutations were identified in *HERG* throughout the gene, including missense mutations, intragenic deletions, stop codons, and splicing mutations *(27,37,38)*. Currently, this gene is thought to be the second most common gene mutated in LQTS (second to *KVLQT1*). As with *KVLQT1*, "private" mutations that are scattered throughout the entire gene without clustering preferentially are seen.

HERG consists of 16 exons and spans 55 kb of genomic sequence *(37)*. The predicted topology of *HERG* is similar to *KVLQT1*. Unlike *KVLQT1*, *HERG* has extensive intracellular amino- and carboxyl termini, with a region in the carboxyl-terminal domain having sequence similarity to nucleotide binding domains.

Electrophysiological and biophysical characterization of expressed *HERG* in *Xenopus oocytes* established that *HERG* encodes the rapidly activating delayed rectifier potassium current I_{Kr} *(39–41)*. Electrophysiological studies of LQTS-associated mutations showed that they act through either a loss-of-function or a dominant-negative mechanism *(41,42)*. In addition, protein trafficking abnormalities have been shown to occur *(43,44)*. This channel has been shown to co-assemble with β subunits for normal function, similar to that seen in I_{Ks}. McDonald et al. *(45)* initially suggested that the complexing of *HERG* with *minK* is needed to regulate the I_{Kr} potassium current. Bianchi et al. *(46)* provided confirmatory evidence that *minK* is involved in regulation of both I_{Ks} and I_{Kr}. Abbott et al. *(47)* identified MiRP1 as a β-subunit for *HERG* (*see* Section 2.3.5. on *MiRP1*).

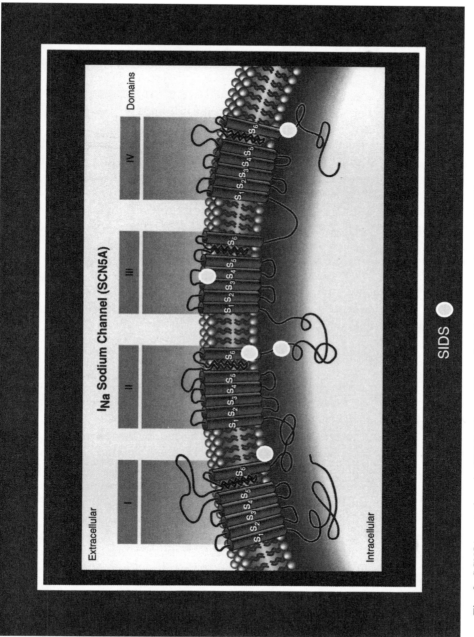

Fig. 3. *SCN5A* mutations in SIDS. The position of the known mutations in *SCN5A* reported to date to cause SIDS.

2.3.3. SCN5A: *The LQT3 Gene*

The positional candidate gene approach was also used to establish that the gene responsible for chromosome 3-linked LQTS (*LQT3*) is the cardiac sodium channel gene *SCN5A (48,49)* (Table 1). *SCN5A* is highly expressed in human myocardium and brain but not in skeletal muscle, liver or uterus *(50–52)*. It consists of 28 exons that span 80 kb and encodes a protein of 2016 amino acids with a putative structure that consists of four homologous domains (DI–DIV), each of which contains six membrane-spanning segments (S1–S6) similar to the structure of the potassium channel α subunits *(27,39)*. Linkage studies with *LQT3* families and *SCN5A* initially demonstrated linkage to the *LQT3* locus on chromosome 3p21-24 *(50,51)*, and multiple mutations were subsequently identified. Biophysical analysis of the initial three mutations were expressed in *Xenopus oocytes*, and it was found that all mutations generated a late phase of inactivation-resistant, mexiletine-, and tetrodotoxin-sensitive whole-cell currents through multiple mechanisms *(53,54)*. Two of the three mutations showed dispersed reopening after the initial transient, but the other mutation showed both dispersed reopening and long-lasting bursts *(54)*. These results suggested that *SCN5A* mutations act through a gain-of-function mechanism (the mutant channel functions normally, but with altered properties such as delayed inactivation) and that the mechanism of chromosome 3-linked LQTS is persistent noninactivated sodium current in the plateau phase of the action potential. Later, An et al. *(55)* showed that not all mutations in *SCN5A* are associated with persistent current and demonstrated that *SCN5A* interacted with β subunits.

2.3.4. minK *or* KCNE1: *The* LQT5 *Gene*

minK (lsK, or *KCNE1*) was initially localized to chromosome 21 (21q22.1) and found to consist of three exons that span approx 40 kb (Table 1). It encodes a short protein consisting of 130 amino acids and has only one transmembrane-spanning segment with small extracellular and intercellular regions *(30,31,56)*. When expressed in *Xenopus oocytes*, it produces potassium current that closely resembles the slowly activating delayed-rectifier potassium current I_{Ks} in cardiac cells *(56,57)*. The fact that the *minK* clone was only expressed in *Xenopus oocytes* and not in mammalian cell lines raised the question whether *minK* is a human channel protein. With the cloning of *KVLQT1* and coexpression of *KVLQT1* and *minK* in both mammalian cell lines and *Xenopus oocytes*, however, it became clear that *KVLQT1* interacts with *minK* to form the cardiac slowly activating delayed-rectifier I_{Ks} current *(28,29)*; *minK* alone cannot form a functional channel but induces the I_{Ks} current by interacting with endogenous *KVLQT1* protein in *Xenopus oocytes* and mammalian cells. Bianchi et al. *(46)* showed that mutant *minK* results in abnormalities of I_{Ks}, I_{Kr}, and protein trafficking abnormalities. McDonald et al. *(45)* showed that *minK* also complexes with *HERG* to regulate the I_{Kr} potassium current. Splawski et al. *(31)* demonstrated that *minK* mutations cause *LQT5* when they identified mutations in two families with LQTS. In both cases, missense mutations (S74L, D76N) were identified which reduced I_{Ks} by shifting the voltage dependence of activation and accelerating channel deactivation. This was supported by the fact that a mouse model of *minK*-defective LQTS was also created *(58)*. The functional consequences of these mutations includes delayed cardiac repolarization and, hence, an increased risk of arrhythmias.

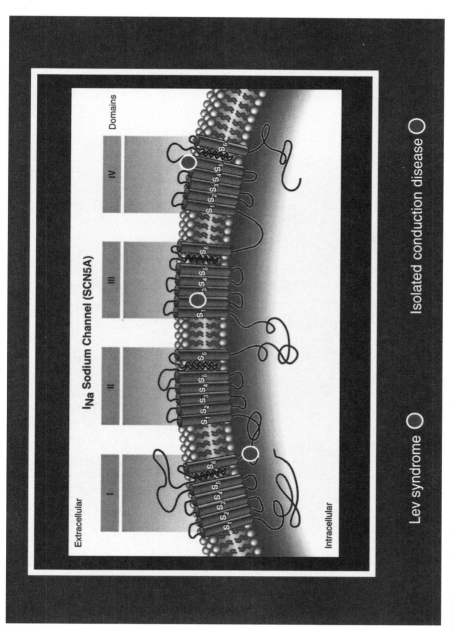
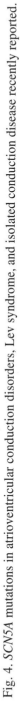

Fig. 4. *SCN5A* mutations in atrioventricular conduction disorders, Lev syndrome, and isolated conduction disease recently reported.

2.3.5. MiRP1 *or* KCNE2: *The* LQT6 *Gene*

MiRP1, the *minK*-related peptide 1, or *KCNE2* (Table 1), is a novel potassium channel gene recently cloned and characterized by Abbott and colleagues *(47)*. This small integral membrane subunit protein assembles with *HERG* (*LQT2*) to alter its function and enable full development of the I_{Kr} current. *MiRP1* is a 123 amino acid channel protein with a single predicted transmembrane segment similar to that described for *minK (56)*. Chromosomal localization studies mapped this *KCNE2* gene to chromosome 21q22.1, within 79kb of *KCNE1* (*minK*), and arrayed in opposite orientation *(47)*. The open reading frames of these two genes share 34% identity and both are contained in a single exon, suggesting that they are related through gene duplication and divergent evolution.

Three missense mutations associated with LQTS and ventricular fibrillation were identified in KCNE2 by Abbott et al. *(47)* and biophysical analysis demonstrated that these mutants form channels that open slowly and close rapidly, thus diminishing potassium currents. In one case, the missense mutation, a C to G transversion at nucleotide 25, which produced a glutamine (Q) to glutamic acid (E) substitution at codon 9 (Q9E) in the putative extracellular domain of *MiRP1*, led to the development of torsade de pointes and ventricular fibrillation after intravenous clarithromycin infusion (i.e., drug-induced).

Therefore, like *minK*, this channel protein acts as a β subunit but, by itself, leads to ventricular arrhythmia risk when mutated. These similar channel proteins (i.e., *minK* and *MiRP1*) suggest that a family of channels exist that regulate ion channel α subunits. The specific role of this subunit and its stoichiometry remains unclear and is currently being hotly debated.

2.3.6. Genetics and Physiology of Autosomal-Recessive LQTS (JLNS)

Neyroud et al. *(59)* reported the first molecular abnormality in patients with JLNS when they reported on two families in which three children were affected by JLNS and in whom a novel homozygous deletion-insertion mutation of *KVLQT1* in three patients was found. A deletion of 7 bp and an insertion of 8 bp at the same location led to premature termination at the C-terminal end of the *KVLQT1* channel. At the same time, Splawski et al. *(60)* identified a homozygous insertion of a single nucleotide that caused a frameshift in the coding sequence after the second putative transmembrane domain (S2) of *KVLQT1*. Together, these data strongly suggest that at least one form of JLNS is caused by homozygous mutations in *KVLQT1* (Table 1). This has been confirmed by others *(27,30,61,62)*.

As a general rule, heterozygous mutations in *KVLQT1* cause Romano–Ward syndrome (LQTS only), whereas homozygous (or compound heterozygous) mutations in *KVLQT1* cause JLNS (LQTS and deafness). The hypothetical explanation suggests that although heterozygous *KVLQT1* mutations act by a dominant-negative mechanism, some functional *KVLQT1* potassium channels still exist in the stria vascularis of the inner ear. Therefore, congenital deafness is averted in patients with heterozygous *KVLQT1* mutations. For patients with homozygous *KVLQT1* mutations, no functional *KVLQT1* potassium channels can be formed. It has been shown by *in situ* hybridization that *KVLQT1* is expressed in the inner ear *(60)*, suggesting that homozygous *KVLQT1* mutations can cause the dysfunction of potassium secretion in the inner ear and lead to deafness. However, it should be noted that incomplete penetrance exists and not all heterozygous or homozygous mutations follow this rule *(11,22)*.

As with Romano–Ward syndrome, if *KVLQT1* mutations can cause the phenotype, it could be expected that *minK* mutations could also be causative of the phenotype (JLNS). Schulze–Bahr et al. *(63)*, in fact, showed that mutations in *minK* result in JLNS syndrome as well, and this was confirmed subsequently (Table 1; ref. *60*). Hence, abnormal I_{Ks} current, whether it occurs because of homozygous or compound heterozygous mutations in *KVLQT1* or *minK* result in LQTS and deafness.

3. GENOTYPE–PHENOTYPE CORRELATIONS IN LQTS

3.1. Clinical Features

To a significant extent, the clinical features of LQTS depend on the gene mutated as well as the intragenic position of the mutation and its effect on the channel protein. Several studies have clarified the specific associations including clinical severity of probands, their parents and siblings, as well as modifying influences on severity.

Kimbrough et al. *(64)* recently reported on the study of 211 probands with LQTS and classified the severity of the probands, affected parents, and siblings. Importantly, they showed that the severity of the disease in the proband did not correlate with the clinical severity seen in first-degree relatives, specifically their parents and siblings. In fact, variable intrafamily penetrance was noted, consistent with other genetic and environmental factors playing a role in modulating and modifying clinical manifestations in members of the same family. However, several stratifiers were identified as important. The length of the QTc in affected parents and siblings was shown to be associated with significant risk of LQTS-related cardiac events. They also confirmed that genotype, age, and sex influence the course of disease in affected family members. For instance, male probands were found to have their first cardiac event at younger mean age than female probands (13 vs 19 yr) but female probands had a higher frequency of cardiac arrest or LQTS-related death by 40 yr of age. For affected parents, they found that female sex and QTc length were risk factors for events whereas QTc duration was the only risk factor for siblings. Affected mothers of LQTS probands displayed an ongoing cardiac event risk well after the birth of the proband but affected fathers did not display this ongoing risk.

These findings complement the findings previously described by Zareba et al. *(65)*. In this study, the authors provided evidence of clinical outcome, age of onset, and frequency of events based on genotype. Patients with mutations in LQT1 had the earliest onset of events and the highest frequency of events followed by mutations in *LQT2*. The risk of sudden death in these two groups was relatively low for any event. Mutations in LQT3 resulted in a paucity of syncopal events but the events commonly resulted in sudden death. In addition, mutations in LQT3 resulted in the longest QTc duration. Mutations in LQT1 and *LQT2* appeared to be associated with stress-induced symptoms *(66)*, with LQT1 associated with exercise and swimming *(67,68)* and *LQT2* associated with auditory triggers *(68–71)*. LQT3 appeared to be associated with sleep-associated symptoms and events.

3.2. Electrocardiographic and Biophysical Features

In 1995, Moss and colleagues *(72)* provided the first evidence that mutations in different genes cause differing EKG features. Specifically, the authors focused on the different types of T waves seen in patients with LQT1 vs *LQT2* vs LQT3. EKGs of

LQT1 patients were shown to display broad-based T waves, *LQT2* patients had low-amplitude T waves, and those with LQT3 mutations had distinctive T waves with late onset. More recently, Zhang et al. *(73)* showed that there are actually four different ST–T wave patterns. Using these definitions, they were able to identify 88% of LQT1 and *LQT2* patients accurately by surface ECG and 65% of LQT3 carriers. Prospectively,, these authors correctly predicted genotype in 100% of patients.

Further insight into EKG findings and genotype were reported by Lupoglazoff et al. *(74)* using Holter monitor analysis. Analysis of 133 LQT1 patients and 57 *LQT2* carriers, as well as 100 control individuals led the authors to conclude that T wave morphology was normal in most LQT1 patients (92%) and normal controls (96%), but the vast majority of *LQT2* patients had abnormal T waves (19% normal, 81% abnormal). In the largest percentage of *LQT2* patients, T-wave notching was identified in which the T-wave protuberance is above the horizontal whereas another subset had a bulge at or below the horizontal. In the former case, young age, missense *LQT2* mutations, and mutations in the core domain of *HERG* predicted morphology, whereas potential diagnostic clues gained by the latter morphology included amino-terminal or carboxy-terminal mutations or frameshifts in *HERG*.

3.3. Animal Models of LQTS

Using an arterially perfused canine left ventricular wedge preparation developed pharmacologically, induced animal models of LQT1, *LQT2*, and LQT3 have been created *(75,76)*. Using chromanol 293B, a specific I_{Ks} blocker, a model that mimics LQT1 was produced *(75)*. In this model, I_{Ks} deficiency alone was not enough to induce torsade de pointes, but addition of β adrenergic influence (i.e., isoproterenol) predisposed the myocardium to torsade by increasing transmural dispersion of repolarization. Addition of β blocker or mexiletine reduced the ability to induce torsade, suggesting that these medications might improve patient outcomes.

Models for *LQT2* and LQT3 were created by using *d*-sotalol (*LQT2*) or ATX-II (*LQT3*) in this wedge preparation *(76)*. Both of these drugs preferentially prolong M cell action potential duration, with ATX-II also causing a sharp rise in transmural dispersion. Mexiletine therapy abbreviated the QT interval prolongation in both models, as well as reducing dispersion. Spontaneous torsade de pointes was suppressed, and the vulnerable window during which torsade de pointes induction occurs was also reduced in both models. These models support the current understanding of the different subtypes of LQTS and provide an explanation for potential therapies.

4. THERAPEUTIC OPTIONS IN LQTS

Currently, the standard therapeutic approach in LQTS is the initiation of {b} blockers at the time of diagnosis *(7)*. Recently, Moss et al. *(77)* demonstrated significant reduction in cardiac events using β blockers. However, syncope, aborted cardiac arrest, and sudden death do continue to occur. In cases in which β blockers cannot be used, such as in patients with asthma, other medications have been tried, such as mexiletine *(78)*. When medical therapy fails, left sympathectomy or implantation of an automatic cardioverter defibrillator has been used *(7)*.

Genetic-based therapy has also been described. Schwartz et al. *(78)* showed that sodium channel blocking agents (i.e., mexiletine) shorten the QTc in patients with

LQT3, whereas exogenous potassium supplementation *(79)* or potassium channel openers *(80)* have been shown to be potentially useful in patients with potassium channel defects. However, long-term potassium therapy with associated potassium-sparing agents has been unable to keep the serum potassium above 4 m*M* because of renal potassium homeostasis. This suggests that potassium therapy may not be useful in the long term. In addition, no definitive evidence that these approaches (i.e., sodium channel blockers, exogenous potassium, or potassium channel openers) improve survival has been published.

5. BRUGADA SYNDROME

5.1. Clinical Aspects of Brugada Syndrome

The first identification of the EKG pattern of right bundle branch block (RBBB) with ST-elevation in leads V1–V3 was reported by Osher and Wolff *(81)*. Shortly thereafter, Edeiken *(82)* identified persistent ST-elevation without RBBB in 10 asymptomatic males, and Levine et al. *(83)* described ST-elevation in the right chest leads and conduction block in the right ventricle in patients with severe hyperkalemia. The first association of this EKG pattern with sudden death was described by Martini et al. *(84)* and later by Aihara et al. *(85)*. This association was further confirmed in 1991 by Pedro and Josep Brugada *(86)*, who described four patients with sudden and aborted sudden death who had EKGs demonstrating RBBB and persistent ST-elevation in leads V1–V3 (Fig. 5). In 1992, these authors characterized what they believed to be a distinct clinical and electrocardiographic syndrome *(3)*.

The finding of ST-elevation in the right chest leads has been observed in a variety of clinical and experimental settings and is not unique or diagnostic of Brugada syndrome by itself *(87)*. Situations in which these EKG findings occur include electrolyte or metabolic disorders, pulmonary or inflammatory diseases, and abnormalities of the central or peripheral nervous system. In the absence of these abnormalities, the term idiopathic ST-elevation is often used and may identify Brugada syndrome patients.

The EKG findings and associated sudden and unexpected death have been reported as a common problem in Japan and Southeast Asia, where it most commonly affects men during sleep *(88)*. This disorder, known as Sudden and Unexpected Death Syndrome or Sudden Unexpected Nocturnal Death Syndrome (SUNDS), has many names in Southeast Asia, including bangungut (to rise and moan in sleep) in the Philippines, non-laitai (sleep-death) in Laos, lai-tai (died during sleep) in Thailand, and pokkuri (sudden and unexpectedly ceased phenomena) in Japan. General characteristics of SUNDS include young, healthy males in whom death occurs suddenly with a groan, usually during sleep late at night. No precipitating factors are identified, and autopsy findings are generally negative *(89)*. Life-threatening ventricular tachyarrhythmias as a primary cause of SUNDS has been demonstrated, with ventricular fibrillation (VF) occurring in most cases *(90)*.

The risk of sudden death associated with Brugada syndrome and SUNDS reported for European and Southeast Asian individuals has been reported to be extremely high; approx 75% of patients reported by Brugada et al. *(3,86,91)* survived cardiac arrest. In addition, symptomatic and asymptomatic patients have been considered to be at equal risk. However, Priori et al. *(92)* have disputed this claim. In a study of 60 patients with Brugada syndrome, asymptomatic patients had no episodes or events. The importance

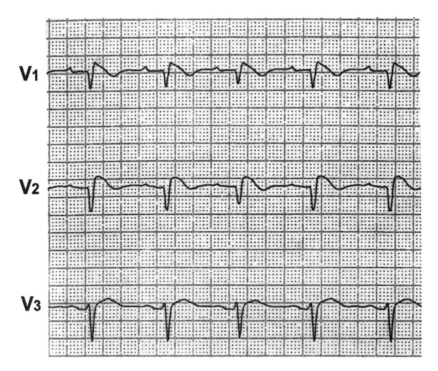

Fig. 5. EKG features of Brugada syndrome. Note the ST-segment elevation (cove-type) in leads V₁ and V₂.

of this difference is its impact on therapeutic decision making because currently all patients receive implantable cardioverter defibrillator (ICD) therapy.

Should the data of Priori et al. *(92)* hold up, selective use of ICDs would be used. If selective use of ICDs were to be considered, other diagnostic tests for risk stratification would be necessary. Kakishita et al. *(93)* studied a high-risk group of patients with 37% having spontaneous episodes of VF. As the majority of patients had ICD placement, the authors were able to show that 65% of episodes were preceded by PVCs, which were essentially identical to the initiating PVCs of VF in morphology. In fact, the PVCs initiating all VF episodes arose from terminal portions of the T-wave and pause-dependent arrhythmias were rare. This suggests that vigilant evaluation by Holter monitoring could identify at-risk patients. In addition, the authors suggested that the use of radiofrequency ablation targeting the initiating premature ventricular complexes (PVCs) could be helpful in reducing risk and reducing the need for ICD placement.

5.2. Clinical Genetics of Brugada Syndrome

Most of the families thus far identified with Brugada syndrome have apparent autosomal dominant inheritance *(94–96)*. In these families, approx 50% of offspring of affected patients develop the disease. Although the number of families reported has been small, it is likely that this is caused by underrecognition as well as premature and unexpected death *(87,97,98)*.

5.3. Molecular Genetics of Brugada Syndrome

In 1998, our laboratory reported the findings on six families and several sporadic cases of Brugada syndrome *(96)*. The families were initially studied by linkage analysis using markers to the known ARVD loci, and LQT loci and linkage was excluded. Candidate gene screening using the mutation analysis approach of single-strand conformation polymorphism analysis and DNA sequencing was performed, and *SCN5A* was chosen for study based on the suggestions of Antzelevitch *(87,95,97–99)*. In three families, mutations in *SCN5A* were identified (Table 1; *96)* including (1) a missense mutation (C-to-T base substitution) causing a substitution of a highly conserved threonine by methionine at codon 1620 (T1620M) in the extracellular loop between transmembrane segments S3 and S4 of domain IV (DIVS3–DIVS4), an area important for coupling of channel activation to fast inactivation; (2) a two nucleotide insertion (AA), which disrupts the splice-donor sequence of intron 7 of *SCN5A*; and (3) a single nucleotide deletion (A) at codon 1397, which results in an in-frame stop codon that eliminates DIIIS6, DIVS1–DIVS6, and the carboxy-terminus of *SCN5A* (Fig. 6). Mutations have also been found in *SCN5A* in children with sudden cardiac death *(100)*.

Biophysical analysis of the mutants in *Xenopus oocytes* demonstrated a reduction in the number of functional sodium channels in both the splicing mutation and one-nucleotide deletion mutation, which should promote development of reentrant arrhythmias. In the missense mutation, sodium channels recover from inactivation more rapidly than normal. Subsequent experiments conducted in modified human embryonic kidney cells revealed that at physiological temperatures (37°C), reactivation of the T1620M mutant channel was actually slower whereas inactivation of the channel was importantly accelerated. These alterations leave the transient outward current unopposed and thus able to effect an all-or-none repolarization of the action potential at the end of phase 1 *(101)*. Failure of the sodium channel to express, as with the insertion and deletion mutations, results in similar electrophysiological changes. Reduction of the sodium channel I_{Na} current causes heterogeneous loss of the action potential dome in the right ventricular epicardium, leading to a marked dispersion of depolarization and refractoriness, an ideal substrate for development of reentrant arrhythmias. Phase 2 reentry produced by the same substrate is believed to provide the premature beat necessary for initiation of the ventricular tachycardia (VT) and VF responsible for symptoms in these patients.

Interestingly, however, Kambouris et al. *(102)* identified a mutation in essentially the same region of *SCN5A* as the T1620M mutation (R1623H), but the clinical and biophysical features of this mutation was found to be consistent with LQT3 and not Brugada syndrome *(102)*. More recently, mutations in *SCN5A* in which both Brugada syndrome and LQT3 features were seen in the same patient has been described *(103)*. Hence, there clearly remains a gap in our understanding of these entities.

6. RISK STRATIFICATION IN BRUGADA SYNDROME

Most symptomatic or at-risk patients with Brugada syndrome manifest an EKG with a "coved-type" ST-segment elevation with or without provocation using sodium channel blocking agents, such as ajmaline or flecainide *(104)*. The other form of ST-segment elevation, the so-called "saddle-type," is not associated with definitive Brugada syndrome unless it transitions into a "coved-type" by provocation or independently.

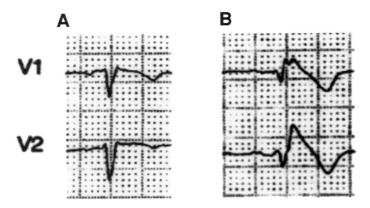

Fig. 6. Ajmaline provocation in Brugada syndrome. (**A**) demonstrates normal electrocardiogram of leads V_1 and V_2 in an individual with asymptomatic concealed Brugada syndrome and an *SCN5A* mutation. (**B**) demonstrates the response to ajmaline, identifying ST-segment elevations in leads V_1 and V_2.

Brugada et al. *(86,91,104)* have suggested, however, that the risk of sudden death is not different between symptomatic patients and asymptomatic patients, including those with concealed forms of disease.

A variety of other risk stratifiers have also been identified *(105–108)*. Assessment of noninvasive markers by Ikeda et al. *(106)* demonstrated that late potentials noted using signal-averaged EKGs were present in 24 of 33 patients (73%) with a history of syncope or aborted sudden death. Using multivariate logistic regression, the authors showed that the presence of late potentials was significantly correlated with the occurrence of life-threatening events in patients with Brugada syndrome. The evaluation of these same patients with microvolt T-wave alternans and corrected QT-interval dispersion failed to correlate with outcome. Others supported these findings as well *(108)*.

Finally, spontaneous episodes of VF in patients with Brugada syndrome were shown to be triggered by PVCs with specific morphologies, and Kakishita et al. *(93)* suggested that the use of ICD therapy not only could be life saving but also could record the specific triggering events. They suggested that this knowledge could define risk and potentially lead to either ablative therapy or the ability to stratify risk of sudden death.

Hence, the identification of "coved-type" ST-segment elevation on surface EKG, the identification of late potentials on signal-average EKG, and the finding of triggering PVCs could provide insight into those patients with Brugada syndrome at high risk. Addition of family history could allow for further improvements of risk stratification.

7. CARDIAC CONDUCTION DISEASE

Syncope and sudden death may also occur as the result of bradycardia. The most common form of life-threatening bradycardias includes disorders in which complete atrioventricular block occurs *(109)*. These disorders require pacemaker implantation for continued well being. Two major forms of conduction system disease in which no congenital heart disease is associated include isolated forms of conduction disease and conduction disease *(109,110)* associated with dilated cardiomyopathy *(111)*.

Progressive cardiac conduction defect, also known as Lev–Lenegre disease, is one of the most common cardiac conduction disorders *(109,112)*. This disorder is characterized by progressive alteration of conduction through the His-Purkinje system with development of RBBB or left-bundle branch block with widening of the QRS complexes.

Ultimately, complete atrioventricular block occurs, resulting in syncope and sudden death. Lev–Lenegre disease represents the most common cause of pacemaker implantation worldwide, accounting for 0.15 implants per 1000 population yearly in developed countries. This disorder has been considered to be a primary degenerative disease, an exaggerated aging process with sclerosis of the conduction system, or an acquired disease. The first gene identified for Lev–Lenegre disease was reported in 1999 by Schott et al. *(112)*, who identified a missense mutation and deletion mutation, respectively, in *SCN5A* (Table 1), the cardiac sodium channel gene, in two families with autosomal-dominant inheritance. Although the authors suggested that the biophysical abnormality was channel loss-of-function, no electrophysiologic analysis was provided. As *SCN5A* also causes LQT3 *(50)*, Brugada syndrome *(61,103,113)*, and SIDS *(114)*, all diseases in which ventricular tachyarrhythmias result in syncope and sudden death *(110)*, the association of conduction disturbance with *SCN5A* mutations was initially surprising. However, it is now known that conduction disturbance occurs in these disorders as well.

A similar disorder, known as isolated cardiac conduction disease, also results in complete atrioventricular block, syncope, and sudden death. This disorder has been considered to be genetically inherited (autosomal-dominant trait) and not acquired. Brink et al. *(115)* and de Meeus et al. *(116)* independently mapped a gene to chromosome 19q13.3 in families with isolated conduction disturbance in 1995, but the gene has remained elusive (Table 1). Recently, however, Tan and colleagues *(110)* identified a mutation in *SCN5A* in this disorder and also presented biophysical analysis (Table 1). This mutation, a G to T transversion in exon 12 of *SCN5A*, resulted in a change from glycine to cysteine at position 514 (G514C) encoding an amino acid within the DI–DII intercellular linker of the cardiac sodium channel. Biophysical characterization of the mutant channel demonstrated abnormalities in voltage-dependent gating behavior. The sodium current (I_{Na}) was found to decay more rapidly than the wild-type channel. In the mutant, open-state inactivation was hastened whereas closed-state inactivation was reduced and destabilized. Computational analysis predicted that the gating defects selectively slowed myocardial conduction without provoking the rapid cardiac arrhythmias seen in LQTS and Brugada syndrome. When comparing Brugada syndrome, LQT3, and conduction disease biophysics, the following findings are notable. In Brugada syndrome, *SCN5A* mutations cause reduction in I_{Na}, hastening epicardial repolarization and causing the development of VT and VF. In contradistinction, LQT3 mutations in *SCN5A* result in excessive I_{Na}, delaying repolarization and torsade de pointes VT. Importantly, the G514C mutation evokes gating shifts reminiscent of both LQT3 and Brugada syndrome, including an activation gating shift responsible for reducing I_{Na} and destabilization of inactivation that causes an increase in I_{Na}. Tan et al. *(110)* showed that these voltage-dependent gating abnormalities may be partially corrected by dexamethasone, consistent with the known salutory effects of glucocorticoids on the clinical phenotype. It is also worth noting again that some patients with LQT3 and Brugada syndrome have been reported to have conduction disturbances.

Finally, patients with conduction disease and dilated cardiomyopathy present a conundrum of what comes first, conduction abnormalities leading to cardiomyopathy or vice versa *(111)*. Clinically, these patients tend to develop variable degrees of atrioventricular block in their teen years or twenties with progression of this block over another one or two decades before developing the signs and symptoms of heart failure consistent with the cardiomyopathic phenotype. To date, only the gene lamin A/C located on chromosome 1q21 has been confirmed to cause this disease *(117,118)*. Lamins A and C are members of the intermediate filament multigene family, which are encoded by a single gene. Lamins A and C polymerize to form part of the nuclear lamina, a structural filamentous network on the nucleoplasmic side of the inner nuclear membrane. The specific cause of conduction disease and myocardial dysfunction are not currently known but could be the result of progressive degeneration of cardiac tissue analogous to that described in Lev–Lenegre disease.

8. SIDS

SIDS is defined as the sudden death of an infant younger than 1 yr of age that remains unexplained after performance of a complete autopsy, review of clinical and family history, and examination of the death scene. Although the incidence of SIDS has been dramatically reduced from 1.6 per 1000 live births in 1991 to 0.64 per 1000 live births as reported in 1998 in the United States, it is still one of the most common causes of death among children between 1 mo and 6 mo of age. Death usually occurs during sleep *(4,119)*.

The potential causes of sudden death in infants are many, including cardiac disorders, respiratory abnormalities, gastrointestinal diseases, metabolic disorders, traumatic injury, brain abnormality, or child abuse, among others. One of the most referenced etiologic speculations was that described by Schwartz in 1976 *(120)*, in which he proposed that a developmental abnormality in cardiac sympathetic innervation predisposed some infants to lethal cardiac arrhythmias. Specifically, an imbalance in the sympathetic nervous system was speculated to result in prolongation of the QT interval on the EKG and in potentially lethal ventricular arrhythmias *(17,18)*. In 1998, Schwartz et al. *(4)* published data collected between 1976–1994 in which EKGs were recorded on the third or fourth day of life in 34,442 Italian newborns. These babies were followed for 1 yr and during that period, 34 children died. Evaluation of these 34 children demonstrated that 24 died of SIDS. These 24 SIDS victims were found to have longer QTc measurements than controls or other infants dying of other causes. In 12 of these 24 cases, the QTc was clearly prolonged, and the authors suggested that QTc prolongation during the first week of life is associated with SIDS *(4,121)*.

Although this suggestion linking SIDS and LQTS was roundly criticized *(122,128)*, the authors were subsequently able to identify a mutation in *SCN5A* (Table 1) in one patient with aborted SIDS *(114)*. In addition, Priori et al. *(100)* reported the identification of an *SCN5A* mutation in an infant with Brugada syndrome. More recently, Ackerman et al. *(129)* reported a molecular epidemiology study of 95 cases of SIDS in which myocardium obtained at autopsy was screened for ion channel gene mutations. In four of 93 cases, mutations in *SCN5A* were identified postmortem, and the authors suggested that 4.3% of this SIDS cohort was the result of mutations in this known arrhythmia-causing gene. Hence, it appears that ion channel mutations, particularly *SCN5A*, result in SIDS in some infants. Biophysical analysis identified a sodium current characterized by slower delay, and a two to threefold increase in late sodium current similar to that seen in LQTS. The fact that these children die during sleep is consistent with the features seen for this channel when mutations result in LQTS (LQT3). *SCN5A* mutations in SIDS have been further confirmed recently *(130)*. It is likely that other ion channel gene abnormalities will be found in infants with SIDS and that there is wide etiologic heterogeneity.

9. ARVD/CARDIOMYOPATHY (ARVD/C)

ARVD/C is characterized by fatty infiltration of the right ventricle, fibrosis, and ultimately thinning of the wall with chamber dilatation (Fig. 7; *5*). It is the most common cause of sudden cardiac death in the young in Italy *(131)* and is said to account for approx 17% of sudden deaths in the young in the United States *(132)*. Rampazzo et al. *(133)* mapped this disease in two families, one to 1q42-q43, and the other on chromosome 14q23-q24 *(134)*, and a third locus was mapped to 14q12 *(135)* (Fig. 8). A large Greek family with arrhythmogenic right ventricular dysplasia and Naxos disease was recently mapped to 17q21 *(136)*. Two loci responsible for ARVD/C in North America were subsequently mapped at 3p23 *(137)* and the other at 10p12 *(138)*.

ARVD/C is a devastating disease because the first symptom is often sudden death. EKG abnormalities include inverted T waves in the right precordial leads, late potentials, and right ventricular arrhythmias with left bundle branch block. In many cases, the EKG looks similar to that seen in Brugada syndrome, with ST elevation *(139)* in V1–V3. The issue of sudden death is compounded by the great difficulty in making the diagnosis of ARVD/C even when occurring in a family with the disease history. Because the disease affects only the right ventricle, it is difficult to detect by most diagnostic modalities. There is no diagnostic definitive standard at present. The right ventricular biopsy may be definitive when positive but often gives a false-negative diagnosis because the disease initiates in the epicardium and spreads to the endocardium of the right ventricular free wall, making it inaccessible to biopsy. A consensus diagnostic criteria was developed which includes right ventricular biopsy, magnetic resonance imaging, echocardiography, and electrocardiography *(140)*.

The genetic basis of ARVD/C has started to unravel recently. The first gene causing ARVD/C was identified by Tiso et al. *(141)* for the chromosome 1q42-1q43-linked ARVD2 locus in 2001. This gene (Table 1), the cardiac ryanodine receptor gene (RYR2), a 105-exon gene that encodes the 565-kDa monomer of a tetrameric structure interacting with four FK-506 binding proteins called FKBP12.6, is fundamental for intracellular calcium homeostasis and for excitation-contraction coupling. This large protein physically links to the dihydropyridine (DHP) receptor of the t-tubule, where the dihydropyridine receptor protein, a voltage-dependent calcium channel, is activated by plasma membrane depolarization, and induces a calcium influx *(142,143)*. The RYR2 protein, activated by calcium, induces release of calcium from the sarcoplasmic reticulum into the cytosol. Hence, mutations in RYR2 would be expected to cause calcium homeostasis imbalance and result in abnormalities in rhythm as well as excitation-contraction coupling and myocardial dysfunction *(143)*. This causative gene, therefore, is in many ways similar to the mutant genes responsible for the ventricular arrhythmias of LQTS, Brugada syndrome, and SIDS in which ion channel mutations cause the clinical phenotype. In those instances, potassium channel and sodium channel dysfunction occurs while, in ARVD2, calcium channel function plays a central role.

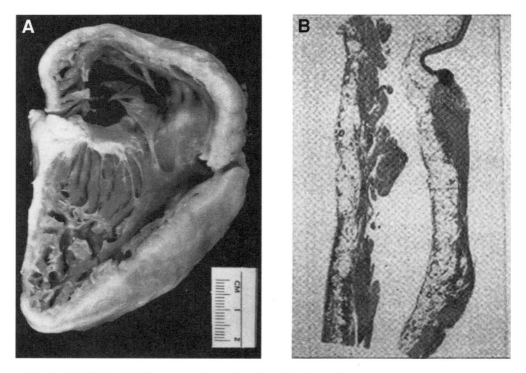

Fig. 7. ARVD/C. (**A**) Heart specimen showing thinning of the right ventricle and fatty infiltration, seen as a white streak on the far left portion to the specimen. (**B**) Histologic section showing fatty infiltration.

Two other genes associated with arrhythmogenic cardiomyopathy have also been described. The first of these, plakoglobin, was shown to cause the chromosome 17q21-linked autosomal-recessive disorder called Naxos disease (Table 1; *144*). This disorder is characterized by ARVD/C in association with abnormalities of skin (palmoplantar keratoderma) and hair (woolly hair) and therefore is not exactly the same as isolated ARVD/C, being a more complex phenotype. Plakoglobin is a cell adhesion protein thought to be important in providing functional integrity to the cell. This protein is found in many tissues, including the cytoplasmic plaque of cardiac junctions and the dermal-epidermal junctions of the epidermis, and it has a potential signaling role in the formation of desmosomal junctions. It is believed that plakoglobin serves as a linker molecule between the inner and outer portions of the desmosomal plaque by binding tightly to the cytoplasmic domains of cadherins. The mutations identified, a homozygous 2 bp deletion, resulted in a frameshift and premature termination of the protein *(144)*. Support for this gene being causative of Naxos disease comes from a mouse model with null mutations, which exhibit the heart and skin abnormalities seen in affected patients. The mutated protein is thought to cause disruption of myocyte integrity, leading to cell death and fibro-fatty replacement with secondary arrhythmias occurring due to the abnormal myocardial substrate.

The last gene identified, desmoplakin *(145)*, is another desmosomal protein with similarities to plakoglobin (Table 1). Homozygous mutations in this gene resulted in a Naxos-like disorder although the cardiac features occurred in the left ventricle instead

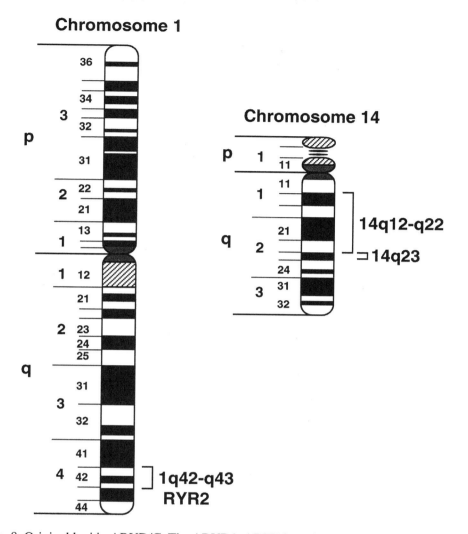

Fig. 8. Original loci in ARVD/C. The ARVD1, ARVD2, and ARVD3 loci on chromosomes 14q23–14q24, 1q42–1q43, and 14q12, respectively, are seen along with the identification of the ARVD2 gene, the cardiac ryanodine receptor, RYR2.

of the right ventricle. The affected protein is an important protein in cell adhesion and appears to function similarly to that described for plakoglobin. Although mutation in this gene and in plakoglobin can easily be speculated to cause the myocardial abnormalities, it remains unclear why differences in ventricular chamber specificity occurs and how the ventricular tachyarrhythmias develop.

10. BRUGADA SYNDROME AND ARVD

Controversy exists concerning the possible association of Brugada syndrome and ARVD, with some investigators arguing that these are the same disorder or at least one is a forme-fruste of the other *(139,146–150)*. However, the classic echocardiographic, angiographic, and magnetic resonance imaging findings of ARVD are not seen in Brugada syndrome patients. In addition, Brugada syndrome patients typically are without the histopathologic findings of ARVD. Further, the morphology of VT/VF differs *(91,139)*. Finally, the genes identified to date differ *(61,141,144,145)*.

11. POLYMORPHIC VT

Familial polymorphic VT, an autosomal-dominant disorder characterized by episodes of bidirectional and polymorphic VT, typically in relation to adrenergic stimulation or physical exercise, was first described by Coumel et al. in 1978 *(151)*. This disorder occurs in childhood and adolescence most commonly, presenting with syncope and sudden death *(6,152)*. Mortality rates of 30–50% by 20–30 yr of age have been reported, suggesting this to be a highly malignant disorder. Autopsy data demonstrate this disorder to have no associated structural cardiac abnormalities.

Mutations in the cardiac ryanodine receptor (RYR2), the same gene responsible for ARVD2, were recently independently identified by Laitinen et al. *(153)* and Priori et al. *(154)* in multiple families linked to chromosome 1q42 (Table 1; *155,156*). Interestingly, ARVD2 typically is considered to be the one form of ARVD/C in which catecholaminergic input is important in the development of symptoms. Why patients with familial polymorphic VT have no associated structural cardiac abnormalities and patients with ARVD/C have classic fibrofatty replacement in the RV is not clear at this time.

Mutations in another member of the ryanodine receptor gene family, RYR1, which is expressed in skeletal muscle, result in malignant hyperthermia and central core disease *(157)*. The mutations in this gene appear to cluster in three regions of the gene, regions similar to the mutations found in RYR2 in the cases of VT reported, suggesting these to be functionally critical regions.

12. WOLFF-PARKINSON-WHITE SYNDROME (WPW)

This disorder is the second most common cause of paroxysmal supraventricular tachycardia (SVT), with a prevalence of 1.5–3.1/1000 individuals *(2)*. In some parts of the world, such as China, WPW is even more common, being responsible for up to 70% of cases of SVT *(158)*. Tachycardia presents typically in a bimodal fashion, with onset common in infancy as well as during the teen years. Symptoms most commonly include syncope, presyncope, shortness of breath, palpitations, and sudden death *(109)*.

WPW has long been described to be caused by accessory pathways derived from muscle fibers providing direct continuity between atrial and ventricular myocardium *(2,159)*. These accessory pathways may be identified by the peculiar EKG findings seen in WPW, including short PR interval, widened QRS complexes, and the classic delta wave in which an abnormal initial QRS vector is notable *(2,159–161)*. In a significant percentage of patients, conduction abnormalities, including high-grade sinoatrial or atrioventricular block, occur *(162)*, necessitating pacemaker implantation. In most patients with WPW and SVT, radiofrequency ablation of the accessory pathway(s) is curative *(163)*.

Some cases of WPW are associated with other primary disorders, such as hypertrophic cardiomyopathy *(162,164)* or left ventricular noncompaction cardiomyopathy

(165), or the congenital cardiac disorder Ebstein's anomaly. Whether the underlying cause of WPW is similar in these cases compared with pure cases of WPW has been discussed for many years, but no definitive answers have been provided.

The first gene in patients with WPW was recently identified by Gollob et al. *(166)* and Blair et al. *(167)* independently in familial forms of WPW. In both reports, autosomal-dominant inheritance was reported. Interestingly, this gene, which maps to chromosome 7q34-7q36 *(164)*, was found to cause WPW and hypertrophic cardiomyopathy in a significant percentage of patients in both reports (Table 1). The gene, the γ2 subunit of adenosine monophosphate-activated protein kinase, consists of 569 amino acids, is 63 kDa in size, and functions as a metabolic sensor in cells, responding to cellular energy demands by regulating ATP production and use *(168–172)*. Confusion exists as to whether this is a primary hypertrophic cardiomyopathy-causing gene or WPW gene, particularly because the initial mapping of this locus was in patients with hypertrophic cardiomyopathy and associated WPW. Clearly, this is not the only gene responsible for WPW and the functional and physiologic abnormalities responsible for the resultant WPW are not yet obvious.

13. FINAL COMMON PATHWAY HYPOTHESIS

Clearly, LQTS is a disease of the ion channel. Similarly, patients with Brugada syndrome, catecholaminergic VT, and conduction abnormalities are primary ion channelopathies. Patients with other cardiac disorders, such as familial dilated cardiomyopathy (FDCM) and familial hypertrophic cardiomyopathy (FHCM) have been shown to have mutations in genes encoding a consistent family of proteins as well. In FDCM, cytoskeletal protein-encoding genes and sarcomeric proteins have been speculated to be causative (i.e., cytoskeletal/sarcomyopathy; *173*). In addition, FHCM has been shown to be a disease of the sarcomere. Hence, the final common pathways of these disorders include the sarcomere and cytoskeletal proteins, similar to the ion channelopathy in arrhythmias and conduction disease. Intermediate disorders, such as ARVD/C, appear to connect the primary electrical and primary muscle disorders mechanistically. In addition, it appears that cascade pathways are involved directly in some cases (i.e., mitochondrial abnormalities in HCM, DCM) whereas secondary influences are likely to result in the wide clinical spectrum seen in patients with similar mutations. In HCM, mitochondrial and metabolic influences are probably important. Additionally, molecular interactions with such molecules as calcineurin, sex hormones, growth factors, amongst others, are probably involved in development of clinical signs, symptoms, and age of presentation. In the future, these factors are expected to be uncovered, allowing for development of new therapeutic strategies.

14. RELEVANCE

The relevance of the hypothesis is its ability to classify disease entities on a molecular and mechanistic basis. This reclassification of disorders on the basis of molecular abnormalities such as "ion channelopathies," "sarcomyopathies," or "cytoskeletopathies" could lead to more focused approaches to gene discovery and future therapeutic interventions. For instance, on the basis of the understanding of the molecular aspects of LQTS, we considered the possibility that all ventricular arrhythmias are the result of ion channel abnormalities. On the basis of the hypothesis, we studied the possibility that the cardiac sodium channel gene (*SCN5A*) was mutated in patients with the idiopathic ventricular fibrillation disorder called Brugada syndrome, identifying mutations in three separate, unrelated families. Use of this hypothesis for disorders, such as inherited DCM, is likely to more narrowly focus efforts at gene identification. In the near future, when the human genome project is completed, this will allow for investigators to more rapidly identify disease responsible genes. Once the genes are known, and the mechanisms causing the clinical phenotype and natural history are known, improved pharmacologic therapies based on the actual disease mechanism can be produced and used. At that time, the impact of molecular genetics on clinical practice and patient care will become fully evident.

15. SUMMARY

Ventricular arrhythmias appear to result from ion channel abnormalities. Whether this is necessarily a primary abnormality or can occur secondary is becoming better understood as the genes responsible for ARVD/C are identified. Therapeutic options are likely to be expanded once this knowledge has matured. Similarly, conduction system abnormalities have been shown to occur secondary to mutations in the ion channel gene *SCN5A*, as well as a result of mutations in the intermediate filament protein lamin A/C. The recent finding of Malhotra et al. *(174)* that *SCN5A*, the α subunit of the cardiac sodium channel, interacts with accessory subunits β1 and β2, which act as a junction protein interactor, could explain how these apparently disparate genes (*SCN5A*, lamin A/C) result in similar clinical findings. The unraveling of these questions will lead to improved ability to develop rational therapies in the future.

REFERENCES

1. Priori, S. G., Barhanin, J., Hauer, R. N. W., Haverkamp, W., Jongsma, H. J., Kleber, A. G., et al. (1999) Genetic and molecular basis of cardiac arrhythmias: Impact on clinical management (Parts I and II). *Circulation* **99,** 518–528.
2. Al-Khatib, S. M. and Pritchett, E. L. (1999) Clinical features of Wolff-Parkinson-White syndrome. *Am. Heart J.* **138,** 403–413.
3. Brugada, P. and Brugada, J. (1992) Right bundle-branch block, persistent ST segment elevation and sudden cardiac death: A distinct clinical and electrocardiographic syndrome. A multicenter report. *J. Am. Coll. Cardiol.* **20,** 1391–1396.
4. Schwartz, P. J., Stramba-Badiale, M., Segantini, A., Austoni, P., Bosi, G., Giorgetti, R., et al. (1997)Prolongation of the QT interval and the sudden infant death syndrome. *N. Engl. J. Med.* **338,** 1709–1714.
5. Thiene, G., Basso, C., Danieli, G., Rampazzo, A., Corrado, D., and Nava, A. (1997)Arrhythmogenic right ventricular cardiomyopathy. *Trends Cardiovasc. Med.* **7,** 84–90.
6. Fisher, J. D., Krikler, D., and Hallidie-Smith, K. A. (1999) Familial polymorphic ventricular arrhythmias: A quarter century of successful medical treatment based on serial exercise-pharmacologic testing. *J. Am. Coll. Cardiol.* **34,** 2015–2022.
7. Schwartz, P. J., Locati, E. H., Napolitano, C., and Priori, S. G. (1996) The long QT syndrome, in *Cardiac Electrophysiology: From Cell to Bedside,* Chapter 72 (Zipes, D. P. and Jalife, J., eds.), W. B. Saunders Co., Philadelphia, PA, pp. 788–811.
8. Romano, C., Gemme, G., and Pongiglione, R. (1963) Antmie cardiache rare in eta pediatrica. *Clin. Pediatr.* **45,** 656–683.

9. Ward, O. C. (1964) A new familial cardiac syndrome in children. *J. Ir. Med. Assoc.* **54,** 103–106.
10. Napolitano, C., and Schwartz, P. J. (1999) Low penetrance in the long-QT syndrome. Clinical impact. *Circulation* **99,** 529–533.
11. Singer, P. A., Crampton, R. S., and Bass, N. H. (1974) Familial Q-T prolongation syndrome: Convulsive seizures and paroxysmal ventricular fibrillation. *Arch. Neurol.* **31,** 64–66.
12. Ratshin, R. A., Hunt, D., Russell, R. O. Jr., and Rackley, C. E. (1971) QT-interval prolongation, paroxysmal ventricular arrhythmias, and convulsive syncope. *Ann. Intern. Med.* **75,** 19–24.
13. Bellavere, F., Ferri, M., Guarini, L., Bax, G., Piccoli, A., Cardone, C., et al. (1988) Prolonged QT period in diabetic autonomic neuropathy: A possible role in sudden cardiac death. *Br. Heart J.* **59,** 379–383.
14. Ewing, D. J., Boland, O., Neilson, J. M. M., Cho, C. G., and Clarke, B. F. (1991) Autonomic neuropathy, QT interval lengthening, and unexpected deaths in male diabetic patients. *Diabetologia* **34,** 182–185.
15. Weintraub, R. G., Gow, R. M., and Wilkinson, J. L. (1990) The congenital long QT syndromes in children. *J. Am. Coll. Cardiol.* **16,** 674–680.
16. Marks. M. L., Trippel, D. L., and Keating, M. T. (1995) Long QT syndrome associated with syndactyly identified in females. *Am. J. Cardiol.* **10,** 744–745.
17. Schwartz, P. J. and Segantini, A. (1988) Cardiac innervation, neonatal electrocardiography and SIDS. A key for a novel preventive strategy? *Ann. NY Acad. Sci.* **533,** 210–220.
18. Schwartz, P. J., Stramba-Badiale, M., Segantini, A., Austoni, P., Bosi, G., Giorgetti, R., et al. (1998) Prolongation of the QT tnterval and the sudden infant death syndrome. *N. Engl. J. Med.* **338,** 1709–1714.
19. Jervell, A. and Lange-Nielsen F. (1957) Congenital deaf-mutism, function heart disease with prolongation of the Q-T interval and sudden death. *Am. Heart J.* **54,** 59–68.
20. Jervell, A. (1971) Surdocardiac and related syndromes in children. *Adv. Intern. Med.* **17,** 425–438.
21. James, T. N. (1967) Congenital deafness and cardiac arrhythmias. *Am. J. Cardiol.* **19,** 627–643.
22. Priori, S. G., Schwartz, P. J., Napolitano, C., Bianchi, L., Dennis, A., DeFusco, M., et al. (1998) A recessive variant of the Romano-Ward long-QT syndrome. *Circulation* **97,** 2420–2425.
23. Keating, M. T., Atkinson, D., Dunn, C., Timothy, K., Vincent, G. M., and Leppert, M. (1991) Linkage of a cardiac arrhythmia, the long QT syndrome, and the Harvey ras-1 gene. *Science* **252,** 704–706.
24. Wang, Q., Curran, M. E., Splawski, I., Burn, T. C., Millholland, J. M., Van Raay, T. J., et al. (1996) Positional cloning of a novel potassium channel gene: KVLQT1 mutations cause cardiac arrhythmias. *Nat. Genet.* **12,** 17–23.
25. Li, H., Chen, Q., Moss, A. J., Robinson, J., Goytia, V., Perry, J. C., et al. (1998) New mutations in the KVLQT1 potassium channel that cause long QT syndrome. *Circulation* **97,** 1264–1269.
26. Choube, C., Neyroud, N., Guicheney, P., Lazdunski, M., Romey, G., and Barhanin, J. (1997) Properties of KVLQTI K+ channel mutations in Romano-Ward and Jervell and Lange-Nielsen inherited cardiac arrhythmias. *EMBO J.* **16,** 5472–5479.
27. Chiang, C. E. and Roden, D. M. (2000) The long QT syndromes: Genetic basis and clinical implications. *J. Am. Coll. Cardiol.* **36,** 1–12.
28. Barhanin, J., Lesage, F., Guillemare, E., Finc, M., Lazdunski, M., and Romey G. (1996) KVLQT1 and IsK (minK) proteins associate to form the IKs cardiac potassium current. *Nature* **384,** 78–80.
29. Sanguinetti, M. C., Curran, M. E., Zou, A., Shen, J., Spector, P. S., Atkinson, D. L., et al. (1996) Coassembly of KvLQT1 and minK (IsK) proteins to form cardiac IKs potassium channel. *Nature* **384,** 80–83.

30. Wollnick, B., Schreeder, B. C., Kubish, C., Esperer, H. D., Wieacker, P., and Jensch, T. J. (1997) Pathophysiological mechanisms of dominant and recessive KVLQTI K+ channel mutations found in inherited cardiac arrhythmias. *Hum. Mol. Genet.* **6,** 1943–1949.

31. Splawski, I., Tristani-Firouzi, M., Lehmann, M. H., Sanguinetti, M. C., and Keating, M. T. (1997) Mutations in the minK gene cause long QT syndrome and suppress IKs function. *Nat. Genet.* **17,** 338–340.

32. Jiang, C., Atkinson, D., Towbin, J. A., Splawski, I., Lehmann, M. H., Li, H., et al. (1994) Two long QT syndrome loci map to chromosome 3 and 7 with evidence for further heterogeneity. *Nat. Genet.* **8,** 141–147.

33. Warmke, J. E. and Ganetzky, B. (1994) A family of potassium channel genes related to eag in Drosophila and mammals. *Proc. Natl. Acad. Sci. USA* **91,** 3438–3442.

34. Arcangeli, A., Rosati, B., Cherubini, A., Crociani, O., Fontana, L., Ziller, C., et al. (1997) *HERG*- and IRK-like inward rectifier currents are sequentially expressed during neuronal crest cells and their derivatives. *Eur. J. Neurosci.* **9,** 2596–2604.

35. Pennefather, P. S., Zhou, W., and Decoursey, T. E. (1998) Idiosyncratic gating of *HERG*-like K$^+$ channels in microglia. *J. Gen. Physiol.* **111,** 795–805.

36. Bianchi, L., Wible, B., Arcangeli, A., Taglialatela, M., Morra, F., Castaldo, P., et al. (1998) *HERG* encodes a K$^+$ current highly conserved in tumors of different histogenesis: A selective advantage for cancer cells? *Cancer Res.* **58,** 815–822.

37. Curran, M. E., Splawski, I., Timothy, K. W., Vincent, G. M., Green, E. D., and Keating, M. T. (1995) A molecular basis for cardiac arrhythmia: *HERG* mutations cause long QT syndrome. *Cell* **80,** 795–803.

38. Schulze-Bahr, E., Haverkamp, W., and Funke, H. (1995) The long-QT syndrome. *N. Engl. J. Med.* **333,** 1783–1784.

39. Sanguinetti, M. C., Jiang, C., Curran, M. E., and Keating, M. T. (1995) A mechanistic link between an inherited and an acquired cardiac arrhythmia: *HERG* encodes the I$_{Kr}$ potassium channel. *Cell* **81,** 299–307.

40. Trudeau, M. C., Warmke, J., Ganetzky, B., and Robertson, G. (1995) *HERG*, a human inward rectifier in the voltage-gated potassium channel family. *Science* **269,** 92–95.

41. Sanguinetti, M. C., Curran, M. E., Spector, P. S., and Keating, M. T. (1996) Spectrum of *HERG* K+-channel dysfunction in an inherited cardiac arrhythmia. *Proc. Natl. Acad. Sci. USA* **93,** 2208–2212.

42. Roden, D. M. and Balser, J. R. (1999) A plethora of mechanisms in the *HERG*-related long QT syndrome genetics meets electrophysiology. *Cardiovasc. Res.* **44,** 242–246.

43. Furutani, M., Trudeau, M. C., Hagiwara, N., Seki, A., Gong, Q., Zhou, Z., et al. (1999) Novel mechanism associated with an inherited cardiac arrhythmia. Defective protein trafficking by the mutant *HERG* (G601S) potassium channel. *Circulation* **99,** 2290–2294.

44. Zhou, Z., Gong, Q., Epstein, M. L., and January, C. T. (1998) *HERG* channel dysfunction in human long QT syndrome. *J. Biol. Chem.* **263,** 21,061–21,066.

45. McDonald, T. V., Yu, Z., Ming, Z., Palma, E., Meyers, M. B., Wang, K. W., et al. (1997) A *minK-HERG* complex regulates the cardiac potassium current IKr. *Nature* **388,** 289–292.

46. Bianchi, L., Shen, Z., Dennis, A. T., Priori, S. G., Napolitano, C., Ronchetti, E., et al. (1999) Cellular dysfunction of *LQT5-minK* mutants: abnormalities of I$_{Ks}$, I$_{Kr}$ and trafficking in long QT syndrome. *Hum. Mol. Genet.* **8,** 1499–1507.

47. Abbott, G. W., Sesti, F., Splawski, I., Buck, M. E., Lehmann, M. H., Timothy, K. W., et al. (1999) *MiRP1* forms I$_{Kr}$ potassium channels with *HERG* and is associated with cardiac arrhythmia. *Cell* **97,** 175–187.

48. Gellens, M., George, A. L., Chen, L., Chanine, M., Horn, R., Barch, R. L., et al. (1992) Primary structure and functional expression of the human cardiac tetrodotoxin-insensitive voltage-dependent sodium channel. *Proc. Natl. Acad. Sci. USA* **89,** 54–558.

49. George, A. L., Varkony, T. A., Drakin, H. A., Han, J., Knops, J. F., Finley, W. H., et al. (1995) Assignment of the human heart tetrodotoxin-resistant voltage-gated Na channel-subunit gene (*SCN5A*) to band 3p21. *Cytogenet. Cell Genet.* **68,** 67–70.

50. Wang, Q., Shen, J., Splawski, I., Atkinson, D., Li, Z., Robinson, J. L., et al. (1995) *SCN5A* mutations associated with an inherited cardiac arrhythmia, long QT syndrome. *Cell* **80,** 805–811.

51. Wang, Q., Shen, J., Li, Z., Timothy, K., Vincent, G. M., Priori, S. G., et al. (1995) Cardiac sodium channel mutations in patients with long QT syndrome, an inherited cardiac arrhythmia. *Hum. Mol. Genet.* **4,** 1603–1607.

52. Hartmann, H. A., Colom, L. V., Sutherland, M. L., and Noebels, J. L. (1999) Selective localization of cardiac *SCN5A* sodium channels in limbic regions of rat brain. *Nat. Neurosci.* **2,** 593–595.

53. Bennett, P. B., Yazawa, K., Makita, N., and George, A. L., Jr. (1995) Molecular mechanism for an inherited cardiac arrhythmia. *Nature* **376,** 683–685.

54. Dumaine, R., Wang, Q., Keating, M. T., Hartmann, H. A., Schwartz, P. J., Brown, A. M., et al. (1996) Multiple mechanisms of sodium channel-linked long QT syndrome. *Circ. Res.* **78,** 916–924.

55. An, R. H., Wang, X. L., Kerem, B., Benhorin, J., Medina, A., Goldmit, M., et al. (1998) Novel LQT-3 mutation affects Na^+ channel activity through interactions between alpha- and beta 1-subunits. *Circ. Res.* **83,** 141–146.

56. Honore, E., Attali, B., Heurteaux, C., Ricard, P., Lesage, F., Lazdunski, M., et al. (1991) Cloning, expression, pharmacology and regulation of a delayed rectifier K^+ channel in mouse heart. *EMBO J.* **10,** 2805–2811.

57. Arena, J. P. and Kass, R. S. (1988) Block of heart potassium channels by clofilium and its tertiary analogs: relationship between drug structure and type of channel blocked. *Mol. Pharmacol.* **34,** 60–66.

58. Vetter, D. E., Mann, J. R., Wangemann, P., Liu, J., McLaughlin, K. J., Lesage, F., et al. (1996) Inner ear defects induced by null mutation of the isk gene. *Neuron* **17,** 1251–1264.

59. Neyroud, N., Tesson, F., Denjoy, I., Leiboovic, M., Donger, C., Barhanin, J., et al. (1997) A novel mutation in the potassium channel gene *KVLQT1* causes the Jervell and Lange-Nielsen cardioauditory syndrome. *Nat. Genet.* **15,** 186–189.

60. Splawski, I., Timothy, K. W., Vincent, G. M., Atkinson, D. L., and Keating, M. T. (1997) Brief report: Molecular basis of the long-QT syndrome associated with deafness. *N. Engl. J. Med.* **336,** 1562–1567.

61. Chen, Q., Zhang, D., Gingell, R. L., Moss, A. J., Napolitano, C., Priori, S. G., et al. (1999) Homozygous deletion in KVLQTI associated with Jervell and Lange-Nielsen syndrome. *Circulation* **99,** 1344–1347.

62. Tyson, J., Tranebjaerg, L., Bellman, S., Wren, C., Taylor, J. F., Bathen, J., et al. (1997) IsK and KVLQTI: Mutation in either of the two subunits of the slow component of the delayed rectifier potassium channel can cause Jervell and Lange-Nielsen syndrome. *Hum. Mol. Genet.* **12,** 2179–2185.

63. Schulze-Bahr, E., Wang, Q., Wedekind, H., Haverkamp, W., Chen, Q., Sun, Y., et al. (1997) *KCNE1* mutations cause Jervell and Lange-Nielsen syndrome. *Nat. Genet.* **17,** 267–268.

64. Kimbrough, J., Moss, A. J., Zareba, W., Robinson, J. L., Hall, J., Benhorin, J., et al. (2001) Clinical implications for affected parents and siblings of probands with long-QT syndrome. *Circulation* **104,** 557–562.

65. Zareba, W., Moss, A. J., Schwartz, P. J., Vincent, G. M., Robinson, J. L., Priori, S. G., et al. (1998) Influence of the genotype on the clinical course of the long-QT syndrome. *N. Engl. J. Med.* **339,** 960–965.

66. Tanabe, Y., Inagaki, M., Kurita, T., Nagaya, N., Taguchi, A., Suyama, K., et al. (2001) Sympathetic stimulation produces a greater increase in both transmural and spatial dispersion of repolarization in LQT1 than *LQT2* forms of congenital long QT syndrome. *J. Am. Coll. Cardiol.* **37,** 911–9919.

67. Ackermann, M. J., Tester, D. J., and Porter, C. J. (1999) Swimming, a gene-specific arrhythmogenic trigger for inherited long QT syndrome. *Mayo Clin. Proc.* **74,** 1088–1094.

68. Moss, A. J., Robinson, J. L., Gessman, L., Gillespie, R., Zareba, W., Schwartz, P. J., et al. (1999) Comparison of clinical and genetic variables of cardiac events associated with loud noise versus swimming among subjects with the long QT syndrome. *Am. J. Cardiol.* **84,** 876–933.

69. Wilde, A. A. M., Jongbloed, R. J. E., Doevendans, P. A., Duren, D. R., Hauer, R. N., van Langen, I. M., et al. (1999) Auditory stimuli as a trigger for arrhythmic events differentiate *HERG*-related (LQTS2) patients from *KVLQT1*-related patients (LQTS1). *J. Am. Coll. Cardiol.* **33,** 327–332.

70. Wilde, A. A. M. and Roden, D. M. (2000) Predicting the long-QT genotype from clinical data: From sense to science. *Circulation* **102,** 2796–2798.

71. Ali, R. H., Zareba, W., Moss, A. J., Schwartz, P. J., Benhorin, J., Vincent, G. M., et al. (2000) Clinical and genetic variables associated with acute arousal and nonarousal-related cardiac events among subjects with the long QT syndrome. *Am. J. Cardiol.* **85,** 457–461.

72. Moss, A. J., Zareba, W., Benhorin, J., Locati, E. H., Hall, W. J., Robinson, J. L., et al. ECG T-wave patterns in genetically distinct forms of the hereditary long-QT syndrome. *Circulation* **92,** 2929–2934.

73. Zhang, L., Timothy, K. W., Vincent, G. M., Lehmann, M. H., Fox, J., Giuli, L. C., et al. (2000) Spectrum of ST-T-wave patterns and repolarization parameters in congenital long-QT syndrome: ECG findings identify genotypes. *Circulation* **102,** 2849–2855.

74. Lupoglazoff, J. M., Denjoy, I., Berthet, M., Neyroud, N., Demay, L., Richard, P., et al. (2001) Notched T waves on Holter recordings enhance detection of patients with *LQT2* (*HERG*) mutations. *Circulation* **103,** 1095–1101.

75. Shimizu, W. and Antzelevitch, C. (1997) Sodium channel block with Mexiletine is effective in reducing dispersion of repolarization and preventing torsade de pointes in *LQT2* and LQT3 models of the long-QT syndrome. *Circulation* **96,** 2038–2047.

76. Shimizu, W. and Antzelevitch, C. (2000) Differential effects of beta-adrenergic agonists and antagonists in LQT1, *LQT2,* and LQT3 models of the long QT syndrome. *J. Am. Coll. Cardiol.* **35,** 778–786.

77. Moss, A. J., Zareba, W., Hall, W. J., Schwartz, P. J., Crampton, R. S., Benhorin, J., et al. (2000) Effectiveness and limitations of beta-blocker therapy in congenital long-QT syndrome. *Circulation* **101,** 616–623.

78. Schwartz, P. J., Priori, S. G., Locati, E. H., Napolitano, C., Cantu, F., Towbin, J. A., et al. (1995) Long-QT syndrome patients with mutations of the *SCN5A* and *HERG* genes have differential responses to Na$^+$ channel blockade and to increases in heart rate: Implications for gene-specific therapy. *Circulation* **92,** 3381–3386.

79. Compton, S. J., Lux, R. L., Ramsey, M. R., Strelich, K. R., Sanguinetti, M. C., Green, L. S., et al. (1996) Genetically defined therapy of inherited long-QT syndrome: Correction of abnormal repolarization by potassium. *Circulation* **94,** 1018–1022.

80. Shimizu, W., Kurita, T., Matsuo, K., Suyama, K., Aihara, N., Kamakura, S., et al. (1998) Improvement of repolarization abnormalities by K$^+$ channel opener in the long QT syndrome. *Circulation* **97,** 1581–1588.

81. Osher, H. L. and Wolff, L. (1953) Electrocardiographic pattern simulating acute myocardial injury. *Am. J. Med. Sci.* **226,** 541–545.

82. Edeiken, J. (1954) Elevation of RS-T segment, apparent or real in right precordial leads as probable normal variant. *Am. Heart J.* **48,** 331–339.

83. Levine, H. D., Wanzer, S. H., and Merrill, J. P. (1956) Dialyzable currents of injury in potassium intoxication resembling acute myocardial infarction or pericarditis. *Circulation* **13,** 29–36.

84. Martini, B., Nava, A., Thiene, G., Buja, G. F., Canciani, B., Scognamiglio, R., Daliento, L., and Dalla Volta, S. (1989) Ventricular fibrillation without apparent heart disease. Description of six cases. *Am. Heart J.* **118,** 1203–1209.

85. Aihara, N., Ohe, T., and Kamakura, S. (1990) Clinical and electrophysiologic characteristics of idiopathic ventricular fibrillation. *Shinzo* **22**, 80–86.

86. Brugada, P. and Brugada, J. (1991) A distinct clinical and electrocardiographic syndrome: right bundle-branch block, persistent ST segment elevation with normal QT interval and sudden cardiac death. *PACE* **14**, 746.

87. Antzelevitch, C., Brugada, P., and Brugada, J. (1999) *The Brugada Syndrome.* Futura Publishing Company, Inc, Armonk, NY.

88. Nademanee, K., Veerakul, G., Nimmannit, S., Chaowakul, V., Bhuripanyo, K., Likittanasom, K., et al. (1997) Arrhythmogenic marker for the sudden unexplained death syndrome in Thai men. *Circulation* **96**, 2595–2600.

89. Gotoh, K. (1976) A histopathological study on the conduction system of the so-called Pokkuri disease (sudden unexpected cardiac death of unknown origin in Japan). *Jpn. Circ. J.* **40**, 753–768.

90. Hayashi, M., Murata, M., Satoh, M., Aizawa, Y., Oda, E., Oda, Y., et al. (1985) Sudden nocturnal death in young males from ventricular flutter. *Jpn. Heart J.* **26**, 585–591.

91. Brugada, J. and Brugada, P. (1997) Further characterization of the syndrome of right bundle branch block, ST segment elevation, and sudden death. *J. Cardiovasc. Electrophysiol.* **8**, 325–331.

92. Priori, S. G., Napolitano, C., Gasparini, M., Pappone, C., Bella, P. D., Brignole, M., et al. (2000) Clinical and genetic heterogeneity of right bundle branch block and ST-segment elevation syndrome: A prospective evaluation of 52 families. *Circulation* **102**, 2509–2515.

93. Kakishita, M., Kurita, T., Matsuo, K., Taguchi, A., Suyama, K., Shimizu, W., et al. (2000) Mode of onset of ventricular fibrillation in patients with Brugada syndrome detected by implantable cardioverter defibrillator therapy. *J. Am. Coll. Cardiol.* **36**, 1647–1653.

94. Kobayashi, T., Shintani, U., Yamamoto, T., Shida, S., Isshiki, N., Tanaka, T., et al. (1996) Familial occurrence of electrocardiographic abnormalities of the Brugada-type. *Intern. Med.* **35**, 637–640.

95. Gussak, I., Antzelevitch, C., Bjerregaard, P., Towbin, J. A., and Chaitman, B. R. (1999) The Brugada syndrome: clinical, electrophysiological, and genetic considerations. *J. Am. Coll. Cardiol.* **33**, 5–15.

96. Chen, Q., Kirsch, G. E., Zhang, D., Brugada, R., Brugada, J., Brugada, P., et al. (1998) Genetic basis and molecular mechanism for idiopathic ventricular fibrillation. *Nature* **392**, 293–296.

97. Antzelevitch, C. (1998) The Brugada Syndrome. *J. Cardiovasc. Electrophys.* **9**, 513–516.

98. Antzelevitch, C. (2001) The Brugada syndrome: Diagnostic criteria and cellular mechanisms. *Eur. Heart J.* **22**, 356–363.

99. Antzelevitch, C. (1999) Ion channels and ventricular arrhythmias: Cellular and ionic mechanisms underlying the Brugada syndrome. *Curr. Opin. Cardiol.* **14**, 274–279.

100. Priori, S. G., Napolitano, C., Giordano, U., Collisani, G., and Memmi, M. (2000) Brugada syndrome and sudden cardiac death in children. *Lancet* **355**, 808–809.

101. Dumaine, R., Towbin, J. A., Brugada, P., Vatta, M., Nesterenko, D. V., Nesterenko, V. V., Brugada, J., et al. (1999) Ionic mechanisms responsible for the electrocardiographic phenotype of the Brugada syndrome are temperature dependent. *Circ. Res.* **85**, 803–809.

102. Kambouris, N. G., Nuss, H. B., Johns, D. C., Tomaselli, G. F., Marban, E., and Balser, J. R. (1998) Phenotypic characterization of a novel long-QT syndrome mutation (R1623Q) in the cardiac sodium channel. *Circulation* **97**, 640–644.

103. Bezzina, C., Veldkamp, M. W., van Den Berg, M. P., Postma, A. V., Rook, M. B., Viersma, J. W., et al. (1999) A single Na(+) channel mutation causing both long-QT and Brugada syndromes. *Circ. Res.* **85**, 1206–1213.

104. Brugada, R., Brugada, J., Antzelevitch, C., Kirsch, G. E., Potenza, D., Towbin, J. A., et al. (2000) Sodium channel blockers identify risk for sudden death in patients with ST

segment elevation and right bundle branch block but structurally normal heart. *Circulation* **101,** 510–515.

105. RuDusky, B. M. (1998) Right bundle branch block, persistent ST-segment elevation, and sudden death. *Am. J. Cardiol.* **82,** 407–408.

106. Ikeda, T., Sakurada, H., Sakabe, K., Sakata, T., Takami, M., Tezuka, N., et al. (2001) Assessment of noninvasive markers in identifying patients at risk in the Brugada syndrome: Insight into risk stratification. *J. Am. Coll. Cardiol.* **37,** 1628–1623.

107. Remme, C. A., Wever, E. F. D., Wilde, A. A. M., Derksen, R., and Hauer, R. N.W. (2001) Diagnosis and long-term follow-up of Brugada syndrome in patients with idiopathic ventricular fibrillation. *Eur. Heart J.* **22,** 400–409.

108. Gussak, I., Bjerregaard, P., and Hammill, S. C. (2001) Clinical diagnosis and risk stratification in patients with Brugada syndrome. *J. Am. Coll. Cardiol.* **37,** 1635–1638.

109. Zipes, D. P. and Wellens, H. J. J. (1998) Clinical cardiology: New frontiers. Sudden cardiac death. *Circulation* **98,** 2334–2351.

110. Tan, H. L., Bink-Boelkens, M. T. E., Bezzina, C. R., Viswanathan, P. C., Beaufort-Krol, G. C. M., van Tintelen, P. J., et al. (2001) A sodium-channel mutation causes isolated cardiac conduction disease. *Nature* **409,** 1043–1047.

111. Kass, S., MacRae, C., Graber, H. L., Sparks, E. A., McNamara, D., Boudoulas, H., et al. (1994) A gene defect that causes conduction system disease and dilated cardiomyopathy maps to chromosome 1p1–1q1. *Nat. Genet.* **7,** 546–551.

112. Schott, J. J., Alshinawi, C., Kyndt, F., Probst, V., Hoorntje, T. M., Hulsbeek, M., et al. (1999) Cardiac conduction defects associate with mutations in *SCN5A. Nat. Genet.* **23,** 20–21.

113. Deschenes, I., Baroudi, G., Berthet, M., Barde, I., Chalvidan, T., Denjoy, I., et al. (2000) Electrophysiological characterization of *SCN5A* mutations causing long QT (E1784K) and Brugada (R1512W and R1432G) syndromes. *Cardiovasc. Res.* **46,** 55–65.

114. Schwartz, P. J., Priori, S. G., Dumaine, R., Napolitano, C., Antzelevitch, C., Stramba-Badiale, M., et al. (2000) A molecular link between the sudden infant death syndrome and the long QT syndrome. *N. Engl. J. Med.* **343,** 262–267.

115. Brink, P. A., Ferreira, A., Moolman, J. C., Weymar, H. W., van der Merwe, P. L., and Corfield, V. A. (1995) Gene for progressive familial heart block type I maps to chromosome 19q13. *Circulation* **91,** 1633–1640.

116. de Meeus, A., Stephan, E., Debrus, S., Jean, M. K., Loiselet, J., Weissenbach, J., et al. (1995) An isolated cardiac conduction disease maps to chromosome 19q. *Circ. Res.* **77,** 735–740.

117. Fatkin, D., MacRae, C., Sasaki, T., Wolff, M. R., Porcu, M., Frenneaux, M., et al. (1999) Missense mutations in the rod domain of the lamin A/C gene as causes of dilated cardiomyopathy and conduction system disease. *N. Engl. J. Med.* **341,** 1715–1724.

118. Brodsky, G. L., Muntoni, F., Miocic, S., Sinagra, G., Sewry, C., and Mestroni, L. (2000) Lamin A/C gene mutation associated with dilated cardiomyopathy with variable skeletal muscle involvement. *Circulation* **101,** 473–476.

119. Towbin, J. A. and Ackerman, M. J. (2001) Cardiac sodium channel gene mutations and SIDS. [editorial] *Circulation* **104,** 1092–1093.

120. Schwartz, P. J. (1976) Cardiac sympathetic innervation and the sudden infant death syndrome. A possible pathogenetic link. *Am. J. Med.* **60,** 167–172.

121. Towbin, J. A. and Friedman, R. A. Prolongation of the QT interval and the sudden infant death syndrome. *N. Engl. J. Med.* **338,** 1760–1761.

122. Lucey, J. F. (1999) Comments on a sudden infant death article in another journal. *Pediatrics* **103,** 812.

123. Martin, R. J., Miller, M. J., and Redline, S. (1999) Screening for SIDS: A neonatal perspective. *Pediatrics* **103,** 812–813.

124. Guntheroth, W. G. and Spiers, P. S. (1999) Prolongation of the QT interval and the sudden infant death syndrome. *Pediatrics* **103,** 813–814.

125. Hodgman, J. E. (1999) Prolonged QTc as a risk factor for SIDS. *Pediatrics* **103**, 814–815.
126. Hoffman, J. I. E. and Lister, G. (1999) The implications of a relationship between prolonged QT interval and the sudden infant death syndrome. *Pediatrics* **103**, 815–817.
127. Shannon, D. C. (1999) Method of analyzing QT interval can't support conclusions. *Pediatrics* **103**, 819.
128. Southall, D. P. (1999) Examine data in Schwartz article with extreme care. *Pediatrics* **103**, 819–820.
129. Ackerman, M. J., Siu, B., Sturner, W. Q., Tester, D. J., Valdivia, C. R., Makielski, J. C., et al. (2001) Postmortem molecular analysis of *SCN5A* defects in sudden infant death syndrome. *JAMA* **286**, 2264–2269.
130. Wedekind, H., Smits, J. P. P., Schulze-Bahr, E., Arnold, R., Veldkamp, M. W., Bajanowski, T., et al. (2001) De novo mutation in the *SCN5A* gene associated with early onset of sudden infant death. *Circulation* **104**, 1158–1164.
131. Thiene, G., Nava, A., Corrado, D., Rossi, L., and Pennelli, N. (1988) Right ventricular cardiomyopathy and sudden death in young people. *N. Engl. J. Med.* **318**, 129–133.
132. Shen, W. K., Edwards, W. D., and Hammill, S. C. (1994) Right ventricular dysplasia: A need for precise pathological definition for interpretation of sudden death. *J. Am. Coll. Cardiol.* **23**, 34.
133. Rampazzo, A., Nava, A., Erne, P., Eberhard, M., Vian, E., Slomp, P., et al. (1995) A new locus for arrhythmogenic right ventricular cardiomyopathy (ARVD2) maps to chromosome 1q42-q43. *Hum. Mol. Genet.* **4**, 2151–2154.
134. Rampazzo, A., Nava, A., Danieli, G. A., Buja, G., Daliento, L., Fasoli, G., et al. (1994) The gene for arrhythmogenic right ventricular cardiomyopathy maps to chromosome 14q23-q24. *Hum. Mol. Genet.* **3**, 959–962.
135. Severini, G. M., Krajinovic, M., Pinamonti, B., Sinagra, G., Fioretti, P., Brunazzi, M. C., et al. (1996) A new locus for arrhythmogenic right ventricular dysplasia on the long arm of chromosome 14. *Genomics* **31**, 193–200.
136. Coonar, A. S., Protonotarios, N., Tsatsopoulou, A., Needham, E. W., Houlston, R. S., Cliff, S., et al. (1998) Gene for arrhythmogenic right ventricular cardiomyopathy with diffuse nonepidermolytic palmoplantar keratoderma and woolly hair (Naxos disease) maps to 17q21. *Circulation* **97**, 2049–2058.
137. Ahmad, F., Li, D., Karibe, A., Gonzalez, O., Tapscott, T., Hill, R., et al. (1998) Localization of a gene responsible for arrhythmogenic right ventricular dysplasia to chromosome 3p23. *Circulation* **98**, 2791–2795.
138. Li, D., Ahmad, F., Gardner, M. J., Weilbaecher, D., Hill, R., Karibe, A., et al. (2000) The locus of a novel gene responsible for arrhythmogenic right ventricular dysplasia characterized by early onset and high penetrance maps to chromosome 10p12-p14. *Am. J. Hum. Genet.* **66**, 148–56.
139. Corrado, D., Nava, A., Buja, G., Martini, B., Fasoli, G., Oselladore, L., et al. (1996) Familial cardiomyopathy underlies syndrome of right bundle branch block, ST segment elevation and sudden death. *J. Am. Coll. Cardiol.* **27**, 443–448.
140. McKenna, W. J., Thiene, G., Nava, A. A., Fontaliran, F., Blomstrom-Lundqvist, C., Fontaine, G., et al. (1994) Diagnosis of arrhythmogenic right ventricular dysplasia/ cardiomyopathy. *Br. Heart J.* **71**, 215–218.
141. Tiso, N., Stephan, D. A., Nava, A., Bagattin, A., Devaney, J. M., Stanchi, F., et al. (2001) Identification of mutations in cardiac ryanodine gene in families affected with arrhythmogenic right ventricular cardiomyopathy type 2 (ARVD2). *Hum. Mol. Genet.* **10**, 189–194.
142. Stokes, D. L. and Wagenknecht, T. (2000) Calcium transport across the sarcoplasmic reticuluum—Structure and function of Ca2+-ATPase and the ryanodine receptor. *Eur. J. Biochem.* **267**, 5274–5279.

143. Missiaen, L., Robberecht, W., Van Den Bosch, L., Callewaert, G., Parys, J. B., Wuytack, F., et al. (2000) Abnormal intracellular Ca^{2+} homeostasis and disease. *Cell Calcium* **28**, 1–21.

144. McKoy, G., Protonotarios, N., Crosby, A., Tsatsopoulou, A., Anastasakis, A., Coonar, A., et al. (2000) Identification of a deletion in plakoglobin in arrhythmogenic right ventricular cardiomyopathy with palmoplantar keratoderma and woolly hair (Naxos disease). *Lancet* **355**, 2119–2124.

145. Norgett, E. E., Hatsell, S. J., Carvajal-Huerta, L., Ruiz Cabezas, J-C., Common, J., Purkis, P. E., et al. (2000) Recessive mutation in desmoplakin disrupts desmoplakin-intermediate filament interactions and causes dilated cardiomyopathy, woolly hair and keratoderma. *Hum Mol Genet* **9**, 2761–2766.

146. Naccarella, F. (1993) Malignant ventricular arrhythmias in patients with a right bundle-branch block and persistent ST segment elevation in V1-V3: A probable arrhythmogenic cardiomyopathy of the right ventricle. [editorial comment] *G. Ital. Cardiol.* **23**, 1219–1222.

147. Fontaine, G. (1996) Familial cardiomyopathy associated with right bundle branch block, ST segment elevation and sudden death [Letter] *J. Am. Coll. Cardiol.* **28**, 540.

148. Scheinman, M. M. (1997) Is Brugada syndrome a distinct clinical entity? *J. Cardiovasc. Electrophysiol.* **8**, 332–336.

149. Ohe, T. (1996) Idiopathic ventricular fibrillation of the Brugada type - an atypical form of arrhythmogenic right ventricular cardiomyopathy. [editorial] *Intern. Med.* **35**, 595.

150. Fontaine, G., Piot, O., Sohal, P., Issi, Y., Fontaliran, F., Pettelot, G., et al. (1996) Right precordial leads and sudden death. Relation with arrhythmogenic right ventricular dysplasia. *Arch. Mal. Coeur Vaiss.* **89**, 1323–1329.

151. Coumel, P., Fidelle, J., Lucet, V., et al. (1978) Catacholaminergic-induced severe ventricular arrhythmias with Adams-Stokes syndrome in children: Report of four cases. *Br. Heart J.* **40(Suppl)**, 28–37.

152. Leenhardt, A., Lucet, V., Denjoy, I., Grau, F., Ngoc, D. D., and Coumel, P. (1995) Catecholaminergic polymorphic ventricular tachycardia in children: A 7-year follow-up of 21 patients. *Circulation* **91**, 1512–1519.

153. Laitinen, P. J., Brown, K. M., Piippo, K., Swan, H., Devaney, J. M., Brahmbhatt, B., et al. (2001) Mutations of the cardiac ryanodine receptor (RyR2) gene in familial polymorphic ventricular tachycardia. *Circulation* **103**, 485–490.

154. Priori, S. G., Napolitano, C., Tiso, N., Memmi, M., Vignati, G., Bloise, R., et al. (2001) Mutations in the cardiac ryanodine receptor gene (hRyR2) underlie catecholaminergic polymorphic ventricular tachycardia. *Circulation* **103**, 196–200.

155. Swan, H., Piippo, K., Viitasalo, M., Heikkila, P., Paavonen, T., Kainulainen, K., et al. (1999) Arrhythmic disorder mapped to chromosome 1q42-q43 causes malignant polymorphic ventricular tachycardia in structurally normal hearts. *J. Am. Coll. Cardiol.* **34**, 2035–2042.

156. Bauce, B., Nava, A., Rampazzo, A., Daliento, L., Muriago, M., Basso, C., et al. (2000) Familial effort polymorphic ventricular arrhythmias in arrhythmogenic right ventricular cardiomyopathy map to chromosome 1q42–43. *Am. J. Cardiol.* **85**, 573–579.

157. McCarthy, T. V., Quane, K. A., and Lynch, P. J. (2000) Ryanodine receptor mutations in malignant hyperthermia and central core disease. *Hum. Mutat.* **15**, 410–417.

158. Wan, Q., Wu, N., Fan, W., Tang, Y. Y., Jin, L., and Fang, Q. (1992) Clinical manifestations and prevalence of different types of supraventricular tachycardia among Chinese. *Chin. Med. J.* **105**, 284–288.

159. Gollob, M. H., Bharati, S., and Swerdlow, C. D. (2000) Accessory atrioventricular node with properties of a typical accessory pathway: Anatomic-electrophysiologic correlation. *J. Cardiovasc. Electrophysiol.* **11**, 922–926.

160. Packard, J. M., Graettinger, J. S., and Graybiel, A. (1954) Analysis of the electrocardiograms obtained from 1000 young healthy aviators: Ten year follow-up. *Circulation* **10**, 384–400.

161. Hejtmancik, M. R., and Hermann, G. R. (1957) The electrocardiographic syndrome of short P-R interval and broad QRS complexes: A clinical study of 80 cases. *Am. Heart J.* **54,** 708–721.

162. Khair, G. Z., Soni, J. S., and Bamrah, V. S. (1985) Syncope in hypertrophic cardiomyopathy. II. Coexistence of atrioventricular block and Wolff-Parkinson-White syndrome. *Am. Heart J.* **110,** 1083–1086.

163. Jackman, W. M., Wang, X., Friday, K. J., Roman, C. A., Moulton, K. P., et al. (1991) Catheter ablation of accessory atrioventricular pathways (Wolff-Parkinson-White syndrome) by radiofrequency current. *N. Engl. J. Med.* **324,** 1605–1611.

164. MacRae, C. A., Ghaisas, N., Kass, S., Donnelly, S., Basson, C. T., Watkins, H. C., et al. (1995) Familial hypertrophic cardiomyopathy with Wolff-Parkinson-White syndrome maps to a locus on chromosome 7q3. *J. Clin. Invest.* **96,** 1216–1220.

165. Ichida, F., Hamamichi, Y., Miyawaki, T., Ono, Y., Kamiya, T., Akagi, T., et al. (1999) Clinical features of isolated noncompaction of the ventricular myocardium: Long-term clinical course, hemodynamic properties, and genetic background. *J. Am. Coll. Cardiol.* **34,** 233–240.

166. Gollob, M. H., Green, M. S., Tang, A. S-L, Gollob, T., Karibe, A., Hassan, A-S., et al. (2001) Identification of a gene responsible for familial Wolff-Parkinson-White syndrome. *N. Engl. J. Med.* **344,** 1823–1831.

167. Blair, E., Redwood, C., Ashratian, H., Oliveira, M., Broxholme, J., Kerr, B., et al. (2001) Mutations in the (2 subunit of AMP-activated protein kinase cause familial hypertrophic cardiomyopathy: Evidence for the central role of energy compromise in disease pathogenesis. *Hum. Mol. Genet.* **10,** 1215–1220.

168. Lang, T., Yu, L., Tu, Q., Jiang, J., Chen, Z., Xin, Y., et al. (2000) Molecular cloning, genomic organization, and mapping of PRKAG2, a heart abundant γ_2 subunit of 5'-AMP-activated protein kinase, to human chromosome 7q36. *Genomics* **70,** 258–263.

169. Hardie, D. G. and Carling, D. (1997) The AMP-activated protein kinase—fuel gauge of the mammalian cell? *Eur. J. Biochem.* **246,** 259–273.

170. Kemp, B. E., Mitchelhill, K. I., Stapleton, D., Michell, B. J., Chen, Z. P., and Witters, L. A. (1999) Dealing with energy demand: The AMP-activated protein kinase. *Trends Biochem. Sci.* **24,** 22–25.

171. Winder, W. W., Holmes, B. F., Rubink, D. S., Jensen, E. B., Chen, M., and Holloszy, J. O. (2000) Activation of AMP-activated protein kinase increases mitochondrial enzymes in skeletal muscle. *J. Appl. Physiol.* **88,** 2219–2226.

172. Cheung, P. C., Salt, I. P., Davies, S. P., Hardie, D. G., and Carling, D. (2000) Characterization of AMP-activated protein kinase gamma-subunit isoforms and their role in AMP binding. *Biochem. J.* **346,** 659–669.

173. Bowles, N. E., Bowles, K. R., and Towbin, J. A. (2000) The "Final Common Pathway" hypothesis and inherited cardiovascular disease: The role of cytoskeletal proteins in dilated cardiomyopathy. *Herz* **25,** 168–175.

174. Malhotra, J. D., Chen, C., Rivolta, I., Abriel, H., Malhotra, R., Mattei, L. N., et al. (2001) Characterization of sodium channel α and β subunits in rat and mouse cardiac myocytes. *Circulation* **103,** 1301–1310.

17

Myocardial Adenoviral Vector Delivery for Cardiovascular Gene Therapy

Hendrik T. Tevaearai, Andrea D. Eckhart, and Walter J. Koch

CONTENTS

1. INTRODUCTION

Cardiovascular disease remains the leading cause of death in industrialized countries and despite major progress in drug development, morbidity and mortality has not significantly changed over the last couple of decades. Today, still more than half a million people are diagnosed with chronic heart failure (HF) each year in the United States (1,2). Interestingly, efforts to reduce risk factors have not yet lead to major reductions in the incidence of cardiovascular disease and HF in particular. However, for some probable high-risk factors, more long-term studies may be required. Nevertheless, new therapeutic strategies are clearly needed to help combat cardiovascular disease and more importantly, HF.

One interesting novel therapeutic approach that has shown recent promise in the myocardium has been that of genetic modulation (3). Over the last 10 yr, the dramatic progress made in molecular and biological technologies has permitted major advances in the basic knowledge of numerous pathologies, including diseases of the cardiovascular system. The results of these efforts, including the recent description of the human genome, have broadened our understanding of cardiovascular disease and provided novel insights into mechanism of myocardial pathology. Consequently, novel targets in the heart have been elucidated that can be manipulated either via gene therapy or can

From: Cardiac Drug Development Guide
Edited by: M. K. Pugsley © Humana Press Inc., Totowa, NJ

also spur the future development of pharmaceutical-grade small molecule chemical modulators *(3,4)*.

The concept of cardiovascular gene therapy implies the delivery of a designated DNA sequence into cardiovascular tissue to provide significant expression of a specific protein with therapeutic consequences. In addition, negative aspects of the method need to be few for such an innovative therapy. As gene therapy has attempted to move from "bench to bedside" in the cardiovascular arena, certain disadvantages have came to the surface and, for HF gene therapy in particular, there are several hurdles that still limit the reality of such treatment. Efficiency of myocardial gene delivery and control of expression remain the leading technical challenge. For example, the choice for short- or long-term expression may differ depending on the specific therapeutic goal to achieve and whether the targeted HF patient population needs temporary or prolonged treatment.

This chapter will include discussion on adenoviral-mediated gene therapy approaches that have recently been applied to the heart and heart diseases. Methods of transgene delivery to cardiac tissue will be presented, followed by applications in animal models and existing human trials for ischemic heart disease. To illustrate the wide potential of adenoviral vectors as tools to study cardiac pathology and to investigate possible future therapeutic modalities, we will detail current knowledge in HF focusing on the modulation of excitation-contraction coupling as well as β-adrenergic receptor (βAR) signaling.

2. ADENOVIRUS AS A VECTOR FOR MYOCARDIAL GENE THERAPY

Even though a number of viral and nonviral vectors are now available and can be used for myocardial gene delivery (Table 1), adenovirus is the most widely employed both in animal models and current human trials *(5–7)*. Importantly, for all these vectors, including adenoviruses, several limitations remain (Table 1) and are the subject of ongoing and, no doubt, intensive future research. Transfection efficiency, organ specificity, immune reactions, duration, and control of transgene of expression are all problems that have to be improved for viral vectors to become commonplace in the therapeutic arsenal of the cardiologist or cardiac surgeon *(8,9)*.

Specifically for adenoviruses, human serotypes 2 and 5 are the most commonly used, although they typically trigger severe immune reaction to host encoded proteins because of pre-existing exposure. As a result, the inflammatory reaction may impair efficiency of gene transfection, and long-term expression is certainly compromised *(7)*. Moreover, a second administration of the adenoviral–transgene package is precluded. Extensive research is being performed to identify novel human and nonhuman adenoviral serotypes with potential advantages for human clinical use, and also studies are being directed to modify the viral backbone that may also prove beneficial in terms of reducing the immune response *(7–9)*.

The adenoviral 35-kb genome is composed of early and late genes with the early regions being necessary for replication and transcription *(8)*. To use adenoviruses as gene vectors, modification of the genomic structure is required so that the organism is rendered replication-deficient. Deletion of the early region 1 (*E1*) gene formed the first-generation of adenoviral vectors.

Table 1
Advantages and Disadvantages of Vectors
Commonly Used for Myocardial Gene Therapy

	Advantages	Disadvantages
Plasmid DNA	Easy to produce Episomal incorporation Low immune reaction	Low efficiency Transient expression

Retrovirus	Efficient transduction
	Easy to manipulate
		Transfection only to
		  proliferating cells
		Random chromosomal
		  incorporation and potential
		  insertional mutagenesis
		Low titers

Adenovirus	Highly efficient transduction Episomal incorporation Transfection of replicating and nonreplicating cells Early gene expression Can be produced in high titers	Induce immune reaction Time limited gene expression

Adeno-associated virus	Transfection of replicating and
	  nonreplicating cells
	Can be produced in high titers
	Low immune reaction
	Long-term expression
		Limit size of DNA inserts
		Delay before gene expression
		Random DNA incorporation and
		  potential for insertional
		  mutagenesis

Currently, most investigators use second- or third-generation vectors with *E1*, *E2*, and/or E4 deletions *(8)*. Importantly, besides providing replication deficiency, the removal of these early genes provide additional space for DNA inserts, which size can range up to 10 kb. Production of replication-deficient adenoviral-transgene packages usually involves recombination in mammalian cell lines with DNA sequence complementing the defective adenoviral genome as for example HEK 293 or 911 cells *(8)*.

3. MYOCARDIAL DELIVERY TECHNIQUES

Direct injection into the heart muscle is the simplest technique for myocardial gene transfer. This technique, however, can be quite traumatic because the needle itself creates significant local injury and can evoke inflammation *(10–12)*. Importantly, this method of cardiac gene delivery is being used clinically in trials for neovascularization in ischemic heart disease. Adenoviral preparations of vascular growth factors, such as vascular endothelial growth factor (VEGF), are being directly injected in affected areas as an adjunct to coronary artery bypass grafting *(10–12)*. However, this technique only supports local transgene expression at the injection site and, therefore, one cannot achieve global and homogeneous gene expression using this method of gene delivery, which is required for modulation of the contractile function of the heart *(13)*. A pericardial gene delivery approach also has been investigated. However, myocardial expression is generally poor, and this results in significant expression in several noncardiac tissues, including lung and liver *(14,15)*.

The most efficient and promising gene delivery approach to the myocardium appears to be intracoronary delivery of adenoviral transgenes. First, ex vivo intracoronary delivery of donor hearts of heterotopic transplant models using retrograde aortic perfusion of adenoviral solutions has been used in rat and rabbit models. This method can result in global transgene delivery that can induce functional changes in the transplanted heart *(16–18)*. An in vivo intracoronary approach that has been successful in several studies using rats and rabbits involves a thoracotomy and injection of an adenoviral solution into the left ventricular (LV) cavity while the ascending aorta is cross-clamped *(19,20)*. Consequently, the adenoviral solution is forced to perfuse the coronary arteries, resulting in global transgene expression. In the rat, the pulmonary artery is also cross-clamped *(19)*. In the rabbit, 45 s of aortic cross-clamping does not affect ventricular function, and it permits significant global gene expression *(20–22)*. Importantly, this in vivo intracoronary delivery technique has been successfully used in rabbits with both acute and chronic LV dysfunction *(21,22)*.

Although producing robust and global transgene delivery, the above methods are not necessary easily translatable to the clinic. Thus, more clinically applicable methods have recently been used in animal models with promising success. Recently, we have taken advantage of cardiopulmonary bypass during cardiac surgery to perform in vivo intracoronary delivery of adenoviral–transgenes to the hearts of piglets *(23)*. This technique is clinically relevant especially because we are seeing increased patients undergoing cardiac surgery with significant LV dysfunction. Most recently, a noninvasive technique that has shown great promise for delivery of adenoviruses to the heart in vivo has been percutaneous subselective coronary artery catheterization and injection *(24–26)*. This technique results in efficient transgene delivery in a ventricular-specific manner depending on which coronary artery is catheterized *(24)*.

It is apparent that a few of these methods of gene delivery may potentially be adapted for clinical use for HF gene therapy because coronary perfusion of an explanted heart before its transplantation, perfusion during cardiopulmonary bypass, and selective coronary delivery via percutaneous catheterization may all be clinically applicable techniques for gene therapy to improve the function of the failing heart. Importantly, as discussed above focal delivery via direct injection of adenoviruses to the heart is being used in angiogenesis trials.

4. MYOCARDIAL GENE THERAPY
OF VENTRICULAR CONTRACTILE DYSFUNCTION

HF is a widespread disease that can result from acute or chronic events or even be inherited. It is a progressive disease that is characterized by different stages of evolution and, thus, patients can have different degrees of ventricular dysfunction. Therefore, HF per se can be viewed as a chronic condition but it may also be transient, such as in acute temporary myocardial ischemia. Studies in genetically engineered mice and larger animal models of disease have recently led to the elucidation of novel molecular targets for potential treatment of the failing heart, which includes specific genetic manipulation of the myocardial βAR system *(4)*. Moreover, intracellular calcium handling and homeostasis appear to be an attractive novel HF target *(27)*. It appears, through several animal studies, that the molecular, biochemical, histological, and functional alterations that take place in the failing heart can be reversed or improved via targeted genetic manipulations of these signaling pathways *(4,27)*.

5. ADENOVIRAL-MEDIATED GENE MODULATION OF MYOCARDIAL CALCIUM HOMEOSTASIS

Figure 1 illustrates calcium (Ca^{2+}) handling in the cardiomyocyte *(27)*. Normal depolarization of cardiomyocytes induces a Ca^{2+} influx from the extracellular milieu via the voltage-dependent L-type Ca^{2+} channel, which in turn activates ryanodine receptors (RyR). RyRs are channels located on sarcoplasmic reticulum (SR) membranes and release Ca^{2+} into the cytoplasm. This results in an acute cytosolic increase in Ca^{2+} (the Ca^{2+} transient) and subsequent induction of contraction. Relaxation is marked by SR Ca^{2+} reuptake via the SR Ca^{2+}-ATPase, SERCA2a, the predominant isoform in cardiomyocytes. Activity of SERCA2a is closely regulated by phospholamban (PLB). The unphosphorylated form of PLB is an inhibitor of SERCA2a activity, whereas its phosphorylation by protein kinase A (PKA) and/or Ca^{2+}–calmodulin-dependent protein kinase causes disinhibition of PLB's negative effect on SERCA2a. Ca^{2+} can also be removed from the cytosolic compartment via the transsarcolemmal Na^+/Ca^{2+} exchanger (NCX; Fig. 1).

Several changes in this system occur in failing cardiomyocytes *(27–29)*. Reduction in SERCA2a activity is consistently observed in addition to a decrease in SERCA2a mRNA and protein. The level of PLB expression is not significantly altered; however it has been shown that its phosphorylation state can be. Thus, the ratio of PLB to SERCA2a is increased in the failing heart and, importantly, the relative inhibitory effect of PLB is augmented *(28,29)*. Accordingly, gene therapy protocols have logically attempted to target SERCA2a and PLB, although other aspects of the Ca^{2+} handling have also been studied, including modulation of NCX activity *(29)*.

First, using neonatal myocytes exposed to phorbol-12-myristate-13-acetate, which decreases endogenous expression of SERCA2 and subsequent prolongation of the Ca^{2+} transient, it was shown that adenoviral-mediated transfer of the SERCA2a transgene allowed normalization of SERCA2a protein levels, shortening of the Ca^{2+} transient, and improvement in SR Ca^{2+} uptake *(30)*. Several other studies have since confirmed the normalization of intracellular Ca^{2+} homeostasis in failing cardiomyocytes from neonatal rats or chick embryos using adenoviral-mediated SERCA2a gene transfer *(31–34)*. More importantly, several studies have now demonstrated the physiologic benefit of overexpressing SERCA2a in normal and failing hearts both in vitro and in vivo using various models of HF *(33–37)*. Interestingly, this functional benefit was also verified in human cardiomyocytes isolated from failing ventricles *(38)*.

Targeted reduction of PLB activity is another approach to modulate myocardial Ca^{2+} metabolism in HF conditions. Even though PLB mRNA and protein levels are unchanged in HF, reduction of PLB activity may be beneficial, as the PLB-SERCA2a ratio would be reduced. This gene transfer approach has been triggered by the finding in PLB knockout mice that showed the loss of PLB expression resulted in a mouse model of heightened cardiac contractility *(39)*. Moreover, cross-breeding of PLB knockout mice has led to the rescue of different murine models of HF *(40,41)*. Furthermore, the deleterious hyperactivity of PLB has also been confirmed in transgenic mice and several studies involving adenoviral-mediated PLB overexpression *(33,42,43)*. Specifically, cardiomyocyte shortening in vitro and LV contractility in vivo were both impaired after myocardial delivery of the PLB transgene *(33,42,43)*. Accordingly, mutant forms of PLB acting as a dominant-negative and antisense RNA constructs of PLB have been engineered into adenoviral vectors *(44,45)*. Delivery of these transgenes

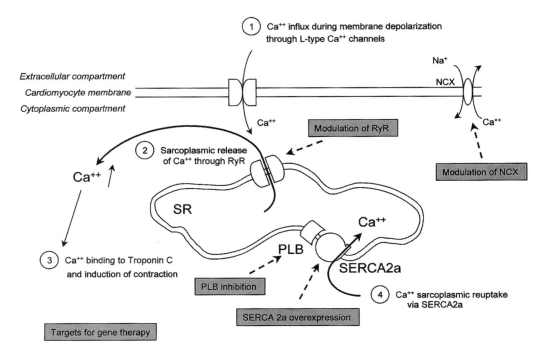

Fig. 1. Schematic overview of myocardial Ca²⁺ handling during excitation-contraction coupling (for review, *see* ref. *27*). Steps 1–4 represent the successive stages starting with the initial Ca²⁺ influx via voltage-dependent L-type Ca²⁺ channels after membrane depolarization. This Ca²⁺ entry triggers activation of RyR and subsequent Ca²⁺ release from the SR. This rapid increase in Ca²⁺ further evokes the generalized scheme of excitation–contraction coupling. Ca²⁺ removal from the cytosolic compartment during cardiac relaxation is primarily via the SR Ca²⁺ ATPase (SERCA2a), which is under control of the phosphorylation state of PLB. NCX can also contribute to cytosolic elimination of Ca²⁺. As indicated in the shaded boxes, targets for HF gene therapy include overexpression of SERCA2a, inhibition of PLB, and modulation of RyR and NCX.

targeting a reduction of PLB expression and/or activity have shown some recent therapeutic promise as contractile function can be improved by this technique in animal models of HF *(44,45)*.

Importantly, other possible ways to effectively improve myocardial contractility involve modulation of RyR or NCX. A recent study showed that overexpressing FKBP12.6, a protein tightly bound to RyR, leads to a significant increase in contractility *(46)*. On the other hand, NCX overexpression altered shortening of cultured cardiomyocytes in a negative fashion *(47,48)*. These targets will no doubt be the subjects of several new studies in the near future.

6. ADENOVIRAL-MEDIATED GENE MODULATION OF MYOCARDIAL βAR SIGNALING

Figure 2 illustrates the classic βAR signaling system in the cardiomyocyte *(4)*. Agonist activation of βARs triggers activation and dissociation of the heterotrimeric Gs

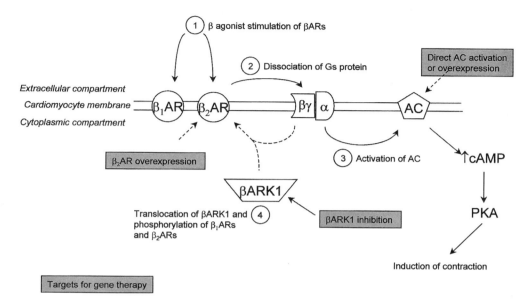

Fig. 2. An overview of myocardial β adrenergic signaling is illustrated via the successive steps 1–4 (for review, *see* ref. *4*). Agonist (norepinephrine or epinephrine) activation of myocardial (βARs) of both the β_1 and β_2 AR subtypes triggers dissociation of Gs proteins into Gsα and Gβγ activated subunits. This leads to the activation of adenylyl cyclase (AC) and intracellular increases in cAMP. The βAR-AC-cAMP cascade activates cAMP-dependent protein kinase, which phosphorylates several downstream targets including sarcolemmal L-type Ca^{2+} channels and PLB, inducing the contraction–relaxation cycle. The Gβγ subunits direct the membrane translocation of the cytoplasmic βAR kinase (βARK1), which phosphorylates βARs and interdicts further signaling (desensitization). As indicated in the shaded boxes, targets for HF gene therapy include selective overexpression of β_2 ARs, inhibition of βARK1 and manipulation of AC.

protein complex into Gsα and Gβγ subunits. The Gsα subunit activates adenylyl cyclase with subsequent intracellular increases of cyclic adenosine monophosphate and protein kinase A.

Interestingly, one of the targets of the βAR-PKA pathway is PLB. One major regulatory mechanism of the βAR signaling pathway involves the phosphorylation of activated βARs following Gβγ-facilitated membrane translocation of the cytoplasmic βAR kinase (βARK1, also named GRK2). Phosphorylation of activated βARs by βARK1 and other G protein-coupled receptor kinases (GRKs) results in desensitization of the receptor, impairing its ability to couple to the G protein. In the failing heart, β_1 ARs are selectively downregulated whereas remaining β_1 and β_2ARS are uncoupled *(49)*. This enhanced βAR desensitization appears to be the result of enhanced GRK activity because βARK1 is upregulated at the mRNA and protein levels in HF *(50)*.

The role of the different components of the βAR signaling system as possible gene therapy targets was initially elucidated in studies involving genetically engineered mice. Transgenic mice with modest to high β_2AR overexpression in the heart initially suggested the inotropic benefit of overexpressing β_2ARs *(51,52)*. In fact, β_2AR overexpression has led to the rescue of a transgenic mouse model of cardiac hypertrophy and ventricular decompensation *(53)*. Interestingly, transgenic mice overexpressing β_1ARs present with opposite effects as these mice developed early cardiomyopathy and HF *(54)*. These critical studies in transgenic mice have led to several recent studies demonstrating that signaling through myocardial β_1 and β_2ARs is qualitatively different and for the most part, results appear to support a therapeutic effect of β_2AR-selective signaling enhancement *(4)*.

Adenoviral-mediated β_2AR overexpression has increased LV contractility in several animal models *(16,17,20,55,56)*. Importantly, functional improvement has also occurred in HF models *(57,58)*. More recently, we have been able to demonstrate improved myocardial recovery of failing hearts when β_2AR gene transfer was combined with mechanical unloading as compared to unloading alone (Tevaearai, Eckhart and Koch, unpublished data). Accordingly, modulation of βAR level specific for the β_2ARsubtype may represent an ideal target for gene manipulation in the failing heart.

Targeting βARK1 is an interesting alternative to β_2AR overexpression for the treatment of HF *(4,59)*. Transgenic mouse models have demonstrated the negative functional effect of overexpressing βARK1 in the heart *(60,61)*. Reciprocally, inhibiting βARK1 appears to be clearly beneficial *(4,60–62)*. A 194-amino acid peptide consisting of the carboxyl terminal portion of βARK1 (βARKct) has been extensively used by our laboratory to inhibit the activity of βARK1 via inhibition of G$\beta\gamma$-mediated membrane translocation, a process required for βARK1 activation *(60)*. The G$\beta\gamma$ binding domain is located in the carboxyl terminus of this GRK, and the βARKct competes with endogenous βARK1, thus inhibiting its activation. Use of the βARKct has shown that it is an effective βARK1 inhibitor in vitro and in vivo. Transgenic mice with myocardial-targeted βARKct expression demonstrated increased entropy as well as an augmented functional response to βAR stimulation *(60)*. Interestingly, cross-breeding of βARKct transgenic mice have led to the functional rescue of several murine models of HF and cardiomyopathy *(41,63,64)*. Functional rescue of these mouse models of HF have included significantly improved survival that actually was potentiated by βAR blockade *(64)*.

In addition to the striking findings in transgenic mice demonstrating the potential beneficial cardiac effects of the βARKct, adenoviral-mediated delivery of the βARKct transgene to the heart has been used in several larger animal models, including a rabbit model of ventricular dysfunction and HF and βARKct expression does promote enhanced in vivo cardiac function *(21,22,25,26)*. Moreover, myocardial delivery of βARKct adenovirus to the heart at the time of myocardial infarction significantly delays development of HF *(21)*, whereas delivery via percutaneous coronary artery catheterization 3 wk after myocardial infarction reverses ventricular dysfunction *(25)*. Adenoviral-βARKct delivery to the heart and myocardial expression also prevents acute contractile dysfunction in clinically relevant models of acute transient failure, such as those observed after cardioplegic arrest *(22)* or even during acute coronary occlusion *(65)*. In fact, the characteristic short-term expression of adenoviral transgenes may emerge as being advantageous in certain clinical applications, such as ischemia–reperfusion situations where myocardial dysfunction is typically transient and, therefore, the need for hemodynamic support is temporary. Importantly, in several studies overall using functionally relevant adenoviral-βARKct, gene transfer has been achieved via different delivery techniques to the heart, either ex vivo during cardiac transplantation, or in vivo by global or selective coronary perfusion, that have supported the hypothesis that inhibition of βARK1 activity in the heart is a worthwhile and novel target for HF therapy.

Delivery of the adenylyl cyclase enzyme itself is another approach of modulating the βAR signaling pathway in the failing heart that has shown promising effects in animal models *(66,67)*. In addition, delivery of a noncardiac receptor, such as the vasopressin V2 receptor, that can directly activate adenylyl cyclase independent of the βAR system has been hypothesized as a novel HF treatment *(68,69)*. Recent studies have indicated that this may represent an interesting novel inotropic strategy *(68,69)*.

7. GENE THERAPY FOR ISCHEMIC HEART DISEASE

The identification and characterization of angiogenic growth factors have created unique opportunities for gene therapy in the neovascularization of ischemic tissues, including the myocardium *(10–12)*. VEGF and the fibroblast growth factor family (FGF1 and FGF2) have received the most attention as potential therapeutic agents. These proteins have been shown to result in new vessels by stimulating endothelial cell proliferation and migration, and gene therapy for ischemic heart disease using these angiogenic factors has theoretical advantages because they are secreted proteins which can act in a paracrine manner. Therefore, transfection of tissues at a lower efficiency is probably adequate to achieve new vessel growth and prolonged transgene expression is probably not necessary since these factors only trigger vascular growth. Thus, current available adenoviruses are perhaps ideal for this type of gene therapy. Moreover, it is suitable for the low-efficiency focal delivery provided by direct intramyocardial injection. Accordingly, clinical trials have been initiated over the last couple of years.

Regarding preclinical large animal studies, direct injection of a VEGF adenovirus succeeded in improving regional myocardial perfusion and ventricular wall motion in ischemic pig myocardium *(70)*. Interestingly, other investigators have used VEGF gene transfer with transmyocardial laser revascularization (TMR; ref. *71)*. TMR consists of laser-induced channels generally created from the epicardial surface to the endocardium and this appears to stimulate inflammation and a general healing process, which includes neovascularization. The combination of TMR with angiogenic growth factor gene therapy couples nonspecific activation of blood vessel growth with specific increases in important factors (i.e., VEGF).

Neovascularization trials were initially started delivering the growth factor peptides themselves to the ischemic heart via intracoronary or intravenous injections. The initial target population has consisted of patients who have regions of ischemic myocardium, which are not amenable to conventional revascularization. Efforts using recombinant growth factor proteins include two larger, phase II trials that have resulted in negative results with no real benefit gained by VEGF or FGF2 delivery *(72,73)*. These negative results using recombinant protein delivery emphasize the importance of directed delivery of adequate doses of the angiogenic growth factors to the ischemic myocardium. Systemic administration of recombinant protein, which was used in these trials, may not have achieved adequate delivery to ischemic regions of the heart *(74)*.

Injection of adenoviral preparations coding for vascular growth factors would appear to offer an advantage in terms of directing therapy to ischemic myocardium and thus, trials have begun in patients. To date, published reports of gene transfer for therapeutic angiogenesis in human subjects are limited to phase I dose-escalating, nonrandomized trials. nterestingly, Rosengart et al. *(75)* reported a group of patients in which the VEGF coding sequence was administered in a first-generation adenoviral vector as an intramyocardial injection into the ischemic region. In this study, one group of patients received simultaneous coronary artery bypass graft and VEGF gene therapy, while another group of patients underwent only VEGF gene therapy. No significant adverse reactions were noted, which is extremely important. These results warrant future trials.

8. CONCLUSIONS

Over the last decade, the concept of gene therapy has evolved from the dream of a new means to cure inherited pathologies to treatment of complex acquired disorders such as cardiovascular disease, including HF. Importantly, however, limitations have brought initial fantasies back to reality. Numerous drawbacks have become evident, and several concerns about gene therapy in general need to be addressed before there is widespread use of vectors such as adenovirus. Accordingly, several delivery systems and techniques and various vectors have been developed and improved upon with the same goals of initiating gene therapy trials in human HF. Certainly, as outlined in this chapter, the use of adenoviral-mediated gene transfer technology has proven its value as an exciting and important molecular tool to study mechanisms and development of cardiovascular pathologies. Moreover, it has allowed the intensive investigations of potential novel targets for the treatment of HF, including the genetic manipulation of SERCA2a, PLB, or βARK1. These studies may further help define future novel therapeutic strategies and new small molecule chemical compounds. Gene modulation may also be used directly as an alternative therapeutic modality and recent clinical trials involving adenoviral-mediated vascular growth factors encourage this approach. In conclusion, recent research has continued to make the prospects for cardiac gene therapy, especially HF, a very promising topic that certainly deserves more attention.

REFERENCES

1. American Heart Association. 2002 Heart and Stroke Statistical Update. http://www.americanheart.org.
2. Cohn, J. N., Bristow, M. R., Chien, K. R., Colucci, W. S., Frazier, O. H., Leinwand, L. A., et al. (1997) Report of the National Heart, Lung, and Blood Institute Special Emphasis Panel on Heart Failure Research. *Circulation* **95,** 766–770.
3. Isner, J. M. (2002) Myocardial gene therapy. *Nature* **415,** 234–239.
4. Rockman, H. A., Koch, W. J., and Lefkowitz, R. J. (2002) Seven membrane spanning receptors and heart function. *Nature* **415,** 206–212.
5. Kay, M. A., Glorioso, J. C., and Naldini, L. (2001) Viral vectors for gene therapy: The art of turning infectious agents into vehicles of therapeutics. *Nat. Med.* **7,** 33–40
6. Ylä-Herttuala, S. and Martin, J. F. (2000) Cardiovascular gene therapy. *Lancet* **355,** 213–222.
7. Duckers, H. J. and Nabel, E. G. (2000) Prospects for genetic therapy of cardiovascular disease. *Med. Clin. North Am.* **84,** 199–213.
8. Benihoud, K., Yeh, P., and Perricaudet, M. (1999) Adenovirus vectors for gene delivery. *Curr. Opin. Biotechnol.* **10,** 440–447.
9. Wattanapitayakul, S. K. and Bauer, J. A. (2000) Recent developments in gene therapy for cardiac disease. *Biomed. Pharmacother.* **54,** 487–504.

10. Losordo, D. W., Vale, P. R., Symes, J. F., Dunnington, C. H., Esakof, D. D., Maysky, M., et al. (1998) Gene therapy for myocardial angiogenesis: Initial clinical results with direct myocardial injection of phVEGF165 as sole therapy for myocardial ischemia. *Circulation* **98,** 2800–2804.

11. Patel, S. R., Lee, L. Y., Mack, C. A., Polce, D. R., El-Sawy, T., Hackett, N. R., et al. (1999) Safety of direct myocardial administration of an adenovirus vector encoding vascular endothelial growth factor 121. *Hum. Gene Ther.* **10,** 1331–1348.

12. Symes, J. F., Losordo, D. W., Vale, P. R., Lathi, K. G., Esakof, D. D., Mayskiy, M., et al. (1999) Gene therapy with vascular endothelial growth factor for inoperable coronary artery disease. *Ann. Thorac. Surg.* **68,** 830–836.

13. White, D. C. and Koch, W. J. (2001) Myocardial gene transfer. *Curr. Cardiol. Rep.* **3,** 37–42.

14. Fromes, Y., Salmon, A., Wang, X., Collin, H., Rouche, A., Hagege, A., et al. (1999) Gene delivery to the myocardium by intrapericardial injection. *Gene Ther.* **4,** 683–688.

15. March, K. L., Woody, M., Mehdi, K., Zipes, D. P., Brantly, M., and Trapnell, B. C. (1999) Efficient in vivo catheter-based pericardial gene transfer mediated by adenoviral vectors. *Clin. Cardiol.* **22,** I23–I29.

16. Kypson, A. P., Peppel, K., Akhter, S. A., Lilly, R. E., Glower, D. D., Lefkowitz, R. J., et al. (1998) Ex vivo adenoviral-mediated gene transfer to the transplanted adult rat heart. *J. Thoracic Cardiovasc. Surg.* **115,** 623–630.

17. Kypson, A. P., Hendrickson, S. C., Akhter, S. A., Wilson, K., McDonald, P. H., Lilly, R. E., et al. (1999) Adenoviral-mediated gene transfer of the β2-adrenergic receptor to donor hearts enhances cardiac function. *Gene Ther.* **6,** 1298–1304.

18. Shah, A. S., White, D. C., Tai, O., Hata, J. A., Pippen, A., Kypson, A. P., et al. (2000) Adenovirus-mediated genetic manipulation of the myocardial β-adrenergic signaling system in transplanted hearts. *J. Thorac. Cardiovasc. Surg.* **120,** 581–588.

19. Hajjar, R. J., Schmidt, U., Matsiu, T., Guerrero, J. L., Lee, K. H., Gwathmey, J. K., et al. (1998) Modulation of ventricular function through gene transfer in vivo. *Proc. Natl. Acad. Sci. USA* **95,** 5251–5256.

20. Maurice, J. P., Hata, J. A., Shah, A. S., White, D. C., McDonald, P. H., Dolber, P. C., et al. (1999) Enhancement of cardiac function after adenoviral-mediated in vivo intracoronary β2-adrenergic receptor gene delivery. *J. Clin. Invest.* **104,** 21–29.

21. White, D. C., Hata, J. A., Shah, A. S., Glower, D. D., Lefkowitz, R. J., and Koch. W. J. (2000) Preservation of myocardial β-adrenergic receptor signaling delays the development of heart failure following myocardial infarction. *Proc. Natl. Acad. Sci. USA* **97,** 5428–5433.

22. Tevaearai, H. T., Eckhart, A. D., Shotwell, K. F., Wilson, K., and Koch, W. J. (2001) Ventricular dysfunction after cardioplegic arrest is improved after myocardial gene transfer of a -adrenergic receptor kinase inhibitor. *Circulation* **104,** 2069–2074.

23. Davidson, M. J., Jones, J. M., Emani, S. M., Wilson, K. H., Jaggers, J., Koch, W. J., et al. (2001) Cardiac gene delivery with cardiopulmonary bypass. *Circulation* **104,** 131–133.

24. Shah, A. S., Lilly, R. E., Kypson, A. P., Tai, O., Hata, J. A., Pippen, A., et al. (2000) Intracoronary adenovirus-mediated delivery and overexpression of the β2-adrenergic receptor in the heart: prospects for molecular ventricular assistance. *Circulation* **101,** 408–414.

25. Shah, A. S., White, D. C., Emani, S., Kypson, A. P., Lilly, R. E., Wilson, K., et al. (2001) In vivo ventricular gene delivery of a β-adrenergic receptor kinase inhibitor to the failing heart reverses cardiac dysfunction. *Circulation* **103,** 1311–1316.

26. Emani, S. M., Shah, A. S., White, D. C., Glower, D. D., and Koch, W. J. (2001) Right ventricular gene therapy with a beta-adrenergic receptor kinase inhibitor improves survival after pulmonary artery banding. *Ann. Thorac. Surg.* **72,** 1657–1661.

27. Marks, A. R. (2000) Cardiac intracellular calcium release channels: Role in heart failure. *Circ. Res.* **87,** 8–11.

28. Houser, S. R., Piacentino, V. III, and Weisser, J. (2000) Abnormalities of calcium cycling in the hypertrophied and failing heart. *J. Mol. Cell Cardiol.* **32,** 1595–1607.

29. Bers, D. M. (2002) Cardiac excitation-contraction coupling. *Nature* **415,** 198–205.

30. Giordano, F. J., He, H., McDonough, P., Meyer, M., Sayen, M. R., and Dillmann, W. H. (1997) Adenovirus-mediated gene transfer reconstitutes depressed sarcoplasmic reticulum Ca2+-ATPase levels and shortens prolonged cardiac myocyte Ca2+ transients. *Circulation* **96,** 400–403.

31. Hajjar, R. J., Kang, J. X., Gwathmey, J. K., and Rosenzweig, A. (1997) Physiological effects of adenoviral gene transfer of sarcoplasmic reticulum calcium ATPase in isolated rat myocytes. *Circulation* **95,** 423–429.

32. Inesi, G., Lewis, D., Sumbilla, C., Nandi, A., Strock, C., Huff, K. W., et al. (1998) Cell-specific promoter in adenovirus vector for transgenic expression of SERCA1 ATPase in cardiac myocytes. *Am. J. Physiol.* **274,** C645–C653.

33. Meyer, M., Bluhm, W. F., He, H., Post, S. R., Giordano, F. J., Lew, W. Y., et al. (1999) Phospholamban-to-SERCA2 ratio controls the force-frequency relationship. *Am. J. Physiol.* **276,** H779–H785.

34. Sumbilla, C., Cavagna, M., Zhong, L., Ma, H., Lewis, D., Farrance, I., et al. (1999) Comparison of SERCA1 and SERCA2a expressed in COS-1 cells and cardiac myocytes. *Am. J. Physiol.* **277,** H2381–H2391.

35. Miyamoto, M. I., del Monte, F., Schmidt, U., DiSalvo, T. S., Kang, Z. B., Matsui, T., et al. (2000) Adenoviral gene transfer of SERCA2a improves left-ventricular function in aortic-banded rats in transition to heart failure. *Proc. Natl. Acad. Sci. USA* **97,** 793–798.

36. del Monte, F., Williams, E., Lebeche, D., Schmidt, U., Rosenzweig, A., Gwathmey, J. K., et al. (2001) Improvement in survival and cardiac metabolism after gene transfer of sarcoplasmic reticulum Ca2+-ATPase in a rat model of heart failure. *Circulation* **104,** 1424–1429.

37. Schmidt, U., del Monte, F., Miyamoto, M. I., Matsui, T., Gwathmey, J. K., Rosenzweig, A., et al. (2000) Restoration of diastolic function in senescent rat hearts through adenoviral gene transfer of sarcoplasmic reticulum Ca2+-ATPase. *Circulation* **101,** 790–796.

38. del Monte, F., Harding, S. E., Schmidt, U., Matsui, T., Kang, Z. B., Dec, G. W., Gwathmey, J. K., Rosenzweig, A., et al. (1999) Restoration of contractile function in isolated cardiomyocytes from failing human hearts by gene transfer of SERCA2a. *Circulation* **100,** 2308–2311.

39. Luo, W., Grupp, I. L., Harrer, J., Ponniah, S., Grupp, G., Duffy, J. J., et al. (1994) Targeted ablation of the phospholamban gene is associated with markedly enhanced myocardial contractility and loss of beta-agonist stimulation. *Circ. Res.* **75,** 401–409.

40. Minamisawa, S., Hoshijima, M., Chu, G., Ward, C. A., Frank, K., Gu, Y., et al. (1999) Chronic phospholamban-sarcoplasmic reticulum calcium ATPase interaction is the critical calcium cycling defect in dilated cardiomyopathy. *Cell* **99,** 313–322.

41. Freeman, K., Lerman, I., Kranias, E. G., Bohlmeyer, T., Bristow, M. R., Lefkowtiz, R. J., et al. (2001) Alterations in cardiac adrenergic signaling and calcium cycling differentially affect the progression of cardiomyopathy. *J. Clin. Invest.* **107,** 967–974.

42. Hajjar, R. J., Schmidt, U., Kang, J. X., Matsui, T., and Rosenzweig, A. (1997) Adenoviral gene transfer of phospholamban in isolated rat cardiomyocytes. Rescue effects by concomitant gene transfer of sarcoplasmic reticulum Ca2+-ATPase. *Circ. Res.* **81,** 145–153.

43. Davia, K., Hajjar, R. J., Terracciano, C. M., Kent, N. S., Ranu, H. K., O'Gara, P., et al. (1999) Functional alterations in adult rat myocytes after overexpression of phospholamban with use of adenovirus. *Physiol. Genomics* **1,** 41–50.

44. He, H., Meyer, M., Martin, J. L., McDonough, P. M., Ho, P., Lou, X., et al. (1999) Effects of mutant and antisense RNA of phospholamban on SR Ca2+-ATPase activity and cardiac myocyte contractility. *Circulation* **100,** 974–980.

45. Eizema, K., Fechner, H., Bezstarosti, K., Schneider-Rasp, S., van der Laarse, A., Wang, H., et al. (2000) Adenovirus-based phospholamban antisense expression as a novel approach to improve cardiac contractile dysfunction: comparison of a constitutive viral versus an endothelin-1-responsive cardiac promoter. *Circulation* **101,** 2193–2199.

46. Prestle, J., Janssen, P. M., Janssen, A. P., Zeitz, O., Lehnart, S. E., Bruce, L., et al. (2001) Overexpression of FK506-binding protein FKBP12.6 in cardiomyocytes reduces ryanodine receptor-mediated Ca2+ leak from the sarcoplasmic reticulum and increases contractility. *Circ. Res.* **88,** 188–194.

47. Schillinger, W., Janssen, P. M., Emami, S., Henderson, S. A., Ross, R. S., Teucher, N., et al. (2000) Impaired contractile performance of cultured rabbit ventricular myocytes after adenoviral gene transfer of Na+-Ca2+ exchanger. *Circ. Res.* **87,** 581–587.

48. Zhang, X. Q., Song, J., Rothblum, L. I., Lun, M., Wang, X., Ding, F., et al. (2001) Overexpression of Na+/Ca2+ exchanger alters contractility and SR Ca2+ content in adult rat myocytes. *Am. J. Physiol.* **281,** H2079–H2088.

49. Bristow, M. R., Minobe, W., Raynolds, M. V., Port, J. D., Rasmussen, R., Ray, P. E., et al. (1993) Reduced β1 receptor messenger RNA abundance in the failing human heart *J. Clin. Invest.* **92,** 2737–2745.

50. Ungerer, M., Parruti, G., Bohm, M., Puzicha, M., DeBlasi, A., Erdmann, E., et al. (1994) Expression of β-arrestins and β-adrenergic receptor kinases in the failing human heart. *Circ. Res.* **74,** 206–213.

51. Milano, C. A., Allen, L. F., Rockman, H. A., Dolber, P. C., McMinn, T. R., Chien, K. R., et al. (1994) Enhanced myocardial function in transgenic mice overexpressing the β2-adrenergic receptor. *Science* **264,** 582–586.

52. Liggett, S. B., Tepe, N. M., Lorenz, J. N., Canning, A. M., Jantz, T. D., Mitarai, S., et al. (2000) Early and delayed consequences of β2-adrenergic receptor overexpression in mouse hearts: Critical role for expression level. *Circulation* **101,** 1707–1714.

53. Dorn, G. W., Tepe, N. M., Lorenz, J. N., Koch, W. J., and Liggett, S. B. (1999) Low- and high-level transgenic expression of β2-adrenergic receptors differentially affect cardiac hypertrophy and function in Gαq-overexpressing mice. *Proc. Natl. Acad. Sci. USA* **96,** 6400–6405.

54. Engelhardt, S., Hein, L., Wiesmann, F., and Lohse, M. J. (1999) Progressive hypertrophy and heart failure in β1-adrenergic receptor transgenic mice. *Proc. Natl. Acad. Sci. USA* **96,** 7059–7064.

55. Drazner, M. H., Peppel, K. C., Dyer, S., Grant, A. O., Koch, W. J., and Lefkowitz, R. J. (1997) Potentiation of β-adrenergic signaling by adenoviral-mediated gene transfer in adult rabbit ventricular myocytes. *J. Clin. Invest.* **99,** 288–296.

56. Kawahira, Y., Sawa, Y., Nishimura, M., Sakakida, S., Ueda, H., Kaneda, Y., et al. (1999) Gene transfection of β2-adrenergic receptor into the normal rat heart enhances cardiac response to beta-adrenergic agonist. *J. Thorac. Cardiovasc. Surg.* **118,** 446–451.

57. Akhter, S. A., Skaer, C. A., Kypson, A. P., McDonald, P. H., Peppel, K. C., Glower, D. D., et al. (1997) Restoration of β-adrenergic signaling in failing cardiac ventricular myocytes via adenoviral-mediated gene transfer. *Proc. Natl. Acad. Sci. USA* **94,** 12,100–12,105.

58. Kawahira, Y., Sawa, Y., Nishimura, M., Sakakida, S., Ueda, H., Kaneda, Y., et al. (1998) In vivo transfer of a β2-adrenergic receptor gene into the pressure-overloaded rat heart enhances cardiac response to β-adrenergic agonist. *Circulation* **98,** II262–II267.

59. Lefkowitz, R. J., Rockman, H. A., and Koch, W. J. (2000) Catecholamines, cardiac "β" adrenergic receptors and heart failure. *Circulation* **101,** 634–1637.

60. Koch, W. J., Rockman, H. A., Samama, P., Hamilton, R. A., Bond, R. A. and Milano, C. A., et al. (1995) Cardiac function in mice overexpressing the β-adrenergic receptor kinase or a βARK inhibitor. *Science* **268,** 1350–1353.

61. Akhter, S. A., Eckhart, A. D., Rockman, H. A., Shotwell, K. F., Lefkowitz, R. J., and Koch, W. J. (1999) In vivo inhibition of elevated myocardial β-adrenergic receptor kinase activity in hybrid transgenic mice restores normal β-adrenergic signaling and function. *Circulation* **100,** 648–653.

62. Rockman, H. A., Choi, D. J., Akhter, S. A., Jaber, M., Giros, B., and Lefkowitz, R. J. (1998) Control of myocardial contractile function by the level of β-adrenergic receptor kinase 1 in gene-targeted mice. *J. Biol. Chem.* **273,** 18,180–18,184.

63. Rockman, H. A., Chien, K. R., Choi, D. J., Iaccarino, G., Hunter, J. J., and Ross, J. Jr. (1998) Expression of a β-adrenergic receptor kinase 1 inhibitor prevents the development of myocardial failure in gene-targeted mice. *Proc. Natl. Acad. Sci. USA* **95,** 7000–7005.

64. Harding, V. B., Jones, L. R., Lefkowitz, R. J., Koch, W. J., and Rockman, H. A. (2001) Cardiac βARK1 inhibition prolongs survival and augments β blocker therapy in a mouse model of severe heart failure. *Proc. Natl. Acad. Sci. USA* **98,** 5809–5814.

65. Tevaearai, H. T., Walton, G. B., Keys, J. R., Eckhart, A. D., Shotwell, K. F., and Koch, W. J. (2001) Acute ischemic myocardial dysfunction is attenuated by inhibiting β-adrenergic receptor kinase (βARK1). *Circulation* **104,** II–36.

66. Roth, D. M., Gao, M. H., Lai, N. C., Drumm, J., Dalton, N., Zhou, J. Y., et al. (1999) Cardiac-directed adenylyl cyclase expression improves heart function in murine cardiomyopahty. *Circulation* **99,** 3099–3102.

67. Lai, N. C., Roth, D. M., Gao, M. H., Fine, S., Head, B. P., Zhu, J., McKirnan, M. D., et al. (2000) Intracoronary delivery of adenoviruses encoding adenylyl cyclase VI increases left ventricular function and cAMP-generating capacity. *Circulation* **102,** 2396–2401.

68. Laugwitz, K. L., Ungerer, M., Schoneberg, T., Weig, H. J., Kronsbein, K., Moretti, A., et al. (1999) Adenoviral gene transfer of the human V2 vasopressin receptor improves contractile force of rat cardiomyocytes. *Circulation* **99,** 925–933.

69. Weig, H, J., Laugwitz, K. L., Moretti, A., Kronsbein, K., Stadele, C., Bruning, S., et al. (2000) Enhanced cardiac contractility after gene transfer of V2 vasopressin receptors In vivo by ultrasound-guided injection or transcoronary delivery. *Circulation* **101,** 1578–1585.

70. Mack, C. A., Patel, S. R., Schwarz, E. A., Zanzonico, P., Hahn, R. T., Ilercil, A., et al. (1998) Biologic bypass with the use of adenovirus mediated gene transfer of the cDNA for Vascular Endothelial Growth Factor 121 improves myocardial perfusion and function in ischemic porcine heart. *J. Thorac. Cardiovasc. Surg.* **115,** 168–176.

71. Sayeed-Shah, U., Mann, M. J. Martin, J., Garchev, S., Reimold, S., Laurence, R., et al. (1998) Complete reversal of ischemic wall motion anormalities by combined use of gene therapy with transmyocardial laser revascularization. *J. Thorac. Cardiovasc. Surg.* **116,** 763–769.

72. Henry, T, D., Annex, B. H., and Azrin, M. A. (1999) Final results of the VIVA trial of rhVEGF for human therapeutic angiogenesis. *Circulation* **100,** I–476.

73. Kleiman, N. S. and Califf, R. M. (2000) Results from late-breaking clinical trials sessions at ACCIS 2000 and ACC 2000. *J. Am. Coll. Cardiol.* **36,** 310–311.

74. Freedman, S. B. and Isner, J. M. (2001) Therapeutic angiogenesis for ischemic cardiovscular disease. *J. Mol. Cell. Cardiol.* **33,** 379–393.

75. Rosengart, T. K., Lee, L. Y., Patel, S. R., Sanborn, T. A., Parikh, M., Bergman, G. W., et al. (1999) Angiogenesis gene therapy: Phase I assessment of direct intramyocardial dministration of an adenovirus vector expressing VEGF121 cDNA to individuals with clinically significant coronary artery disease. *Circulation* **100,** 468–474.

18

The Role of Pharmacometrics
in Cardiovascular Drug Development

Paul J. Williams, Amit Desai, and Ene Ette

CONTENTS

1. INTRODUCTION

Minto and Schnider *(1)* have pointed out that "Rapidly evolving changes in health care economics and consumer expectation make it unlikely that traditional drug development approaches will succeed in the future. A shift away from the narrow focus on rejecting the null hypothesis toward a broader focus on seeking to understand the factors that influence the dose–response relationship together with the development of the next generation of software based on population models (*see* Section 2.5. for the definition of population models) should permit a more efficient and rational drug development programme." Their comments are further supported by the fact that the direct cost of drug development has continued to escalate at two and one half times the rate of inflation. The cost of introducing a drug to the market was $802 million in 2000 compared with $237 million in 1987 *(2)*. As an indirect cost, it takes 7–12 yr for a drug to move through development to the final Food and Drug Administration approval *(2)*. Several factors have influenced the escalation in the cost of drug development, including more rigorous approval standards. Regulatory standards are not likely to become less rigorous; therefore, one must look elsewhere to improve the process.

From: *Cardiac Drug Development Guide*
Edited by: M. K. Pugsley © Humana Press Inc., Totowa, NJ

The drug development process can be improved by implementing knowledge driven drug-development strategies that result in powerful, informative, and robust clinical trials. A survey of drugs approved during 1994 and 1995 noted that the typical drug spent over 7 yr in development and required more than 60 clinical trials *(3)*. It was noted that for the drug approved with the least number of clinical trials 23 studies were executed, with only two confirmatory studies in phase III. The greatest number of studies for a drug were 150 and 25% of all drugs required 75 or more clinical studies.

One source of failed drug-development strategies has been failed individual studies. Studies often fail because they are underpowered, inappropriate patient populations are chosen, the dosing strategy for the study is wrong, the duration of the study is too short, patients fail to comply with the administration strategy, and dropout rates are greater than a priori estimates. Many of these problems could be circumvented if antecedent studies were constructed to be more informative and adequate knowledge were generated and created from existing data. The design of any study can be no better than the knowledge on which it is based. Without adequate knowledge, it is impossible to have a thorough understanding of one's drug and, therefore, optimal study decision-making is compromised.

It must be stated that in the current climate insufficient attention is given to knowledge-based drug development. Drug-development knowledge must begin with a thorough understanding of the pathophysiology and biochemical pathways of the disease. The pharmacology of the drug must be understood in terms of where the drug intervenes in the disease process. Pharmacometrics then adds value to the above information by providing quantitative descriptions of drug actions.

2. PHARMACOMETRICS

2.1. Definition

Pharmacometrics (PM) is the science of developing and applying mathematical and statistical methods to characterize, understand, and predict a drug's pharmacokinetic and pharmacodynamic behavior, quantify uncertainty of information about that behavior, and rationalize knowledge-driven decision-making in the process. It is dependent on knowledge discovery; the application of informative graphics; and an understanding of biomarkers/surrogate endpoints. When applied to drug development, PM often involves the development or estimation of pharmacokinetic, pharmacodynamic, pharmacodynamic-outcomes linking, and disease progression models. These models can be linked and applied to competing study designs to aid in understanding the impact of varying dosing strategies, patient selection criteria, and different study endpoints.

2.2. Pharmacokinetics (PK)

PK is the development of mathematical models that describe the time course of drug and metabolite levels in various regions of a subject's body as a function of some drug input function, most often route and dose. Pharmacokinetic models are often represented as compartments with figures illustrating the location of each compartment, as a geometric shape, and drug movement between compartments represented by arrows (Fig. 1). Most models are parameterized in terms of clearances, apparent volumes, and rate constants; other models may not be founded on compartments; and still others may be physiologically based. Once data are assembled, the PK modeler determines which

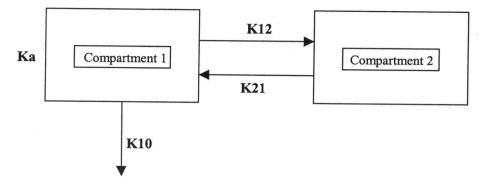

Fig. 1. An example of a diagrammatic representation of a PK model.

model best describes the data and this may involve the determination of the number of compartments that should be applied to the model or whether the model follows dose dependent PK. These models can then be used to estimate the expected drug levels that would be the result of competing dosing strategies. PK models have their greatest utility when they are employed in conjunction with pharmacodynamic models.

2.3. Pharmacodynamics (PD)

PD models are mathematical representations of the relationship between either the drug input function (dose and route), the drug level and time; and some response variable, such as heart rate, blood pressure, or corrected QT interval (QTc). When selecting a PD model one must address the following:

1. What is the shape of the drug level–response relationship?
2. How long does the response take to develop; is the PD effect immediate, delayed, or cumulative?
3. Should the response be related to dose or concentration?

Commonly employed models include the simple E_{max} model (Eq. 1); the sigmoid E_{max} model (Hill equation); and indirect pharmacologic response models (4). Here, E_{max} represents the maximum effect that a drug is capable of eliciting, that is, as the drug level (level) approaches infinity, the effect approaches E_{max}; EC_{50} is the drug level at which one half of E_{max} is observed and is a measure of the sensitivity of the response to the drug. The lower the EC_{50}, the more sensitive the response. Figure 2 presents a plot of the level vs effect for this type of model.

$$\text{Effect} = (E_{max} * \text{Drug Level})/(EC_{50} + \text{Drug Level}) \tag{1}$$

A modification of the simple E_{max} model is the sigmoid E_{max} model, which is sometimes referred to as the Hill equation. This model adds an exponential component to the drug level and the EC_{50} (Eq. 2). Figure 3 shows the shape of a model where the EC_{50} is 20, E_{max} is 100, and gamma (the exponential) is 3.5. Sigmoid E_{max} (Hill Equation) Model is shown as follows:

$$\text{Effect} = (E_{max} * \text{Conc}^{\gamma})/(EC_{50}{}^{\gamma} + \text{Conc}^{\gamma}) \tag{2}$$

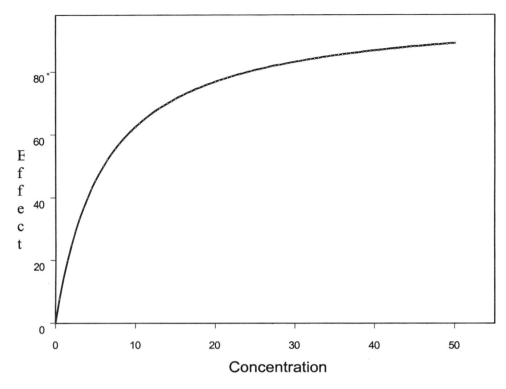

Fig. 2. Concentration (level) vs effect for a simple E_{max} model. Concentration and effect E_{max} model: $EC_{50} = 20$; $E_{max} = 100$.

The most useful PD models are those that relate the entire time course of drug level to the time course of drug effect. Dyneka et al. *(5,6)* have described useful PD models that have been labeled indirect pharmacodynamic response models. These models are appealing because they provide a mathematical description of mechanisms for many drugs. There are four basic types of these models that are presented in Fig. 4.

When effects are delayed relative to drug level, models have been developed that have delayed distribution to a hypothetical effect site *(7)*. This model assumes that the onset and offset of effect is governed by the rate of drug distribution to and from a hypothetical effect site. The model is used to estimate concentrations at the effect site that are immediately related to a PD response (model), usually an E_{max} model. This type of model is often referred to as a link model because PD response is directly linked to a concentration at the hypothetical effect site. One problem with the effect compartment model is that it has not extrapolated well. The indirect pharmacodynamic response models also can account for delayed effects. They have the advantage that they often parallel the proposed mechanism of action of a drug *(8)*.

Careful consideration must be given when selecting a PD model. Although the above approaches to modeling PD responses are appealing, real-life pharmacology is more complex than described by formula. Additional factors that must be considered in the model are tolerance effects, placebo effects, circadian rhythms, and drug interactions *(9,10)*.

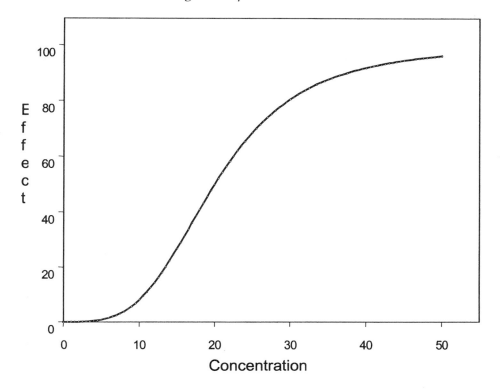

Fig. 3. Concentration–effect relationship for a sigmoidal E_{max} (Hill equation) model. Concentration and effect Hill Equation: $EC_{50} = 20$; $E_{max} = 100$; gamma = 3.5.

2.4. Outcomes Models

An outcomes model translates some surrogate endpoint or biomarker (QTc, blood pressure, and international normalized ratio) into a terminal subject effect, such as cure or no cure, improved vs worsened, survival, or disease progression. Although outcomes models are important, they are less often available for use or application than are PK or PD models and therefore their development is one of the greatest areas of need in PM. Outcomes models can be time to event models, such as Kaplan–Meier curves for which hazard functions can be estimated. The hazard function is a differential equation that when integrated links the PD biomarker to the outcome in a time dependent manner. Discrete outcomes can also be modeled as logistic regression or discriminant function models where the biomarker at some exact moment in time is related to an outcome. The disease progression model has recently been shown to be useful in relating drug administration to outcomes *(11)*. Other models that should be considered are disease tolerance models that can be applied to such outcomes as tumor or viral load.

2.5. Population Models

In recent years, population models have become popular because of their broad applicability to drug development *(12–14)*. As with other models typical values for subjects are estimated, but most significantly with population models the between and

I. INHIBITION - k_{in}

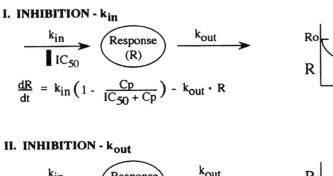

$$\frac{dR}{dt} = k_{in}\left(1 - \frac{Cp}{IC_{50} + Cp}\right) - k_{out} \cdot R$$

II. INHIBITION - k_{out}

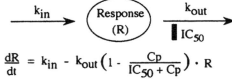

$$\frac{dR}{dt} = k_{in} - k_{out}\left(1 - \frac{Cp}{IC_{50} + Cp}\right) \cdot R$$

III. STIMULATION - k_{in}

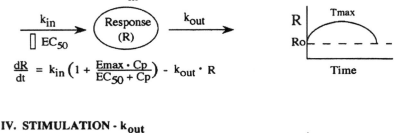

$$\frac{dR}{dt} = k_{in}\left(1 + \frac{Emax \cdot Cp}{EC_{50} + Cp}\right) - k_{out} \cdot R$$

IV. STIMULATION - k_{out}

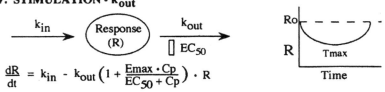

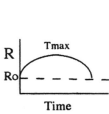

$$\frac{dR}{dt} = k_{in} - k_{out}\left(1 + \frac{Emax \cdot Cp}{EC_{50} + Cp}\right) \cdot R$$

Fig. 4. The four fundamental types of PD indirect response models. Here, k_{in} is an input function and k_{out} is an output function in the differential equation that controls the response variable, R. The response variable, R, is influenced by the inhibition (IC_{50}) or stimulation (EC_{50}) of k_{in} or k_{out} in relation to the drug level (Cp). Reprinted from ref. *6* with permission from Elsevier Science.

residual random effects are also estimated. Population models attempt to explain the between subject random effects by relating covariates to PK or PD parameters, such as relating subject size or renal function to drug clearance or drug effect to age. Three approaches to estimating population models have been described.

The standard two-stage approach involves estimating the individual model parameters for each subject *(14–16)*. To implement this approach several observations per subject (usually six or more) must be obtained and the individual parameters of the model estimated in the first of the two stages under the assumption that the same structural model describes the data across individuals. In the second stage, the population parameters are estimated as the mean of all the individual parameters, the dependencies of the parameters on covariates can also be estimated by standard statistical approaches (stepwise regression and cluster analysis), and in the final step the between subject variability is estimated. When this approach is taken, the typical population parameter estimates are usually without bias; however, the variance and covariance parameters are overestimated *(15)*. Approaches have been proposed (the global two-stage approach) to improve the two-stage approach through bias correction for the random effects covariance and differential weighting of individual data according to the data's quality and quantity *(16)*. When this approach is taken it is important to estimate the covariance matrix describing the distribution of the parameters.

The naïve pooled data approach is simple and involves pooling all the data across individuals to estimate the population parameters *(17,18)*. This approach does not yield a characterization of the between individual variability and therefore its ability to project the range of expected outcomes is limited. Although the naïve pooled data has worked well for population PK model estimation, it has not been valid for the E_{max} PD model because it does not account for the fact that different patients have different EC_{50} values and that for the sigmoid E_{max} PD model, the estimate of γ is low *(19,20)*.

An approach that has great utility for population model estimation is the nonlinear mixed effects approach *(12–15)*. The nonlinear mixed-effects approach to population modeling can be used to obtain typical parameter estimates, between subject variability, unexplained residual variability, and relate PM parameters to covariates. It has great value when only sparse data have been or can be obtained and the standard two-stage approach cannot be used because individual parameter estimates cannot be estimated directly. However, Bayesian estimates of individual subjects parameters can be generated from this approach. The nonlinear mixed effects approach was developed from the recognition that if PM models were to be developed in populations of investigated patients, practical considerations dictate that data should be collected under conditions that are not as restrictive as traditional study designs. This approach considers the study group as the unit of analysis rather than the individual and it functions even when data are sparse, fragmentary, and unbalanced. This approach has been used successfully to estimate PK, PD, and outcomes models of many different types. A general scheme for the implementation of this approach is presented in Table 1 and is explained, in detail, in the knowledge discovery section that follows *(21)*.

Valid PM models developed from the nonlinear mixed effects approach are especially useful for extrapolation to help understand the results of various competing study strategies. With these types of models the expected range of results of competing dosing strategies, differing patient populations, duration of study, and so on can be investigated by Monte Carlo simulations.

3. ROLE OF KNOWLEDGE DISCOVERY

At each step of drug development all previous knowledge should be used in construction of the processes that are to follow. The more that is known about the drug of interest, the more powerful and efficient remaining segments of development can become. Knowledge must come from an understanding of data and when knowledge is generated, then a clear comprehension of directions of development and use is pos-

Table 1
Steps to be Used in the Population Pharmacometric Knowledge Discovery (PHARKNOWDISC) Process

1. Defining or stating the objective of the PHARKNOWDISC process.
2. Creating a data set on which knowledge will be performed. (Data preparation step is a very critical step in the PHARKNOWDISC. Sometimes more effort can be expended in preparing data than in analysis.)
3. Data quality analysis (i.e., cleaning and processing the data; refs. *8,9*).
4. Data structure analysis: exploratory examination of raw data (dose, exposure, response, and covariates) for hidden structure and the reduction of the dimensionality of the covariate vector.
5. Determining the basic PK model that best describes the data and generating post-hoc empiric individual Bayesian parameter estimates.
6. Searching for patterns and relationships between parameters and parameters and covariates through graphical displays and visualization.
7. Exploratory modeling using modern statistical modeling techniques such as multiple linear regression, generalized additive modeling *(10)*, cluster analysis, and tree-based modeling to reveal structure in the data and initially select explanatory covariates.
8. Consolidating the discovered knowledge in *(7)* into irreducible form, that is, developing a population PK–PD model using the nonlinear mixed effects modeling approach.
9. Determining model robustness through sensitivity analysis, examination of parametric/ nonparametric standard errors, stability checking with or without predictive performance depending on the objective of the PHARKNOWDISC.
10. Interpreting the results: the PHARKNOWDISC process prescribes that the model developed is interpreted in a relational manner. That is, do the findings of the PHARKNOWDISC make sense in the domain in which they will be used? Can the results be communicated in a manner that they can be used? Only if they make sense can the results be considered as "knowledge" (which is viewed pragmatically here).
11. Applying (or using) the discovered knowledge: The pragmatic view of knowledge implies that the results of the PHARKNOWDISC process must have some impact on the way individuals act. Thus, the discovered knowledge must be applied to demonstrate how it can be used.
12. Communicating the discovered knowledge.

sible. In fact, huge amounts of data are generated from modern clinical trials, observational studies, and clinical practice, but at the same time there is an acute widening gap between data collection, knowledge, and comprehension. Therefore, it is important to extract as much knowledge, which often lies hidden, from all existing data as is possible. Knowledge discovery is an energetic and active process whereby one attempts to identify valid, understandable, and useful patterns from the data *(21)*. It can be formalized into a number of steps: (1) creation of a data set for PM knowledge discovery; (2) data quality assurance; (3) data structure analysis; (4) determination of the basic PM model that best describes the data; (5) the search for patterns and relationships between parameters of the model and covariates; (6) the use of statistical modeling techniques for data structure revelation and covariate selection; (7) consolidation of discovered knowledge into irreducible form; and (8) the communication and integration of the discovered PM knowledge. Some modern graphical and statistical procedures that are useful in knowledge discovery include histogram and density plots, pairs plots, multiple linear regression, generalized additive modeling, box plots, nonparametric smooth plots, and tree models *(22,23)*.

4. IMPORTANCE OF REAL-TIME MODELING

The steps to the development of population models as presented in Table 1 can be time consuming. It is important that PM knowledge be discovered in a timely manner so that downstream elements of drug development strategy can be impacted. Real-time data analysis and model development can also result in expeditious knowledge discovery and can help identify potential problems in the analysis at an early stage of data collection *(24,25)*.

5. IMPORTANCE OF PLANNING

The complexities of drug development and the pivotal role of PM models point to the importance of planning *(24,25)*. There are two levels at which planning relative to PM must occur. There is an overall plan for the entire drug development process and a local plan for individual projects or studies. The overall plan would (1) identify important questions that need to be answered; (2) identify the application and intended use of the PM model; (3) identify which covariates need to be studied; and 4) identify possible drug–drug interactions.

Planning at the level of the individual project or study must also take place. Plans must be in place for data management, data collection, quality assurance of the data, and staff training for data collection. A plan for data analysis and model validation must also be in place.

6. SIMULATIONS AND DRUG DEVELOPMENT

Monte Carlo simulation is a technique that has been used extensively in engineering intense industries and has recently been identified as a useful tool for the construction of efficient, powerful, informative, and robust clinical trials in drug development *(26)*. Recent advances in computational performance, the appearance of new simulation software targeting clinical trials, and improved methods for estimating PM models support this technological advancement. Simulation provides an excellent avenue for application of the developed PM models. Simulation of clinical trials provides a means of evaluation of the impact of various dosing strategies on outcomes, patient-selection strategies, competing designs, competing outcomes measures, and competing statistical methods with all stochastic elements in the trial execution model. Recently, one large pharmaceutical company reported that the early integration of PM models via simulation resulted in development time savings, regulatory concurrence, and perceived value that outweighed costs *(27)*.

For a simulation, three types of models must be defined; the covariate model, the input-output model, and the execution model. The covariate model creates simulated individuals by defining the distribution of variables such as age, gender, weight, and renal function. The input–output models are the main place where the PM models enter into the simulation process. Here the PK, PD, and outcomes models are defined in terms of both their typical parameter values and the variability of the parameters and also the residual random variability of the model. The execution model for a simulation deals with patient and practitioner behaviors during the execution of the trial; describing dropouts, compliance and missing samples.

7. LEARN: CONFIRM–LEARN APPROACH

At the local level each element (PK, PD, outcomes models) of study during the drug development process is important. Each of these elements is permeated by a philosophy of drug development, and one's philosophy will always affect one's attitude and approach to any individual study. A very useful and promising philosophy of drug development has been described by Sheiner *(28)* termed the learn–confirm approach. As described by Sheiner, drug development ought to consist of alternating elements of learning from experience and then confirming what has been learned. We have modified this concept slightly by naming the second phase confirm–learn because we are always interested in learning even when confirming is the primary objective of a study.

The earliest parts of the process of clinical drug development should emphasize learning but all later stages should emphasize the confirm–learn process. Thus, learning and confirming become a part of each clinical trial, although their relative emphasis changes as the drug progresses toward approval. Although learning and confirming can be performed to varying degrees on the same data set, their goals are quite different. Clinical trial structures that optimize confirming often inhibit learning, though never completely. The focus of commercial drug development on confirmation is understandable as this immediately precedes and justifies regulatory approval. However, the focus on confirming has led to a less than desirable level of learning which has in turn led to a predictable result that drug development is often inefficient and inadequate.

The goal of confirming is to falsify the hypothesis that efficacy is absent and the only question that it aims to answer is "is the null hypothesis true or false." Therefore, factors that increase learning such as administering differing dose levels and enrolling a variety of subjects are often eliminated from confirming studies. Confirming studies proceed by contrasting the average outcomes between two study groups.

Learning has as its objective answering many questions, such as the relationship between dose, prognostic variables, and outcome. Learning is often model based and focuses on building a model between outcome and many variables such as dosing strategy, exposure, patient type and prognostic variables. The model that is built here is the defining of the response surface. The response surface can be thought of as three-dimensional. On one axis are the input variables (controllable factors), such as dosage regimen and concurrent therapies. Another axis incorporates patient characteristics, which summarizes all the important ways patients can differ that affect the benefit to toxic ratio. The final axis represents the benefit to toxicity ratio. Sheiner has stated, "... the real surface is neither static, nor is all information about a patient conveyed by his initial prognostic status, nor are exact predictions possible. A realistically useful response ... must include the elements of variability, uncertainty and time..." *(7)*. The response surface deals with a complex of relationships to answer the question of what is the relationship between input profile and dose magnitude to beneficial and harmful pharmacological effects and how does this relationship vary with individual patient characteristics and time to explain tolerance or sensitivity? For rational drug development and the optimization of individual therapy, this response surface must be mapped for the target population. These models then allow extrapolation beyond the immediate study subjects to predict the effect of competing dosing strategies, patient type selection, competing study structures, endpoints; and therefore aid in the construction of future studies. One important feature of model based learning is that models increase the signal:noise ratio because they can translate some of the noise in a data set to signal. This is important because the information content of a data set is proportional to the signal:noise ratio. For the learning study, which attempts to define the dose–concentration–effect model, PK delineates the dose–concentration component and PD defines the concentration–effect component of the model.

Although the latter stages of drug development emphasize confirming, learning can still be pursued because the cost of adding several more observations per subject is small compared to the cost of the fixed overhead of these late studies. If confirmation fails and learning is targeted during the confirming study then one must plan a future diagnosis of why the study failed. If learning types of data are not collected, then this becomes unlikely. For example one may not be able to confirm efficacy, not because the drug does not work but because there was a high degree of noncompliance that could be remediated. If the confirming study does not have some learning aspects then correction of the components that resulted in inefficacy cannot be performed.

8. CLINICAL TRIAL STRUCTURE

The learn: confirm–learn process emphasizes the dose–concentration–effect or the dose–effect relationship and, therefore, one of the most important components of learning is the dose ranging study. Most dose ranging studies have a single goal of simply finding a reasonable initial dose (and sometimes an effective dose). However, this goal is narrow and ought to be expanded to include identification of the dose increment after the initial dose and the estimation of population models that could be employed to design subsequent clinical drug trials. These goals depend on the shape of the individual dose response curves and the between subject and residual variability relative to these curves. The initial goal of the dose ranging study is to quantify these curves. The common approaches to the dose ranging study are the parallel dose, the crossover, and the dose-escalation designs. The most common approach to dose ranging is the parallel dose design in which each subject receives a single level of dosing chosen from one of several possible levels of dosing. The crossover and dose-escalation designs involve several levels of dosing to each subject and therefore these designs allow the estimation of the individual response curves. A problem with the parallel dose design is that it provides poor information about the distribution of the response curves, biased estimates of the typical curve, and little information of patient variability. The crossover and dose-escalation designs provide better information about the response curves than the parallel dose design and the dose-escalation design has the advantage that it mimics clinical practice.

Sheiner et al. *(19,20)* have presented an individual dose response curve (Fig. 5A). Here, the dose is plotted on the abscissa and the response, blood pressure, on the ordinate. The curve shown is for a hypothetical antihypertensive drug where the drug lowers patient blood pressure to some minimum value (E_{max}). The parameters of the model as shown are E_{max}, the maximum decrease in blood pressure that the drug can effect as the dose becomes very high, D_{50}, which is the dose at which the blood pressure is

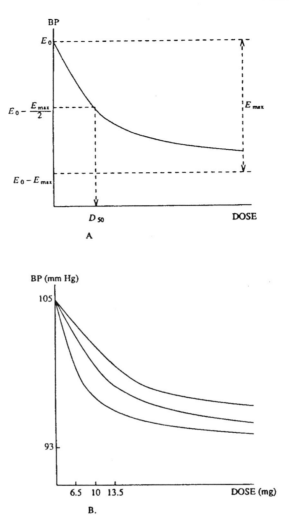

Fig. 5. A possible dose–response curve according to Sheiner et al. *(19)*. Drug response (BP) vs dose according to E_{max} model. (**A**) depicts the baseline response, E_0, maximum response is $E_0 - -E_{max}$; half of this response occurs at a dose = D_{50}. In (**B**), the curve of A is interpreted as a population curve. The central line is the response of the mean subject; the outer lines delimit ± 1 SD of curves about the mean curve (assuming interindividual variability only in D_{50}). Reprinted from ref. *19* with permission from Elsevier Science.

decreased by half of E_{max}, and, E_0 is the baseline blood pressure. In the figure the authors assumed that only D_{50} varied between subjects; $E_0 = 105$ mmHg, $E_{max} = 12$ mmHg, and mean $D_{50} = 10$ mg/d with a coefficient of variation (CV) of 35%. Figure 5B shows the typical curve with the outer curves being ±1 SD results of the D_{50}. When these parameters (E_{max}, D_{50}, and E_0) with their variability (CV) are known the mean response of a typical patient can be constructed and also the response of atypical patients can be estimated (those 1 and 2 SD from the mean). Now using the estimated

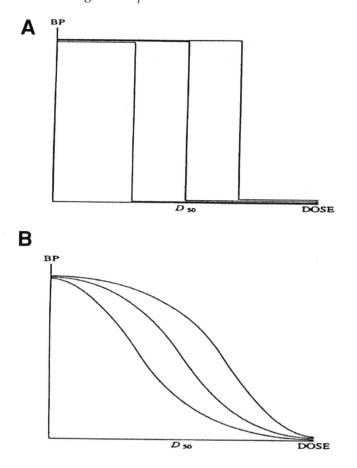

Fig. 6. Another possible dose–response curve. Now the effect occurs abruptly and switches from "none" to "all" at a characteristic value, D_{50}. (**A**) depicts model viewed as a population curve. (Inner and outer lines, *see* legend to Fig. 5B.) In (**B**), center line is mean ($\pm$ 1SD – outer lines) of response observed in study group at various doses for the model of A. Note that this curve is not the same as that of A because ordinate does not indicate response of the mean subject. Rather, at any dose value, E_0 minus the ordinate (center line), divided by $E_0 - E_{max}$ is equal to the fraction of subjects with D_{50} values less than or equal to the value on the abscissa. Reprinted from ref. *19* with permission from Elsevier Science.

parameters a new approach to the initial dose can be redefined as the dose that produces some specified degree of response in a percentage of the target population.

An important concept here is the difference between the mean parameter and mean response curves. Both the upper and lower figures (*see* Fig. 6) have the same E_{max} but in Fig. 6A, the D_{50} is different for each curve with each patient responding in an all or none manner at the D_{50} dose. The center line in the upper diagram and the outer lines show the mean $\pm$ 1 SD limits of the patient specific curves. Figure 6B shows the corresponding mean response curve (mean $\pm$ 1 SD). These curves display very different shapes. In the lower curve the ordinate is proportional to the fraction of subjects with $D_{50} > D$. Therefore, the response curve is deficient because if it is misinterpreted as the mean parameter curve, it can be misleading.

The parallel-dose design results in biased individual parameter estimates which, when used to calculate population parameters, also results in biased population parameter estimates. These problems are either not present or present to a small extent for the crossover design and the dose-escalation design. These characteristics become important when the model is to be extrapolated to design subsequent studies. It is hoped that knowledge from the dose ranging study can be applied by Monte Carlo simulation to investigate the dosing strategy implications for subsequent studies. If the population parameters are not estimated accurately then this promising approach to study design will be less valuable. Dose escalation with population parameter estimates also allows interpolation of the expected outcomes of doses that have not been administered.

9. APPLYING PM MODELS TO DRUG DEVELOPMENT

It is not sufficient simply to derive and estimate PM models but the intended use and application of the model must be kept in mind during the entire model development process. The intended use of a model should influence the attitude and modeling approaches used by the pharmacometrician at the various stages of the modeling process. This would determine what covariates are considered important and which parameters are of primary concern.

Models can be applied in several ways. Typical or average parameter estimates from models can be used to estimate typical values for dependent variables such as serum drug concentrations, typical pharmacodynamic parameter effects, such as QT interval or blood pressure, or parameters such as area under the concentration time curve. Issues that could be addressed with this type of model would be as follows:

1. What would be the typical concentration–time profile for several different dosing approaches or for different types of patients?
2. What would be the typical pharmacodynamic biomarker as a function of patient type or differing dosing strategies?
3. What would be the expected concentration–time area under the curve for a capsule to be swallowed vs a buccal preparation designed to avoid first-pass metabolism?

To estimate these types of variables from the model, one simply estimates the typical model parameters then plugs in the missing elements, such as dose and/or time, to estimate the typical dependent variable.

Models characterized by only typical value and applications estimating only average outcomes, lack broad applicability and result in suboptimal understanding of the variable being studied (e.g., dose). Models containing random effects in addition to typical values have broader application when compared with the models without random effects. These are the population models mentioned previously, which contain typical values, between subject, and residual random effects. With these models not only can the typical result be projected but also the range of expected outcomes. These projections require not only models but also the implementation of Monte Carlo simulations *(26)*. Simulations can be implemented in any of a number of software programs such as the Pharsight Trial Simulator® or the NONMEM program with the simulation subroutine. These are implemented by supplying the software with the typical PM model values along with the random effects. In the end a vector of concentrations or biomarkers is generated, and at each time point these could be ranked as the 10th, median and 90th percentile concentrations observed. So rather than estimate the typical concentration as a function of dose, one could go further and suggest a dosing strategy, then estimate the typical concentration, the 90th percentile concentration and the 10th percentile concentration and even plot these as a function of time after dose.

A powerful use of PM models is their application for evaluation of the structure and strategy of confirming clinical drug trials. The PK, PD, and outcomes links models can be applied to understand the implications of various dosing strategies, patient population selection, drop out rates, duration of the study, and so on; on the power, robustness, efficiency, and informativeness of the trial. One may be interested in such a study to estimate the effect on power of adopting three levels of dosing (placebo, a low dose, and a high dose) instead of two levels (placebo and high) in a confirming study. Adopting three levels of dosing has the advantage of adding a learning element to the confirming study. This may be valuable because one would not like the dose to be lowered after the drug has already entered the market place and studying several levels of dosing ought to result in choosing the optimal dose. If the lower dose is as equally effective as the higher dose, then it would be chosen as the standard of care. If the lower dose is less effective than the high dose, the administration of the low dose would be unethical because the documentation of the inappropriateness of the lower dose has occurred. In the simulation, one would specify in the software program of the typical and random effects for the PK, PD, and linking parameters; an execution model would be used by specifying the number of subject, drop out rates, duration of the study, and so on; and finally a covariate model (distribution of gender, weights) would be assumed. Power would then be calculated by determining how often the treatment was superior to the placebo.

The cost of drug development has continued to escalate and is currently very high with no prospect of decreasing. PM offers an opportunity for knowledge based drug development by developing models and applying them to clinical trial construction via Monte Carlo simulation. Application of knowledge-based PM models will result in powerful, efficient, informative and robust clinical trials.

10. AN INFORMATIVE EXAMPLE

PM methods and models have been applied to cardiovascular drugs. Csajka et al. *(29)* used phase I data obtained over several years at their institutions to refine the "response surface" to gain better insight into the dose-concentration-effect relationship for angiotensin II receptor antagonists. These insights into the response surface were used to better understand the expected response to various dosing strategies.

The PK and PD data were obtained from 13 phase I studies, which enrolled 151 subjects for 10 angiotensin II receptor antagonists. There were 2685 drug concentrations, 900 metabolite concentrations, and 7360 blood pressure measurements. The clinical testing of the effect of the antagonist was performed using the exogenous challenges of angiotensin II. This method is considered as a surrogate for the therapeutic target. The pharmacodynamic effect was expressed as the reduction of blood pressure from baseline, which was obtained from the Finapress® device.

First, a PK model was determined, and two drugs were best characterized as one compartment and the others were all two-compartment PK models. For two drugs, a two-compartment model also provided the best fit not only for the parent compound but also for the metabolite. There were a variety of absorption patterns between the drugs, covariates were tested for inclusion in the PK model, and none could be included for any of the drugs. Interindividual variability was included in the models when it was

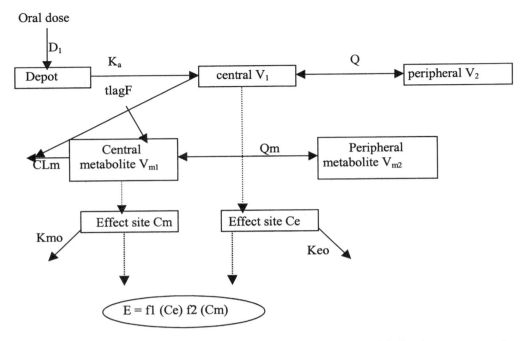

Fig. 7. Compartmental representation of the common PK–PD model. Cn, drug concentration the effect compartment; CL, clearance; CLm, clearance of the metabolite; Cm, metabolite in the effect compartment; D_1, duration of the zero-order absorption rate process; E, effect; F, bioavailability; f1 and f2, functions linking effect to concentration for drug and metabolite respectively; K_a, first-order absorption rate constant; Kdm, transfer rate constant of drug to metabolite; Keo, transfer rate constant between plasma and effect compartment; Q, intercompartment clearance; Qm, intercompartmental clearance of the metabolite; tlag, lag time; V_1, apparent volume of the central compartment; V_2, apparent volume of the peripheral compartment; V_{m1}, apparent volume of the metabolite for the central compartment; V_{m2}, apparent volume of the metabolite for the peripheral compartment.

justifiable on a statistical basis and was included for Cl for all drugs. For some drugs interindividual variability was included for intercompartmental clearance, central apparent volume and peripheral volume.

The PD model for blood pressure was performed sequentially with the PK parameters fixed to their individual post-hoc estimates. Systolic and diastolic blood pressures were modeled separately. The relationship was modeled as an E_{max} model:

$$E = Peak_0/[1 + (Ce/EC_{50}) + (Cm/ECm_{50})]$$

Where $Peak_0$ is the baseline increase in blood pressure, Ce is the concentration in the hypothetical effect compartment, EC_{50} is the drug concentration antagonizing the peak by 50%, Cm is the concentration of the metabolite at the effect site, and ECm_{50} is the concentration of the metabolite that accounted for a 50% antagonization of the peak. Here, an effect compartment was created to account for a delayed response between serum concentrations and the hysteresis in blood pressure that resulted.

The data were fitted using the NONMEM program (Globomax LLC, Hanover, MD) using the first-order conditional estimation method. For hierarchical models, improvements in any model were considered to have occurred when the objective function (−2 log likelihood) decreased by four points per additional parameter. A schematic representation of the PK–PD model is illustrated in Fig. 7. The results of the PK and PD modeling are presented in Table 2 and Table 3.

Complex PK–PD models were developed that reflected mechanisms of angiotensin II antagonists. From the complex PK–PD models, the time course of blood pressure was predicted. The relationship between plasma concentration, dose, and time was defined by the PK part of the model whereas the relationship between blood pressure and effect compartment concentrations was defined by the PD part of the model. These models were linked and the expected outcomes (blood pressures) as a function of differing doses were predicted. The blood pressure as a function of drug, dose, and time are presented in Fig. 8. From the figure differences in intensity of effect are primarily a function of dose and higher doses also increase the duration of the effect.

Several important and informed decisions can be inferred from the graphics modeled in Fig. 8 as one proceeds forward with the drug development process. First, it appears that the frequency of drug administration is not uniform across the drugs examined and some drugs could actually be scheduled every 12 h but others would have to be administered every 6 h. For example, it appears that candesartan (Fig. 8A) and losartan (Fig. 8B) could almost certainly be administered every 12 h but that SC-52458 (Fig. 8G) would need to be administered every 6 h. Some other conclusions that can be drawn from the blood pressure vs time graphs is that the initial dose for irbesartan (Fig. 8C) should be 75 mg, or possibly even less. It also appears that, on average, little is to be gained from increasing the dose to those in excess of 75 mg. Model-based blood pressure vs time profiles for irbesartan could be constructed for doses less than 75 mg. A parallel comment may apply to tasosartan (Fig. 8E) for a 100 vs 400 mg dose, SC-52458 (Fig. 8G) for a 100 vs 200 mg dose and TAK-536 (Fig. 8D) for a 5 vs 20 mg dose.

Still more can be inferred from the model-based figure. The initial doses that may result in an average decrease in blood pressure of 10 mmHg can be observed. For example, this dose is 2 mg for candesartan and, therefore, the 1 mg dose would probably be too low for a starting dose. For UP 269-6 (Fig. 8F) initial doses of 5 and 10 mg would also most likely be too low to achieve this therapeutic response.

Another important feature of the model-based approach is that dose interpolation can be made. For the drug TAK-536, for example, it appears that an initial decrease in blood pressure for the 0.3 mg dose is less than 10 mmHg, and for the 1 mg dose is significantly greater than a reduction of 10 mmHg (Fig. 8D). With the model-based approach, it would be possible to apply doses between 0.3 mg and 1.0 mg and assess the expected typical decrease in blood pressure.

The graphs presented in Fig. 8 are the model-based predictions of a single dose. However, from the models, predictions of the expected blood pressure changes based on multiple doses can also be estimated and graphed. This would be of importance because it would aid in visualizing the effect of differing dosing levels and differing dosing intervals for multiple dose studies. From these types of graphics, the dosing levels and intervals of interest could be selected for the next phase of drug development.

It is significant that the authors estimated PK and PD models that include the variability of the parameters and that all models estimated the variability of clearance, $Peak_0$, and residual variability. This is important because with the estimation of typical parameter value and associated variability, a Monte Carlo simulation can be performed and

Table 2
PK Modeling: Population Parameter Estimates

Drug	Ka Value (h^{-1})	Ka Variability (CV%)	D1 Value (h)	D1 Variability (CV%)	CL(m) Value (L/h)	CL(m) Variability (CV%)	$V_1(V_{m1})$ Value (L)	$V_1(V_{m1})$ Variability (CV%)
Losartan	4.9 (57)				124 (8)	24 (32)	131 (13)	27 (65)
E-3147					1.0 (28)		4 (28)	28 (89)
Tasortan	1.6 (17)	41 (90)	0.7 (17)	78 (35)	29.2 (7)	23 (69)	15 (7)	
Enoltasortan					0.06 (125)		4 (14)	
TAK-536	0.9 (9)	37 (32)	0.2 (43)	153 (37)	1.4 (10)	25 (49)	7 (8)	21 (48)
Candesartan	0.9 (21)	51 (58)	26 (12)	9.2 (27)	32 (34)	60 (12)	35 (41)	4.9 (27)
Irbesartan	0.8 (9)			17.6 (8)	22 (43)	33 (13)		7.2 (17)
L-159,282			2.9 (14)		77.2 (32)	16 (99)	28 (71)	
SC-52456	0.8 (7)				40.5 (8)	32 (29)	15 (12)	14 (77)
UP-269-6			1×10^{-6} (55)		46.8 (9)	14 (114)	77 (14)	35 (36)
Olmesartan			1.5 (8)		4.3 (5)	3 (115)	29 (5)	
LRB-081	2.5 (31)		2.4 (13)	70 (129)	98.7 (21)	74 (60)	463 (8)	23 (97)

Continued

Table 2 (*continued*)
PK Modeling: Population Parameter Estimates

Drug	Q(m) Value (L/h)	Q(m) Variability (CV%)	$V_1(V_{m2})$ Value (L)	$V_1(V_{m2})$ Variability (CV%)	K_{dm} (h−1)	Residual variability prop (CV%)	Add (SD)
Losartan	193 (39)	95 (53)	132 (30)		0.04 (9)	42 (18)	8.0[a]
E-3147	0.2 (35)		3 (74)			37 (22)	
Tasortan	23 (11)		13 (15)		0.02 (9)	41 (10)	8.9[a]
Enoltasortan	0.1 (135)		42 (150)			24 (135)	26 (345)
TAK-536	0.7 (7)		6 (11)			16 (32)	0.4 (207)
Candesartan	81 (47)	57 (28)	86 (47)			25 (27)	1.2 (66)
Irbesartan		75 (23)				20 (19)	
L-159,282	7.4 (39)		67 (39)			53 (30)	
SC-52456	6.1 (14)		32 (15)			35 (18)	
UP-269–6	6.7 (19)		68 (14)			44 (167)	2.5[a]
Olmesartan						40 (8)	
LRB-081						47 (14)	2.6 (26)

All parameters are expressed as apparent values except for tasosartan. All values are means, with SE in parentheses. Variability is interindividual variability, expressed as coefficient of variation (CV%); intraindividual variability is expressed as coefficient of variation (prop, CV%) and standard deviation (add, SD μg/L or μmol/L).

[a]Variance fixed at the equal half of the detection limit.

CL, clearance of the drug and the metabolite (CLm); D_1, zero-order absorption constant; Ka, absorption rate constant; V_1, volume of central compartment; V_2, volume of peripheral compartment; Q, intercompartmental clearance for drug and the metabolite (Qm); K_{dm}, transfer rate from drug to metabolite; SE, standard error of the estimates and the variance components take as equation: SEestimate/ expressed as percentage; V_{m1}, volume of central compartment; V_{m2}, volume of peripheral compartment.

Table 3
PD Modeling: Parameter Estimates

Blood pressure	Peak$_0$		Ec(m)$_{50}$		Keo(Kmo)		Residual	t$_{1/2}$
	Value (mmHg)	Interindividual variability (CV%)	Value (µg/L)	Interindividual variability (CV%)	Value (hs-1)	Interindividual variability (CV%)	variability (mmHg)	Ke(m)o (h)
Losartan								
DBP	23.3 (3)	6 (23)	159		6.1 (61)		5.3 (10)	0.1
SBP	27.2	13 (30)	228		5.9 (65)			
E-174								
DBP			20 (7)	33 (29)	0.2 (13)			3.6
SBP			28 (7)	32 (30)	0.2 (19)			3.4
Tasortan								
DBP	22.8 (3)	16 (23)	107 (12)	44 (89)	1.7 (16)		4.4 (6)	0.4
SBP	28.5 (3)	16 (23)	195 (16)	67 (51)	1.7 (18)		6.2 (17)	0.4
Enoltasortan								
DBP			145 (9)	26 (59)	0.2 (11)			2.9 2.3
SBP			297 (14)	43 (61)	0.3 (30)			
Tak-536								
DBP	22.2 (4)	12 (42)	29 (17)	41 (44)	0.3 (13)		4.2 (10)	2.5 2.2
SBP	27.8 (6)	15 (51)	65 (19)	44 (53)	0.3 (24)		7.2 (11)	
Candesartan								
DBP	25.1 (3)	17 (31)	8 (10)	22 (123)	0.3 (10)		4.1 (9)	2.0 1.9
SBP	30.2 (3)	12 (29)	12 (11)	39 (58)	0.4 (13)		5.6 (10)	
Irbesartan								
DBP	26.8 (4)	16 (32)	89 (17)	52 (56)	0.8 (45)	132 (41)	4.1 (14)	
SBP	28.7 (5)	17 (35)	124 (34)	119 (34)	0.8 (51)	137 (53)	6.2 (11)	
L-159,282								
DBP	30.1 (3)	6 (49)	41 (10)	18 (97)	0.4 (8)		4.7 (7)	0.9
SBP	29.2 (5)	13 (66)	63 (15)	28 (71)	0.3 (12)		6.4 (6)	0.6
SC-52458								
DBP	28.0 (3)	12 (31)	119 (31)	109 (45)	0		4.0 (10)	1.7
SBP	31.7 (3)	13 (43)	436 (38)	132 (68)	0		5.5 (9)	1.6

All values are means, with SE in parentheses. DBP indicates diastolic blood pressure and SBP indicates systolic blood pressure.

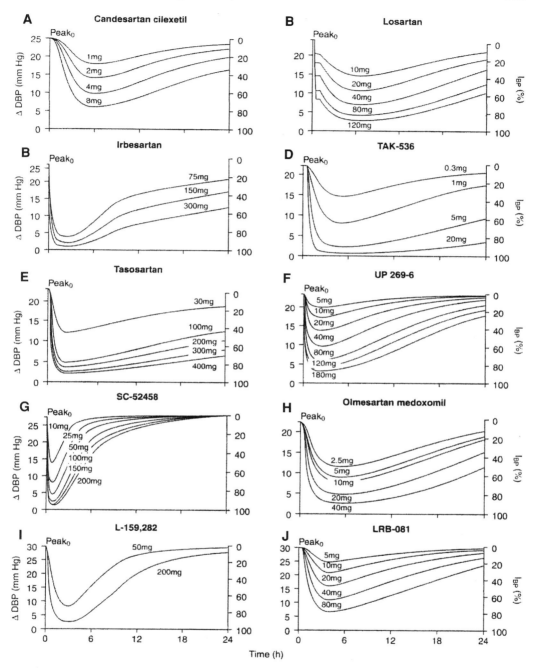

Fig. 8. Model-based predicted decrease in diastolic blood pressure (δDBP) and percentage DBP inhibition (I_{BP}) after administration of all studied doses of the angiotensin II receptor antagonist. The left vertical axis represents the decrease in DBP from baseline (Peak$_0$): (Eq. 10): $BP_{peak} = (BP_{max\ postinjection}) - (BP_{min\ preinjection})$. The right vertical axis represents the percentage of DBP inhibition: (Eq. 11): $1_{BP} = 100 \times [(1 - BP_{peakpostdrug})/BP_{peakpredrug}]$, where BP = blood.

then not only can the typical or average blood pressure changes be estimated and graphed but also the expected range of blood pressure changes for each dosing strategy can be estimated and visualized. For example the 10th, 50th, and 90th percentile of blood pressure changes for a dose of candesartan of 2 mg every 12 h can be generated. Although this was not done in the publication, if this had been done it may have been noted that at the 90th percentile the drop of blood pressure was 25 mmHg, which would be excessive in many patients and therefore a lower starting dose would be needed. When the expected range of blood pressure changes is estimable then one can set very specific criteria for the initial dose, such as "the initial dose should result in a decrease in blood pressure of 10 mmHg in 75% of subjects and no subjects decrease in blood pressure be more than 20 mmHg." A search of the response surface for such a dose is possible with a PK and PD model that has variability of the parameters included in the model.

11. SUMMARY

Drug development has become unacceptably costly both in terms of dollars and time expended. Most of the expenditures (both time and money) are applied to clinical development. One important tool that will aid in decreasing the cost of development is knowledge based/driven development. Without thoroughly applying PM, knowledge driven drug development is not possible. The essential elements of PM have been presented so that they can be applied to knowledge driven drug development in the cardiovascular drug therapeutic arena or any therapeutic class in general.

REFERENCES

1. Minto, C. and Schinder, T. (1998) Expanding clinical applications of population pharmacodynamic modeling. *Br. J. Clin. Pharmacol.* **46,** 321–333.
2. Tufts Center for the Study of Drug Development (2001) Press Release, November 30.
3. Peck, C. C. (1997) Drug development: Improving the process. *Food Drug Law J.* **52,** 163–167.
4. Holford, N. H. and Sheiner, L. B. (1981) Understanding the dose-effect relationship: clinical application of pharmacokinetic-pharmacodynamic models. *Clin. Pharmacokinet.* **6,** 429–453.
5. Dyneka, N. L., Garg, V., and Jusko, W. J. (1993) Comparison of four basic models of indirect pharmacodynamic responses. *J. Pharmacokinet. Biopharm.* **21,** 457–478.
6. Jusko, W. J. and Ko, H. C. (1994) Physiologic indirect response models characterize diverse types of pharmacodynamic effects. *Clin. Pharmacol. Ther.* **56,** 406–419.
7. Sheiner, L. B., Stanski, D. R., Vozeh, S., Miller, R. D., and Ham, J. (1979) Simultaneous modeling of pharmacokinetics and pharmacodynamics: Application to d-tubocurarine. *Clin. Pharmacol. Ther.* **25,** 358–371.
8. Williams, P. J., Lane, J. R., Turkel, C., Capparelli, E. V., Dzewanowska, Z., and Fox, A. (2001) Dichloroacetate: Population pharmacokinetics with a pharmacodynamic sequential link model. *J. Clin. Pharmacol.* **41,** 259–267.
9. Porchet, H. C., Benowitz, N. L., and Sheiner, L. B. (1988) Pharmacodynamic model of tolerance: Application to nicotine. *J. Pharmacol. Exp. Ther.* **244,** 231–236.
10. Derendorf, H., Mollman, H., Hochhaus, G., Meibohm, B., and Barth, J. (1997) Clinical PK/PD modeling as a tool in drug development of cortecosteroids. *Int. J. Clin. Pharmacol. Ther.* **35,** 481–488.
11. Holford, N. H. G. and Peace, K. E. (1992) Results and validation of a population pharmacodynamic model for cognitive effects in Alzheimer patients with tacrine. *Proc. Natl. Acad. Sci. USA* **89,** 11,471–11,475.

12. Sheiner, L. B., Rosenberg, B., and Marathe, V. (1977) Estimation of population characteristics of pharmacokinetic parameters from routine clinical data. *J. Pharmacokinet. Biopharm.* **5,** 445–479.
13. Mandema, J. W., Verotta, D., and Sheiner, L. B. (1992) Building population pharmacokinetic pharmacodynamic models. *J. Pharmacokinet. Biopharm.* **20,** 511–528.
14. Department of Health and Human Services (1999) Guidance for Industry: Population Pharmacokinetics. US Food and Drug Administration, Rockville, MD.
15. Sheiner, L. B. and Beal, S. L. (1980) Evaluation of methods for estimating population pharmacokinetic parameters. *J. Clin. Pharmacokinet.* **9,** 635–651.
16. Steimer, J. L., Mallet, A., and Golmard, J. L. (1984) Alternative approaches to the estimation of population pharmacokinetic parameters: Comparison with the nonlinear mixed effects model. *Drug Metab. Rev.* **15,** 265–292.
17. Egan, T. D., Lemmens, H. J., Fiset, P., Hermann, D. J., Muir, K. T., Stanski, D. R., et al. (1993) The Pharmacokinetics of a new short-acting opioid remifentanil (G187084B) in healthy adult male volunteers. *Anesthesiology* **79,** 881–892.
18. Kataria, B. K., Ved, S. A., Nicodemus, H. F., Hoy, G. R., Lea, D., Dubois, M. Y., et al. (1994) The Pharmacokinetics of propofol in children using three different analysis approaches. *Anesthesiology* **80,** 104–122.
19. Sheiner, L. B., Beal, S. L., and Sambol, N. C. (1989) Study designs for dose-ranging. *Clin. Pharmacol. Ther.* **46,** 63–77.
20. Sheiner, L. B., Hashimoto, Y., and Beal, S. L. (1991) A simulation study comparing designs for dose ranging. *Stats Med.* **10,** 303–321.
21. Ette, E. I., Williams, P. J., Fadiran, E., Ajayi, F. O., and Onyiah, L. C. (2001) The process of knowledge discovery from large pharmacokinetic data sets. *J. Clin. Pharmacol.* **41,** 25–34.
22. Ette, E. I. and Ludden, T. M. (1995) Population pharmacokinetic modeling: The importance of informative graphics. *Pharmaceut. Res.* **12,** 1845–1855.
23. Ette, E. I. (1998) Statistical graphics in pharmacokinetics and pharmacodynamics: A tutorial. *Ann. Pharmacother.* **32,** 818–828.
24. Rombout, F. (1997) Good pharmacokinetic practice (GPP) and logistics: a continuing challenge, in *The Population Approach: Measuring and Managing Variability in Response, Concentration and Dose* (Aarons, L., Balant, L. P., Gundert-Remy, U. A., et al., eds.) Office for Official Publications of the European Communities, Luxemborg, pp. 183–193.
25. Grasela, T. H., Antal, E. J., Fiedler-Kelley, J., et al. (1999) An automated drug concentration screening and quality assurance program for clinical trials. *Drug Info. J.* **33,** 273–279.
26. Holford, N. H., Kimko, H. C., Monteleone, J. P., and Peck, C. C. (2000) Simulation of Clinical Trials. *Annu. Rev. Pharmacol. Toxicol.* **40,** 209–234.
27. Reigner, B. G., Williams, P. E. O., Patel, I. H., et al. (1997) An evaluation of the integration of pharmacokinetic and pharmacodynamic principles in clinical drug development. Experience with Hoffmann La Roche. *Clin. Pharmacokinet.* **33,** 142–152.
28. Sheiner, L. B. (1997) Learning versus confirming in clinical drug development. *Clin. Pharmacol. Ther.* **61,** 275–291.
29. Csajka, C., Buclin, T., Fattinger, K., Brunner, H. R., and Biollaz, J. (2002) Population pharmacokinetic-pharmacodynamic modeling of angiotensin receptor blockade in healthy volunteers. *Clin. Pharmacokinet.* **41,** 137–152.

19

Gender Differences in Heart Failure

Concerns for Drug Development

Mark A. Sussman

CONTENTS

1. INTRODUCTION

Congestive heart failure is a major health problem in terms of morbidity, mortality, increasing prevalence in the population, and economic burden to the health care system. The scope of the problem is evident by looking at the numbers (1): hospital discharges for heart failure increased 155.2% in the 20-yr period from 1979 to 1999, and currently there are about 4.8 million Americans living with congestive heart failure. There are over a half million new cases of congestive heart failure each year, and the incidence approaches 10% of the population after age 65. Heart failure follows a heart attack in 22% of men and 46% of women, and 75% of heart failure cases were preceded by hypertension, indicating a link between development of heart failure and previous myocardial damage or stress. The need for cost-effective therapeutic approaches is further reinforced by the economics of heart failure (Table 1). Ultimately, heart failure can only be treated by cardiac transplantation, which has dramatically increased in recent years (Fig. 1), and current pharmacologic interventions at best can only slow progression of deteriorating heart function and provide symptomatic relief. Our inability to mitigate the progression of congestive heart failure is evident from mortality associated with the syndrome, ending in death within 8 yr for 80% of men and 70% of women. Although survival after diagnosis of congestive heart failure is worse in men than women, fewer than 15% of women survive more than 8–12 yr. Clearly, heart failure is a syndrome affecting both sexes, especially in the aging population, that would benefit tremendously from novel therapeutic approaches to management, particularly

From: *Cardiac Drug Development Guide*
Edited by: M. K. Pugsley © Humana Press Inc., Totowa, NJ

Table 1
Economic Cost of Cardiovascular Disease: Estimated Direct and Indirect Costs (in Billions of Dollars) of Cardiovascular Diseases and Stroke United States, 2002

	Heart disease[b]	Coronary heart disease	Stroke	Hypertensive disease	Congestive heart failure	Total cardiovascular diseases[a]
Direct costs						
Hospital/nursing home	81.0	41.8	24.5	8.6	15.4	126.1
Physicians/other professionals	15.3	8.6	2.4	8.6	1.6	29.9
Drugs/other medical durables	13.5	6.2	0.8	15.5	2.0	31.8
Home health care	5.2	1.6	3.1	1.7	2.4	11.7
Total expenditures[a]	115.0	58.2	30.8	34.4[c]	21.4	199.5
Indirect costs						
Lost productivity/morbidity	19.0	8.4	5.6	6.7	NA	30.9
Lost productivity/mortality[d]	80.0	45.2	13.0	6.1	1.8	98.8
Grand totals	214.0	111.8	49.4	47.2	23.2	329.2

[a] Totals do not add up because of rounding and overlap.
[b] This category includes coronary heart disease, congestive heart failure, part of hypertensive disease, cardiac heart disease, cardiomyopathy, pulmonary heart disease, and other ill-defined "heart" diseases.
[c] Tom Hodgson and Liming estimated that health care expenditures attributed to hypertension that could not be allocated to cardiovascular complications and other diagnoses totaled $108.8 billion in 1998.
[d] Lost future earnings of persons who will die in 2002, discounted at 4%.
NA indicates not available.
Sources: Hodgson, T. A. and Cohen, A. J. (1999) Medical care expenditures for selected circulatory diseases: opportunities for reducing expenditures. *Med. Care* **37**, 994–1012.
National Health Expenditures Amounts, and Average Annual Percentage Change, by Type of Expenditures: Selected Calendar Years 1980–1982. (www.hcfa.gov)
Rice, D. P., Hodgson, T. A., and Kopstein, A. N. (1985) The economic cost of illness: a replication and update. *Health Care Financ. Rev.* **7**, 61–80.
Historic Income Tables: www.consensus.gov
Deaths for 282 Selected Causes by 5-Year Age Groups, Race, and Sex, United States.
Unpublished estimates of the present value of lifetime earnings by age and sex, United States, 1998, obtained in 2001 from University of California at San Francisco. All estimates prepared by Thomas Thorn, NHLBI.
Reproduced with permission from the American Heart Association. World Wide Web Site: www.americanheart.org. © 2001, Copyright American Heart Association.

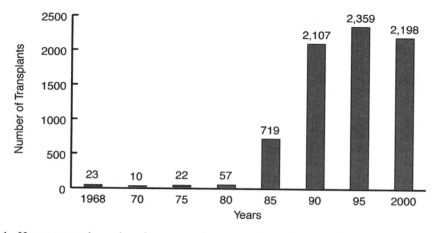

Fig. 1. Heart transplantation frequency by year. Reproduced with permission from the American Heart Association. World Wide Web Site: www.americanheart.org, © 2001, Copyright American Heart Association.

efforts to inhibit the progression of decompensation and restore contractile function. Current research into the possibilities of gene therapy *(2)*, stem cell transplantation *(3)*, or mobilization of endogenous cell populations *(4)* provide exciting new possibilities but the potential of these approaches for therapeutic treatment in the context of human disease remain unclear. Regardless, new pharmacologic approaches for treatment of heart failure to be used alone or in conjunction with other treatment regimens could have a profoundly positive impact for millions of patients diagnosed with this debilitating and often fatal disease.

2. GENDER DIFFERENCES IN CONGESTIVE HEART FAILURE

Evidence that gender influences the development and/or outcome of heart failure has been accumulating for over a decade. Risk of congestive heart failure is comparable regardless of gender until later life (55–64 yr) when men are almost twice as likely to develop heart failure compared with age-matched women (Fig. 2A). In the elderly population above 65 years of age, relative risk for either sex returns to comparable levels. Despite the relative increase in risk for age-matched midlife males vs females, hospital discharges for women with heart failure are growing at a faster rate than men (Fig. 2B). Thus, although on a percentile basis men between 55–64 years of age are more likely to develop congestive heart failure, the total number of women in the population afflicted with this disease is actually higher than men. These statistics have turned increased attention toward the underlying nature of heart failure in women, in part to combat the public perception that heart failure is primarily a disease of men *(5–8)*. Researchers and clinicians have called for increasing awareness of potential differences that exist in etiology, presentation, progression, and treatment of heart failure in women. To date, a majority of published literature has highlighted the increased risk of heart failure associated with the male gender relative to age-matched women (Table 2). However, heightened interest in the cardioprotective role of estrogenic stimulation has led to an expansion of research in female myocardial biology that will be discussed later in this chapter.

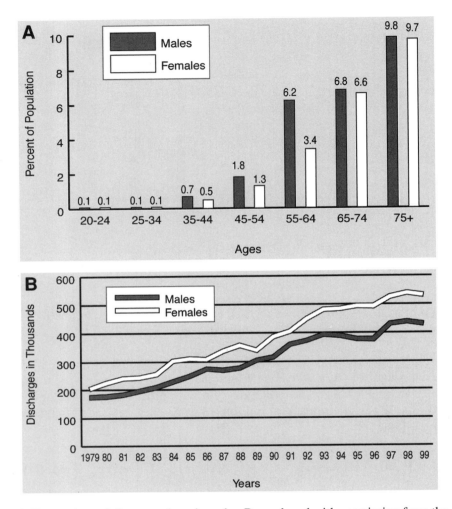

Fig. 2. Human heart failure trends and gender. Reproduced with permission from the American Heart Association. World Wide Web Site: www.americanheart.org, © 2001, Copyright American Heart Association.

Multiple studies have found that men have a higher incidence of heart failure and heart failure-associated mortality than age-matched women (Table 2). The first National Health and Nutrition Examination Survey (NHANES I) follow-up study found the incidence of congestive heart failure was positively and significantly associated with male sex, with a relative risk of 1.24 compared with women *(9)*. Once admitted to the hospital for treatment, elderly women live longer than men *(10)*, and the risk of mortality for women treated with diuretics and angiotensin-converting enzyme inhibitors was reduced by 36% compared with men *(11)*. After onset of heart failure, the risk of mortality is doubled for men compared with similarly afflicted women within a comparable time period *(12–14)*. On average, the onset of hypertrophic cardiomyopathy symptoms in women occurs at an older age than in men, in agreement with the idea that maladaptive cardiac remodeling begins earlier in men *(15)*. Ventricular hypertrophic remodeling is an important factor to consider in the development of heart fail-

Table 2
Association of Male Gender with Increased Risk of Heart Failure: Human Studies

Group examined	Outcome	Ref.
National Health and Nutrition Examination Study (NHANES I), 19-yr follow up	Incidence of congestive heart failure positively and significantly associated with male sex	*9*
Elderly patients	Women live longer than men in cases involving hospitalization for heart failure as part of treatment	*10*
Cardiac Insufficiency Bisoprol Study (CIBIS)	Probability of mortality significantly reduced by 36% in women compared with men	*11*
NHANES I, 55 yr and older	15-yr mortality rate was 39.1% for women and 71.8% for men	*12*
Flohan International Randomized Survival Trial (FIRST)	Risk of death for men vs women was 2.18, women have significantly better survival than men	*13*
United Kingdom	Risk of dying from congestive heart failure double in men vs women, but effect of age on mortality stronger in women than men	*14*
Various age groups	Delayed onset of hypertrophic cardiomyopathy symptoms in women compared with men as a function of age	*15*
Egyptian National Hypertension Project	Elevation of resting heart rate in hypertensive females is associated with concentric left ventricular remodeling and hypertrophy	*21*
Elderly heart failure patients	Incidence of heart failure greater in men than women	*110*

ure because increased left ventricular mass is associated with a higher relative risk for death from cardiovascular disease *(16)*. The underlying cause(s) that could account for this gender bias remain poorly understood from examination of human samples because heart failure is a complex disease with multifaceted etiology. Differential factors between the sexes touted as potential contributory agents in the increased risk of heart failure for men (Table 3) include decreased systolic chamber function and higher diastolic compliance *(17)*, stronger nighttime pulse pressure *(18)*, heightened heart rate *(19–21)*, decreased phospholamban phosphorylation *(22)*, and lower activation levels of the phosphatidylinositol 3-kinase–Akt (protein kinase B) pathway *(23)*. However, limited availability of samples, a myriad of pharmacologic interventions, and the inability to experimentally manipulate the system hampers the use of human tissue for understanding the molecular mechanism for differential gender risk. Therefore, research has turned to animal models for additional insight that cannot be gathered from analysis of human samples.

With the connection between male gender and increased risk of congestive heart failure in humans established, researchers assessed their animal models to determine

Table 3
Specific Observations of Human Male
vs Female Biology, Pharmacology, or Physiology

Group examined	Outcome	Ref.
Normal patients	Greater systolic chamber function and lower diastolic compliance in women vs men	17
Dialysis for nondiabetic patients	Men show significant relationship between left ventricular mass index and pulse pressure that was stronger at nighttime relative to women	18
Heart failure patients	Heart rate variability shows women have attenuated sympathetic activation and parasympathetic withdrawl compared with men	19
Myocardial samples from both normal and failing hearts	Decreased phospholamban phosphorylation in failing male hearts compared with normal or female samples	22
Normal subjects	Increased myocardial activation of Akt kinase in women vs men	23
Normal volunteers	Gender differences in pharmacokinetics of metoprolol resulting in greater drug exposure in females	83
Heart failure patients	Surviving women have less improvement in physical health status and perceive quality of care to be lower	111
Heart failure patients	Tolerance to high-dose angiotensin-converting enzyme comparable between gender, although women continued to be more symptomatic than men	112

whether similar sex-linked risks could be identified. In fact, differential susceptibility to heart failure associated with gender has been found in a variety of experimental animal models (Table 4). The spontaneous hypertensive heart failure (SHHF) rat is a genetically based animal model that has been extensively characterized with respect to remodeling and molecular signaling. Studies using the SHHF rat revealed that cardiomyocytes in males are larger than in age-matched females and that males possess a reduced adaptive hypertrophic response *(24)*. Some component of the compromised response in male SHHF rats could be to the result of paracrine signaling, where males show early activation of the renin–angiotensin axis vs females, who show activation of the endothelin vasopressor system *(25)*. Consistent with these observations from the SHHF rat, a transgenic rat model of hypertension showed increased cardiac hypertrophy in males relative to females *(26)*. Even normal male rats show increased susceptibility to heart failure after surgical intervention to cause pressure overload in the myocardium: adult female rats show preservation of contractile reserve relative to males *(27)*, and induction of pressure overload in young rats leads to accelerated heart failure in males *(28)*. Experimental mouse models also show a correlation between male gender and increased frequency of heart failure. Modeling the human genetic

Table 4
Association of Male Gender with Increased Risk of Heart Failure: Animal Studies

Group examined	Outcome	Ref.
Spontaneous hypertensive heart failure rats	Males show larger myocyte volume and cross-sectional area than age-matched females; reduced adaptive hypertrophic reserve observed in males	24
Spontaneous hypertensive heart failure rats	Males show early activation of the renin–angiotensin system, whereas females show early activation of the endothelin vasopressor system	25
Hypertensive transgenic rats	Increased cardiac hypertrophy in males relative to females	26
Normal adult rats	Contractile reserve preserved in female vs male rats after pressure overload aortic stenosis	27
Normal young rats	Males show accelerated progression into heart failure compared to females	28
Familial hypertrophic cardiomyopathy transgenic mouse model	Males show increased electrophysiologic abnormalities compared with females	29
Hypertrophic cardiomyopathy transgenic mouse model	Males show accelerated progression of functional impairment compared with females	30
Phospholamban-overexpressing transgenic mice	Males show accelerated progression of heart failure compared with females	31
Peroxisome proliferator-activated receptor α-deficient mice	Death in 100% of males but only 25% of females	32
Rats of varying ages	Males show decrease in telomerase activity compared with females in ventricular myocytes	33

condition, known as familial hypertrophic cardiomyopathy in transgenic mice, demonstrated that males possess increased electrophysiologic abnormalities *(29)* and accelerated progression of functional impairment *(30)*. Another transgenic mouse line created with overexpression of phospholamban specifically in the myocardium shows faster progression of heart failure in males relative to females *(31)*. A knockout mouse model possessing a metabolic disorder in cellular lipid use shows death resulting from heart failure in 100% of males but only 25% of females *(32)*. Collectively, these studies show that animal models can be valuable tools to recapitulate and study increased susceptibility of males to heart failure. Recent studies have revealed molecular differences between the sexes that could potentially account, at least in part, for why female hearts are more resistant to cardiomyopathic challenge. Both studies point to preservation of cardiomyocytes as a potential mechanism: telomerase activity in male myocytes decreased with aging whereas it increased with aging in females *(33)*, and female mice show enhanced activation of Akt kinase *(23)*, which has been shown to protect cardiomyocytes from apoptotic cell death. The activation of Akt kinase has been liked with estrogenic stimulation *(34–36)*, providing a gender-linked molecular basis for the heightened activation of this protective kinase in females.

3. ESTROGEN AND MYOCARDIAL FAILURE

Association of gender with differential susceptibility to cardiovascular disease inevitably led to examination of the role that sex hormones could play in modulating cardiac remodeling, cell signaling, and survival. A significant debate erupted over the last few years regarding the efficacy of postmenopausal hormone replacement therapy in prevention of heart disease because of the Heart and Estrogen/Progestin Replacement Study (HERS) that was primarily concerned with coronary heart disease *(37–40)*. Despite the HERS controversy, epidemiological results from human population studies link estrogen supplementation with decreased mortality from heart failure. Postmenopausal estrogen use in women exhibiting symptoms of congestive heart failure significantly decreased mortality with a relative risk of 0.68 compared with women without estrogen supplementation *(41)*. Estrogen supplementation after a heart attack does not increase the risk of reinfarction or mortality *(42)* and does not increase the risk of stroke in postmenopausal women with coronary disease *(43)*.

4. ESTROGENIC SIGNALING IN THE MYOCARDIUM

To identify mechanisms responsible for the beneficial effects of estrogen, researchers have turned to animal and cell culture models to dissect the myocardial response to stimulation on organ, cellular, and molecular levels (Table 5). In vivo, estradiol treatment of the SHHF rat model before the development of hypertension prevented cardiac remodeling and hypertension *(44)*. Curiously, a different report suggests that the ability of the heart to undergo hypertrophy is related to the presence of estrogen in both normotensive and hypertensive rats *(45)*. Estrogen supplementation in ovariectomized rats protected hearts from damage caused by global myocardial ischemia–reperfusion *(46)*. Implantation of estradiol release pellets in rats before coronary artery ligation resulted in reduction of preload and afterload pressures and restored the vasodilator role of basal nitric oxide *(47)*. A canine model of ischemia–reperfusion damage showed protection from endothelial and myocardial dysfunction mediated by estrogen supplementation *(48)*. Very compelling evidence for a role of estrogen signaling in cardiac resistance to damage was found using knockout mice lacking estrogen receptor, which showed increased injury after ischemia–reperfusion treatment in comparison with normal mice *(49)*. Ex vivo, estrogen treatment reduced heart rate and output pressure in isolated perfused hearts treated with isoproterenol *(50)*. In vitro, estrogen treatment of isolated cardiomyocytes inhibits apoptosis *(51)*, protects against hypoxia–reoxygenation injury *(52)* and hyperkalemia-induced calcium overload *(53)*, activates selected mitogen-activated protein kinase pathways *(54)* and Akt kinase *(23)*, and modulates hypertrophic responsiveness *(55)*. Cardiac myocytes possess functional estrogen receptors *(56)* and respond to incubation with estrogen precursors by expression of α and β receptors in a gender-specific fashion, prompting speculation regarding the role of local estrogen synthesis in cardiac signaling *(57)*. Cardiac fibroblasts, like cardiomyocytes, also possess functional estrogen receptors *(56)* and respond to

Table 5
Results of Estrogenic Stimulation in the Context of the Myocardium and Cardiac Cells

Group examined	Outcome	Ref.
Mouse and rat myocardial cells	Increased activation of Akt kinase in female vs male hearts, cultured cells respond to estrogenic stimulation by Akt activation	23
Ovariectomized rats with heart failure	17β estradiol treatment given before development of hypertension prevented hypertension and heart failure	44
Ovariectomized rats with heart failure	17β estradiol reduces preload and afterload, restores the vasodilator role of basal nitric oxide in ovariectomized rats	47
Dogs	Estrogen treatment protects against myocardial dysfunction resulting from ischemia–reperfusion	48
Isolated rat hearts	17β estradiol reduced heart rate and developed pressure in perfused hearts treated with isoproterenol	50
Cultured cardiomyocytes	17β estradiol treatment inhibits apoptosis	51
Isolated cardiomyocytes	17β estradiol protects cardiac cells against hypoxia–reoxygenation injury	52
Isolated cardiomyocytes	17β estradiol prevents hyperkalemia-induced Ca^{2+} loading and hypercontracture	53
Rat cardiomyocytes	Mitogn activated protein kinase pathways are activated by estrogen	54
Cardiac fibroblasts	17β estradiol inhibits fibroblast growth	58
Rat cardiac fibroblasts	Female cells resistant to hypoxia relative to males; estrogen treatment alters responsiveness to hypoxia	59
Phytoestrogens and SERMs		
Isolated hearts from ovariectomized female rats	Diet high in phytoestrogen content protects against damage from global ischemia–reperfusion	65
Rats subjected to ischemia–reperfusion injury	Genistein limits the inflammatory response and protects against myocardial damage	66
Isolated cardiomyocytes	Tamoxifen inhibits Ca^{2+} uptake by the sarcoplasmic reticulum	69
Isolated cardiomyocytes	Tamoxifen blocks the delayed rectifier potassium current, IKr	70
Isolated cardiomyocytes	Tamoxifen inhibits gap juction communication	71
Female rats	Tamoxifen decreases conversion of doxorubicin to toxic metabolite doxorubicinol (implications for cardiotoxicity)	72
Dogs subjected to ischemia–reperfusion injury	Raloxifene reduces myocardial infarct size	73
Ventricular tissue	SERMs inhibit Ca^{2+} uptake by the sarcoplasmic reticulum	113
Coronary arteries	Estrogen increases artery diameter, tamoxifen increases constriction	114

estrogenic stimulation with decreased proliferation *(58)* and gender-specific alterations in DNA synthesis *(59)*. It is possible that estrogenic modulation of angiotensin receptor expression could also contribute to differences in remodeling between the sexes *(60)*, but the relevance of this observation in the context of the myocardium remains unresolved. From these multiple characterizations, it is clear the heart is an estrogen-sensitive organ that has the potential for responding to estrogenic stimulation by activating a variety of molecular signaling pathways that are known to influence the remodeling process and cell survival. Manipulation of these estrogenic pathways may be useful in the design of therapeutic interventions to treat heart failure, as well as an important factor to consider for agents that exert antiestrogenic effects. Development of compounds that modulate estrogenic signaling, particularly for treatment of breast cancer, need to be considered in the context of myocardial signaling. So too, "natural" hormone replacements derived from dietary soy-based products are likely to influence signaling in the myocardium.

5. PHYTOESTROGENS AND SELECTIVE ESTROGEN RECEPTOR MODULATORS

If estrogenic stimulation of the myocardium affects signaling and remodeling, then it is reasonable to expect that related compounds with estrogen agonist activities could also exert similar effects. In fact, the cardiovascular benefits of phytoestrogens have been touted for many years, although primarily in the area of decreasing serum cholesterol and altering lipid profiles *(61–63)*. Phytoestrogens are plant-derived compounds of natural origin with nonsteroidal structure that can act as estrogen mimics (reviewed in ref. *64*). As might be expected, phytoestrogens have been found to exert similar effects for cardiac remodeling and protection to those described for estrogen (Table 5). A diet high in phytoestrogen content can protect the myocardium against damage from ischemia–reperfusion injury *(65)*, and treatment with a purified phytoestrogen, genistein, also prevents ischemia–reperfusion damage as well as limiting inflammatory response *(66)*. Genistein also induces activation of the antiapoptotic kinase Akt in hearts of treated mice as well as in cultured cardiomyocytes after overnight exposure *(23)*. We have also found that administration of genistein before development of cardiomyopathic changes can inhibit the progression of heart failure in our transgenic mouse models (unpublished observations). Thus, phytoestrogens, such as genistein and its metabolites, possess estrogenic signaling properties that can influence the myocardium. The presence of high phytoestrogen content in some laboratory rodent dietary formulas *(67)* may affect myocardial signaling and could be a factor in myocardial research involving rat, mouse, and rabbit model systems.

Phytoestrogens belong to a larger category of molecules that function as selective estrogen receptor modulators (SERMs) that exert estrogen agonist and/or antagonist properties. SERMs, such as tamoxifen and raloxifene, have become popular therapeutic drug agents for combating the growth of estrogen-sensitive breast cancers *(68)* and, as might be expected, these SERMs have effects upon the myocardium and cardiomyocytes as well. In cultured cardiomyocytes, tamoxifen inhibits calcium resequestration in the sarcoplasmic reticulum *(69)*, blocks the IKr potassium channel *(70)*, and inhibits gap junction communication *(71)*. Tamoxifen may also be useful in combinatorial chemotherapeutic treatment with doxorubicin owing to the ability of tamoxifen to inhibit the production of the cardiotoxic metabolite doxorubicinol *(72)*. Another SERM, raloxifene, reduces myocardial infarct size in a canine model of ischemic injury *(73)*. Building upon findings such as these, the prevailing opinion of the research community could be characterized as cautiously optimistic with regard to the salutary effects of tamoxifen *(74–78)* and raloxifene *(79,80)* upon the myocardium. Raloxifene is currently undergoing evaluation in large-scale clinical trials to assess cardiovascular effects *(81,82)*.

6. FUTURE DIRECTIONS FOR RESEARCH ON GENDER, HEART FAILURE, AND DRUG DEVELOPMENT

Results of epidemiological analysis of human populations, together with years of laboratory research, support the idea that men and women differ with respect to myocardial signaling, remodeling, and risk for development of congestive heart failure. In addition, research has shown that the sexes differ in response to drug treatments *(83–85)* or operations *(86)* designed to interrupt the progression of heart disease, raising the possibility of "gender-specific therapy" for treatment of congestive heart failure *(87)*. With the realization that the heart is an estrogen-responsive organ, research has been directed at understanding the role of estrogenic signaling for prevention of cardiovascular disease *(88,89)* and the ability of SERMs to provide an alternative to estrogen replacement therapy while also conferring side benefits of improved cardiovascular health *(90–92)*. The success of SERMs like tamoxifen and raloxifene has prompted development of new SERMs, increased interest in defining the mechanism of SERM biological activity, and new so-called antiestrogens *(93–96)*. Although estrogen and SERM therapies continue to be developed with women, testosterone is also being evaluated for cardioprotective and functional activities upon the heart *(97,98)*.

The advent of genomic and proteomic approaches has revolutionized the way researchers think about studying the molecular biology of heart failure *(99,100)*. Current research has predominantly been directed at defining differences in transcriptional and protein profiles between normal and diseased tissue, but similar approaches could also be used to examine the molecular basis for gender difference in signaling, particularly regarding response to estrogenic stimulation. The information gleaned from these screening approaches could be used to identify novel targets for pharmacologic intervention by gene discovery or can be used in pharmacogenomic studies designed to evaluate drug response and/or efficacy *(101,102)*. Proteomic science is potentially even more valuable by revealing post-translational modifications to signaling proteins that are so important to cardiac remodeling pathways that would be missed by genomic analyses. Although currently challenged by the complexity and subtlety of pathophysiologic changes in the myocardium, proteomic investigation of heart failure has already shown promising early results *(103,104)*.

We are just beginning to drill down beneath the surface of phenomenologic observations to understand the molecular basis of estrogenic signal transduction and impact upon cardiovascular function. Survival pathways, such as Akt kinase *(23)*, or gender-based differences in telomerase activity *(33)* open intriguing possibilities for downstream targets that could, at least in part, explain the beneficial effect of estrogen and higher risk of congestive heart failure in men. Of course, heart failure is a multifaceted syndrome with many contributory factors rooted in both biology *(105)* and sociology

(106–109). Research has shown that heart failure is an equal opportunity killer, but sex does matter. The future of cardiac pharmacologic intervention should try to take note of these gender-based differences and use them to gain the advantage for inhibiting progression of heart failure.

REFERENCES

1. American Heart Association. (2002) Heart and Stroke Statistical Update. American Heart Association, Dallas, 2001.
2. Isner, J. M. (2002) Myocardial gene therapy. *Nature* **415,** 234–239.
3. Orlic, D., Kajstura, J., Chimenti, S., Jakoniuk, I., Anderson, S. M., Li, B., et al. (2001) Bone marrow cells regenerate infarcted myocardium. *Nature* **410,** 701–705.
4. Orlic, D., Kajstura, J., Chimenti, S., Limana, F., Jakoniuk, I., Quaini, F., et al. (2001) Mobilized bone marrow cells repair the infarcted heart, improving function and survival. *Proc. Nat. Acad. Sci. USA* **98,** 10,344–10,349.
5. Morgan, N. A., Colling, C. L., and Fye, C. L. (1996) Cardiovascular diseases in women: An equal opportunity killer. *J. Am. Pharm. Assoc. (Wash).* **NS36,** 360–369.
6. Halm, M. A. and Penue, S. (2000) Heart failure in women. *Prog. Cardiovasc. Nurs.* **15,** 121–133.
7. Giardina, E. G. (2000) Heart disease in women. *Int. J. Fertil. Womens Med.* **45,** 350–357.
8. Richardson, L. G. and Rocks, M. (2001) Women and heart failure. *Heart Lung* **30,** 87–97.
9. He, J., Ogden, L. G., Bazzano, L. A., Vupputuri, S., Loria, C., and Whelton, P. K. (2001) Risk factors for congestive heart failure in US men and women: NHANES I epidemiologic follow-up study. *Arch. Intern. Med.* **161,** 996–1002.
10. Vaccarino, V., Chen, Y. T., Wang, Y., Radford, M. J., and Krumholz, H. M. (1999) Sex differences in the clinical care and outcomes of congestive heart failure in the elderly. *Am. Heart J.* **138,** 835–842.
11. Simon, T., Mary-Krause, M., Funck-Brentano, C, and Jaillon, P. (2001) Sex differences in the prognosis of congestive heart failure: Results from the Cardiac Insufficiency Bisoprol Study (CIBIS II). *Circulation* **103,** 375–380.
12. Schocken, D. D., Arieta, M. I., Leaverton, P. E., and Ross, E. A. (1992) Prevalence and mortality rate of congestive heart failure in the United States. *J. Am. Coll. Cardiol.* **20,** 301–306.
13. Adams, K. F. Jr., Sueta, C. A., Gheorghiade, M., O'Conner, C. M., Schwartz, T. A., Koch, G. G., et al. (1999) Gender differences in survival in advanced heart failure. Insights from the FIRST study. *Circulation* **99,** 1816–1821.
14. Ruigomez, A., Johansson, S., Wallander, M. A., and Garcia Rodriguez, L. A. (2001) Gender and drug treatment as determinants of mortality in a cohort of heart failure patients. *Eur. J. Epidemiol.* **17,** 329–335.
15. Dimitrow, P. P., Czarnecka, D., Jaszcz, K. K., and Dubiel, J. S. (1997) Sex differences in age at onset of symptoms in patients with hypertrophic cardiomyopathy. *J. Cardiovasc. Res.* **4,** 33–35.
16. Levy, D., Garrison, R. J., Savage, D. D., Kannel, W. B., and Castelli, W. P. (1990) Prognostic implications of echocardiographically determined left ventricular mass in the Framingham Heart Study. *N. Engl. J. Med.* **322,** 1561–1566.
17. Hayward, C. S., Kalnins, W. V., and Kelly, R. P. (2001) Gender-related differences in left ventricular chamber function. *Cardiovasc. Res.* **49,** 340–350.
18. Savage, T., Giles, M., Tomson, C. V., and Raine, A. E. (1998) Gender differences in mediators of left ventricular hypertrophy in dialysis patients. *Clin. Nephrol.* **49,** 107–112.
19. Aronson, D. and Burger, A. J. (2000) Gender-related differences in modulation of heart rate in patients with congestive heart failure. *J. Cardiovasc. Electrophysiol.* **11,** 1071–1077.

20. Palatini, P. (2001) Heart rate as a cardiovascular risk factor: Do women differ from men? *Ann. Med.* **33,** 213–221.

21. Saba, M. M., Ibrahim, M. M., and Rizk, H. H. (2001) Gender and the relationship between resting heart rate and left ventricular geometry. *J. Hypertens.* **19,** 367–373.

22. Dash, R., Frank, K. F., Carr, A. N., Moravec, C. S., and Kranias, E. G. (2001) Gender influences on sarcoplasmic reticulum Ca^{2+}-handling in failing human myocardium. *J. Mol. Cell. Cardiol.* **33,** 1345–1353.

23. Camper-Kirby, D., Welch. S., Walker, A., Shiraishi, I., Setchell, K. D., Schaefer, E., et al. (2001) Myocardial Akt activation and gender: increased nuclear activity in females versus males. *Circ. Res.* **88,** 1020–1027.

24. Tamura, T., Said, S., and Gerdes, A. M. (1999) Gender-related differences in myocyte remodeling in progression to heart failure. *Hypertension* **33,** 676–680.

25. Radin, M. J., Holycross, B. J., Sharkey, L. C., Shiry, L., and McCune, S. A. (2002) Gender modulates activation of renin-angiotensin an endothelin systems in hypertension and heart failure. *J. Appl. Physiol.* **92,** 935–940.

26. Brosnan, M. J., Devlin, A. M., Clark, J. S., Mullins, J. J., and Dominiczak, A. F. (1999) Different effects of anti-hypertensive agents on cardiac and vascular hypertrophy in the transgenic rat line TGR(mBen2)27. *Am. J. Hypertens.* **12,** 724–731.

27. Weinberg, E. O., Thienelt, C. D., Katz, S. E., Bartunek, J., Tajima, M., Rohrbach, S., et al. (1999) Gender differences in molecular remodeling in pressure overload hypertrophy. *J. Am. Coll. Cardiol.* **34,** 267–273.

28. Douglas P. S., Katz, S. E., Weinberg, E. O., Chen, M. H., Bishop, S. P., and Lorell, B. H. (1998) Hypertrophic remodeling: gender differences in the early response to left ventricular pressure overload. *J. Am. Coll. Cardiol.* **32,** 1118–1125.

29. Berul, C. I., Christe, M. E., Aronovitz, M. J., Maguire, C. T., Seidman, C. E., Seidman, J. G., et al. (1998) Familial hypertrophic cardiomyopathy mice display gender differences in electrophysiological abnormalities. *J. Interven. Card. Electrophysiol.* **2,** 7–14.

30. Olsson, M. C., Palmer, B. M., Leinwand, L. A., and Moore, R. L. (2001) Gender and aging in a transgenic mouse model of hypertrophic cardiomyopathy. *Am. J. Physiol. Heart Circ. Physiol.* **280,** H1136–1144.

31. Haghighi, K., Schmidt, A. G., Hoit, B. D., Brittsan, A. G., Yatani, A., Lester, J. W., et al. (2001) Superinhibition of sarcoplasmic reticulum function by phospholamban induces cardiac contractile failure. *J. Biol. Chem.* **276,** 24,145–24,152.

32. Djouadi, F., Weinheimer, C. J., Saffitz, J. E., Pitchford, C., Bastin, J., Gonzalez, F. J., et al. (1998) A gender-related defect in lipid metabolism and glucose homeostasis in peroxisome proliferator-activated receptor alpha- deficient mice. *J. Clin. Invest.* **102,** 1083–1091.

33. Leri, A., Malhotra, A., Liew, C. C., Kajstura, J., and Anversa, P. (2000) Telomerase activity in rat cardiac myocytes is age and gender dependent. *J. Mol. Cell. Cardiol.* **32,** 385–390.

34. Haynes, M. P., Sinha, D., Russel, K. S., Collinge, M., Fulton, D., Morales-Ruiz, M., et al. (2000) Membrane receptor estrogen engagement activates endothelial nitric oxide synthase via the PI3-K-Akt pathway in human endothelial cells. *Circ. Res.* **87,** 677–682.

35. Simoncini, T., Hafezi-Moghadam, A., Brazil, D. P., Ley, K., Chin, W. W., and Liao, J. K. (2000) Interaction of the oestrogen receptor with the regulatory subunit of phosphatidylinositol-3-OH kinase. *Nature* **407,** 538–541.

36. Tsai, E. M., Wang, S. C., Lee, J. N., and Hung, M. C. (2001) Akt activation by estrogen in estrogen receptor-negative breast cancer cells. *Cancer Res.* **61,** 8390–8392.

37. Herrington, D. M., Fong, J., Sempos, C. T., Black, D. M., Schrott, H. G., Rautaharju, P., et al. (1998) Comparison of the Heart and Estrogen/Progestin Replacement Study (HERS) cohort with women with coronary disease from the National Health and Nutrition Examination Survey II (NHANES III). *Am. Heart. J.* **136,** 115–124.

38. Bush, T. (2001) Beyond HERS: Some (not so) random thoughts on randomized clinical trials. *Int. J. Fertil. Womens Med.* **46,** 55–59.

39. Wells, G. and Herrington, D. M. (1999) The Heart and Estrogen/Progestin Replacement Study: what have we learned and what questions remain? *Drugs Aging* **15,** 419–422.

40. Blumenthal, R. S., Zacur, H. A., Reis, S. E., and Post, W. S. (2000) Beyond the null hypothesis—do the HERS results disprove the estrogen/coronary heart disease hypothesis? *Am. J. Cardiol.* **85,** 1015–1017.

41. Reis, S. E., Holubkov, R., Young, J. B., White, B. G., Cohn, J. N., and Feldman, A. M. (2000) Estrogen is associated with improved survival in aging women with congestive heart failure: Analysis of the vesnarinone studies. *J. Am. Coll. Cardiol.* **36,** 529–533.

42. Newton, K. M., LaCroix, A. Z., McKnight, B., Knopp, R. H., Siscovick, D. S., Heckbert, S. R., et al. (1997) Estrogen replacement therapy and prognosis after first myocardial infarction. *Am. J. Epidemiol.* **145,** 269–277.

43. Simon, J. A., Hsia, J., Cauley, J. A., Richards, C., Harris, F., Fong, J., et al. (2001) Post-menopausal hormone therapy and risk of stroke: The Heart and Estrogen-progestin Replacement Study (HERS). *Circulation* **103,** 638–642.

44. Sharkey, L. C., Holycross, B. J., Park, S., Shiry, L. J., Hoepf, T. M., McCune, S. A., et al. (1999) Effect of ovariectomy and estrogen replacement on cardiovascular disease in heart failure prone SHHF/Mcc-fa cp rats. *J. Mol. Cell. Cardiol.* **31,** 1527–1537.

45. Wallen, W. J., Cserti, C., Belanger, M. P., and Wittnich, C. (2000) Gender-differences in myocardial adaptation to afterload in normotensive and hypertensive rats. *Hypertension* **36,** 774–779.

46. Zhai, P., Eurell, T. E., Cotthaus, R., Jeffery, E. H., Bahr, J. M., and Gross, D. R. (2000) Effect of estrogen on global myocardial ischemia-reperfusion injury in female rats. *Am. J. Physiol. Heart Circ. Physiol.* **279,** H2766–2775.

47. Nekooeian, A. A. and Pang, C. C. (1998) Estrogen restores role of basal nitric oxide in control of vascular tone in rats with chronic heart failure. *Am. J. Physiol.* **274,** H2094–2099.

48. Kim, Y. D., Chen, B., Beauregard, J., Kouretas, P., Thomas, G., Farhat, M. Y., et al. (1996) 17β estradiol prevents dysfunction of canine coronary endothelium and myocardium and reperfusion arrhythmias after brief ischemia/reperfusion. *Circulation* **94,** 2901–2908.

49. Zhai, P., Eurell, T. E., Cooke, P. S., Lubahn, D. B., and Gross, D. R. (2000) Myocardial ischemia-reperfusion injury in estrogen receptor alpha knockout and wild-type mice. *Am. J. Physiol. Heart Circ. Physiol.* **278,** H1640–H1647.

50. Li, H. Y., Bian, J. S., Kwan, Y. W., and Wong, T. M. (2000) Enhanced responses to 17β estradiol in rat hearts treated with isoproterenol: Involvement of a cyclic AMP-dependent pathway. *J. Pharmacol. Exp. Ther.* **293,** 592–598.

51. Pelzer, T., Schumann, M., Neumann, M., de Jager, T., Stimpel, M., Serfling, E., et al. (2000) 17β-estradiol prevents programmed cell death in cardiac myocytes. *Biochem. Biophys. Res. Commun.* **268,** 192–200.

52. Jovanovic, S., Jovanovic, A., Shen, W. K., and Terzic, A. (2000) Low concentrations of 17β-estradiol protect single cardiac cells against metabolic stress-induced Ca^{2+} loading. *J. Am. Coll. Cardiol.* **36,** 948–952.

53. Jovanovic, S., Jovanovic, A., Shen, W. K., and Terzic, A. (1998) Protective action of 17β-estradiol in cardiac cells: Implications for hyperkalemic cardioplegia. *Ann. Thorac. Surg.* **66,** 1658–1661.

54. Nuedling, S., Kahlert, S., Loebbert, K., Meyer, R., Vetter, H., and Grohe C. (1999) Differential effects of 17β-estradiol on mitogen-activated protein kinase pathways in rat cardiomyocytes. *FEBS Lett.* **454,** 271–276.

55. Pelzer, T., Shamim, A., Wolfges, S., Schumann, M., and Neyses, L. (1997) Modulation of cardiac hypertrophy by estrogens. *Adv. Exp. Med. Biol.* **432,** 83–89.

56. Grohe, C., Kahlert, S., Lobbert, K., Stimpel, M., Karas, R. H., Vetter, H., et al. (1997) Cardiac myocytes and fibroblasts contain functional estrogen receptors. *FEBS Lett.* **416,** 107–112.

57. Grohe, C., Kahlert, S., Lobbert, K., and Vetter, H. (1998) Expression of oestrogen receptor α and β in rat heart: Role of local oestrogen synthesis. *J. Endocrinol.* **156,** R1–R7.
58. Dubey, R. K., Gillespie, D. G., Jackson, E. K., and Keller, P. J. (1998) 17β-estradiol, its metabolites, and progesterone inhibit cardiac fibroblast growth. *Hypertension* **31,** 522–528.
59. Griffin, M., Lee, H. W., Hao, L., and Eghbali-Webb, M. (2000) Gender-related differences in proliferative response of cardiac fibroblasts to hypoxia: effects of estrogen. *Mol. Cell. Biochem.* **215,** 21–30.
60. Krishnamurthi, K., Verbalis, J. G., Zheng, W., Wu, Z., Clerch, L. B., and Sandberg, K. (1999) Estrogen regulates angiotensin AT1 receptor expression via cytosolic proteins that bind to the 5' leader sequence of the receptor mRNA. *Endocrinology* **140,** 5435–5438.
61. Anderson, J. W., Smith, B. M., and Washnock, C. S. (1999) Cardiovascular and renal benefits of dry bean and soybean intake. *Am. J. Clin. Nutr.* **70,** 464S–474S.
62. Cassidy, A. and Griffin, B. (1999) Phyto-oestrogens: A potential role in the prevention of CHD? *Proc. Nutr. Soc.* **58,** 193–199.
63. Lissin, L. W. and Cooke, J. P. (2000) Phytoestrogens and cardiovascular health. *J. Am. Coll. Cardiol.* **35,** 1403–1410.
64. Setchell, K. D. R. (1998) Phytoestrogens: The biochemistry, physiology, and implications for human health of soy isoflavones. *Am. J. Clin. Nutr.* **68(Suppl),** 1333S–1346S.
65. Zhai, P., Eurell, T. E., Cotthaus, R. P., Jeffery, E. H., Bahr, J. M., and Gross, D. R. (2001) Effects of dietary phytoestrogen on global myocardial ischemia-reperfusion injury in isolated female rat hearts. *Am. J. Physiol. Heart Circ. Physiol.* **281,** H223–232.
66. Deodato, B., Altavilla, D., Squadrito, G., Campo, G. M., Arlotta, M., Minutoli, L., et al. (1999) Cardioprotection by the phytoestrogen genistein in experimental myocardial ischaemia-reperfusion injury. *Br. J. Pharmacol.* **128,** 1683–1690.
67. Thigpen, J. E., Setchell, K. D. R., Ahlmark, K. B., Locklear, J., Spahr, T., Caviness, G. F., et al. (1999) Phytoestrogen content of purified, open- and closed-formula laboratory animal diets. *Lab. Animal Sci.* **49,** 530–536.
68. MacGregor, J. I. and Jordan, V. C. (1998) Basic guide to the mechanisms of antiestrogen action. *Pharmacol. Rev.* **50,** 151–196.
69. Kargacin, M. E., Ali, Z., Ward, C. A., Pollock, N. S., and Kargacin, G. J. (2000) Tamoxifen inhibits Ca^{2+} uptake by the cardiac sarcoplasmic reticulum. *Pflugers Arch.* **440,** 573–579.
70. Liu, X. K., Katchman, A., Ebert, S. N., and Woosley, R. L. (1998) The antiestrogen tamoxifen blocks the delayed rectifier potassium current, IKr, in rabbit ventricular myocytes. *J. Pharmacol. Exp. Ther.* **287,** 877–883.
71. Verrecchia, F. and Herve, J. (1997) Reversible inhibition of gap junctional communication by tamoxifen in cultured cardiac myocytes. *Pflugers Arch.* **434,** 113–116.
72. Vaidyanathan, S. and Boroujerdi, M. (2000) Effect of tamoxifen pretreatment on the pharmocokinetics, metabolism and cardiotoxicity of doxirubicin in female rats. *Cancer Chemother. Pharmacol.* **46,** 185–192.
73. Ogita, H., Node, K., Asanuma, H., Sanada, S., Takashima. S., Asakura. M., et al. (2002) Amelioration of ischemia- and reperfusion-induced myocardial injury by the selective estrogen receptor modulator, raloxifene, in the canine heart. *J. Cardiol.* **39,** 55–56.
74. Wiseman, H. (1995) Taking tamoxifen to heart. *Nat. Med.* **1,** 1226.
75. Wiseman, H. (1995) Tamoxifen as an antioxidant and cardioprotectant. *Biochem. Soc. Symp.* **61,** 209–219.
76. Weitzman, J. (2001) Tamoxifen is good for the heart. *Trends Mol. Med.* **7,** 150.
77. Love, R. R., Wiebe, D. A., Feyzi, J. M., Newcomb, P. A., and Chappel, R. J. (1994) Effects of tamoxifen on cardiovascular risk factors in postmenopausal women after 5 years of treatment. *J. Natl. Cancer Inst.* **86,** 1534–1539.
78. Reis, S. E., Constantino, J. P., Wickerham, D. L., Tan-Chiu, E., Wang, J., and Kavanah, M. (2001) Cardiovascular effects of tamoxifen in women with and without heart disease:

Breast cancer prevention trial. National Surgical Adjuvant Breast and Bowel Project Breast Cancer Prevention Trial Investigators. *J. Natl. Cancer Inst.* **93,** 16–21.

79. Gustafsson, J. A. (1998) Raloxifene: Magic bullet for heart and bone? *Nat. Med.* **4,** 152–153.

80. Walsh, B. W. (2001) The effects of estrogen and selective estrogen receptor modulators on cardiovascular risk factors. *Ann. N. Y. Acad. Sci.* **949,** 163–167.

81. Mosca, L. (2001) Rationale and overview of the Raloxifene Use for the Heart (RUTH) trial. *Ann. N. Y. Acad. Sci.* **949,** 181–185.

82. Mosca, L., Barrett-Conner, E., Wenger, N. K., Collins, P., Grady, P., Kornitzer, M., et al. (2001) Design and methods of the Raloxifene for The Heart (RUTH) study. *Am. J. Cardiol.* **88,** 392–395.

83. Luzier, A. B., Killian, A., Wilton, J. H., Wilson, M. F., Forrest, A., and Kazierad, D. J. (1999) Gender-related effects on metoprolol pharmacokinetics and pharmacodynamics in healthy volunteers. *Clin. Pharmacol. Ther.* **66,** 594–601.

84. Klassen, G. A., Yeung, P. K., Barclay, K. D., Pollak, P. T., Hung, O. R., and Buckley S. J. (1997) Effect of diltiazem on intraarterial blood pressure and heart rate during stress testing in patients with angina: a gender comparison study. *J. Clin. Pharmacol.* **37,** 297–303.

85. Woodfield, S. L., Lundergan, C. F., Reiner, J. S., Thompson, M. A., Rohrbeck, S. C., Deychak Y., et al. (1997) Gender and acute myocardial infarction: Is there a different response to thrombolysis? *J. Am. Coll. Cardiol.* **29,** 35–42.

86. Capdeville, M., Chamogeogarkis, T., and Lee, J. H. (2001) Effect of gender on outcomes of beating heart operations. *Ann. Thorac. Surg.* **72,** S1022–1025.

87. Schwartz, J. B. (2000) Congestive heart failure medications: Is there a rationale for sex-specific therapy? *J. Gend. Specific Med.* **3,** 17–22.

88. Nair, G. V., Klien, K. P., and Herrington, D. M. (2001) Assessing the role of oestrogen in the prevention of cardiovascular disease. *Ann. Med.* **33,** 305–312.

89. Herrington, D. (2000) Role of estrogens, selective estrogen receptor modulators and phytoestrogens in cardiovascular protection. *Can. J. Cardiol.* **16(Suppl E),** 5E–9E.

90. Tinelli, A., Perrone, A., and Tinelli, F. G. (2001) An alternative to postmenopausal hormone replacement therapy? Selective Estrogen Receptors Modulators (SERMs). *Minerva Ginecol.* **53,** 127–135.

91. Fitzpatrick, L. A. (1999) Selective estrogen receptor modulators and phytoestrogens: new therapies for the postmenopausal women. *Mayo Clin. Proc.* **74,** 601–607.

92. Bryant, H. U. and Dere, W. H. (1998) Selective estrogen receptor modulators: An alternative to hormone replacement therapy. *Proc. Soc. Exp. Biol. Med.* **217,** 45–52.

93. Anthony, M., Williams, J. K., and Dunn, B. K. (2001) What would be the properties of an ideal SERM? *Ann. N. Y. Acad. Sci.* **949,** 261–278.

94. O'Reagan, R. M. and Jordan, V. C. (2001) Tamoxifen to raloxifene and beyond. *Semin. Oncol.* **28,** 260–273.

95. Dhingra, K. (1999) Antiestrogens—tamoxifen, SERMs and beyond. *Invest. New Drugs* **17,** 285–311.

96. Poletti, A. (1999) Searching for the ideal SERM. *Pharmacol. Res.* **39,** 333.

97. Shapiro, J., Christiana, J., and Frishman, W. H. (1999) Testosterone and other anabolic steroids as cardiovascular drugs. *Am. J. Ther.* **6,** 167–174.

98. Pugh, P. J., English, K. M., Jones, T. H., and Channer, K. S. (2000) Testosterone: A natural tonic for the failing heart? *Quart. J. Med.* **93,** 689–694.

99. Hwang, J. J., Dzau, V. J., and Liew, C. C. (2001) Genomics and the pathophysiology of heart failure. *Curr. Cardiol. Rep.* **3,** 198–207.

100. Jiang, L., Tsubakihara, M., Heinke, M. Y., Yao, M., Dunn, M. J., Phillips, W., et al. (2001) Heart failure and apoptosis: electrophoretic methods support data from micro- and macro-arrays. A critical review of genomics and proteomics. *Proteomics* **1,** 1481–1488.

101. Mehraban, F. and Tomlinson, J. E. (2001) Application of industrial scale genomics to discovery of therapeutic targets in heart failure. *Eur. J. Heart. Fail.* **3,** 641–650.

102. Winkelmann, B. R., Marz, W., Boehm, B. O., Zotz, R., Hager, J., Hellstern, P., Senges, J., and LURIC Study Group (LUdwigshafen RIsk and Cardiovascular Health) (2001) Rationale and design of the LURIC study—a resource for functional genomics, pharmacogenomics and long term prognosis of cardiovascular disease. *Pharmacogenomics* **2(Suppl 1),** S1–73.

103. Van Eyk, J. E. (2001) Proteomics: Unraveling the complexity of heart disease and striving to change cardiology. *Curr. Opin. Mol. Ther.* **3,** 546–553.

104. Macri, J. and Rapundalo, S. T. (2001) Application of proteomics to the study of cardiovascular biology. *Trends Cardiovasc. Med.* **11,** 66–75.

105. Hayward, C. S., Kelly, R. P., and Collins, P. (2000) The roles of gender, the menopause and hormone replacement on cardiovascular function. *Cardiovasc. Res.* **46,** 28–49.

106. Weidner, G. (2000) Why do men get more heart disease than women? An international perspective. *J. Am. Coll. Health* **48,** 291–294.

107. Hood, S., Taylor, S., Roeves, A., Crook, A. M., Tlusty, P., Cohen, J., et al. (2000) Are there age and sex differences in the investigation and treatment of heart failure? A population-based study. *Br. J. Gen. Pract.* **50,** 559–563.

108. Harjai, K. J., Nunez, E., Stewart A., Humphrey, J., Turgut, T., Shah, M., et al. (2000) Does bias exist in the medical management of heart failure? *Int. J. Cardiol.* **75,** 65–69.

109. Mejhert, M., Holmgren, J., Wandell, P., Persson, H., and Edner, M. (1999) Diagnostic tests, treatment and follow-up in heart failure patients—is there a gender bias in coherence to guidelines? *Eur. J. Heart Fail.* **1,** 407–410.

110. Chin, N. H. and Goldman, L. (1998) Gender differences in 1-year survival and quality of life among patients admitted with congestive heart failure. *Med. Care* **36,** 1033–1046.

111. Gottdiener, J. S., Arnold, A. M., Aurigemma, G. P., Polak, J. F., Tracy, R. P., Kitzman, D. W., et al. (2000) Predictors of congestive heart failure in the elderly: the cardiovascular health study. *J. Am. Coll. Cardiol.* **35,** 1628–1637.

112. Levine, T. B., Levine, A. B., Kaminski, P., and Stommel R. J. (2000) Reversal of heart failure remodeling in women. *J. Womens Gend. Based Med.* **9,** 513–519.

113. Dodds, M. L., Kargacin, M. E., and Kargacin, G. J. (2001) Effects of anti-oestrogens and beta-estradiol on calcium uptake by cardiac sarcoplasmic reticulum. *Br. J. Pharmacol.* **132,** 1374–1382.

114. Wellman, G. C., Bonev, A. D., Nelson, M. T., and Brayden, J. E. (1996) Gender differences in coronary artery diameter involve estrogen, nitric oxide, and Ca(2+)-dependent K+ channels. *Circ Res.* **79,** 1024–1030.

20

Angiogenesis Therapies for Coronary Artery Disease

Trials and Tribulations

Michael Simons

1. INTRODUCTION

The development of therapeutic angiogenesis promises to revolutionize the treatment of coronary artery disease (CAD) by providing, for the first time, means to medically restore circulation to ischemic areas of the heart. Because of such promise, this area of therapeutics has undergone rapid development over the last decade. Much has been learned, both in terms of biology of angiogenesis and the development strategies. This chapter will attempt to summarize some of these lessons. It will begin with a historical background and then will consider key issues related to therapeutic angiogenesis: the choice of therapeutic agent, delivery strategy, selection of patient population, assessment of therapeutic benefit, and the placebo effect.

2. HISTORICAL BACKGROUND

Several different threads of investigations have converged in the mid-1980s to launch the field of therapeutic cardiovascular angiogenesis. The pioneering works of Judah Folkman and colleagues have brought the concept of angiogenesis as an important biological process that can be harnessed for therapeutic processes into the consciousness of the biomedical community. At the same time, long-standing efforts of Wolfgang

From: *Cardiac Drug Development Guide*
Edited by: M. K. Pugsley © Humana Press Inc., Totowa, NJ

Schaper and his colleagues have resulted in thorough anatomical and physiological characterization of collateral development in various animal models and demonstrated the functional impact of this process in chronic myocardial ischemia.

Simultaneously, groundbreaking efforts in several laboratories have resulted in isolation, purification, and cloning of several angiogenic growth factors, including fibroblast growth factor (FGF), vascular endothelial growth factor (VEGF), platelet-derived growth factor (PDGF), and their receptors. The availability of molecular probes led to rapid realization that both normal and ischemic tissues contain growth factors *(1)* and that the expression of some of them is upregulated in ischemic tissues *(2–9)*. These developments made it inevitable that sooner or late these agents would be tested for their ability to induce therapeutic angiogenesis.

The attempts to study whether FGF2, VEGF, or other angiogenic growth factors could be effective in chronic ischemia, soon resulted in publication of a number of studies showing increased tissue perfusion and improved function in the ischemic heart *(10–13)* or hindlimb *(14–18)*. All of these studies were characterized by a remarkably robust effect achieved with various regimens, doses, and means of administration. At the same time, investigators working in the limb ischemia models reported beneficial therapeutic effects of FGF2 and VEGF$_{165}$ administration.

In parallel with the studies using protein therapies, a number of investigators used gene transfer to stimulate therapeutic angiogenesis. Successful results were reported using a variety of vectors, including plasmid and adenoviral injections into skeletal and cardiac muscle as well into the bloodstream. Remarkably, intramuscular plasmid injections were reported to produce high levels of expression, sufficient enough to increase plasma levels of the growth factor, that remained elevated for an extended period of time.

Naturally, such findings have raised high hopes that therapeutic induction of vessel growth cannot be far behind, given how easy it was to achieve seemingly remarkable results in animals. Little consideration was given to the fact that these preclinical studies tended to use juvenile animals, that these animals were free of atherosclerosis, that the time course of angiogenesis is likely to be very different between small animals and patients, and that given these differences, single-dose therapies, so effective in animal models, may not be effective in humans.

The early trials investigated single therapy with a growth factor delivered as a protein or by means of gene transfer. Because there was little information to guide the investigators with regard to choice of dose or potential toxicities, open-label dose escalation format was commonly used. Very soon, all trials began reporting remarkable results with marked improvements in patients symptoms, exercise capacity, and even resolution of large perfusion defects. Unfortunately, there was little previous clinical experience with the kind of patients that were now being enrolled in clinical trials and, consequently, the rate of spontaneous improvements in the extent and manifestations of coronary or peripheral vascular disease, placebo effect, or reproducibility of single photon emission computed tomography (SPECT) scans in the presence of advanced CAD were not known.

The overwhelmingly negative results of the first double-blind, randomized control trial of VEGF (VIVA) and ambiguous results of following trials forced reassessment of therapeutic angiogenesis strategies. Much has been learned since then, and now we are in a better position to rationally develop therapeutic angiogenesis product.

3. THE CHOICE OF THERAPEUTIC AGENT

Quite a few growth factors are reported to have angiogenic activity, that is, the ability to induce proliferation and/or migration of endothelial cells in vitro. A number of factors have been also shown to have the ability to induce formation of vascular structures in vivo in a variety of models, including Matrigel™, chronic allantoic membrane (CAM), and corneal implant assays, as well as ischemic heart or hindlimb assays. These factors can be broadly divided in to the VEGF family (VEGF A, B, and C; placenta growth factor [PLGF]), FGF family (FGF1, 2, 4, and 5), platelet-derived growth factor (PDGF), and hepatpcyte growth factor (HGF) *(19,20)*.

In addition, several other genes, including a transcription factor HIF-1α *(21)* and macrophage-derived PR39 peptide *(22)*, have the ability to induce multiple angiogenic pathways. Initial enthusiasm for VEGF as a principle therapeutic agent was based on observations of embryonic lethality in mice with a deletion of a single VEGF gene *(23,24)* and presumed endothelial cell specificity of VEGF (thereby minimizing bystander effects). However, neither of these arguments really makes a strong case for VEGF as a therapeutic agent. Embryonic lethality in VEGF gene deletions occurs for a number of different reasons, not all of which are related to growth of new vessels. Furthermore, no data exist showing that a comparable effect would be seen in adult tissues. The so-called selectivity of effect argument is a curious one because the blood vessels consist of more then endothelial cells. Indeed, experience with VEGF has shown that it induces formation of capillary-like leaky vessels that are not very effective in carrying bulk flow *(25)*. The other drawback of VEGF is its induction of vessel permeability as well as profound hypotension. The latter side effects effectively limits its administration to local protein delivery or gene therapy approaches. Finally, recent reports have suggested that VEGF, perhaps because of its ability to promote monocyte recruitment, increases growth of atherosclerotic plaques *(26)*.

By the same token, FGFs have been looked at with suspicion because of their pluripotent spectrum of activity and, in case of FGF1 and FGF2, lack of the signal peptide. At the same time, FGFs are much more potent endothelial mitogens than VEGF and appear to induce growth of larger vessels, more suitable as native bypasses around sites of arterial occlusion than capillaries *(27,28)*.

FGFs also have less systemic toxicity with prominent exception of their ability to induce renal protein loss in patients with pre-existing kidney disease. However, like VEGF, FGFs induce only a single signaling cascade and thus may not be ideal for stimulating a robust sustained neovascularization that likely requires coordinate actions of numerous growth factors.

The angiogenic abilities of PDGF-BB and HGF are just beginning to be appreciated and little is yet known about them. One attractive feature of HGF is its ability to stimulate VEGF synthesis, in addition to its own proliferative activity, thereby potentially providing for activation of at least two distinct angiogenic signaling cascades *(29)*. PDGF-BB is particularly interesting because its activity has been linked to blood vessel maturation, a process at least as important as the initial vessel growth *(30)*.

Of the past individual growth factors, two proteins have been shown to have a broad-spectrum "master switch" effect. The transcription factor HIF-1α was initially identified as the gene responsible for increase in erythropoietin production in anemic animals.

It was rapidly shown to function as an oxygen sensor (in as yet undefined manner) and to induce expression of a number of angiogenesis related genes, including VEGF-A, its receptor Flt-1, inducible nitric oxide synthase, and angiopoietin-2, a protein involved in vessel maturation *(31,32)*. This is a very desirable transcription profile from a therapeutic angiogenesis point of view because a combination of VEGF and angiopoietin-2 has been shown to produce mature, nonleaky, long-living vessels.

PR39 is another master switch gene with less precisely determined properties *(22,33)*. This short, highly positively charged peptide induces expression of HIF-1α and, in addition, stimulates expression of FGF receptors FGF R1 and syndecan-4.

This ability to induce the FGF signaling cascade (primarily regulated at the level of receptor expression) in addition to stimulating VEGF and angiopoietin II expression may be particularly effective. In summary, given that angiogenesis and arteriogenesis in mature cardiac tissues involve numerous events from initial proliferation of endothelial cells to maturation and retention of newly formed vessels and that these processes are regulated by different growth factors, combination therapy approach should be more effective than monotherapy.

4. DELIVERY OF ANGIOGENIC AGENTS

Several considerations are involved in decisions regarding optimal delivery strategy. On the practical side, the ease of administration is clearly appealing from a marketing perspective. Thus, an agent that can be administered orally or intravenously likely expands the potential patient population willing to undergo treatment and, more importantly, from a pharmaceutical company perspective, extends the number of physicians that can prescribe and administer the treatment. However, a complex invasive delivery procedure, such as an intramyocardial injection, reduces the number of patients, and the number of times the treatment can be given per patient, and limits the treatment to a select group of physicians able to administer it.

Ease of administration notwithstanding, the delivery modality needs to be effective, and this effectiveness should be achieved with the simplest regimen and/or formulation. Minimization of systemic toxicity is another important consideration. Interestingly, until very recently, it was not clear what the requirements for effective delivery were. The success of single bolus administration of proteins in a number of animal models *(34)* led to an understandable belief that the same strategy can be effective in patients, even though the mechanism of the effectiveness of this delivery strategies were not obvious. Quantitative studies in animals demonstrated that only a small fraction of the dose localized to the myocardium immediately after an intracoronary infusion and that fraction was much smaller after an intravenous infusion. Furthermore, by 24 h essentially all of the dose was no longer in the myocardium *(35)*. Because the process of angiogenesis (and arteriogenesis) takes much longer than that, it was postulated that such an infusion triggered a self-amplifying process that was responsible for the observed neovascularization. The absence of dose–response after ic or iv administrations of growth factors further supports this concept.

The nature of such a process is unclear but may involve local accumulation of circulation monocytes and/or endothelial precursor cells *(19)*. However, when tested in clinical trials, such a delivery strategy met with largely negative results in case of both VEGF *(36)* and FGF2 *(37)*. In retrospect, it seems clear that inducing angiogenesis in juvenile healthy animals (ameroid pigs model, hindlimb rabbit ischemia model) is much easier than in older, sick individuals *(38)*. Indeed, one likely explanation of failure of this approach in older patients is a rapid decline in circulation of pro-endothelial stem cells with age.

An alternative strategy to the single bolus therapy is a prolonged systemic or local presence of the growth factors. Because prolonged systemic exposure to an angiogenic growth factor is likely undesirable from the safety perspective, efforts of many investigators have centered on local delivery of growth factors *(39)*. Simple means of local delivery, such as intramyocardial protein injections, provide better initial retention of material and a slower washout. However, even with this strategy, most of the growth factor is gone by 7 d. Although such a regimen is effective in animal models, it does not necessarily predict human effectiveness because the limited time of exposure and because the time of course of angiogenesis in humans have not been established.

Alternatives to simple protein injections include polymer-based protein delivery and gene therapy. Although polymer-based delivery strategy is simplest from the conceptual point of view (a known dose is administered with well-defined pharmacokinetics), in practice polymer delivery to the heart cannot be yet achieved in catheter-based manner. A requirement for open-chest approach greatly diminishes the appeal of this approach. Nevertheless, polymer-based delivery of FGF2 has been shown to be effective in a small double-blind clinical trial *(40)*.

As already mentioned, gene therapy provides another alternative to polymer-based delivery *(41,42)*. Numerous gene transfer vectors with various characteristics of expression are available. Plasmid- and adenoviral-based systems have received the most exposure and study in angiogenesis trials. Plasmid-based vectors offer simplicity of construction, low cost, and presumed low toxicity. Unfortunately, the magnitude of expression for most plasmid vectors is very low and the duration of expression is fairly short (< 7–10 d).

Adenoviruses provide for much higher level of expression and the duration of expression is longer, averaging ~14 d. However, the use of adenoviruses is associated with systemic toxicity concerns and is marred by unpredictability of expression levels (i.e., the amount of expressed protein does not correlate well with the amount of adenoviruses injected). The latter consideration leads to great difficulties in effective study design. An additional consideration is the fact that a considerable portion of patient population has significant titers of antiadenoviral antibodies. Clinical experience suggests that adenoviruses are ineffective in such patients *(43)*. Nevertheless, some progress has been achieved with adenoviral therapies, and currently this strategy seems the only viable alternative to polymer-based protein therapies. It should be noted that other viral vectors, most notably adeno-associated virus (AAV) and lentiviruses, in addition to newer generations of adenoviruses, are entering clinical practice, and it is hoped that we will have an effective gene transfer agent before long.

As already emphasized, the duration of expression is an important parameter in determining angiogenic efficacy. An additional consideration, however, is the vessel stability. Although it was appreciated for some time that newly formed vessel tend to regress once the stimulation is withdrawn (as is the case for CAM and cornea implant models), it was argued that once vessels have formed in tissues and began carrying blood, they would persist. A recent study shows that is not necessarily the case. Dor and colleagues *(44)* have shown that a 2-wk induction of VEGF expression in the mouse heart resulted in production of new vessels. However, all of these vessels regressed once VEGF was withdrawn. However, VEGF withdrawal after 6 wk of stimulation did not produce regression of newly formed vasculature *(44)*. This is a very important result and the implications for human studies have not yet been examined. If indeed 6 wk of continuous VEGF presence is required for formation of stable vasculature in a mouse, the time requirement in patients could considerably greater (in the order of months).

5. CHOICE OF PATIENT POPULATION

One of the major challenges in therapeutic angiogenesis field, is the choice of patient population suitable for demonstration of benefit of such therapy. Traditionally, testing of new therapies have been reserved for patients not well served by the existing treatments. In the case of therapeutic angiogenesis, this meant so-called no option patients, that is, symptomatic patients with advanced CAD that could not be effectively treated by means of coronary bypass or percutaneous interventions. However, such individuals likely represent failures of natural angiogenic responses and, thus, can be particularly resistant to stimulation of neovascularization. This can happen because of genetic factors or other reasons, such as high circulating levels of angiogenesis inhibitors *(45,46)*. Therefore, this may not be the optimal population suitable for proof-of-concept for growth factor therapy.

Until recently, little information has been available regarding prognosis and natural history of disease among these patients. It was assumed that mortality would be high and the incidence of other major adverse events, such as infarctions and strokes, would also be significant. It now appears that this may not be the case. Although clearly symptomatic, these patients have mortality rates no higher than patients suitable for conventional therapies and the incidence of myocardial infarction and stroke is also similar to that of the general CAD population *(47)*.

The choice of a homogenous patient group is a very important consideration. Initially, the investigators relied on the Canadian Cardiac Society (CCS) anginal class to select patients with a similar degree of angina. The experience in coronary angiogenesis trials has clearly shown that this does not select a sufficiently homogenous group. Thus, in the FIRST trial, despite 88% of patients being CCS class II or III, the symptomatic benefit of FGF2 did not correlate with baseline CCS class whereas it correlated very tightly with baseline Seattle Angina Questionnaire scores *(37)*. Another interesting observation has been the lack of correlation between exercise performance as judged by treadmill testing and the magnitude of angina symptoms (Simons and Chronos, unpublished observations; ref. *48*). Finally, anatomical considerations (extent of coronary disease, feeder vessels, etc.) to date have largely not being taken into account in design and randomization of clinical trials. This may be a mistake because it is hard to expect an adequate collateral development when there are no plausible proximal sources of blood flow. Although we lack definitive animal or clinical trial data, the ideal candidate may be a patient with a long-standing single occlusion of a proximal coronary artery subtending viable myocardium. For example, a patient with an occluded right coronary artery, normal left anterior descending and left circumflex coronary arteries, and evidence of viability in the inferior wall would be an ideal substrate for a trail of angiogenic therapy. Unfortunately, although very attractive from a proof of concept point of view, such patients are too rare to form a basis for a clinical trial. They may, however, be very valuable for clinical experimentation, a concept that has not been used effectively in recent times. The downside, of course, is the relative paucity of such patients.

Clinical observations have clearly hinted that the ability to form collateral circulation is different among different patients. Thus, anecdotally practitioners have observed individuals with an occluded coronary who have extensive collateral at the site of occlusion and individuals who do not. Unfortunately, we do not understand what genetic and biological factors account for this difference. A better knowledge of collateral circulation biology seems mandatory for rapid advancement of therapeutic angiogenesis field.

Another consideration in choosing clinical population that has received little attention is the concurrent medical therapy these patients are receiving. A number of anecdotal observations have suggested that certain frequently used medications, including COX-2 inhibitors, captopril, and furosemide, may inhibit collateral development.

6. ASSESSMENT OF THERAPEUTIC BENEFIT

Therapeutic angiogenesis can be positioned as the symptomatic treatment strategy aimed at ameliorating angina symptoms in patients with coronary disease similar to other anti-anginal medications. Alternatively, this therapy may change the natural history of CAD by reducing the risk of death and myocardial infarction. To date, all trials of therapeutic angiogenesis have focused on the symptomatic benefits strategy because it is felt that the trial of sufficient size to demonstrate mortality differences would require too many patients at this stage of drug development. In the absence of the firm mortality end point, we are left with various measures designed to assess functional status and quality of life. It should also be noted that a purely palliative treatment would be expected to show a substantial improvement in quality of life that is sufficiently significant to justify expensive, invasive therapy with uncertain safety record. At the same time, a life-prolonging therapy would justify greater treatment-associated risks and discomforts.

Another consideration is the need to demonstrate a mechanism of therapeutic benefit that will be necessary to gain acceptance in the medical community. At a minimum, this must include demonstration of improved myocardial perfusion and, possibly, improvement in global and/or regional left ventricular function or increased collateral vessels on coronary angiography. Traditionally, exercise testing has been used as a primary endpoint to demonstrate symptomatic benefits of anti-anginal therapies. However, exercise testing has never been used in the kind of no-option patients that form the basis of angiogenesis trials. A significant number of these patients are unable to exercise for reasons unrelated to the extent of CAD, such as such as claudication, pulmonary disease, and motivation, among others, thereby reducing the sensitivity of this measure.

The limitations of maximal treadmill time as a trial end point are underscored by clinical studies of therapeutics for heart failure. Agents with consistently proven favorable effects on long-term outcomes, such as angiotensin-converting enzyme inhibitors and beta-adrenergic blockers, have not shown consistent positive effects on maximal treadmill time, whereas other therapies with an adverse effect on survival (such as milrinone) may improve exercise time. Thus, although exercise duration is often used as the primary efficacy endpoint in angiogenesis trials, it is unclear whether this will prove to be a robust measure that reflects clinical improvement resulting from therapeutic angiogenesis. Coupled with inherent variability of exercise testing employed in a serial manner over time, this has led many investigators to question the usefulness of this endpoint.

The alternative endpoints involve assessments of quality of life. Such endpoints are gaining widespread acceptance in cardiovascular studies. In paticular, improvement in health-related quality of life is an important therapeutic objective for patients with chronic ischemic heart disease that may be well suited to serve as an end point in therapeutic angiogenesis trials. An important advantage is that improvements in health status tend to be realized in the relatively short time frames that are required for Phase II and III studies *(46)*. However, these endpoints lack a long-term track record in CAD trials. Furthermore, there no uniformly accepted single definition of quality of life.

Other approaches to health status assessment include disease-specific Measures, such as the CCS Anginal Classification or the Seattle Angina Questionnaire *(49,50)*. In the case of the latter, only certain domains, including functional limitations and symptoms, such as angina and dyspnea, are particularly relevant. The disease-specific measures tend to be more responsive to modest changes in health than generic measures *(51)* and thus can be an efficient study endpoint. Generic health status measures, such as SF-36 or SF-12 questionnaires or the Sickness Impact Profile that are designed to summarize a spectrum of concepts of health and quality of life issues, may be too insensitive to modest improvements in cardiovascular function.

The use of surrogate markers of biological efficacy has a long history in clinical research, and the validity and desirability of such markers are firmly established. Unfortunately, to date no such markers have been described or validated for CAD therapeutic angiogenesis trials. The development of such markers is of the highest importance.

The other challenge of the therapeutic angiogenesis field is the demonstration of physiologic benefit. Because the primary driver of anginal symptoms is, presumably, tissue hypoxia, the demonstration of improved oxygenation in ischemic beds would be the most direct way of establishing a therapeutic benefit. Unfortunately, no techniques for such measurement are currently available. Therefore, investigators have resorted to the use of more derived parameters, such as myocardial perfusion and function. Although functional benefits (i.e., improvement in ejection fraction or local wall motion) remain the ultimate goal of restoration of flow to an ischemic area of the heart, the experience has shown that this is not a sensitive measure. Indeed, significant improvement in perfusion can occur before any functional benefits are seen. This leads us, therefore, to assessment of myocardial perfusion.

Nuclear myocardial perfusion imaging in the form of SPECT has been the most established tool for the diagnosis of ischemic heart disease and for detecting improved blood flow after revascularization of epicardial coronary arteries. However, the usefulness of this imaging modality in detecting improved perfusion secondary to enhanced collateral supply has not been established. Several considerations come into play, including relatively poor spatial resolution of the technique, the relative assessment of perfusion (that is, the perfusion in the ischemic bed is assessed relative to that of the nonischemic bed and an equal improvement in flow to both territories would leave the apparent flow deficit intact), and the poor reproducibility of SPECT imaging over time in this patient population.

Other confounding problems involve the choice of stressor agent. The advanced extent of CAD in patients enrolled in angiogenesis trials and frequent concomitant diseases lead to the inability to attain a maximal heart rate with exercise, thereby limiting assessment of the extent of myocardial ischemia. Because it is virtually impossible to match levels of myocardial demand on repeat exercise tests, serial comparison over time becomes difficult and inaccurate *(46)*. This limitation can potentially be overcome with the use of pharmacologic stress (dipyridamole, adenosine, and dobutamine). Because collateral-dependent myocardium has limited flow reserve, this may not be an effective means of quantification. Furthermore, we do not know whether these drugs will equally affect newly formed vessels and the pre-existing native vessels. The possibility of coronary steal is another important consideration. Given these considerations in mind, increased perfusion may more accurately assessed by measuring changes in resting perfusion *(46)*. However, there is limited experience in tracking changes in resting perfusion.

Positron emission tomography (PET) may overcome some of the limitations of SPECT imaging. In particular, the spatial resolution of PET imaging is much higher and it provides quantitative (rather than qualitative as with SPECT) assessment of perfusion. Its ability to demonstrate subtle changes in myocardial perfusion has been demonstrated in studies of coronary flow reserve in patients treated with lipid-lowering therapy *(52,53)*. Unfortunately, there is a very limited experience with PET imaging before and after angiogenic therapy, and there are currently no clinical trial data using this technique.

Magnetic resonance imaging (MRI) in theory can provide so-called one-stop shopping for the assessment of myocardial function and blood flow *(54)*. MRI functional assessment of ventricular performance can be regarded as a gold standard. At the same time, MRI perfusion assessment is still an evolving tool, albeit with a lot of promise. Because there are no MRI perfusion agents that are retained by the myocardium, MRI assessment of perfusion is based on the quantification of first-pass contrast appearance and washout rates. MRI offers exceptional spatial resolution, allowing assessment of transmural flow gradients, subendocardial perfusion, and perfusion reserve *(54,55)*. Animal models of coronary stenosis have validated MRI measurement of late contrast appearance as a measure of collateral-dependent myocardium, which has been reduced with VEGF administration *(13,56,57)*. Several clinical trials have demonstrated significant improvement in delayed contrast arrival after angiogenic therapies *(40,58,59)*, suggesting that this imaging modality may be sensitive enough to show the benefits of angiogenic agents.

7. PLACEBO EFFECT

The initial excitement over positive results in open-label angiogenesis trials soon gave way to realization that significant improvements occur in placebo-treated patients in this population. The full extent of the placebo effect in these trials and its causes are still not well understood. Likely, a number of factors play a role. On the one hand, there is genuine improvement in myocardial perfusion and function in placebo-treated patients as can be documented by MRI, SPECT, and PET imaging. This is probably caused by the more meticulous care these patients are receiving as a part of the trial and better compliance with medication regimen. Indeed, a recent study has shown the reversibility of SPECT defect after effective lipid-lowering therapy. On the other hand, improved exercise regiment and high hopes for cure may also play a role. Remarkably, it is the most symptomatic patients that show placebo effect, whereas those who have lesser symptoms do not show as much improvement *(37)*. Another interesting feature of the placebo effect in these trials is its long duration *(37)*. Clearly, given the magnitude and duration of the placebo response, no therapeutic angiogenesis agent can be evaluated in the open-label trial format.

8. SUMMARY AND CONCLUSION

The field of therapeutic angiogenesis has traveled a long way since the initial studies a decade ago. Many issues have been brought into sharp focus, including the existence of large and persistent placebo effect, the need for prolonged therapy, the concept of synergistic growth factor activity, vessel stability, and many others. We also have a much better handle on patient selection and the means of assessment of therapeutic benefit. Therefore, there is every reason to think that we will be able to develop effective therapeutic angiogenesis agents, thereby ushering a new era of cardiovascular therapeutics.

REFERENCES

1. Casscells, W., Speir, E., Sasse, J., Klagsbrun, M., Allen, P., Lee, M., et al. (1990) Isolation, characterization, and localization of heparin-binding growth factors in the heart. *J. Clin. Invest.* **85,** 433–441.
2. Sharma, H. S., Wunsch, M., Schmidt, M., Schott, R. J., Kandolf, R., and Schaper, W. (1992) Expression of angiogenic growth factors in the collateralized swine myocardium. *Exs* **61,** 255–260.
3. Shweiki, D., Itin, A., Soffer, D., and Keshet, E. (1992) Vascular endothelial growth factor induced by hypoxia may mediate hypoxia-initiated angiogenesis. *Nature* **359,** 843–845.
4. Speir, E., Tanner, V., Gonzalez, A. M., Farris, J., Baird, A., and Casscells, W. (1992) Acidic and basic fibroblast growth factors in adult rat heart myocytes. Localization, regulation in culture, and effects on DNA synthesis. *Circ. Res.* **71,** 251–259.
5. Berse, B., Brown, L. F., Van de Water, L., Dvorak, H. F., and Senger, D. R. (1992) Vascular permeability factor (vascular endothelial growth factor) gene is expressed differentially in normal tissues, macrophages, and tumors. *Mol. Biol. Cell* **3,** 211–220.
6. Fallon, J. H., Di Salvo, J., Loughlin, S. E., Gimenez-Gallego, G., Seroogy, K. B., Bradshaw, R. A., et al. (1992) Localization of acidic fibroblast growth factor within the mouse brain using biochemical and immunocytochemical techniques. *Growth Factors* **6,** 139–157.
7. Bernotat-Danielowski, S., Sharma, H. S., Schott, R. J., and Schaper, W. (1993) Generation and localisation of monoclonal antibodies against fibroblast growth factors in ischaemic collateralised porcine myocardium. *Cardiovasc. Res.* **27,** 1220–1228.
8. Ladoux, A. and Frelin, C. (1993) Hypoxia is a strong inducer of vascular endothelial growth factor mRNA expression in the heart. *Biochem. Biophys. Res. Commun.* **195,** 1005–1010.
9. Banai, S., Shweiki, D., Pinson, A., Chandra, M., Lazarovici, G., and Keshet, E. (1994) Upregulation of vascular endothelial growth factor expression induced by myocardial ischaemia: implications for coronary angiogenesis. *Cardiovasc. Res.* **28,** 1176–1179.
10. Banai, S., Jaklitsch, M. T., Shou, M., Lazarous, D. F., Scheinowitz, M., Biro, S., et al. (1994) Angiogenic-induced enhancement of collateral blood flow to ischemic myocardium by vascular endothelial growth factor in dogs. *Circulation* **89,** 2183–2189.
11. Unger, E. F., Banai, S., Shou, M., Lazarous, D. F., Jaklitsch, M. T., Scheinowitz, M., et al. (1994) Basic fibroblast growth factor enhances myocardial collateral flow in a canine model. *Am. J. Physiol.* **266,** H1588–H1595.

12. Harada, K., Grossman, W., Friedman, M., Edelman, E. R., Prasad, P. V., Keighley, C. S., et al. (1994) Basic fibroblast growth factor improves myocardial function in chronically ischemic porcine hearts. *J. Clin. Invest.* **94,** 623–630.

13. Pearlman, J. D., Hibberd, M. G., Chuang, M. L., Harada, K., Lopez, J. J., Gladstone, S. R., et al. (1995) Magnetic resonance mapping demonstrates benefits of VEGF-induced myocardial angiogenesis. *Nat. Med.* **1,** 1085–1089.

14. Baffour, R., Berman, J., Garb, J. L., Rhee, S. W., Kaufman, J., and Friedmann, P. (1992) Enhanced angiogenesis and growth of collaterals by in vivo administration of recombinant basic fibroblast growth factor in a rabbit model of acute lower limb ischemia: Dose-response effect of basic fibroblast growth factor. *J. Vasc. Surg.* **16,** 181–191.

15. Pu, L. Q., Sniderman, A. D., Brassard, R., Lachapelle, K. J., Graham, A. M., Lisbona, R., et al. (1993) Enhanced revascularization of the ischemic limb by angiogenic therapy. *Circulation* **88,** 208–215.

16. Pu, L. Q., Sniderman, A. D., Arekat, Z., Graham, A. M., Brassard, R., and Symes, J. F. (1993) Angiogenic growth factor and revascularization of the ischemic limb: Evaluation in a rabbit model. *J. Surg. Res.* **54,** 575–583.

17. Bauters, C., Asahara, T., Zheng, L. P., Takeshita, S., Bunting, S., Ferrara, N., et al. (1994) Physiological assessment of augmented vascularity induced by VEGF in ischemic rabbit hindlimb. *Am. J. Physiol.* **267,** H1263–H1271.

18. Takeshita, S., Pu, L. Q., Stein, L. A., Sniderman, A. D., Bunting, S., Ferrara, N., et al. (1994) Intramuscular administration of vascular endothelial growth factor induces dose-dependent collateral artery augmentation in a rabbit model of chronic limb ischemia. *Circulation* **90,** II228–II234.

19. Ware, J. A. and Simons, M. (1997) Angiogenesis in ischemic heart disease. *Nat. Med.* **3,** 158–164.

20. Carmeliet, P. (2000) Mechanisms of angiogenesis and arteriogenesis. *Nat. Med.* **6,** 389–395.

21. Semenza, G. L. (2000) HIF-1: Mediator of physiological and pathophysiological responses to hypoxia. *J. Appl. Physiol.* **88,** 1474–1480.

22. Li, J., Post, M., Volk, R., Gao, Y., Li, M., Metais, C., et al. (2000) PR39, a peptide regulator of angiogenesis. *Nat. Med.* **6,** 49–55.

23. Ferrara, N., Carver-Moore, K., Chen, H., Dowd, M., Lu, L., O'Shea, K. S., et al. (1996) Heterozygous embryonic lethality induced by targeted inactivation of the VEGF gene. *Nature* **380,** 439–442.

24. Carmeliet, P., Ferreira, V., Breier, G., Pollefeyt, S., Kieckens, L., Gertsenstein, M., et al. (1996) Abnormal blood vessel development and lethality in embryos lacking a single VEGF allele. *Nature* **380,** 435–439.

25. Carmeliet, P. and Collen, D. (2000) Molecular basis of angiogenesis. Role of VEGF and VE-cadherin. *Ann. N Y Acad. Sci.* **902,** 249–262; discussion 262–264.

26. Celletti, F. L., Waugh, J. M., Amabile, P. G., Brendolan, A., Hilfiker, P. R., and Dake, M. D. (2001) Vascular endothelial growth factor enhances atherosclerotic plaque progression. *Nat. Med.* **7,** 425–429.

27. Parsons-Wingerter, P., Elliott, K. E., Clark, J. I.. and Farr, A. G. (2000) Fibroblast growth factor-2 selectively stimulates angiogenesis of small vessels in arterial tree. *Arterioscler. Thromb. Vasc. Biol.* **20,** 1250–1256.

28. Simons, M., Laham, R. J., Post, M. J., and Sellke, F. W. (2000) Therapeutic angiogenesis: Potential role of basic FGF in patients with severe ischemic heart disease. *BioDrugs* **14,** 13–20.

29. Gille, J., Khalik, M., Konig, V., and Kaufmann, R. (1998) Hepatocyte growth factor/scatter factor (HGF/SF) induces vascular permeability factor (VPF/VEGF) expression by cultured keratinocytes. *J. Invest. Dermato.* **111,** 1160–1165.

30. Hellstrom, M., Gerhardt, H., Kalen, M., Li, X., Eriksson, U., Wolburg, H., et al. (2001) Lack of pericytes leads to endothelial hyperplasia and abnormal vascular morphogenesis. *J. Cell. Biol.* **153,** 543–553.

31. Semenza, G. L. (1998) Hypoxia-inducible factor 1: Master regulator of O2 homeostasis. *Curr. Opin. Genet. Dev.* **8,** 588–594.

32. Semenza, G. L. (2000) HIF-1 and human disease: One highly involved factor. *Genes Dev.* **14,** 1983–1991.

33. Gao, Y., Lecker, S., Post, M. J., Hietaranta, A. J., Li, J., Volk, R., et al. (2000) Inhibition of ubiquitin-proteasome pathway-mediated IkappaBalpha degradation by a naturally occurring antibacterial peptide. *J. Clin. Invest.* **106,** 439–448.

34. Post, M. J., Laham, R., Sellke, F. W., and Simons, M. (2001) Therapeutic angiogenesis in cardiology using protein formulations. *Cardiovasc. Res.* **49,** 522–531.

35. Laham, R. J., Rezaee, M., Post, M., Sellke, F. W., Braeckman, R. A., Hung, D., et al. (1999) Intracoronary and intravenous administration of basic fibroblast growth factor: Myocardial and tissue distribution. *Drug Metab. Dispos.* **27,** 821–826.

36. Henry, T., Annex, B., Azrin, M., McKendall, G., Willerson, J., Hendel, R., et al. (1999) Final results of the VIVA trial of rhVEGF human therapeutic angiogenesis. *Circulation* **100,** I–476.

37. Simons, M., Annex, B. H., Laham, R. J., Kleiman, N., Henry, T., Dauerman, H., et al. (2002) Pharmacological treatment of coronar artery disease with recombinant fibroblast growth factor-2: Double-blind, randomized, controlled clinical trial. *Circulation* **105,** 788–793.

38. Simons, M. (2001) Therapeutic coronary angiogenesis: A fronte praecipitium a tergo lupi? *Am. J. Physiol.* **280,** H1923–H1927.

39. Kornowski, R., Fuchs, S., Leon, M. B., and Epstein, S. E. (2000) Delivery strategies to achieve therapeutic myocardial angiogenesis. *Circulation* **101,** 454–458.

40. Laham, R. J., Sellke, F. W., Edelman, E. R., Pearlman, J. D., Ware, J. A., Brown, D. L., et al. (1999) Local perivascular delivery of basic fibroblast growth factor in patients undergoing coronary bypass surgery: Results of a phase I randomized, double-blind, placebo-controlled trial. *Circulation* **100,** 1865–1871.

41. Yla-Herttuala, S. and Martin, J. F. (2000) Cardiovascular gene therapy. *Lancet* **355,** 213–222.

42. Hammond, H. K. and McKirnan, M. D. (2001) Angiogenic gene therapy for heart disease: A review of animal studies and clinical trials. *Cardiovasc. Res.* **49,** 561–567.

43. Grines, C. L., Watkins, M. W., Helmer, G., Penny, W., Brinker, J., Marmur, J. D., et al. (2002) Angiogenic Gene Therapy (AGENT) trial in patients with stable angina pectoris. *Circulation* **105,** 1291–1297.

44. Dor, Y., Djonov, V., Abramovitch, R., Itin, A., Fishman, G. I., Carmeliet, P., et al. (2002) Conditional switching of VEGF provides new insights into adult neovascularization and pro-angiogenic therapy. *EMBO J.* **21,** 1939–1947.

45. Schultz, A., Lavie, L., Hochberg, I., Beyar, R., Stone, T., Skorecki, K., et al. (1999) Interindividual heterogeneity in the hypoxic regulation of VEGF: Significance for the development of the coronary artery collateral circulation. *Circulation* **100,** 547–552.

46. Simons, M., Bonow, R. O., Chronos, N. A., Cohen, D. J., Giordano, F. J., Hammond, H. K., et al. (2000) Clinical trials in coronary angiogenesis: Issues, problems, consensus: An expert panel summary. *Circulation* **102,** E73–E86.

47. Mukherjee, D., Comella, K., Bhatt, D. L., Roe, M. T., Patel, V., and Ellis, S. G. (2001) Clinical outcome of a cohort of patients eligible for therapeutic angiogenesis or transmyocardial revascularization. *Am. Heart J.* **142,** 72–74.

48. Wiklund, I., Comerford, M. B., and Dimenas, E. (1991) The relationship between exercise tolerance and quality of life in angina pectoris. *Clin. Cardiol.* **14,** 204–208.

49. Spertus, J. A., Winder, J. A., Dewhurst, T. A., Deyo, R. A., Prodzinski, J., McDonell, M., et al. (1995) Development and evaluation of the Seattle Angina Questionnaire: A new functional status measure for coronary artery disease. *J. Am. Coll. Cardiol.* **25,** 333–341.

50. Dougherty, C. M., Dewhurst, T., Nichol, W. P., and Spertus, J. (1998) Comparison of three quality of life instruments in stable angina pectoris: Seattle Angina Questionnaire, Short

Form Health Survey (SF-36), and Quality of Life Index-Cardiac Version III. *J. Clin. Epidemiol.* **51**, 569–575.

51. Spertus, J. A., Winder, J. A., Dewhurst, T. A., Deyo, R. A., and Fihn, S. D. (1994) Monitoring the quality of life in patients with coronary artery disease. *Am. J. Cardiol.* **74**, 1240–1244.

52. Gould, K. L., Martucci, J. P., Goldberg, D. I., Hess, M. J., Edens, R. P., Latifi, R., et al. (1994) Short-term cholesterol lowering decreases size and severity of perfusion abnormalities by positron emission tomography after dipyridamole in patients with coronary artery disease. A potential noninvasive marker of healing coronary endothelium. *Circulation* **89**, 1530–1538.

53. Baller, D., Notohamiprodjo, G., Gleichmann, U., Holzinger, J., Weise, R., and Lehmann, J. (1999) Improvement in coronary flow reserve determined by positron emission tomography after 6 months of cholesterol-lowering therapy in patients with early stages of coronary atherosclerosis. *Circulation* **99**, 2871–2875.

54. Pearlman, J. D., Laham, R. J., Post, M., Leiner, T., and Simons, M. (2002) Medical imaging techniques in the evaluation of strategies for therapeutic angiogenesis. *Curr. Pharm. Des.* **8**, 1467–1496.

55. Wilke, N. M., Zenovich, A. G., Jerosch-Herold, M., and Henry, T. D. (2001) Cardiac magnetic resonance imaging for the assessment of myocardial angiogenesis. *Curr. Interv. Cardiol. Rep.* **3**, 205–212.

56. Harada, K., Friedman, M., Lopez, J. J., Wang, S. Y., Li, J., Prasad, P. V., et al. (1996) Vascular endothelial growth factor administration in chronic myocardial ischemia. *Am. J. Physiol.* **270**, H1791–H1802.

57. Lopez, J. J., Laham, R. J., Stamler, A., Pearlman, J. D., Bunting, S., Kaplan, A., et al. (1998) VEGF administration in chronic myocardial ischemia in pigs. *Cardiovasc. Res.* **40**, 272–281.

58. Laham, R. J., Chronos, N. A., Pike, M., Leimbach, M., Udelson, J. E., Pearlman, J. D., et al. (2000) Intracoronary basic fibroblast growth factor (FGF-2) in patients with severe ischemic heart disease: Results of a Phase I open-label dose escalation study. *J. Am. Coll. Cardiol.* **36**, 2132–2139.

59. Laham, R. J., Simons, M., Pearlman, J. D., Ho, K. K., and Baim, D. S. (2002) Magnetic resonance imaging demonstrates improved regional systolic wall motion and thickening and myocardial perfusion of myocardial territories treated by laser myocardial revascularization. *J. Am. Coll. Cardiol.* **39**, 1–8.

Index